VOLUME NINETY FIVE

ADVANCES IN PHARMACOLOGY

Pharmacology and Toxicology of Cytochrome P450 – 60th Anniversary

VOLUME NINETY FIVE

ADVANCES IN PHARMACOLOGY

Pharmacology and Toxicology of Cytochrome P450 – 60th Anniversary

Edited by

HIROSHI YAMAZAKI
Showa Pharmaceutical University,
Machida, Tokyo, Japan

ELSEVIER

ACADEMIC PRESS
An imprint of Elsevier

Academic Press is an imprint of Elsevier
50 Hampshire Street, 5th Floor, Cambridge, MA 02139, United States
525 B Street, Suite 1650, San Diego, CA 92101, United States
The Boulevard, Langford Lane, Kidlington, Oxford OX5 1GB, United Kingdom
125 London Wall, London, EC2Y 5AS, United Kingdom

First edition 2022

ISBN: 978-0-323-91109-2
ISSN: 1054-3589

For information on all Academic Press publications
visit our website at https://www.elsevier.com/books-and-journals

Publisher: Zoe Kruze
Developmental Editor: Jhon Michael Peñano
Production Project Manager: Vijayaraj Purushothaman
Cover Designer: Matthew Limbert

Typeset by STRAIVE, India

Contents

Contributors

Pamela Bachour-El Azzi
Biopredic International SARL, Saint Grégoire, France

Eric Chun Yong Chan
Department of Pharmacy, Faculty of Science, National University of Singapore, Singapore, Singapore

Christophe Chesné
Biopredic International SARL, Saint Grégoire, France

Stephlina A. D'Cunha
School of Chemistry & Molecular Biosciences, The University of Queensland, Brisbane, QLD, Australia

Ann K. Daly
Translational and Clinical Research Institute, Newcastle University, Newcastle Upon Tyne, United Kingdom

M. Denise Dearing
School of Biological Sciences, University of Utah, Salt Lake City, UT, United States

Xinxin Ding
Department of Pharmacology and Toxicology, Ken R. Coit College of Pharmacy, The University of Arizona, Tucson, AZ, United States

Chie Emoto
Laboratory of Drug Metabolism and Pharmacokinetics, Showa Pharmaceutical University; Translational Research Division, Chugai Pharmaceutical Co., Ltd., Tokyo, Japan

Elizabeth M.J. Gillam
School of Chemistry & Molecular Biosciences, The University of Queensland, Brisbane, QLD, Australia

F. Peter Guengerich
Department of Biochemistry, Vanderbilt University School of Medicine, Nashville, TN, United States

James R. Halpert
Department of Pharmacology and Toxicology, College of Pharmacy, University of Arizona, Tucson, AZ, United States

Sarrah L. Hannon
Department of Pharmacology and Toxicology, Ken R. Coit College of Pharmacy, The University of Arizona, Tucson, AZ, United States

Martin A. Hayes
Compound Synthesis and Management, Discovery Sciences, BioPharmaceuticals R&D AstraZeneca, Mölndal, Sweden

W. Griffith Humphreys
Aranmore Pharma Consulting, Lawrenceville, NJ, United States

Magnus Ingelman-Sundberg
Department of Physiology and Pharmacology, Section of Pharmacogenetics, Karolinska Institute, Stockholm, Sweden

Trevor N. Johnson
Certara UK Limited, Sheffield, United Kingdom

Jacqueline Wen Hui Leow
Department of Pharmacy, Faculty of Science, National University of Singapore, Singapore, Singapore

Michele M. Skopec
Department of Zoology, Weber State University, Ogden, UT, United States

Marlaina R. Stocco
Department of Psychological and Brain Sciences, University of California, Santa Barbara, Santa Barbara, CA, United States

Hiroshi Suemizu
Central Institute for Experimental Animals, Kawasaki, Kanagawa, Japan

Lloyd Wei Tat Tang
Department of Pharmacy, Faculty of Science, National University of Singapore, Singapore, Singapore

Raine E.S. Thomson
School of Chemistry & Molecular Biosciences, The University of Queensland, Brisbane, QLD, Australia

Rachel F. Tyndale
Department of Pharmacology and Toxicology; Campbell Family Mental Health Research Institute, CAMH; Department of Psychiatry, University of Toronto, Toronto, ON, Canada

Shotaro Uehara
Central Institute for Experimental Animals, Kawasaki, Kanagawa; Showa Pharmaceutical University, Machida, Tokyo, Japan

Yasuhiro Uno
Joint Faculty of Veterinary Medicine, Kagoshima University, Kagoshima, Japan

Hiroshi Yamazaki
Showa Pharmaceutical University, Machida, Tokyo, Japan

Preface

The year 2022 represents the 60th anniversary since the first article on cytochrome P450 (P450) was published by Omura and Sato (1962). It is a pleasure to celebrate 60 years of meaningful research on many forms of P450 that exist in microorganisms, plants, animals, and humans. P450s have been a focus of attention in many industrial bioengineering applications and the syntheses of unique human drug metabolites in pharmaceutical development. Research on P450s in animal models with introduced human *P450 (CYP)* genes or transplanted humanized liver and with nonhuman primates has extended into different fields, from molecules to in vivo situations, by attracting pharmacologists, toxicologists, and biochemists.

P450 electron transport is mediated by a multicomponent monooxygenase system with reduced nicotinamide adenine dinucleotide phosphate (NADPH). Microsomal P450s receive electrons from NADPH-cytochrome P450 reductase. The catalytic cycle of P450 involves the activation of molecular oxygen to a reactive form (see Fig. 3 in Chapter 1). In addition to the basic science, research on drug metabolism in liver and extrahepatic organs (e.g., brain) in animal models and humans has expanded to one of important areas in clinical pharmacology and toxicology. P450 research has developed from the studies with rat liver in the 1960s to personalized medicine, mediated by studies of polymorphic P450s in individual patients including pediatrics and the elderly in the 21st century, as discussed in this book series.

The extensive contributions of scientists throughout the world to the P450 research field over past six decades should be noted. The success of P450 research has had implications in fields such as herbal medicine, drug interactions, pharmacogenetics, pharmacogenomics, and physiologically based pharmacokinetic modeling. The basic principle for this book series comprises three parts: (i) collection of a comprehensive coverage of major progress in 60 years in pharmacology and toxicology, (ii) discussion for future directions of the research on P450s (especially for better pharmacotherapy in humans), and (iii) the invitation to young scientists to join this important and exciting basic and advanced world of P450.

The volumes in *Advances in Pharmacology* are part of a series. I hope that this book series will stimulate and encourage many young scientists in P450 research to try new methods and approaches. Historical achievements on

P450 research in former times cannot be dismissed in new studies. For example, human drug-metabolizing P450s (in phospholipid membranes) require another protein, NADPH-cytochrome P450 reductase, in appropriate ionic strength environments to exert their catalytic functions of aerobic metabolism in the presence of NADPH. As the volume editor, I will be delighted if our book series can extensively facilitate new research.

Hiroshi Yamazaki
Showa Pharmaceutical University, Tokyo, Japan

Reference

Omura, T., & Sato, R. (1962). A new cytochrome in liver microsomes. *Journal of Biological Chemistry*, *237*, 1375–1376.

In Memoriam—Tsuneo Omura

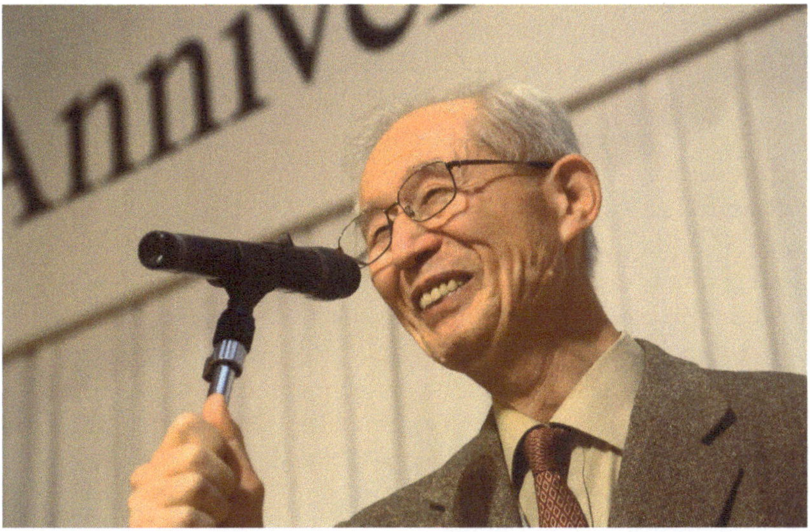

(by F. Peter Guengerich, Bettie Sue S. Masters, Ken-Ichirou Morohashi, Masahiko Negishi, and Hiroshi Yamazaki)

The biochemical community, especially his colleagues in the field of cytochrome P450, lost one of its true pioneers with the death of Prof. Tsuneo Omura on January 29, 2022. He discovered cytochrome P450 in his work with the late Prof. Ryo Sato at Osaka University, and a Clarivate search indicates that a *JBC* paper (*J. Biol. Chem.* 239, 2370–2378, 1964) describing the work has been cited at least 12,700 times. Tsuneo Omura was Honorary Member of the ASBMB, a distinct honor.

Tsuneo Omura was born on July 29, 1930, in Shizuoka Prefecture, Japan. He graduated from the University of Tokyo with a BS in chemistry. He then worked as an instructor and lecturer in chemistry at Shizuoka University. The course of his doctoral work and advancement was rather unique compared to our current systems, but in 1960 he joined Prof. Ryo Sato's laboratory at the Osaka University Institute for Protein Research as Associate Professor. In 1961, he was awarded a DSc in biochemistry from the University of Tokyo, based on the work he had performed at Shizuoka University. It was during the early 1960s in Osaka that Omura and Sato published three major papers about the discovery of P450 (including the most highly cited one in the *JBC*), plus seven others in related areas. From 1964 to 1966, Omura was a visiting scientist at the Johnson Foundation of the University of Pennsylvania (with Ronald W. Estabrook) and then Rockefeller University (with Philip Siekevitz). He returned to the Osaka Institute for Protein Research and then moved in 1970 to the position of Professor of Biology and Molecular Biology at Kyushu University, a position he held throughout his career until he assumed Emeritus status in 1994. From 1995 to 1997, he was Visiting Professor of Biochemistry at Vanderbilt University (with Michael R. Waterman and others).

Prof. Omura made many contributions to the field of P450 research throughout his career. These include studies on the regulation of P450s and, in particular, trafficking of P450s in both the endoplasmic reticulum and mitochondria. His studies with mitochondrial P450s, specifically the cholesterol side chain cleavage enzyme, led to an enhanced understanding of the regulation of these P450s by proteins such as Ad4BP/SF-1, a steroidogenic transcription factor.

Not surprisingly, Prof. Omura was a leading figure in biochemistry in Japan, and many of his students went on to very productive careers. Along with Honorary ASBMB Membership, Omura received the first R.T. Williams Award from the International Society for the Study of Xenobiotics in 2001, and he was also honored at the 1994 International Microsomes and Drug Oxidations (MDO) meeting. Omura continued to attend and actively participate in meetings many years after his retirement. He presented a plenary lecture at the 2018 MDO meeting in Kanazawa. Tributes were also made to him at a special 2012 meeting in Fukuoka, commemorating 50 years since his discovery of cytochrome P450.

Tsuneo Omura will be remembered as a humble and very thoughtful man. He was very friendly, communicative, and always very anxious to help young scientists and lend his advice. His laboratory was always open to visitors from abroad, and he was very happy to help people throughout the 91-plus years of his life. Many visitors recall his joy in driving his guests all around Kyushu with many stops at pottery-making artisans and notable sites, including the active volcano, Mt. Aso. Due to his warm personality and erudite knowledge, many students were attracted to him. During 24 years of his tenure in Kyushu University, 112 undergraduate students and 42 graduate students joined his laboratory, and 33 of them took PhD degrees under his thoughtful and persistent guidance. All the students spent meaningful and valuable time in Prof. Omura's laboratory, and he created an atmosphere of camaraderie and mutual respect. He was a true *sensei* in every sense of this Japanese title of honor.

Prof. Omura was preceded in death by his wife, Yone (December 9, 2000), and is survived by their three children. Obviously, he was loved by many scientists in the field, and he will be missed.

CHAPTER ONE

Roles of cytochrome P450 enzymes in pharmacology and toxicology: Past, present, and future

F. Peter Guengerich*
Department of Biochemistry, Vanderbilt University School of Medicine, Nashville, TN, United States
*Corresponding author: e-mail address: f.guengerich@vanderbilt.edu

Contents

Advances in Pharmacology, Volume 95
ISSN 1054-3589
https://doi.org/10.1016/bs.apha.2021.12.001

Abstract

The development of the cytochrome P450 (P450) field has been remarkable in the areas of pharmacology and toxicology, particularly in drug development. Today it is possible to use the knowledge base and relatively straightforward assays to make intelligent predictions about drug disposition prior to human dosing. Much is known about the structures, regulation, chemistry of catalysis, and the substrate and inhibitor specificity of human P450s. Many aspects of drug-drug interactions and side effects can be understood in terms of P450s. This knowledge has also been useful in pharmacy practice, as well as in the pharmaceutical industry and medical practice. However, there are still basic and practical questions to address regarding P450s and their roles in pharmacology and toxicology. Another aspect is the discovery of drugs that inhibit P450 to treat diseases.

Abbreviations

Adx	adrenodoxin
AhR	aryl hydrocarbon receptor
AO	aldehyde oxidase
ARNT	aryl hydrocarbon receptor nuclear transferase
AUC	area-under-the-curve
b_5	cytochrome b_5
CAR	constitutively active receptor
COMT	catechol *O*-methyl transferase
DDI	drug-drug interactions
EGFR	epidermal growth factor receptor
FDA	(United States) Food and Drug Administration
FMO	flavin-containing monooxygenase
HNF	hepatic nuclear factor
IND	Investigational New Drug (application)
K_d	dissociation constant
K_i	inhibition constant
K_m	Michaelis constant
LC-MS	combined liquid chromatography-mass spectrometry
MIST	metabolites in safety testing
NME	new molecular entity
NMR	nuclear magnetic resonance (spectroscopy)
NC	non-classical (congenital adrenal hyperplasia)
P450 or CYP	cytochrome P450
PDB	Protein Data Bank
Pgp	P-glycoprotein
POR	NADPH-cytochrome P450 oxidoreductase
PPAR	peroxisome proliferator-activated receptor
PXR	pregnane X receptor
RAR	retinoic acid receptor
RXR	retinoid X receptor

SNV	single nucleotide variant
SV	simple virile (congenital adrenal hyperplasia)
SW	salt-wasting (congenital adrenal hyperplasia)
TCPOBOP	1,4-*bis*[2-(3,5-dichloropyridyloxy)]benzene
UGT	uridine diphosphate glucuronosyl transferase

1. Introduction

The field of cytochrome P450 (P450 or CYP) research had its origin in studies on the metabolism of drugs, steroids, and carcinogens in the middle of the 20th Century (Axelrod, 1955; Mueller & Miller, 1948; Ryan, 1959). However, the discovery of P450 as such did not occur until a few years later (Klingenberg, 1958; Omura & Sato, 1962, 1964). The evidence for a role as the terminal oxidase in a hydroxylation developed with the 17α-hydroxylation of a steroid (Cooper, Levine, Narasimhulu, Rosenthal, & Estabrook, 1965). Studies on a bacterial P450 by Gunsalus developed independently (Hedegaard & Gunsalus, 1965; Katagiri, Ganguli, & Gunsalus, 1968), and that system ($P450_{cam}$, or CYP101A1) served as a useful model for many years (Mueller, Loida, & Sligar, 1995). Two papers in 1968 and 1969 by Lu and Coon established the identity of the liver microsomal P450 system involved in oxidations, consisting of three components: a P450, NADPH-P450 reductase (POR), and phospholipid (Lu & Coon, 1968; Lu, Junk, & Coon, 1969).

More about the historical development of the field was described in a recent review (Guengerich, 2019a). With considerable effort, many liver P450s (and some extrahepatic ones) were purified by conventional chromatography methods and characterized. Progress was also made in terms of mechanisms of catalysis and gene regulation. The introduction of recombinant DNA technology led to cloning of cDNAs, expression of P450s in heterologous systems, and ultimately a better understanding of the complexity of the P450 Superfamily with the completion of the Human Genome Project. Today the field of P450 research must be considered as mature, but that is not to say that all important questions have been answered. As a field matures, the background knowledge and the research tools improve and more important questions can be addressed.

The focus of this book is on pharmacology and the roles of P450 enzymes in the metabolism of drugs. However, P450s also have important roles in the metabolism of steroids (some of which are used as drugs), fat-soluble vitamins, fatty acids, chemical carcinogens, pesticides, industrial chemicals, food additives, and other chemicals. Collectively >90% of all oxidations and reductions of chemicals known today are catalyzed by P450s (Rendic & Guengerich, 2015). This high percentage is also in part due to the preponderance of P450 reactions in the biosynthesis of natural products (Guengerich, 2022b), as well as drugs and industrial chemicals. P450s are found throughout nature, with the only current exceptions being some enteric bacteria (e.g., *Escherichia coli*, *Salmonella typhimurium*). The number of *CYP* genes in bacteria and plants probably exceeds the number in mammals, in large part because most plants have hundreds and sometimes >1,000 *CYP* genes (e.g., wheat has 1,285).

2. Where is the P450 field today and what do we know?

This is an introductory chapter, and several other chapters will focus on some detailed aspects of P450 science. The focus here will be on human P450s, although the P450s in experimental animals are also still of great interest in the drug development process.

2.1 Roles of individual human P450s

One of the ways of grouping the 57 human P450s by function is presented in Table 1. Of these, it is not clear that *CYP2A7* is expressed but *CYP4F3* yields two proteins, so the number is still 57. The classification by substrates is not without caveats. Some P450s can be classified under multiple headings (e.g., 1B1 for steroids and xenobiotics, 27A1 for steroids and vitamins). Some of the P450s have moved from "orphan" status (Unknown in Table 1) but it is not clear how important these reactions are (e.g., 2U1, 2S1). P450 4X1 can slowly oxidize anandamide (Stark, Dostalek, & Guengerich, 2008) but has been left in the Unknown column. It is not clear how important most of the reactions of Xenobiotics and Fatty acids are to mammalian physiology. The point can be made that the P450s in the Xenobiotics column have a general function of clearing a wide variety of ingested natural products present in our food (e.g., terpenes, alkaloids) as a general protective mechanism, in the same way that export transporters do. Studies with transgenic mice have shown that the orthologs of many of the P450s listed under the headings of Xenobiotics and Fatty acids are

Table 1 Classification of human P450s based on major substrate class. **Eicosanoids**

Steroids	Xenobiotics	Fatty acids	Eicosanoids	Vitamins	Unknown
1B1*	1A1*	2J2	2U1	2R1*	2A7
7A1*	1A2*	2S1	4F2	24A1**	4X1
7B1	2A6*	2U1	4F3	26A1	20A1
8B1	2A13*	4A11	4F8	26B1	
11A1*	2B6*	4A22	5A1	27A1	
11B1*	2C8*	4B1**	8A1*	27B1	
11B2*	2C9*	4F11		27C1	
17A1*	2C18	4F12			
19A1*	2C19*	4F22			
21A2*	2D6*	4V2			
27A1	2E1*	4Z1			
39A1	2F1				
46A1*	2W1				
51A1*	3A4*				
	3A5*				
	3A7*				
	3A43				

This classification is somewhat arbitrary in some cases, e.g., P450s 1B1 and 27A1 could be grouped in either of two different categories. *Crystal structure available. **Crystal structure of animal orthologue available.

not essential (Bissig et al., 2018; Gonzalez & Kimura, 2003). However, those involved in the metabolism of steroids, eicosanoids, and vitamins generally are essential.

2.2 Abundance of P450s

Of the 57 P450s (Table 1), 50 are expressed mainly in the endoplasmic reticulum and seven are expressed by nuclear genes but transported (following proteolysis) to the mitochondria (11A1, 11B1, 11B2, 24A1, 27A1, 27B1, 27C1). Fractions of some of the endoplasmic reticulum (microsomal) P450s are cleaved and also enter the mitochondria (e.g., 1B1, 2D6, 2E1, 2C8) (Avadhani, Sangar, Bansal, & Bajpai, 2011). The microsomal P450s receive electrons (from NADPH) via the diflavin protein POR and sometimes cytochrome b_5 (b_5). Those in the mitochondria use a system involving the flavoprotein NADPH-adrenodoxin (Adx) reductase and Adx. Although the mitochondrial P450s clearly have important roles in the metabolism of steroids and vitamins (Table 1) (Guengerich, 2015), in some cases they can also be involved in the metabolism of drugs (Zhang et al., 2012) and other chemicals.

In mammalian liver the ratio of total P450 to POR has long been known to be 10–20:1 (Estabrook, Franklin, Cohen, Shigamatzu, & Hildebrandt, 1971). The concentrations of several P450s in human liver have been estimated using immunochemical (Shimada, Yamazaki, Mimura, Inui, & Guengerich, 1994) and, more recently, mass spectrometry proteomic approaches (Achour, Al Feteisi, Lanucara, Rostami-Hodjegan, & Barber, 2017). The results from several studies are summarized in Fig. 1. While it is clear that P450 3A4 and two P450 Subfamily 2C enzymes (2C8, 2C9) are the most abundant, there is a large amount of variability, even in cases

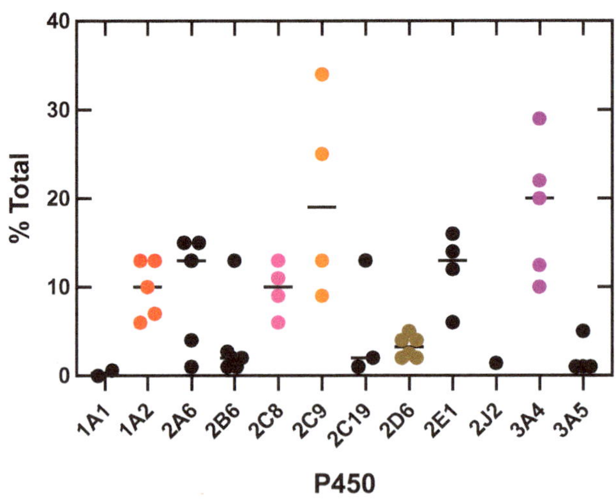

Fig. 1 Percentages of total P450 in human liver samples accounted for by each P450. The data points were compiled (Guengerich, 2022a) from four sets with multiple liver samples (Achour, Russell, Barber, & Rostami-Hodjegan, 2014; Kawakami et al., 2011; Shimada et al., 1994) and one with a single liver sample high in P450 1A1 (Lang, Radtke, & Bairlein, 2019). The estimates were made immunochemically in one case (Shimada et al., 1994) and by LC-MS proteomic methods in the others (Achour et al., 2014; Kawakami et al., 2011; Lang et al., 2019). The value for P450 1A1 is a mean of measurements of 30 samples (Lang et al., 2019). The individual colors have no meaning but are added to facilitate visualization.

where the same liver sets were analyzed (Guengerich, 2015). For instance, it is not clear whether P450s 2A6 and 2B6 should be considered minor or abundant enzymes (Fig. 1) (Guengerich, 2015).

The composition of individual P450s in human small intestine has also been analyzed (Paine et al., 2006). In this organ, the dominance of P450 3A4 is even more striking and this has relevance in considering the disposition of only administered drugs and inhibition of drug metabolism. The total amount of P450 in the small intestine is only a few percent of that in liver, however, and this point needs to be considered in the context of first-pass clearance.

2.3 Regulation

Many of the P450s are subject to enzyme induction, as well as localization in different tissues due to the influence of tissue-specific promoters. A general scheme for induction (Fig. 2) involves binding of a ligand to a receptor, formation of a heterodimeric pair, nuclear transport, and binding to specific sites of the gene to cause (chromosome rearrangement and) enhanced

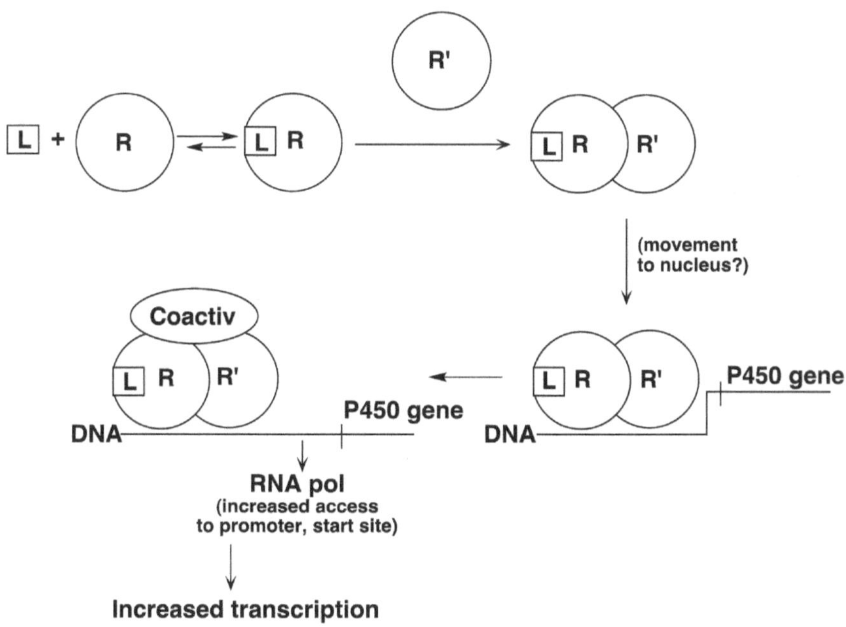

Fig. 2 General scheme for transcriptional regulation of P450s. L: ligand, R: receptor, R′-heterodimeric partner, Coactiv: co-activator protein (e.g., hepatic nuclear factor (HNF) α in the case of P450 3A4), RNA pol: RNA polymerase (Guengerich, 2018a, 2022a).

transcription by RNA polymerase (Fig. 2). This is the general pattern seen for the AhR, PXR, PPARα, and RAR systems of gene regulation. With AhR the heterodimer partner is ARNT. With the bulk of the systems, which use receptors from the steroid nuclear receptor superfamily (PXR, PPARα, ...), the partner is RXR, which is bound to retinoic acid or possibly another ligand. CAR, involved in regulation of P450s 2B6 and 3A4, is different in that while it can bind some ligands (e.g., 1,4-*bis*[2-(3,5-dichloropyridyloxy)]benzene, (TCPOBOP) (Maglich et al., 2003), in most cases the receptor is constitutively active and nuclear import is regulated by a phosphorylation cascade involving EGFR (Mutoh et al., 2013).

Induction by drugs is important for several reasons: (1) It leads to changes in pharmacokinetics when the drug of interest is also an inducer. (2) Drug-drug interactions can be important clinically, as seen in the classic example of enhanced metabolism of 17α-ethnylestradiol (in oral contraceptives) by P450 3A4 inducers (Bolt, Kappus, & Bolt, 1975). (3) In some animal models, enzyme induction is correlated with development of certain cancers, particularly in rodent liver (e.g., barbiturates, PPARα inducers) (Lubet, Nims, Ward, Rice, & Diwan, 1989; Rao & Reddy, 1987). Although this is much less of a regulatory concern than in the past, the development of rodent tumors in the drug development scenario must be explained and regulatory agencies need assurance that this will not be an issue in humans.

The most thoroughly studied model of P450 induction is transcriptional control. However, regulation can also be at the post-translational level, including mRNA and protein stabilization, and epigenetic control. Examples of roles of gene methylation (i.e., 5-methyl deoxycytidine), histone modification (e.g., acetylation), and microRNA involvement are now known for P450s (Guengerich, 2015; Ingelman-Sundberg et al., 2013), although the significance in humans is still not established.

P450 genes can also be regulated by cytokines. Interferons can down-regulate P450s, and the suppression of drug metabolism by interferons has long been known to be associated with colds, flu shots, etc. (Mannering, Renton, el Azhary, & Deloria, 1980; Renton, 1981). Another phenomenon observed in rats is the down-regulation of some P450s by some of the common inducers, e.g. barbiturates and particularly Family 1 inducers, as seen particularly with P450s 2C11 and 2E1 (Dannan, Guengerich, Kaminsky, & Aust, 1983; Guengerich, Dannan, Wright, Martin, & Kaminsky, 1982; Thomas, Bandiera, Maines, Ryan, & Levin, 1987). This suppression has been shown to occur at the transcriptional level (Sawaya & Riddick, 2008) but its relevance in humans is unknown.

Rodents display dramatic sex effects with regard to P450 regulation (Waxman, Dannan, & Guengerich, 1985; Waxman & Holloway, 2009). The basis of this is complex and involves not only androgens and estrogens but also pulsatile patterns of growth hormone and JAK/STAT regulation (Waxman & Holloway, 2009; Wiwi & Waxman, 2005). Although there are some reports of sex differences in some P450s in humans (Wolbold et al., 2003; Zhang et al., 2011), the differences have not been seen by others (Yang et al., 2010) and, at the pharmacokinetic level, may be attributable to body fat. However, knowledge of sex differences in rodent P450s may be important in understanding the results of pre-clinical testing in drug development.

2.4 Catalytic mechanism

Much has been written about chemical mechanisms of catalysis by P450s elsewhere (Guengerich, 2018b; Guengerich & Yoshimoto, 2018; Ortiz de Montellano, 2015).

The catalytic cycle is shown in Fig. 3, where the P450 binds substrate (Step 1), the iron is reduced (Step 2), oxygen binds (Step 3), and the second electron is donated to the iron (Step 4). At this point the intermediates are unstable, and information about them has taken some time to accumulate. The Fe^{3+}-O_2^- form (called Compound 0) becomes protonated (Step 5) and then H_2O is released to leave Compound I (after Step 6). In Step 7 the formal FeO^{3+} complex abstracts a hydrogen atom (or an electron from a heteroatom if the redox potential is low enough) to leave a "caged" radical (Step 7), which undergoes recombination with Compound II ($FeOH^{3+}$) to generate the product in Step 8. Finally, the product (ROH) is released in Step 9.

The P450 can be reduced without having substrates present, at least with some P450s (Guengerich & Johnson, 1997; Johnston et al., 2011). In some cases there is evidence that b_5 provides the second electron (in Step 4) but in other cases b_5 can stimulate P450 reactions without electron transfer (Yamazaki et al., 2002). Another point is that the cycle in Fig. 3 relates only to the electronic changes that occur, but numerous changes in protein structure occur as well, and even binding of a substrate can involve a complex series of steps (Guengerich, Wilkey, Glass, & Reddish, 2019; Guengerich, Wilkey, & Phan, 2019; Isin & Guengerich, 2006).

An appreciation of the catalytic mechanism of P450 is important in understanding the kinds of reactions that P450s can do. In areas such as drug metabolism and natural product biosynthesis, products must be

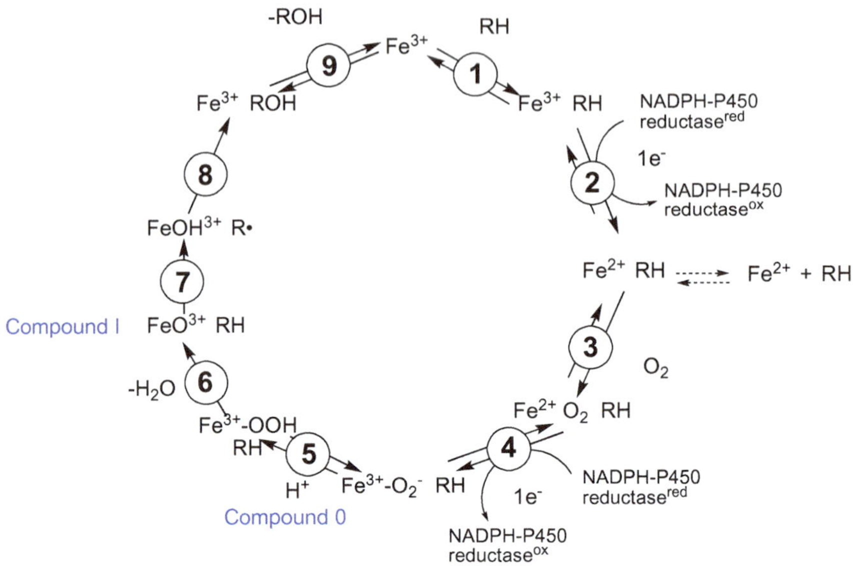

Fig. 3 P450 catalytic cycle. The nine labeled steps show sequential (1) substrate binding, (2) 1-electron reduction, (3) oxygen binding, (4) second 1-electron reduction, (5) protonation of "Compound 0," (6) loss of water to form "Compound I," (7) hydrogen atom abstraction by Compound I, (8) oxygen rebound to form product, and (9) product dissociation. As indicated, ferrous P450 can also bind substrate (Yun, Kim, Calcutt, & Guengerich, 2005). In some cases, b_5 can provide the electron in step 2 or 4. In some sequential reactions, step 9 does not occur and a second oxidation of the initial product is observed (Gonzalez & Guengerich, 2017; Reddish & Guengerich, 2019).

characterized and a knowledge of possible mechanisms is needed to discern possible pathways (Guengerich & Yoshimoto, 2018; Isin & Guengerich, 2007a).

Although possibilities have been raised of various other oxidant forms of P450 in various oxidations, almost all reactions can be explained by involving Compound I reactions. Some proposals for Compound 0 or other species have been re-valuated or analyzed further and re-interpreted in terms of Compound I (Groves, McClusky, White, & Coon, 1978; Guengerich & Yoshimoto, 2018; Huang & Groves, 2017; Krest et al., 2013; Rittle & Green, 2010; Yoshimoto & Guengerich, 2014). Only in a few cases has P450 Compound I been prepared directly and rigorously characterized (by reaction with a peracid) (Krest et al., 2013; Rittle & Green, 2010). Some bona fide Baeyer-Villiger-type oxidations may still prove to involve Compound 0 (Guengerich, 2022b).

2.5 Structures of P450s and binding of ligands

Although X-ray crystallography of P450s was limited to soluble bacterial P450s before 2000, the work of Johnson (Williams, Cosme, Sridhar, Johnson, & MeRee, 2000) and then others has led to a plethora of P450 structures. As of 2021 there were at least 260 structures of mammalian P450s in the Protein Data Bank, and 25 of the 57 human P450s have crystal structures available (plus apparent animal orthologues of P450 4B1 and 24A1).

All P450 structures to date have similar overall folds (Fig. 4). The interaction and movements among the I, F′, and G′ helices are important in modulating ligand specificity.

Some of the human P450s have been crystallized in open, closed, and intermediate forms (Guengerich, Waterman, & Egli, 2016; Poulos & Johnson, 2015). A single structure of a P450 provides useful information about the bonding of a P450 with a substrate but it may not present a picture of how the P450 bound that substrate, i.e. the course of events leading to (productive) binding. Some of the P450s have been found to bind substrates in multiple ways and also to have multiple conformations in the absence of a substrate or other ligand (Ekroos & Sjögren, 2006; Hsu & Johnson, 2019; Porubsky, Battaile, & Scott, 2010).

One hypothesis about how enzymes such as P450s are able to bind so many substrates is that of induced fit (Fig. 5) (Koshland, Nemethy, & Filmer, 1966); i.e. binding of a substrate to an enzyme induces the enzyme

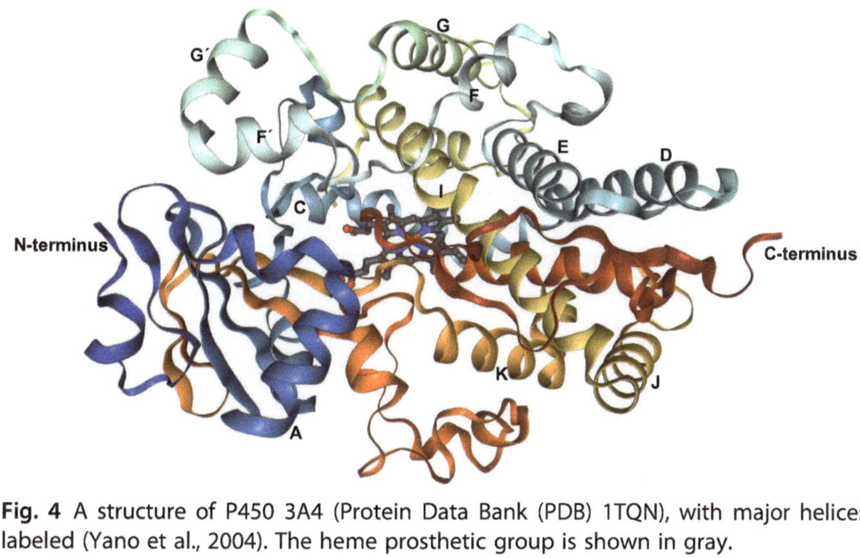

Fig. 4 A structure of P450 3A4 (Protein Data Bank (PDB) 1TQN), with major helices labeled (Yano et al., 2004). The heme prosthetic group is shown in gray.

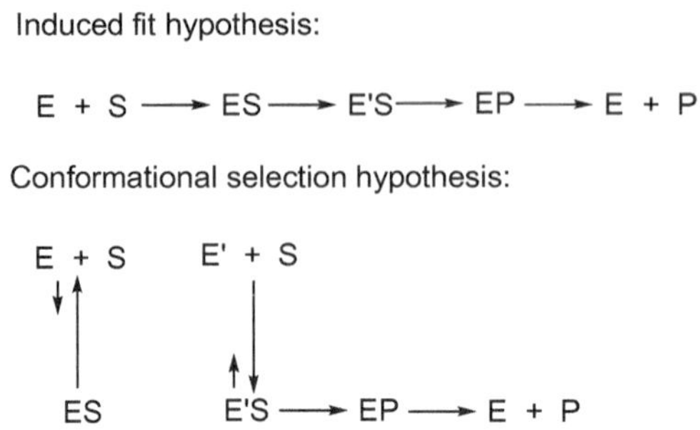

Fig. 5 Hypotheses to explain complex substrate recognition data (Gianni, Dogan, & Jemth, 2014; Vogt & Di Cera, 2012).

to adopt a new conformation that is more favorable for productive catalysis. An alternative mechanism involves conformational selection (Fig. 5), where the enzyme exists in multiple conformations in the absence of ligand, one (or more) of which binds the substrate to yield a productive complex (Fig. 5). These are not necessarily completely distinct phenomena and may occur together. Discerning which course (Fig. 5) is dominant is usually difficult, in that the free energy involved in the route from E to a productive E´S complex is identical regardless of the route (Chakraborty & Di Cera, 2017; Vogt, Pozzi, Chen, & Di Cera, 2014). One hallmark of the presence of complex binding pathways is slow kinetics, i.e. at less than diffusion-limited rates (Johnson, 2019). The two routes (Fig. 5) can be distinguished by measuring the kinetics of binding as a function of varying the concentration of ligand, enzyme, or both (Gianni et al., 2014; Vogt & Di Cera, 2012). Such kinetic studies have been done with several human P450s and indicate the dominance of conformational selection pathways (Guengerich, Wilkey, Glass, & Reddish, 2019; Guengerich, Wilkey, & Phan, 2019). The binding of the preferred substrate camphor to bacterial $P450_{cam}$ (P450 101A1) appears to be an exception (Guengerich, Child, Barckhausen, & Goldfarb, 2021), but the conformational selection mechanism appeared to be more dominant with alternate substrates of $P450_{cam}$.

The binding of inhibitors to P450 3A4 has been shown to be a complex process, with multiple steps and spectrally detectable intermediates (Fig. 6) (Guengerich et al., 2020; Isin & Guengerich, 2007b). Achieving full inhibition requires completion of the steps for P450 3A4 (i.e., the E*I complex in Fig. 6). With P450 17A1, multiple spectral intermediates are seen upon mixing but inhibition occurs immediately, before the spectral changes are

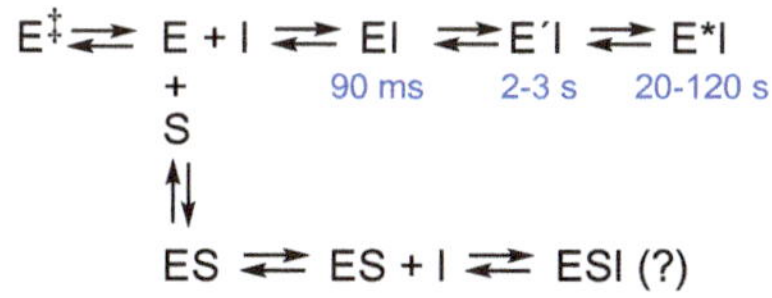

Fig. 6 Scheme summarizing interaction of P450 3A4 with inhibitors. The times of appearance of individual species are indicated in blue (Guengerich, McCarty, & Chapman, 2020).

completed (Fig. 6) (Child & Guengerich, 2020; Guengerich, McCarty, Chapman, & Tateishi, 2021). The difference may be due to the large size of the active site of P450 3A4 ($\sim$1400 $Å^3$ (Yano et al., 2004)), which is able to accommodate two molecules of the inhibitor ketoconazole (Ekroos & Sjögren, 2006). No crystal structure of a P450 containing *both* a substrate and inhibitor has been published but is certainly feasible for P450 3A4 and probably some other P450s.

3. P450s and drug metabolism

In the early history of P450 research, little information was available about how many P450s existed, how many had major roles in drug metabolism, and which of these P450s metabolized individual drugs. Today the human P450s are all known (Table 1), with the completion of the human genome and recognition of the P450 signature sequence:

$$\text{Phe} - \text{X} - \text{X} - \text{Gly} - \text{X} - \text{Arg} - \text{X}_\text{b} - \text{Cys} - \text{X} - \text{Gly}$$

where the Cys is liganded to the heme iron atom and X_b is a basic residue. P450s are involved in the metabolism of $\sim$ ¾ of (small molecule) drugs (Fig. 7), and about five P450s are involved with 90% of the drugs (Guengerich, 2015; Rendic & Guengerich, 2015). Those fractions have remained similar for new drugs, with P450 3A4 playing an even more dominant role (Fig. 7). This trend may be due, at least in part, to (i) a tendency towards larger molecules, in efforts to achieve selectivity and potency, and (ii) efforts to avoid dependence on the P450s showing more genetic polymorphism (e.g., 2C19 and 2D6).

3.1 P450s and pharmacokinetic issues

One issue in drug development is prediction of sites of metabolism. Over the years there has been some progress in the *in silico* prediction of sites

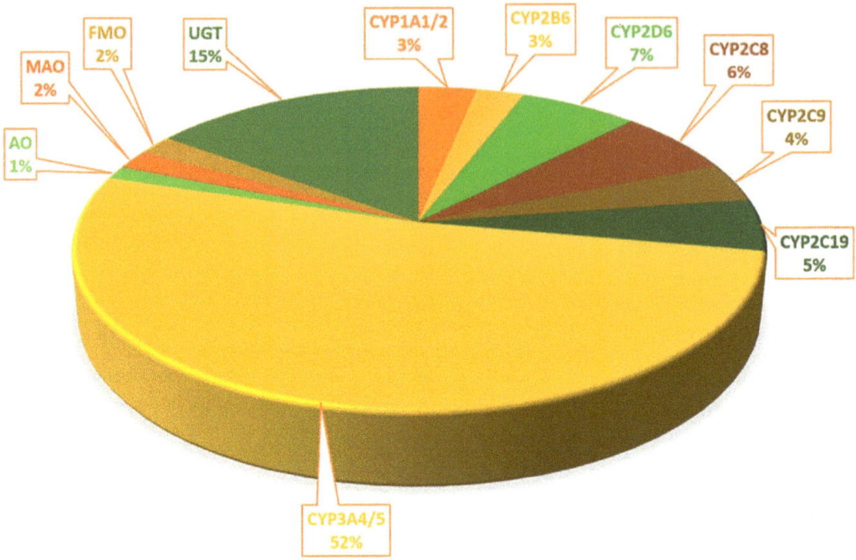

Fig. 7 Fractions of small molecule drugs approved by US FDA in 2015–2020 metabolized by individual enzymes (Bhutani et al., 2021). UGT, uridine diphosphate glucuronosyl transferase; FMO, flavin-containing monooxygenase; AO, aldehyde oxidase. *Reprinted from Bhutani, P., Joshi, G., Raja, N., Bachhav, N., Rajanna, P. K., Bhutani, H., et al. (2021). US FDA approved drugs from 2015-June 2020: A perspective.* Journal of Medical Chemistry, 64*(5), 2339–2381, Copyright (2021), with permission from the American Chemical Society.*

(Afzelius et al., 2007; Boyer et al., 2007; de Bruyn Kops, Sicho, Mazzolari, & Kirchmair, 2021; Ekins et al., 2005; Kirchmair et al., 2015; Martiny & Miteva, 2013; Wilson, White, & Mueller, 2003), especially if the "top three" sites are all predicted. Much of the success has been achieved with algorithms based on prior examples, as opposed to docking into X-ray structures. Nevertheless, there will probably always be some surprises regarding in silico predictions, e.g. testosterone is hydroxylated by P450 3A4 mainly at the 6β (as well as 2β, 1β, and 15β) carbon but 4,5-dihydrotestosterone is hydroxylated at the (chemically more inert) 18- and 19-methyl carbons (Cheng, Sohl, Yoshimoto, & Guengerich, 2012).

As molecules progress in the discovery/development process, they do require the use of analytical chemistry to define structures of metabolites. Progress in the past three decades in LC-MS and NMR has greatly improved the process, and there are novel techniques with possibilities, such as crystallization and X-ray diffraction of trapped compounds (Rosenberger et al., 2020).

What is more difficult is the prediction of rates of metabolism by P450s, although there are claims to be able to do this with artificial intelligence (Xiong et al., 2021). This is probably only realistic in situations where, for instance, rates are known for close analogs and the effects of adding substituents are subject to Hammett analysis or other linear free energy relationships (Burka, Guengerich, Willard, & Macdonald, 1985). Rates of (total) oxidative metabolism can be measured in relatively high throughput assays with liver microsomes and LC-MS, however. Such assays can be done with hepatocytes but not as rapidly or large-scale. The microsomal assays are a rapid means of stratifying for drug stability. However, if pharmacologically active products are formed, the results will be misleading regarding the value of a drug candidate.

3.1.1 Changing molecules to attenuate metabolism

When a lead drug is metabolized too rapidly, there may be possibilities for slowing the metabolism. To do this effectively, the site of oxidation should be known. If the P450 involved in oxidation is known, it is possible to dock the molecule to suggest changes that might prevent metabolism or bioactivation while maintaining pharmacological activity (Brodney et al., 2015). Strategies may involve (i) adding a moiety (at the site) that will resist oxidation or prevent binding to the P450, (ii) substituting deuterium for protium (Gant, 2014; Pirali, Serafini, Cargnin, & Genazzani, 2019; Stringer et al., 2014), or (iii) adding a "soft" site elsewhere in the molecule that "steer" oxidation there. Of these, the first option has been the most useful.

3.1.2 Variations in pharmacokinetics

In an ideal world, a new drug would have the same metabolites, half-life, and clearance in all individuals, and prescriptions would be easy to develop. However, there are several reasons for variable pharmacokinetics.

One issue is genetic inter-individual variability, i.e. genetic differences in the P450 enzymes. This issue is discussed in detail in the chapter "Pharmacogenetics of the cytochromes P450: Selected pharmacological and toxicological aspects" by Daly.

Other issues involve changes due to enzyme induction and inhibition. These can be due to the drug itself or to other drugs, or even chemicals found in foods (e.g., grapefruit) or societal habits (smoking, alcohol). When induction and inhibition are associated with the drug itself, the pharmacokinetics of the drug can be expected to change with time, even in the absence of other drugs.

3.2 Drug-drug interactions

Drug-drug interactions are an important issue and account for both a sizeable fraction of hospitalizations and hospital deaths (Montane, Arellano, Sanz, Roca, & Farre, 2018). These problems are seen with many diseases and therapeutic areas (Fig. 8A) (Yu et al., 2018). A large fraction of the pharmacokinetic drug-drug interactions are seen with P450 3A(4) and some of the drug transporters (Fig. 8B).

The complexity of drug metabolism makes it hard to totally avoid drug-drug interactions and some other toxicity problems, as exemplified in the metabolism of phenacetin and acetaminophen (Fig. 9).

The analgesic phenacetin is no longer in use because it was associated with rat kidney cancers. It undergoes oxidation in several P450-dependent reactions, some of which can lead to the generation of reactive products that can covalently bind to proteins and DNA. The product of *O*-deethylation is acetaminophen, a drug used extensively for fever and pain. Acetaminophen is used therapeutically at least once per week by ~23% of the US population (Larson et al., 2005), with benefit. However, it is also involved in ½ of the cases of drug-induced liver failure.

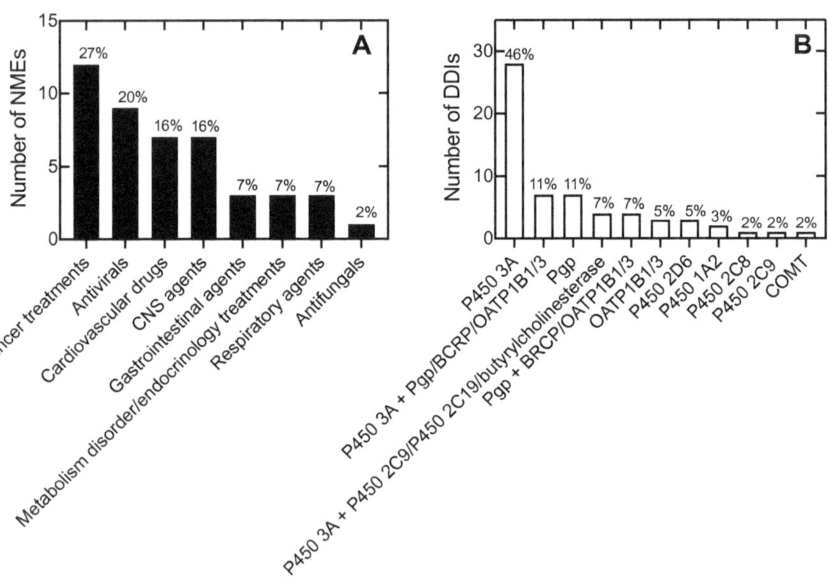

Fig. 8 Frequency of new molecular entities (NMEs, i.e. new drug candidates) in inhibition-based drug-drug interactions (DDIs) with drugs approved by the Food and Drug Administration (FDA) in the United States between 2013 and 2016 (Yu, Zhou, Tay-Sontheimer, Levy, & Ragueneau-Majlessi, 2018). (A) Grouping by therapeutic class. (B) Grouping by enzymes involved. Pgp and OAT1B1 are transporters. COMT, catechol *O*-methyl transferase.

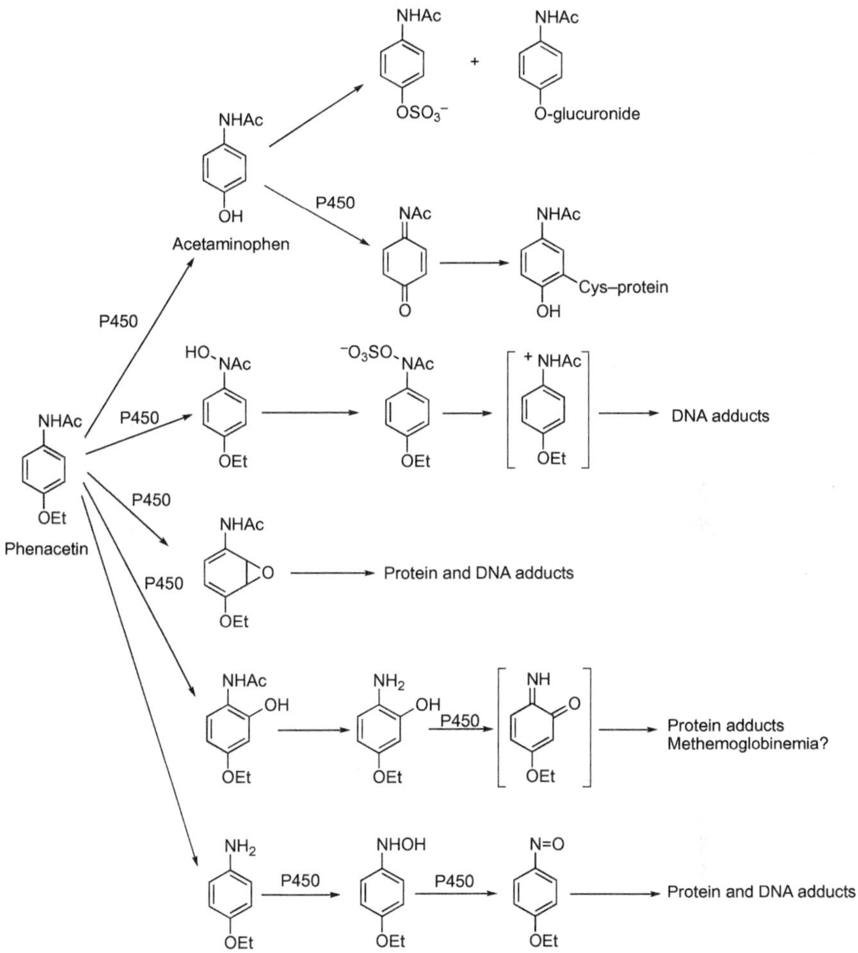

Fig. 9 Roles of P450s in the bioactivation and detoxication of chemicals: the complex example of phenacetin (Guengerich, 2019a). Acetaminophen (paracetamol, Tylenol®) is widely used as an analgesic, safe at low doses and hepatotoxic at high levels (Lee, Buters, Pineau, Fernandez-Salguero, & Gonzalez, 1996). Phenacetin has been classified as a carcinogen and withdrawn from use. The metabolism of acetaminophen has been investigated in detail (Dahlin, Miwa, Lu, & Nelson, 1984; Dahlin & Nelson, 1982; Guengerich, 2022a). Only in a few cases are the structures of the protein and DNA adducts known. Some of the indicated P450s have been identified in different species, including humans (Distlerath et al., 1985; Lee et al., 1996).

The metabolism of phenacetin is induced (at least P450 1A2, the *O*-deethylase) by polycyclic hydrocarbons and other P450 Family 1 inducers (AhR agonists) (Conney et al., 1976; Pantuck et al., 1974). In humans, the oxidation of acetaminophen to a potentially toxic iminoquinone is catalyzed mainly by three P450s—2E1, 1A2, and 3A4 (Patten et al., 1993). P450 2E1 appears to dominate, and induction of P450 2E1 by ethanol is generally considered to be the basis of enhanced hepatotoxicity of acetaminophen in alcoholics (Lee & Kaplowitz, 2021).

Drug-drug interactions can either render a drug ineffective or exaggerate the pharmacology and make it toxic.

3.2.1 Induction

The most common problem with induction is the loss of drug efficacy due to enhanced metabolism of a drug. A classical example involves the induction of P450 3A4 by rifampicin or barbiturates and the ineffectiveness of oral contraceptives due to enhanced clearance of 17α-ethynylestradiol (Bolt, Bolt, & Kappus, 1977; Guengerich, 1988). This phenomenon continues to occur with other barbiturates (Wilbur & Ensom, 2000) and it is also seen with some herbal medicines (Hall et al., 2003), in that St. John's wort contains a potential PXR inducer, hyperforin (Moore et al., 2000).

P450 inducers not only pose problems in the clinic but are also issues in experimental animals in the process of safety assessment. Some chemicals induce animal P450s and can confound pre-clinical pharmacokinetic studies or lead to toxicity problems. Even though the issues may not be relevant to humans, those issues need to be explained to regulatory agencies, and the testing may waste valuable resources. Moreover, some animal tumors are seen with certain modes of induction (e.g., PPARα), even if they are not recognized as being relevant to human medical situations. Overall, it is generally desirable to advance a lead drug that is not an inducer, it there is a choice and other factors are equal.

3.2.2 Inhibition

3.2.2.1 Modes of inhibition

Inhibition is a very important factor in pharmacokinetic drug-drug interactions. The subject has been treated extensively elsewhere, and only a brief treatise will be provided here.

A simple way of dividing P450 inhibitors is among (i) reversible inhibitors, (ii) quasi-reversible inhibitors, and (iii) irreversible inhibitors. Reversible inhibition is the most straight-forward situation. It follows the basic schemes generally taught in introductory biochemistry, i.e. competitive, non-competitive, uncompetitive, and mixed inhibition. In the simplest cases, two drugs are bound to the enzyme at either the same or at different sites. Reversible inhibition can be detected quickly with high throughput screening. The mechanisms may be more complicated than just simple competition for an active site, in that multiple ligand occupancy is possible for some P450s such as 3A4 (Ekroos & Sjögren, 2006). Other complex phenomena have been reported in our own laboratory (Bojic et al., 2014; Shinkyo & Guengerich, 2011).

3.2.2.2 Time-dependent inhibition

The reversible inhibition modes mentioned above occur quickly and are reversed as the inhibitor is removed, most generally by metabolism (sometimes by the same P450 enzyme) (Guengerich, 2019b). There are several modes of time-dependent inhibition, in which the catalytic activity of the P450 is involved in exacerbating the inhibition. Time-dependent inhibition can be divided into three general modes.

(i) Formation of quasi-reversible complexes. The most prominent examples are the oxidation of amines (primary) to C-nitroso compounds and of methylenedioxyphenyls to carbenes. These unstable products bind very tightly to ferrous P450 (Fe^{2+}), yielding complexes with absorption maxima at 455 nm. The binding is very tight. A relevant example is troleandomycin (Pessayre et al., 1983). The rates of breakdown of the complex is slow and takes more than a day in vivo (Delaforge, Jaouen, & Mansuy, 1984).

(ii) Generation of reactive metabolites that bind to P450 covalently to inhibit. The list includes quinones, quinone imines, epoxides, and other species. These are chemical entities that bind irreversibly to P450s (and possibly to other proteins, including other P450s) (Fig. 9).

(iii) True mechanism-based inhibitors, which are compounds that are oxidized to enzyme intermediates (usually species with radical or carbocationic character) that react with groups in the protein—or the heme prosthetic group—to inactivate. Covalent products are formed.

In all three cases the inhibition develops with time, in the presence of POR, NADPH, and oxygen.

Drug candidates that behave in this way can be identified using in vitro screening paradigms, although they are more complex than for single reversible inhibitors and not as adaptable to high-throughput screening. With all three modes of quasi-reversible and irreversible inhibition, the nature of the kinetic constants is more complex than for simple reversible inhibition, and the most valuable parameters are $k_{inactivation}$ (the maximum rate of enzyme inactivation at infinite inhibitor concentration) and K_i, the inhibitor concentration at which half the maximal rate of enzyme inhibition is obtained. In contrast to a K_m value, a K_i in this case is actually a parameter that reflects the dissociation constant (K_d) for the enzyme-inhibitor complex (before activation) (Johnson, 2019; Silverman, 1995).

3.2.2.3 Use of inhibitors to slow drug metabolism

Although the focus is usually on avoiding drug-drug interactions due to inhibition, there are situations in which inhibition of P450 metabolism is desirable. In some cases achieving metabolic stability of drugs is difficult, and the production of complex drugs (especially some natural products) may be expensive, e.g. cyclosporin. This has been an issue with some HIV therapies.

An anecdotal approach to slowing gut metabolism by P450 3A4 (and perhaps some other enzymes) is by ingestion of grapefruit juice (Bailey, Edgar, Spence, Munzo, & Arnold, 1990). The problem is that the content of bergamottin can vary, so the control of exactly how much inhibition occurs may be problematic. The viral protease inhibitor ritonavir is also a potent inhibitor of P450 3A4 (Greenblatt & Harmatz, 2015) and has been used as a "booster" in prescribing information with some P450 3A4 substrates. This is more powerful and, unlike grapefruit juice, inhibits hepatic P450 3A4 as well as intestinal. Rational design methods have been used with P450 3A4 crystal structures to pursue ritonavir analogs for this purpose (Sevrioukova & Poulos, 2014). The drug cobicistat, resembling ritonavir, was developed as a P450 3A4 inhibitor and is FDA approved as a booster drug.

3.2.2.4 Clinical issues

There are numerous examples of P450-based drug-drug interactions. One that is now classic is terfenadine (Fig. 10), the first non-sedating antihistamine on the market. More than 100 million people used the drug (as Seldane®), and for most the drug was very helpful (Guengerich, 2014; Thompson & Oster, 1996). However, deaths were reported beginning in 1990, due to cardiac arrythmia, and eventually at least 25 deaths were attributed to terfenadine (some estimates as high as 125 or more). A major factor was the use of ketoconazole or erythromycin at the same time. Terfenadine is oxidized mainly by P450 3A4 (Yun et al., 1993), a fact which was unknown when the problems began. Normally terfenadine is oxidized rapidly and not found in the plasma; the product fexofenadine (which also has pharmacological activity) is the circulating active drug (Fig. 10). Blocking the metabolism of terfenadine causes it to accumulate, and it binds tightly to the hERG potassium channel receptor and causes torsades de pointes (long QT intervals) and leads to arrhythmias.

With the development of knowledge about human P450 enzymes, it is now fairly routine to establish which P450(s) is involved in the metabolism

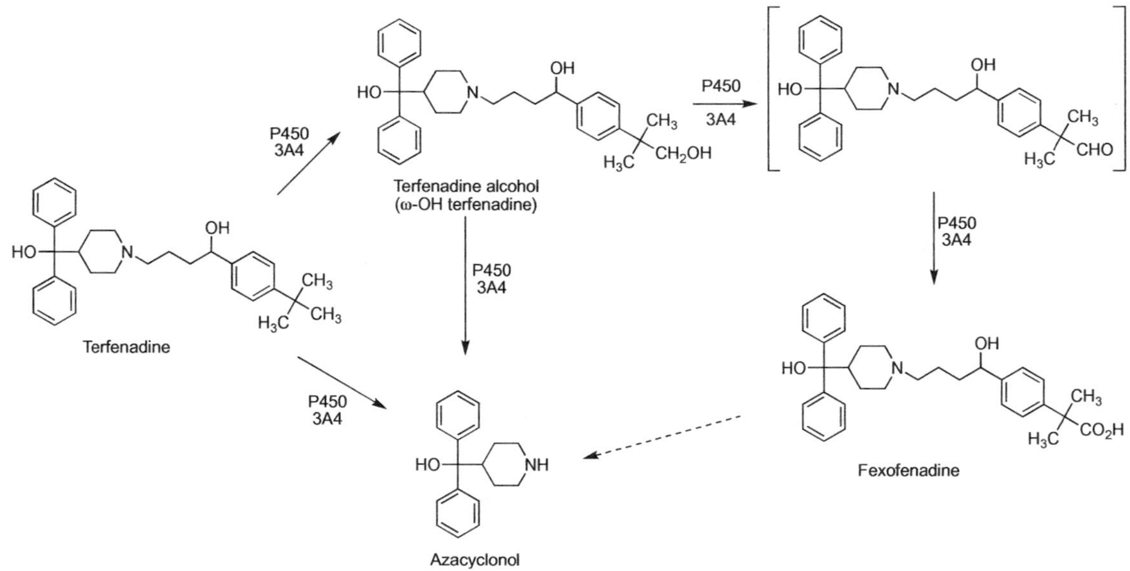

Fig. 10 Metabolism of terfenadine (Guengerich, 2014; Thompson & Oster, 1996; Yun, Okerholm, & Guengerich, 1993). All steps are catalyzed primarily by P450 3A4. Oxidations of the antihistamine terfenadine catalyzed by P450 3A4. The oxidation of terfenadine was attenuated in individuals who have inherently low levels of P450 3A4 (Yang et al., 2010) or used P450 3A4 inhibitors (e.g., erthyromycin, ketoconazole) concomitantly with terfenadine (Guengerich, 2014; Yun et al., 1993).

of a drug (Fig. 7), and regulatory agencies have this expectation at the IND stage (filing of an "Investigational New Drug" application at the U. S. FDA or the equivalent elsewhere, when a new drug candidate is first administered to humans). Tables of known inhibitors of the major human P450s are available (Table 2), and predictions can be made about which drug interactions might be problematic.

Some P450 substrates are more sensitive to inhibition (by other drugs), and some have narrow therapeutic windows (Table 3), e.g. warfarin. If a new drug would be likely to be given in combination with one of these drugs, then a regulatory agency might well require a clinical interaction study.

The US FDA has ranges for the effects of inhibitors. The most general approach is to compare the pharmacokinetic "area-under-the-curve" (AUC) without and with inhibitor (AUC_R). If this value is in the range of 1.25–2.0, then the inhibition is considered "weak" and not expected to be a problem. A value of AUC_R in the range of 2–5 is considered "moderate," and a value >5 is "strong." The latter two groups ($AUC_R > 2$) may require labeling in the form of a contraindication warning.

As mentioned earlier, one of the troublesome issues in drug development has been time-dependent inhibition, particularly with P450 3A4 substrates (Fig. 7) (Zimmerlin, Trunzer, & Faller, 2011). Eng, Tseng, Cerny, Goosen, and Obach (2021) have compared a large series of P450 3A4 substrates for *in vitro* inhibition parameters with clinical AUC_R values (Fig. 11).

Several points are of note. (i) Many drugs show time-dependent inhibition, even drugs that have been on the market for some time, often without major issues. (ii) The assays with hepatocytes showed less-time-dependent inhibition (Fig. 11B) than the assays with microsomes (Fig. 11A). (iii) There is a rough correlation between *in vitro* rates of time-dependent inhibition of P450 3A4 and AUC_R but there are many outliers. (iv) The structures of many of the drugs that show time-dependent inhibition are not obvious as to why they should be (i.e., lack of acetylenes, cyclopropylamines, etc.). The results shown in Fig. 11 indicate that in vitro assays of time-dependent inhibition are still not completely reliable in predicting whether drug-drug interactions will be a problem. In the analysis of Novartis compounds by Zimmerlin et al. (2011), it was noted that the incidence of time-dependent P450 3A4 inhibition—and of strong reversible inhibition—was much lower in drugs that reached the market than in drug candidates, indicative of the liability of time-dependent inhibition (Zimmerlin et al., 2011).

Table 2 Inhibitors of major P450s.

1A2	2C9	2C19	2D6	3A4
Amiodarone	Amiodarone	Chloramphenicol	Amiodarone	Amiodarone
Cimetidine	Capecitabine	Cimetidine	Bupropion	Aprepitant
Ciprofloxacin	Clopidogrel	Citalopram	Celecoxib	Atomoxetine
Citalopram	Crisaborole	Esomeprazole	Chlorpheniramine	Boceprevir
Crisaborole	Efavirenz	Felbamate	Chlorpromazine	Chloramphenicol
Efavirenz	Fenofibrate	Fluoxetine	Cimetidine	Cimetidine
Fluoroquinolone	Fluconazole	Fluvoxamine	Cinacalcet	Ciprofloxacin
Fluvoxamine	Fluvastatin	Indomethacin	Citalopram	Clarithromycin
Furafylline	Fluvoxamine	Isoniazid	Clemastine	Delaviridine
Interferon	Isoniazid	Ketoconazole	Clomipramine	Diethyldithiocarbamate
Methoxsalen	Lovastatin	Lansopraxole	Cocaine	Diltiazem
Mibefradil	Metronidazole	Modafinil	Diphenhydramine	Erythromycin
Ribociclib	Paroxetine	Omeprazole	Doxepin	Esomeprazole
Rucaparib	Phenylbutazone	Oxcarbazepine	Doxorubicin	Fluconazole
Ticlopidine	Probenicid	Pantoprazole	Duloxetine	Fluvoxamine
	Rucaparib	Probenicid	Escitalopram	Gestodene
	Sertraline	Rucaparib	Fluoxetine	Grapefruit juice
	Sulfamethoxazole	Ticlopidine	Halofantrine	Idelalisib
	Sulfaphenazole	Ropiramate	Haloperidol	Imatinib
	Teniposide	Voriconazole	Hydroxyzine	Indinavir
	Voriconazole		Levomepromzaine	Itraconazole
	Zafirlukast		Methadone	Ketoconazole
			Metoclopramide	Lesinurad
			Mibefradil	Mibefradil
			Midodrine	Mifepristone
			Moclobemide	Nefazodone
			Palonosetron	Nelfinavir
			Panobinostat	Netupitant
			Paroxetine	Norfloxacin
			Perphenazine	Norfluoxetine
			Promethazine	Omeprazole

Continued

Table 2 Inhibitors of major P450s.—cont'd

1A2	2C9	2C19	2D6	3A4
			Quinidine	Pantoprazole
			Ranitidine	Regorafenib
			Riclopidine	Ribociclib
			Ritonavir	Ritonavir
			Rolapitant	Saquinavir
			Rucaparib	Starfruit
			Sertraline	Telaprevir
			Terbinafine	Telithromycin
			Tripelennamine	Verapamil
				Voriconazole

Modified from Flockhart, D. A. (2007). Drug interactions: Cytochrome P450 drug interaction table. Indiana University School of Medicine. "https//drug-interactions.medicine.iu.edu" Accessed 19 August 2021.

Table 3 Examples of sensitive *in vivo* P450 substrates and P450 substrates with narrow therapeutic range.

P450 Enzymes	Sensitive substrates	Substrates with narrow therapeutic range
1A2	Alosetron, caffeine, duloxetine, melatonin, ramelteon, tacrin, tizanidine	Theophylline, tizanidine
2B6	Bupropion, efavirenz	
2C8	Repaglinide	Paclitaxel
2C9	Celecoxib	Warfarin, phenytoin
2C19	Clobazam, lansoprazole, omeprazole, (*S*)-mephenytoin	(*S*)-Mephenytoin
3A (4,5)	Alfentanil, aprepitant, budesonide, buspirone, conivaptan, darifenacin, darunavir, dasatinib, dronedarone, eletriptan, eplerenone, everolimus, felodipine, indinavir, fluticasone, lopinavir, lovastatin, lurasidone, maraviroc, midazolam, nisoldipine, quetiapine, saquinavir, sildenafil, simvastatin, sirolimus, tolvaptan, tipranair, triazolam, ticagrelor, vardenafil	Alfentanil, astemizole, cisapride, cyclosporine, dihydroergotamine, ergotamine, fentanyl, pimozide, quinidine, sirolimus, tacrolimus, terfenadine
2D6	Atomoxetine, desipramine, dextromethorphan, metoprolol, nebivolol, perphenazine, tolterodine, venlafaxsine	Thioridazine, pimozide

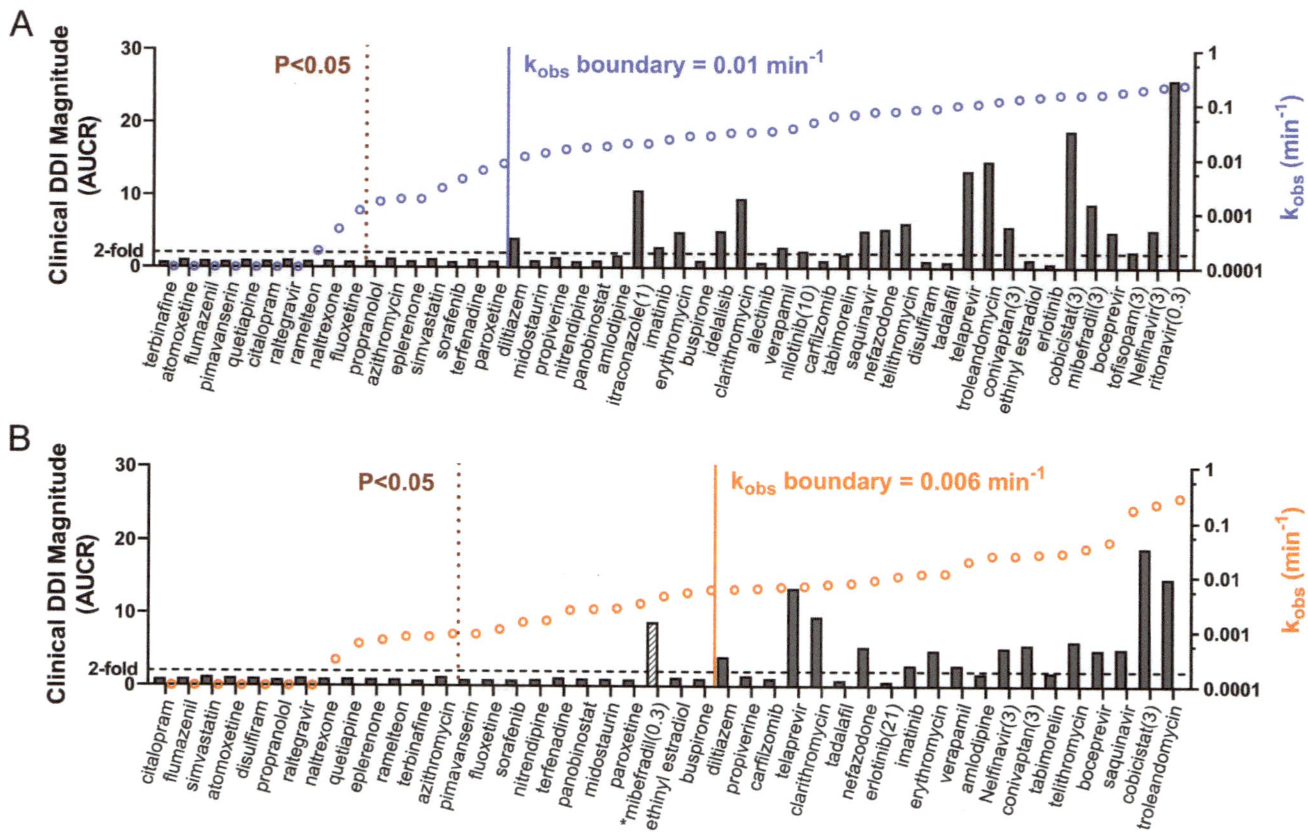

Fig. 11 See figure legend on next page.

3.3 Toxicity issues

3.3.1 Slow metabolism

Rates of drug clearance are generally developed for the majority of patients, and it is the individuals who have unusually slow metabolism who are at the most risk, generally due to either genetic reasons (see other chapters in this treatise) or inhibition (*vide supra*). If an individual with slow metabolism is given the usual dose, then the buildup of drug can (i) yield an exaggerated pharmacological response of the normal target or (ii) alternatively, result in metabolism at a secondary site to produce a toxic product (Fig. 9). Either action can result in toxicity to the patient. For these reasons it is important to define the variability of pharmacokinetic parameters in clinical trials.

3.3.2 Bioactivation

The matter of the potential for generation of reactive metabolites has already been considered in regard to P450 inhibition, but the general issue of bioactivation involves the generation of products that can modify other proteins or nucleic acids to cause toxicity. As indicated with phenacetin and acetaminophen (Fig. 9), there is usually a balance of detoxication and bioactivation reactions occurring, and the net result determines whether a chemical is toxic or not—as well as the dose, of course. Some chemical moieties are more likely to cause problems. There are called "toxicophores," and the list includes hydrazines and hydrazides, aryl acetic and aryl propionic acids, thiophenes, furans, pyrroles, anilines and anilides, quinones and quinone imines, medium chain fatty acids, halogenated hydrocarbons and some halogenated aromatics, nitroaromatics, thiols, thiono compounds and thiazolidinediones, and

Fig. 11 Boundary line for k_{obs} for time-dependent inhibition and relation to *in vivo* drug-drug interactions (DDI) (Eng et al., 2021). (A) Fifty drugs were evaluated for P450 3A4 time-dependent inhibition in human liver microsomes (at 30 μM unless noted otherwise) and ranked by k_{obs}, the first-order rate of inactivation, as judged using midazolam 1′-hydroxylation (○), presented on a $\log_{10}$ scale (right y-axis). The filled bars show the in vivo drug-drug interactions as judged by the AUC_R (AUC with the drug divided by the AUC without the drug, Clinical DDI magnitude). (B) The study in Part *A* was repeated in human hepatocytes. The stippled line indicates a twofold *in vivo* difference. Also indicated are $P < 0.05$ statistical limits and a k_{obs} "boundary" of the lowest *in vitro* value with twofold *in vivo* difference. *Reprinted from Eng, H., Tseng, E., Cerny, M. A., Goosen, T. C., & Obach, R. S. (2021). Cytochrome P450 3A time-dependent inhibition assays are too sensitive for identification of drugs causing clinically significant drug-drug interactions: A comparison of human liver microsomes and hepatocytes and definition of boundaries for inactivation rate constants.* Drug Metabolism & Disposition, 49, *442–450, Copyright (2021), with permission from the American Society for Pharmacology and Experimental Therapeutics.*

moieties that form α,β-unsaturated enol-like compounds (Michael acceptors) (Guengerich, 2021). However, in some therapeutic programs one (or more) of these entities may be needed for the desired pharmacological activity. Also, there are numerous exceptions—e.g., atorvastatin (Lipitor®), which has a masked aniline present but was the best-selling drug in the world for several years.

The finding of toxicity late in a drug development program is highly problematic and expensive, if a drug candidate must be dropped after spending considerable resources. Thus, there is considerable interest in *reliably* identifying bioactivation (and any other toxicity) issues early in the drug development process. The systems differ among pharmaceutical companies but the main elements follow.

(i) *In silico* screening. The most useful systems to date involve genotoxicity. The screens are based largely upon literature bases of results plus structural similarity. Tissue-selective toxicities are more complex and mechanisms are generally not well-described, so these are far less reliable.

(ii) Covalent binding screens. The extent of binding of drug candidates *in vitro* (microsomal and hepatocyte systems) and *in vivo* was proposed and used extensively in some pharmaceutical companies (Evans, Watt, Nicoll-Griffith, & Baillie, 2004). There was never a cut-off parameter but the approach was used to stratify compounds in making decisions as to which to advance. An issue is that compounds must be synthesized with radiolabels early in the process. There are correlations between the level of covalent binding and toxicity but many exceptions, even when accounting for the dose and body burden (Bauman et al., 2009; Dahal, Obach, & Gilbert, 2013; Nakayama et al., 2009; Obach, Kalgutkar, Soglia, & Zhao, 2008; Takakusa et al., 2008; Thompson et al., 2012).

(iii) General cellular toxicity. In some programs, toxicity is measured in cells in culture, particularly in some types of hepatocytes. However, all liver cells in culture have some type of metabolic deficiencies (regarding P450 expression). Even more problematic is the difficulty in using cellular assays to predict what will occur in a tissue.

(iv) Measurement of selective biomarkers. Some assays of interest include gross cell toxicity, mitochondrial toxicity, and inhibition of bile salt exporter protein (BSEP) and the transporter MRP2. Some pharmaceutical companies use a battery of assays, including covalent binding, in order to stratify their new chemical entities (Monroe et al., 2020; Thompson et al., 2012).

(v) Genotoxicity is a particular type of toxicity, and some of the assays are very well developed. The Ames bacterial mutagenicity tests (Ames, Durston, Yamasaki, & Lee, 1973) have been used extensively for 50 years and are almost universally used as the primary screen for genotoxicity, which is an indicator not only for potential carcinogenicity but also other maladies drive by mutation (e.g., teratogenesis). Bacterial mutation results are followed up by mammalian mutagenicity.

3.3.3 Human specific metabolites

Humans and experimental animals have different P450s, even if they are similar in their primary sequences and structures. One of the problems is human-specific (or "disproportionate") metabolites and the MIST issue (Metabolites in Safety Testing) (Guengerich, 2006). The U.S. FDA and the International Commission on Harmonisation of Technical Requirements for Pharmaceuticals for Human Use (ICH) have agreed that if a metabolite is present at >10% of the *in vivo* metabolites of a drug, then it should be tested for safety in animals if the animal test species do not produce it (at the human level of exposure). The analysis generally involves the (*in vivo*) AUC, which is the most appropriate measure of the exposure of an animal or human to a chemical. Further, regulatory agencies are interested in having multiples (AUC) of exposure in animals compared to humans, in order to have more assurance of drug safety, particularly in vulnerable populations.

There are several relevant strategies to deal with the MIST requirements. One point is that in vitro comparisons of human and animal drug metabolism should be done very early in order to make decisions about which animal species in the most appropriate model. Another important early investigation is a human "mass balance" study (with radioactively-tagged drug) to be sure that a large fraction of the metabolites are accounted for.

If there are human-specific metabolites found, there are a few options. (i) If any of the disproportionate human metabolite is formed at all in a test animal, then it may be possible to increase the dose in order to produce the exposure (AUC) that is found in humans (if the drug is not toxic to the animals at the high dose). (ii) Transgenic ("humanized") mice, expressing human P450s or other enzymes, may be used to produce the metabolite. (iii) The most straight-forward approach may be to synthesize the metabolite and administer it to animals, in order to achieve exposure. The synthesis might be difficult (e.g., with a macrolide antibiotic). If long-term testing is in order (e.g. cancer bioassay) then considerable time (and resources) may be required.

3.3.4 Human differences in regulation

One of the problems with the use of animals in risk assessment (or, more properly, risk characterization) is that humans and animals have differences in their regulation of P450s and other genes. As mentioned earlier, this variation makes P450 induction studies in animals less than predictive for humans. Accordingly, the most generally accepted induction assays are done with human hepatocytes. Although assays can be done with reporter constructs in other cells, there are issues regarding the need for co-activators etc. (e.g., HNF-4α with PXR and P450 3A4) (Tirona et al., 2003).

Another issue is that the levels of some of the receptors and their actions are very different in animals. In particular, PPARα agonists can lead to liver tumors in rodents, as do barbiturates in rodents (Rao & Reddy, 1987). In the past, these were considered serious issues but are not today.

4. P450s as drug targets

Much of this chapter has dealt with concerns about avoiding P450 inhibition by drugs (with the exception of the P450 3A4 "booster" drugs). However, in several cases there are P450s that function in normal physiological processes but inhibition can be used therapeutically.

4.1 Current P450 inhibitors in use

Drugs are approved for the inhibition of at least four human P450 targets, namely 5A1, 11B1, 17A1, and 19A1 (Table 4).

P450 5A1 is known by its more common name, thromboxane synthase. This is an unusual P450 that does not require electrons or oxygen; it rearranges prostaglandin H_2, an endoperoxide, to generate thromboxane. The inhibitors (including aspirin) are used to inhibit platelet aggregation in a variety of cardiovascular situations.

Mifepristone (RU-486) is approved for use in inhibiting P450 11B1 for treating Cushing's Disease (Chu et al., 2001).

In castration-resistant prostate cancer, reducing the androgen load is an issue. The only approved drug for inhibiting P450 17A1, the androgen-synthesizing P450, is abiraterone acetate, a pro-drug ester that is cleaved to release abiraterone (Fig. 12A). Although there has been some speculation about how abiraterone works (Cheong et al., 2020), it appears to be simply a very tight-binding direct competitive inhibitor of P450 17A1 ($K_d \sim 1$ nM), the steroid 17α-hydroxylase/lyase (Guengerich, McCarty, et al., 2021).

Table 4 P450s as drug targets.

Currently in clinical practice
- P450 5A1 (anti-platelet drugs, inhibit thromboxane production)
  - Pictamide
  - Riogrel
  - Ozagrel
  - Furegrelate
- P450 11B1 (Cushing's disease)
  - Mifepristone
- P450 17A1 (prostate cancer)
  - Abiraterone
- P450 19A1 (breast and other hormonal cancers)
  - Exemestane
  - Anastrozole
  - Letrozole
- P450 51 (anti-fungal, inhibit fungal P450s)
  - Ketoconazole
  - Fluconazole
  - Itraconazole
  - Vorconazole
  - Posaconazole
  - Isavuconazole
  - Mifepristone
  - *Discovery and development programs*
    - P450 4A11 (hypertension)
    - P450 11A1 (prostate cancer)
    - P450 11B2 (hypertension)
    - P450 24A1 (increase vitamin D_3 levels)
    - P450 26A1 (increase vitamin A levels)
    - P450 26B1 (increase vitamin A levels)

One long-standing goal with this P450 is the selective inhibition of the lyase reaction to block androgen production but not the synthesis of glucocorticoids, i.e. 17α-hydroxylation (Bird & Abbott, 2016; Burris-Hiday & Scott, 2021; Guengerich, McCarty, et al., 2021).

P450 19A1, the steroid aromatase, is involved in estrogen synthesis (Fig. 12B), which is important in cancers of the breast, ovary, and uterus. At least three (third-generation) aromatase inhibitors have been successful and are in current use (Table 4). These are very tight-binding (K_i in low nM range). The major side effects are related to changes in calcium homeostasis, which is an inherent physiological response. Thus, it will probably be difficult to improve on aromatase inhibitors in the future.

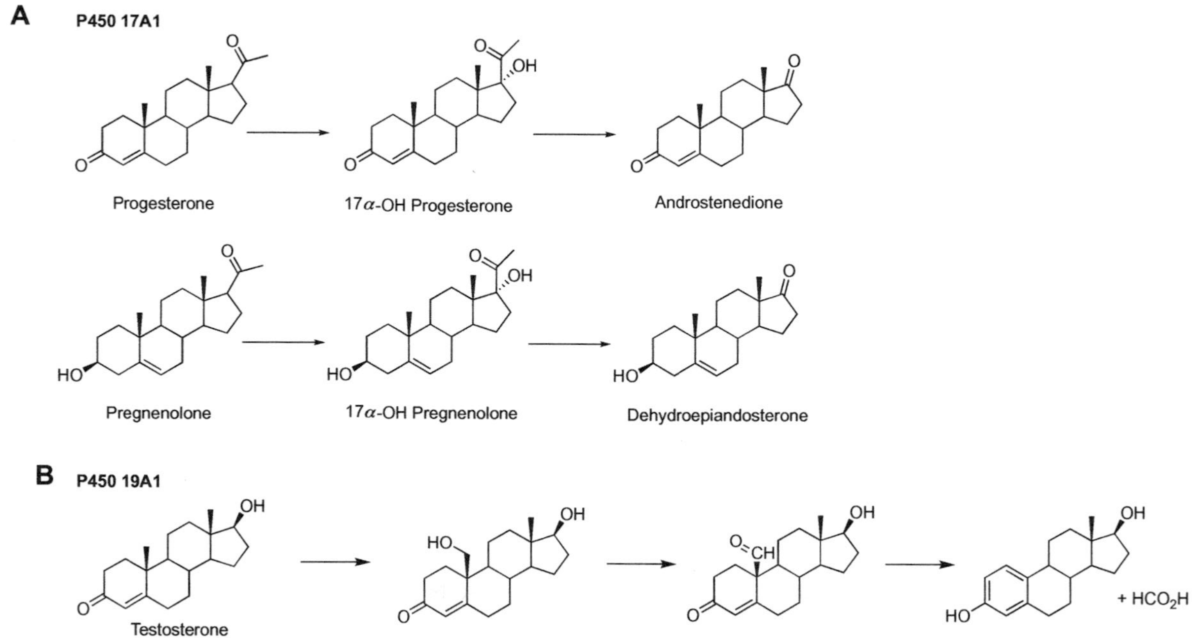

Fig. 12 Some multi-step steroid biosynthetic reactions catalyzed by human P450s that are targets for drugs. (A) P450 17A1; (B) P450 19A1.

4.2 Future prospects for P450 inhibition

Several other human P450s have been considered in the context of inhibition in relationship to other disease (Table 4). Of these, the most viable today may be P450 11B2. P450 11B2 produces aldosterone, a target in some forms of hypertension (Fig. 13).

Although not listed in Table 4, there have been considerations given to the use of P450 inhibitors in cancer prevention, as a means of blocking the bioactivation of chemical carcinogens (Chun, Kim, Kim, Lee, & Guengerich, 2001). However, the approach is difficult in that many of the chemical carcinogens undergo both bioactivation and detoxication by P450s, sometimes even the same P450 (Ueng, Shimada, Yamazaki, & Guengerich, 1995). One target has been P450 2A6, with the goal of blocking the metabolism, of nicotine to decrease the desire to smoke more (Yano et al., 2006).

4.3 Pest control

P450s in microorganisms have also been drug targets. In particular, Family 51 P450s are involved in the 14α-demethylation of lanosterol and the equivalent sterol precursors in several species, and the final sterols (e.g., ergosterol) are needed for membrane integrity in these microorganisms. This is an important target not only for local conditions with troublesome yeasts (e.g., athlete's foot) but serious systemic infections. In addition, CYP51 Family enzymes are targets in serious tropical diseases such as leishmania and sleeping sickness, which are endemic in parts of the world (Emami, Tavangar, & Keighobadi, 2017; Friggeri et al., 2018; Hargrove et al., 2017).

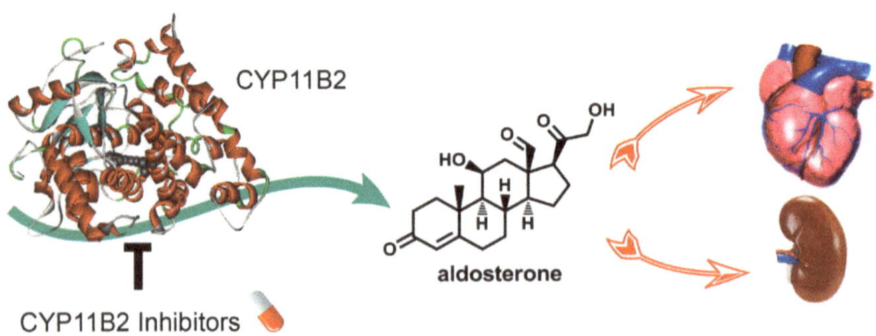

Fig. 13 P450 11B2 oxidation of 11-deoxycorticosterone to aldosterone, a drug target (Hu, Yin, & Hartmann, 2014). *Reprinted from Hu, Q., Yin, L., & Hartmann, R. W. (2014). Aldosterone synthase inhibitors as promising treatments for mineralocorticoid dependent cardiovascular and renal diseases.* Journal of Medicinal Chemistry, *67, 5011–5022, Copyright (2014), with permission from the American Chemical Society.*

The complexity and difficult of developing better inhibitors is exemplified in the case of the antifungal posaconazole (Fig. 14A). During discovery and development his drug showed considerably better activity than a previous lead (SCH 51048) in several fungal species. The structure of the

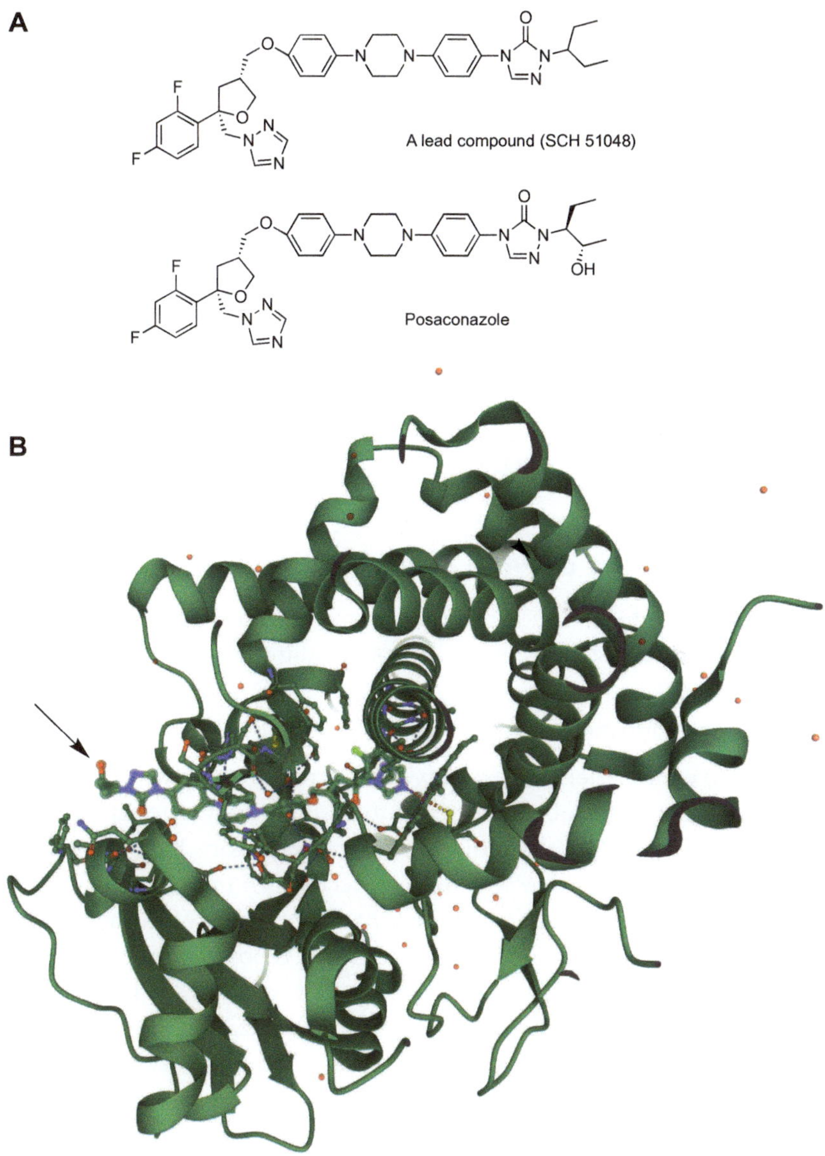

Fig. 14 Posaconazole bound in the *C. albicans* CYP51 active site (Hargrove et al., 2017). (A) An early lead compound in the program (SCH 51048) and posaconazole. (B) X-ray crystal structure of *C. albicans* P450 51A1 bound to posaconazole. The arrow in Part B is pointed to the extra hydroxyl group in posconazole.

Candida albicans P450 51A enzyme crystal structure bound to posaconazole was solved later (Hargrove et al., 2017), after the drug entered the market (Fig. 14B). Although posaconazole had much better intrinsic anti-fungal activity than SCH 51048, the only difference is a hydroxyl on the side chain (Fig. 14A). However, in the crystal structure (Fig. 14B) the moiety containing the hydroxyl is positioned outside of the protein. Thus, rational design using SCH 51048 would almost certainly not have led to a decision to make the molecule now known as posaconazole.

4.4 Targeting accessory enzymes

P450s use several accessory enzymes. The microsomal P450s use POR and sometimes b_5. The seven mitochondrial P450s use Adx and NADPH-Adx reductase, although this latter enzyme does not interact directly with P450s (Lambeth, Seybert, Lancaster Jr., Salerno, & Kamin, 1982). Some drugs have been designed to block allosteric interactions (Busby et al., 2020; Sawyer, 2020), and one effort to screen inhibitors that selectively block interactions with individual P450s has appeared (Jensen et al., 2021) (see also Kim, Kim, McCarty, & Guengerich, 2021).

5. The future of P450 research

Predicting the future is always difficult. Following are some of my own thoughts; I realize that others may have different ones.

5.1 Recent developments

As alluded to earlier, there are extensive efforts to utilize artificial intelligence to better predict both metabolism and toxicology (Xiong et al., 2021). A nagging problem with high-throughput screening efforts has been the need to incorporate enzymes that will mimic metabolism in human liver.

The ability to use transgenic animals has developed. With the advent of CRISPR-Cas9 and newer gene technologies, it is possible to use transgenic rats (and other species) (Yasuda et al., 2021), not only mice. There are other approaches to "humanizing" mouse livers (Yamazaki, Suemizu, Mitsui, Shimizu, & Guengerich, 2016), although these animals are generally not as viable as wild-type mice. Rats offer a number of advantages over mice, particularly when addressing some toxicology questions.

There are also efforts to produce cell lines and model organelles that will better reflect mammalian physiology and human metabolism in vitro (Janssen et al., 2020; Park, Georgescu, & Huh, 2019; Underhill & Khetani, 2018).

5.2 Questions regarding basic research

Six questions are listed (Table 5). Some success has been achieved, although these are difficult topics and considerable resources have been spent. Most of these topics have already been discussed in the chapter and will not be elaborated further. It is noteworthy that the b_5 effect was first reported 50 years ago and many details still remain to be addressed.

5.3 Practical questions to be addressed

A list of questions regarding practical P450 issues is also presented (Table 6). The second item (predicting rates of metabolism) may never happen. The remainder will be commented on.

We know now that we are not dealing with *only* 57 human P450s—each has many SNVs and the list will grow as more human genomic data becomes available. Is it even realistic to try to express all of the SNVs and measure their functions *in vitro*? Are there prospects for using artificial intelligence?

Table 5 Basic questions about P450 to be answered

• Is Compound I the only mechanism?
• How many conformational states exist & how do they relate to ligand recognition?
• Accessory enzymes: structures of binary complexes?
• Structures of the rest (32 more) of the human P450s
• Functions of the orphans (and quasi-orphans)?
• How does "allosteric" regulation work (including b_5)?

Table 6 Practical questions about P450 to be addressed

- Predicting sites of metabolism
- Predicting rates *a priori*
- Predicting functions of SNVs
- Do SNVs affect disease incidence?
  - Cardiovascular
  - Hypertension
  - Cancer
- Can we use SNV data better in clinical practice?
- Better drugs for pests
- Veterinary applications

Is structural biology realistic? To date the only P450 SNV structures are of P450 SNV structures are of P450 2C9 variants (Parikh et al., 2020). The problem of understanding SNV effects is seen in our own work with P450 21A2 (Fig. 15) (Wang et al., 2017). The changes tend to be in certain regions. However, a single SNV can change the catalytic specificity constant (k_{cat}/K_m) a million-fold. However, crystallizing these mutants has been difficult, and several are even hard to express. Moreover, the Eyring equation

$$k_{obs} = (k_B T/h)\ e^{-\Delta G\ddagger/RT}$$

(where k_B is the Boltzman contant, h is Planck's constant, T is the absolute temperature, and R is the gas constant) indicates that a 10-fold change in activity only relates to a free energy ($\Delta\Delta G$) change of 1.3 kcal/mol, less than

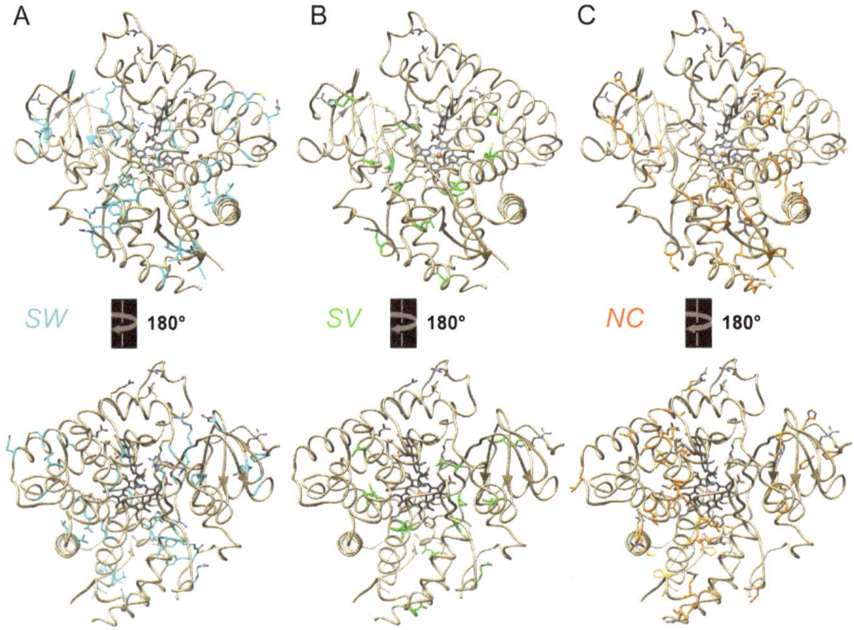

Fig. 15 P450 21A2 variants. Amino acid changes which give rise to the (A) salt-wasting (SW), (B) simple virile (SV), and (C) non-classical (NC) congenital adrenal hyperplasia phenotypes are mapped in the crystal structure of P450 21A2 (Pallan et al., 2015). Carbon atoms of wild type (*1) residues are highlighted in blue (SW), green (SV), and purple (NC). *Reprinted from Pallan, P. S., Lei, L., Wang, C., Waterman, M. R., Guengerich, F. P., & Egli, M. (2015). Research Resource: Correlating human cytochrome P450 21A2 crystal structure and phenotypes of mutations in congenital adrenal hyperplasia.* Molecular Endocrinology, 29, *1375–1384, Copyright (2015), with permission from The Endocrine Society.*

one hydrogen bond. This makes the task of understanding the structural basis of a functional change difficult. Further, a coding region SNV can show different effects with different substrates (or reactions of the same substrate).

Although the effects of SNVs in P450s with roles in steroid biochemistry have been rather obvious in terms of phenotypic endocrinological problems (Auchus & Miller, 2015), these SNV effects have been more subtle in diseases such as hypertension and other cardiovascular problems. Although chemical carcinogenesis was one of the early reasons for emphasis on the study of P450s and there was much interest in SNVs and molecular epidemiology of cancer (Kirk, Bah, & Montesano, 2006; Vineis & Perera, 2007), it is still not very clear what most of the effects are or how important they are.

At the turn of the century, there was considerable enthusiasm for genomic medicine. Today the number of examples of application of P450 SNV knowledge to clinical practice is still small (actually the information has been more useful in drug development). Can this be improved?

The opportunity to use P450 targets in pests still seems enormous. Anti-fungals were discussed but there are also opportunities with tuberculosis (McLean, Dunford, Neeli, Driscoll, & Munro, 2007; Ouellet, Lang, Couture, & Ortiz de Montellano, 2009) and other maladies involving infectious microorganisms.

Finally, there is still considerable opportunity in veterinary medicine. Many of the questions where we have answers about drug-drug interactions are just beginning to be asked in veterinary practice.

6. Conclusion

In a sense, the field of P450 has become a mature one. However, that also means that we have accumulated a large knowledge base and also that we have the tools to cut deeper and address harder questions. In retrospect, the application of biochemical findings to problems in pharmaceutical science has been a true scientific success story. There are still more opportunities.

Acknowledgments

P450 research in the author's laboratory has been supported by United States National Institutes of Health grant R01 GM118122. This content is solely the responsibility of the authors and does not necessarily represent the official views of the National Institutes of Health.

Thanks are extended to K. Trisler for assistance in preparation of the manuscript.

Conflict of interest statement

The author declares no conflicts of interest with the contents of this article.

References

Achour, B., Al Feteisi, H., Lanucara, F., Rostami-Hodjegan, A., & Barber, J. (2017). Global proteomic analysis of human liver microsomes: rapid characterization and quantification of hepatic drug-metabolizing enzymes. *Drug Metabolism and Disposition*, *45*(6), 666–675.

Achour, B., Russell, M. R., Barber, J., & Rostami-Hodjegan, A. (2014). Simultaneous quantification of the abundance of several cytochrome P450 and uridine 5'-diphospho-glucuronosyltransferase enzymes in human liver microsomes using multiplexed targeted proteomics. *Drug Metabolism and Disposition*, *42*, 500–510.

Afzelius, L., Arnby, C. H., Broo, A., Carlsson, L., Isaksson, C., Jurva, U., et al. (2007). State-of-the-art tools for computational site of metabolism predictions: comparative analysis, mechanistical insights, and future applications. *Drug Metabolism Reviews*, *39*(1), 61–86.

Ames, B. N., Durston, W. E., Yamasaki, E., & Lee, F. D. (1973). Carcinogens are mutagens: A simple test system combining liver homogenates for activation and bacteria for detection. *Proceedings of the National Academy of Sciences of the United States of America*, *70*, 2281–2285.

Auchus, R. J., & Miller, W. L. (2015). P450 enzymes in steroid processing. In P. R. Ortiz de Montellano (Ed.), *Vol. 2. Cytochrome P450: Structure, mechanism, and biochemistry* (4th ed., pp. 851–879). New York: Springer.

Avadhani, N. G., Sangar, M. C., Bansal, S., & Bajpai, P. (2011). Bimodal targeting of cytochrome P450s to endoplasmic reticulum and mitochondria: The concept of chimeric signals. *The FEBS Journal*, *278*(22), 4218–4229.

Axelrod, J. (1955). The enzymatic deamination of amphetamine. *The Journal of Biological Chemistry*, *214*, 753–763.

Bailey, D. G., Edgar, B., Spence, J. D., Munzo, C., & Arnold, J. M. O. (1990). Felodipine and nifedipine interactions with grapefruit juice. *Clinical Pharmacology and Therapeutics*, *47*, 180.

Bauman, J. N., Kelly, J. M., Tripathy, S., Zhao, S. X., Lam, W. W., Kalgutkar, A. S., et al. (2009). Can in vitro metabolism-dependent covalent binding data distinguish hepatotoxic from nonhepatotoxic drugs? An analysis using human hepatocytes and liver S-9 fraction. *Chemical Research in Toxicology*, *22*(2), 332–340.

Bhutani, P., Joshi, G., Raja, N., Bachhav, N., Rajanna, P. K., Bhutani, H., et al. (2021). US FDA approved drugs from 2015-June 2020: A perspective. *Journal of Medicinal Chemistry*, *64*(5), 2339–2381.

Bird, I. M., & Abbott, D. H. (2016). The hunt for a selective 17,20 lyase inhibitor; learning lessons from nature. *The Journal of Steroid Biochemistry and Molecular Biology*, *163*, 136–146.

Bissig, K. D., Han, W. G., Barzi, M., Kovalchuk, N., Ding, L., Fan, X. Y., et al. (2018). P450-Humanized and human liver chimeric mouse models for studying xenobiotic metabolism and toxicity. *Drug Metabolism and Disposition*, *46*(11), 1734–1744.

Bojic, M., Barbero, L., Dolgos, H., Freisleben, A., Gallemann, D., Riva, S., et al. (2014). Time- and NADPH-dependent inhibition of cytochrome P450 3A4 by the cyclopentapeptide cilengitide: Significance of the guanidine group and accompanying spectral changes. *Drug Metabolism and Disposition*, *42*(9), 1438–1446.

Bolt, H. M., Bolt, M., & Kappus, H. (1977). Interaction of rifampicin treatment with pharmacokinetics and metabolism of ethinyloestradiol in man. *Acta Endocrinologica*, *85*, 189–197.

Bolt, H. M., Kappus, H., & Bolt, M. (1975). Effect of rifampicin treatment on the metabolism of oestradiol and 17α-ethinyloestradiol by human liver microsomes. *European Journal of Clinical Pharmacology*, *8*, 301–307.

Boyer, S., Arnby, C. H., Carlsson, L., Smith, J., Stein, V., & Glen, R. C. (2007). Reaction site mapping of xenobiotic biotransformations. *Journal of Chemical Information and Modeling*, *47*(2), 583–590.

Brodney, M. A., Beck, E. M., Butler, C. R., Barreiro, G., Johnson, E. F., Riddell, D., et al. (2015). Utilizing structures of CYP2D6 and BACE1 complexes to reduce risk of drug-drug interactions with a novel series of centrally efficacious BACE1 inhibitors. *Journal of Medicinal Chemistry*, *58*(7), 3223–3252.

Burka, L. T., Guengerich, F. P., Willard, R. J., & Macdonald, T. L. (1985). Mechanism of cytochrome P-450 catalysis. Mechanism of *N*-dealkylation and amine oxide deoxygenation. *Journal of the American Chemical Society*, *107*, 2549–2551.

Burris-Hiday, S. D., & Scott, E. E. (2021). Steroidogenic cytochrome P450 17A1 structure and function. *Molecular and Cellular Endocrinology*, *528*, 111261.

Busby, S. A., Carbonneau, S., Concannon, J., Dumelin, C. E., Lee, Y., Numao, S., et al., & S. (2020). Advancements in assay technologies and strategies to enable drug discovery. *ACS Chemical Biology*, *15*(10), 2636–2648.

Chakraborty, P., & Di Cera, E. (2017). Induced fit is a special case of conformational selection. *Biochemistry*, *56*(22), 2853–2859.

Cheng, Q., Sohl, C. D., Yoshimoto, F. K., & Guengerich, F. P. (2012). Oxidation of dihydrotestosterone by human cytochromes P450 19A1 and 3A4. *The Journal of Biological Chemistry*, *287*(35), 29554–29567.

Cheong, E. J. Y., Nair, P. C., Neo, R. W. Y., Tu, H. T., Lin, F., Chiong, E., et al. (2020). Slow-, tight-binding inhibition of CYP17A1 by abiraterone redefines its kinetic selectivity and dosing regimen. *The Journal of Pharmacology and Experimental Therapeutics*, *374*(3), 438–451.

Child, S. A., & Guengerich, F. P. (2020). Multistep binding of the non-steroidal inhibitors orteronel and seviteronel to human cytochrome P450 17A1 and relevance to inhibition of enzyme activity. *Journal of Medicinal Chemistry*, *63*(12), 6513–6522.

Chu, J. W., Matthias, D. F., Belanoff, J., Schatzberg, A., Hoffman, A. R., & Feldman, D. (2001). Successful long-term treatment of refractory Cushing's disease with high-dose mifepristone (RU 486). *The Journal of Clinical Endocrinology and Metabolism*, *86*(8), 3568–3573.

Chun, Y.-J., Kim, S., Kim, D., Lee, S. K., & Guengerich, F. P. (2001). A new selective and potent inhibitor of human cytochrome P450 1B1 and its application to antimutagenesis. *Cancer Research*, *61*(22), 8164–8170.

Conney, A. H., Pantuck, E. J., Hsiao, K.-C., Garland, W. A., Anderson, K. E., Alvares, A. P., et al. (1976). Enhanced phenacetin metabolism in human subjects fed charcoal-broiled beef. *Clinical Pharmacology and Therapeutics*, *20*, 633–642.

Cooper, D. Y., Levine, S., Narasimhulu, S., Rosenthal, O., & Estabrook, R. W. (1965). Photochemical action spectrum of the terminal oxidase of mixed function oxidase systems. *Science*, *147*, 400–402.

Dahal, U. P., Obach, R. S., & Gilbert, A. M. (2013). Benchmarking in vitro covalent binding burden as a tool to assess potential toxicity caused by nonspecific covalent binding of covalent drugs. *Chemical Research in Toxicology*, *26*(11), 1739–1745.

Dahlin, D. C., Miwa, G. T., Lu, A. Y. H., & Nelson, S. D. (1984). *N*-Acetyl-*p*-benzoquinone imine: A cytochrome P-450-mediated oxidation product of acetaminophen. *Proceedings of the National Academy of Sciences of the United States of America*, *81*, 1327–1331.

Dahlin, D. C., & Nelson, S. D. (1982). Synthesis, decomposition kinetics, and preliminary toxicological studies of pure *N*-acetyl-*p*-benzoquinone imine, a proposed toxic metabolite of acetaminophen. *Journal of Medicinal Chemistry*, *25*, 885–886.

Dannan, G. A., Guengerich, F. P., Kaminsky, L. S., & Aust, S. D. (1983). Regulation of cytochrome P-450. Immunochemical quantitation of eight isozymes in liver microsomes of rats treated with polybrominated biphenyl congeners. *The Journal of Biological Chemistry*, *258*(2), 1282–1288.

de Bruyn Kops, C., Sicho, M., Mazzolari, A., & Kirchmair, J. (2021). GLORYx: Prediction of the metabolites resulting from Phase 1 and Phase 2 biotransformations of xenobiotics. *Chemical Research in Toxicology*, *34*(2), 286–299.

Delaforge, M., Jaouen, M., & Mansuy, D. (1984). The cytochrome P-450 metabolite complex derived from troleandomycin: Properties in vitro and stability in vivo. *Chemico-Biological Interactions*, *51*, 371–376.

Distlerath, L. M., Reilly, P. E., Martin, M. V., Davis, G. G., Wilkinson, G. R., & Guengerich, F. P. (1985). Purification and characterization of the human liver cytochromes P-450 involved in debrisoquine 4-hydroxylation and phenacetin *O*-deethylation, two prototypes for genetic polymorphism in oxidative drug metabolism. *The Journal of Biological Chemistry*, *260*(15), 9057–9067.

Ekins, S., Andreyev, S., Ryabov, A., Kirillov, E., Rakhmatulin, E. A., Bugrim, A., et al. (2005). Computational prediction of human drug metabolism. *Expert Opinion on Drug Metabolism & Toxicology*, *1*(2), 303–324.

Ekroos, M., & Sjögren, T. (2006). Structural basis for ligand promiscuity in cytochrome P450 3A4. *Proceedings of the National Academy of Sciences of the United States of America*, *103*(37), 13682–13687.

Emami, S., Tavangar, P., & Keighobadi, M. (2017). An overview of azoles targeting sterol 14α-demethylase for antileishmanial therapy. *European Journal of Medicinal Chemistry*, *135*, 241–259.

Eng, H., Tseng, E., Cerny, M. A., Goosen, T. C., & Obach, R. S. (2021). Cytochrome P450 3A time-dependent inhibition assays are too sensitive for identification of drugs causing clinically significant drug-drug interactions: A comparison of human liver microsomes and hepatocytes and definition of boundaries for inactivation rate constants. *Drug Metabolism and Disposition*, *49*(6), 442–450.

Estabrook, R. W., Franklin, M. R., Cohen, B., Shigamatzu, A., & Hildebrandt, A. G. (1971). Biochemical and genetic factors influencing drug metabolism. Influence of hepatic microsomal mixed function oxidation reactions on cellular metabolic control. *Metabolism*, *20*(2), 187–199.

Evans, D. C., Watt, A. P., Nicoll-Griffith, D. A., & Baillie, T. A. (2004). Drug-protein adducts: An industry perspective on minimizing the potential for drug bioactivation in drug discovery and development. *Chemical Research in Toxicology*, *17*(1), 3–16.

Friggeri, L., Hargrove, T. Y., Rachakonda, G., Blobaum, A. L., Fisher, P. B., de Oliveira, G., et al. (2018). Sterol 14α-demethylase structure-based optimization of drug candidates for human infections with the protozoan trypanosomatidae. *Journal of Medicinal Chemistry*, *61*, 10910–10921.

Gant, T. G. (2014). Using deuterium in drug discovery: Leaving the label in the drug. *Journal of Medicinal Chemistry*, *57*, 3595–3611.

Gianni, S., Dogan, J., & Jemth, P. (2014). Distinguishing induced fit from conformational selection. *Biophysical Chemistry*, *189*, 33–39.

Gonzalez, E., & Guengerich, F. P. (2017). Kinetic processivity of the two-step oxidations of progesterone and pregnenolone to androgens by human cytochrome P450 17A1. *The Journal of Biological Chemistry*, *292*(32), 13168–13185.

Gonzalez, F. J., & Kimura, S. (2003). Study of P450 function using gene knockout and transgenic mice. *Archives of Biochemistry and Biophysics*, *409*(1), 153–158.

Greenblatt, D. J., & Harmatz, J. S. (2015). Ritonavir is the best alternative to ketoconazole as an index inhibitor of cytochrome P450-3A in drug-drug interaction studies. *British Journal of Clinical Pharmacology*, *80*(3), 342–350.

Groves, J. T., McClusky, G. A., White, R. E., & Coon, M. J. (1978). Aliphatic hydroxylation by highly purified liver microsomal cytochrome P-450: Evidence for a carbon radical intermediate. *Biochemical and Biophysical Research Communications*, *81*, 154–160.

Guengerich, F. P. (1988). Oxidation of 17α-ethynylestradiol by human liver cytochrome P-450. *Molecular Pharmacology*, *33*(5), 500–508.

Guengerich, F. P. (2006). Saftey assessment of stable drug metabolites. *Chemical Research in Toxicology*, *19*, 1559–1560.
Guengerich, F. P. (2014). Cytochrome P450-mediated drug interactions and cardiovascular toxicity: The Seldane to Allegra transformation. In J. Wang, & L. Urban (Eds.), *Predictive ADMET: Integrated approaches in drug discovery and development* (1st ed., pp. 523–534). New York: Wiley.
Guengerich, F. P. (2015). Human cytochrome P450 enzymes. In P. R. Ortiz de Montellano (Ed.), *Vol. 2. Cytochrome P450: Structure, mechanism, and biochemistry* (4th ed., pp. 523–785). New York: Springer.
Guengerich, F. P. (2018a). Cytochrome P450 enzymes. In F. P. Guengerich (Ed.), *Vol. 4. of Comprehensive Toxicology (C. A. McQueen, Series Ed.). Biotransformation* (3rd ed., pp. 54–96). Oxford, UK: Elsevier.
Guengerich, F. P. (2018b). Perspective: Mechanisms of cytochrome P450-catalyzed oxidations. *ACS Catalysis*, *8*, 10964–10976.
Guengerich, F. P. (2019a). Cytochrome P450 research and The Journal of Biological Chemistry. *The Journal of Biological Chemistry*, *294*, 1671–1680.
Guengerich, F. P. (2019b). Kinetic modeling of steady-state situations in cytochrome P450 enzyme reactions. *Drug Metabolism and Disposition*, *47*(11), 1232–1239.
Guengerich, F. P. (2021). A history of the role of cytochrome P450 enzymes in the toxicity of drugs. *Toxicological Research*, *37*, 1–23.
Guengerich, F. P. (2022a). Cytochrome P450. In D. S. Riddick (Ed.), *Comprehensive pharmacology (in press)*. New York: Elsevier.
Guengerich, F. P. (2022b). Cytochrome P450 catalysis in natural product biosynthesis. In M. Bollinger, S. Booker, & V. Bandarian (Eds.), *Vol. 5, Radicals and Metalloenzymology, in press. Comprehensive natural products, III: Chemistry and biology*. New York: Elsevier.
Guengerich, F. P., Child, S. A., Barckhausen, I. F., & Goldfarb, M. H. (2021). Kinetic evidence for an induced fit mechanism in the binding of the substrate camphor by cytochrome $P450_{cam}$. *ACS Catalysis*, *11*, 639–649.
Guengerich, F. P., Dannan, G. A., Wright, S. T., Martin, M. V., & Kaminsky, L. S. (1982). Purification and characterization of liver microsomal cytochromes P-450: Electrophoretic, spectral, catalytic, and immunochemical properties and inducibility of eight isozymes isolated from rats treated with phenobarbital or β-naphthoflavone. *Biochemistry*, *21*(23), 6019–6030.
Guengerich, F. P., & Johnson, W. W. (1997). Kinetics of ferric cytochrome P450 reduction by NADPH-cytochrome P450 reductase: Rapid reduction in the absence of substrate and variations among cytochrome P450 systems. *Biochemistry*, *36*(48), 14741–14750.
Guengerich, F. P., McCarty, K. D., & Chapman, J. G. (2020). Kinetics of cytochrome P450 3A4 inhibition by heterocyclic drugs defines a general sequential multistep binding process. *The Journal of Biological Chemistry*, *295*, 100223.
Guengerich, F. P., McCarty, K. D., Chapman, J. G., & Tateishi, Y. (2021). Stepwise binding of inhibitors to human cytochrome P450 17A1 and kinetics of inhibition of androgen biosynthesis. *The Journal of Biological Chemistry*, *297*, 100969.
Guengerich, F. P., Waterman, M. R., & Egli, M. (2016). Recent structural insights into cytochrome P450 function. *Trends in Pharmacological Sciences*, *37*(8), 625–640.
Guengerich, F. P., Wilkey, C. J., Glass, S. M., & Reddish, M. J. (2019). Conformational selection dominates binding of steroids to human cytochrome P450 17A1. *The Journal of Biological Chemistry*, *294*(26), 10028–10041.
Guengerich, F. P., Wilkey, C. J., & Phan, T. T. N. (2019). Human cytochrome P450 enzymes bind drugs and other substrates mainly through conformational-selection modes. *The Journal of Biological Chemistry*, *294*(28), 10928–10941.
Guengerich, F. P., & Yoshimoto, F. K. (2018). Formation and cleavage of C-C bonds by enzymatic oxidation-reduction reactions. *Chemical Reviews*, *118*(14), 6573–6655.

Hall, S. D., Wang, Z., Huang, S. M., Hamman, M. A., Vasavada, N., Adigun, A. Q., et al. (2003). The interaction between St John's wort and an oral contraceptive. *Clinical Pharmacology and Therapeutics*, *74*(6), 525–535.

Hargrove, T. Y., Friggeri, L., Wawrzak, Z., Qi, A., Hoekstra, W. J., Schotzinger, R. J., et al. (2017). Structural analyses of *Candida albicans* sterol 14α-demethylase complexed with azole drugs address the molecular basis of azole-mediated inhibition of fungal sterol biosynthesis. *The Journal of Biological Chemistry*, *292*(16), 6728–6743.

Hedegaard, J., & Gunsalus, I. C. (1965). Mixed function oxidation. IV. An induced methylene hydroxylase in camphor oxidation. *The Journal of Biological Chemistry*, *240*(10), 4038–4043.

Hsu, M. H., & Johnson, E. F. (2019). Active-site differences between substrate-free and ritonavir-bound cytochrome P450 (CYP) 3A5 reveal plasticity differences between CYP3A5 and CYP3A4. *The Journal of Biological Chemistry*, *294*(20), 8015–8022.

Hu, Q., Yin, L., & Hartmann, R. W. (2014). Aldosterone synthase inhibitors as promising treatments for mineralocorticoid dependent cardiovascular and renal diseases. *Journal of Medicinal Chemistry*, *57*(12), 5011–5022.

Huang, X. Y., & Groves, J. T. (2017). Beyond ferryl-mediated hydroxylation: 40 years of the rebound mechanism and C-H activation. *Journal of Biological Inorganic Chemistry*, *22*(2-3), 185–207.

Ingelman-Sundberg, M., Zhong, X.-B., Hankinson, O., Beedanagari, S., Yu, A.-M., Peng, L., et al. (2013). Potential role of epigenetic mechanisms in the regulation of drug metabolism and transport. *Drug Metabolism and Disposition*, *41*(10), 1725–1731.

Isin, E. M., & Guengerich, F. P. (2006). Kinetics and thermodynamics of ligand binding by cytochrome P450 3A4. *The Journal of Biological Chemistry*, *281*(14), 9127–9136.

Isin, E. M., & Guengerich, F. P. (2007a). Complex reactions catalyzed by cytochrome P450 enzymes. *Biochimica et Biophysica Acta*, *1770*(3), 314–329.

Isin, E. M., & Guengerich, F. P. (2007b). Multiple sequential steps involved in the binding of inhibitors to cytochrome P450 3A4. *The Journal of Biological Chemistry*, *282*(9), 6863–6874.

Janssen, A. W. F., Duivenvoorde, L. P. M., Rijkers, D., Nijssen, R., Peijnenburg, A., van der Zande, M., et al. (2020). Cytochrome P450 expression, induction and activity in human induced pluripotent stem cell-derived intestinal organoids and comparison with primary human intestinal epithelial cells and Caco-2 cells. *Archives of Toxicology*, *1-16*.

Jensen, S. B., Thodberg, S., Parween, S., Moses, M. E., Hansen, C. C., Thomsen, J., et al. (2021). Biased cytochrome P450-mediated metabolism via small-molecule ligands binding P450 oxidoreductase. *Nature Communications*, *12*(1), 2260.

Johnson, K. A. (2019). *Kinetic analysis for the new enzymology* (1st ed.). Austin, TX: KinTek.

Johnston, W. A., Hunter, D. J., Noble, C. J., Hanson, G. R., Stok, J. E., Hayes, M. A., et al. (2011). Cytochrome P450 is present in both ferrous and ferric forms in the resting state within intact *Escherichia coli* and hepatocytes. *The Journal of Biological Chemistry*, *286*(47), 40750–40759.

Katagiri, M., Ganguli, B. N., & Gunsalus, I. C. (1968). A soluble cytochrome P450 functional in methylene hydroxylation. *The Journal of Biological Chemistry*, *243*, 3543–3546.

Kawakami, H., Ohtsuki, S., Kamiie, J., Suzuki, T., Abe, T., & Terasaki, T. (2011). Simultaneous absolute quantification of 11 cytochrome P450 isoforms in human liver microsomes by liquid chromatography tandem mass spectrometry with in silico target peptide selection. *Journal of Pharmaceutical Sciences*, *100*(1), 341–352.

Kim, D., Kim, V., McCarty, K. D., & Guengerich, F. P. (2021). Tight binding of cytochrome b_5 to cytochrome P450 17A1 is a critical feature of stimulation of C21 steroid lyase activity and androgen synthesis. *The Journal of Biological Chemistry*, *296*, 100571.

Kirchmair, J., Goeller, A. H., Lang, D., Kunze, J., Testa, B., Wilson, I. D., et al. (2015). Predicting drug metabolism: Experiment and/or computation? *Nature Reviews. Drug Discovery*, *14*(6), 387–404.

Kirk, G. D., Bah, E., & Montesano, R. (2006). Molecular epidemiology of human liver cancer: Insights into etiology, pathogenesis and prevention from The Gambia, West Africa. *Carcinogenesis*, *27*(10), 2070–2082.

Klingenberg, M. (1958). Pigments of rat liver microsomes. *Archives of Biochemistry and Biophysics*, *75*, 376–386.

Koshland, D. E., Jr., Nemethy, G., & Filmer, D. (1966). Comparison of experimental binding data and theoretical models in proteins containing subunits. *Biochemistry*, *5*, 365–385.

Krest, C. M., Onderko, E. L., Yosca, T. H., Calixto, J. C., Karp, R. F., Livada, J., et al. (2013). Reactive intermediates in cytochrome P450 catalysis. *The Journal of Biological Chemistry*, *288*(24), 17074–17081.

Lambeth, J. D., Seybert, D. W., Lancaster, J. R., Jr., Salerno, J. C., & Kamin, H. (1982). Steroidogenic electron transport in adrenal cortex mitochondria. *Molecular and Cellular Biology*, *45*, 13–31.

Lang, D., Radtke, M., & Bairlein, M. (2019). Highly variable expression of CYP1A1 in human liver and impact on pharmacokinetics of riociguat and granisetron in humans. *Chemical Research in Toxicology*, *32*(6), 1115–1122.

Larson, A. M., Polson, J., Fontana, R. J., Davern, T. J., Lalani, E., Hynan, L. S., et al. (2005). Acetaminophen-induced acute liver failure: Results of a United States multicenter, prospective study. *Hepatology*, *42*(6), 1364–1372.

Lee, S. S. T., Buters, J. T. M., Pineau, T., Fernandez-Salguero, P., & Gonzalez, F. J. (1996). Role of CYP2E1 in the hepatotoxicity of acetaminophen. *The Journal of Biological Chemistry*, *271*, 12063–12067.

Lee, W. L. M., & Kaplowitz, N. (2021). Alcohol, fasting, and therapeutic dosing of acetaminophen: A perfect storm. *Hepatology*, *73*(5), 1634–1636.

Lu, A. Y. H., & Coon, M. J. (1968). Role of hemoprotein P-450 in fatty acid ω--hydroxylation in a soluble enzyme system from liver microsomes. *The Journal of Biological Chemistry*, *243*, 1331–1332.

Lu, A. Y. H., Junk, K. W., & Coon, M. J. (1969). Resolution of the cytochrome P-450-containing ω-hydroxylation system of liver microsomes into three components. *The Journal of Biological Chemistry*, *244*, 3714–3721.

Lubet, R. A., Nims, R. W., Ward, J. M., Rice, J. M., & Diwan, B. A. (1989). Induction of cytochrome P-450_b and its relationship to liver tumor promotion. *Journal of the American College of Toxicology*, *8*, 259–268.

Maglich, J. M., Parks, D. J., Moore, L. B., Collins, J. L., Goodwin, B., Billin, A. N., et al. (2003). Identification of a novel human CAR agonist and its use in the identification of CAR target genes. *The Journal of Biological Chemistry*, *278*, 17277–17283.

Mannering, G. J., Renton, K. W., el Azhary, R., & Deloria, L. B. (1980). Effects of interferon-inducing agents on hepatic cytochrome P-450 drug metabolizing systems. *Annals of the New York Academy of Sciences*, *350*, 314–331.

Martiny, V. Y., & Miteva, M. A. (2013). Advances in molecular modeling of human cytochrome P450 polymorphism. *Journal of Molecular Biology*, *425*(21), 3978–3992.

McLean, K. J., Dunford, A. J., Neeli, R., Driscoll, M. D., & Munro, A. W. (2007). Structure, function and drug targeting in *Mycobacterium tuberculosis* cytochrome P450 systems. *Archives of Biochemistry and Biophysics*, *464*(2), 228–240.

Monroe, J. J., Tanis, K. Q., Podtelezhnikov, A. A., Nguyen, T., Machotka, S. V., Lynch, D., et al. (2020). Application of a rat liver drug bioactivation transcriptional response assay early in drug development that informs chemically reactive metabolite formation and potential for drug-induced liver injury. *Toxicological Sciences*, *177*(1), 281–299.

Montane, E., Arellano, A. L., Sanz, Y., Roca, J., & Farre, M. (2018). Drug-related deaths in hospital inpatients: A retrospective cohort study. *British Journal of Clinical Pharmacology*, *84*(3), 542–552.

Moore, L. G., Goodwin, B., Jones, S. A., Wisely, G. B., Serabjit-Singh, C. J., Wilson, T. M., et al. (2000). St. John's wort induces hepatic drug metabolism through activation of the pregnane X receptor. *Proceedings of the National Academy of Sciences of the United States of America, 97*, 7500–7502.

Mueller, E. J., Loida, P. J., & Sligar, S. G. (1995). Twenty-five years of $P450_{cam}$ research–mechanistic insights into oxygenase catalysis. In P. R. Ortiz de Montellano (Ed.), *Cytochrome P450: Structure, mechanism, and biochemistry* (2nd ed., pp. 83–124). New York: Plenum Press.

Mueller, G. C., & Miller, J. A. (1948). The metabolism of 4-dimethylaminoazobenzene by rat liver homogenates. *The Journal of Biological Chemistry, 176*, 535–544.

Mutoh, S., Sobhany, M., Moore, R., Perera, L., Pedersen, L., Sueyoshi, T., et al. (2013). Phenobarbital indirectly activates the constitutive active androstane receptor (CAR) by inhibition of epidermal growth factor receptor signaling. *Science Signaling, 6*(274), ra31.

Nakayama, S., Atsumi, R., Takakusa, H., Kobayashi, Y., Kurihara, A., Nagai, Y., et al. (2009). A zone classification system for risk assessment of idiosyncratic drug toxicity using daily dose and covalent binding. *Drug Metabolism and Disposition, 37*(9), 1970–1977.

Obach, R. S., Kalgutkar, A. S., Soglia, J. R., & Zhao, S. X. (2008). Can in vitro metabolism-dependent covalent binding data in liver microsomes distinguish hepatotoxic from nonhepatotoxic drugs? An analysis of 18 drugs with consideration of intrinsic clearance and daily dose. *Chemical Research in Toxicology, 21*(9), 1814–1822.

Omura, T., & Sato, R. (1962). A new cytochrome in liver microsomes. *The Journal of Biological Chemistry, 237*, 1375–13762.

Omura, T., & Sato, R. (1964). The carbon monoxide-binding pigment of liver microsomes. I. Evidence for its hemoprotein nature. *The Journal of Biological Chemistry, 239*, 2370–2378.

Ortiz de Montellano, P. R. (2015). Substrate oxidation. In P. R. Ortiz de Montellano (Ed.), *Cytochrome P450: Structure, mechanism, and biochemistry* (4th ed., pp. 111–176). New York: Springer.

Ouellet, H., Lang, J., Couture, M., & Ortiz de Montellano, P. R. (2009). Reaction of *Mycobacterium tuberculosis* cytochrome P450 enzymes with nitric oxide. *Biochemistry, 48*(5), 863–872.

Paine, M. F., Hart, H. L., Ludington, S. S., Haining, R. L., Rettie, A. E., & Zeldin, D. C. (2006). The human intestinal cytochrome P450 "pie". *Drug Metabolism and Disposition, 34*(5), 880–886.

Pallan, P. S., Lei, L., Wang, C., Waterman, M. R., Guengerich, F. P., & Egli, M. (2015). Research resource: Correlating human cytochrome P450 21A2 crystal structure and phenotypes of mutations in congenital adrenal hyperplasia. *Molecular Endocrinology, 29*(9), 1375–1384.

Pantuck, E. J., Hsiao, K.-C., Maggio, A., Nakamura, K., Kuntzman, R., & Conney, A. H. (1974). Effect of cigarette smoking on phenacetin metabolism. *Clinical Pharmacology and Therapeutics, 15*, 9–17.

Parikh, S. J., Evans, C. M., Obi, J. O., Zhang, Q. H., Maekawa, K., Glass, K. C., et al. (2020). Structure of cytochrome P450 2C9*2 in complex with losartan: Insights into the effect of genetic polymorphism. *Molecular Pharmacology, 98*(5), 529–539.

Park, S. E., Georgescu, A., & Huh, D. (2019). Organoids-on-a-chip. *Science, 364*(6444), 960–965.

Patten, C. J., Thomas, P. E., Guy, R. L., Lee, M., Gonzalez, F. J., Guengerich, F. P., et al. (1993). Cytochrome P450 enzymes involved in acetaminophen activation by rat and human liver microsomes and their kinetics. *Chemical Research in Toxicology, 6*(4), 511–518.

Pessayre, D., Tinel, M., Larrey, D., Cobert, B., Funck-Brentano, C., & Babany, G. (1983). Inactivation of cytochrome P-450 by a troleandomycin metabolite. Protective role of glutathione. *The Journal of Pharmacology and Experimental Therapeutics, 224*, 685–691.

Pirali, T., Serafini, M., Cargnin, S., & Genazzani, A. A. (2019). Applications of deuterium in medicinal chemistry. *Journal of Medicinal Chemistry*, *62*(11), 5276–5297.

Porubsky, P. R., Battaile, K. P., & Scott, E. E. (2010). Human cytochrome P450 2E1 structures with fatty acid analogs reveal a previously unobserved binding mode. *The Journal of Biological Chemistry*, *285*(29), 22282–22290.

Poulos, T. L., & Johnson, E. F. (2015). Structures of cytochrome P450 enzymes. In P. R. Ortiz de Montellano (Ed.), *Vol. 1. Cytochrome P450: Structure, function, and biochemistry* (4th ed., pp. 3–32). New York: Springer.

Rao, M. S., & Reddy, J. K. (1987). Peroxisome proliferation and hepatocarcinogenesis. *Carcinogenesis*, *8*, 631–636.

Reddish, M. J., & Guengerich, F. P. (2019). Human cytochrome P450 11B2 produces aldosterone by a processive mechanism due to the lactol form of the intermediate 18-hydroxycorticosterone. *The Journal of Biological Chemistry*, *294*(35), 12975–12991.

Rendic, S., & Guengerich, F. P. (2015). Survey of human oxidoreductases and cytochrome P450 enzymes involved in the metabolism of xenobiotic and natural chemicals. *Chemical Research in Toxicology*, *28*(1), 38–42.

Renton, K. W. (1981). Depression of hepatic cytochrome P-450-dependent mixed function oxidases during infection with encephalomyocarditis virus. *Biochemical Pharmacology*, *30*, 2333–2336.

Rittle, J., & Green, M. T. (2010). Cytochrome P450 compound I: Capture, characterization, and C-H bond activation kinetics. *Science*, *330*(6006), 933–937.

Rosenberger, L., von Essen, C., Khutia, A., Kühn, C., Urbahns, K., Georgi, K., et al. (2020). Crystalline sponges as a sensitive and fast method for metabolite identification: Application to gemfibrozil and its Phase I and II metabolites. *Drug Metabolism and Disposition*, *48*(7), 587–593.

Ryan, K. J. (1959). Biological aromatization of steroids. *The Journal of Biological Chemistry*, *234*(2), 268–272.

Sawaya, R. M., & Riddick, D. S. (2008). Cytochrome P450 2C11 5'-flanking region and promoter mediate in vivo suppression by 3-methylcholanthrene. *Drug Metabolism and Disposition*, *36*(9), 1803–1811.

Sawyer, A. (2020). Developing drugs for the 'undruggable'. *BioTechniques*, *69*(4), 239–241.

Sevrioukova, I. F., & Poulos, T. L. (2014). Ritonavir analogues as a probe for deciphering the cytochrome P450 3A4 inhibitory mechanism. *Current Topics in Medicinal Chemistry*, *14*(11), 1348–1355.

Shimada, T., Yamazaki, H., Mimura, M., Inui, Y., & Guengerich, F. P. (1994). Interindividual variations in human liver cytochrome P-450 enzymes involved in the oxidation of drugs, carcinogens and toxic chemicals: Studies with liver microsomes of 30 Japanese and 30 Caucasians. *The Journal of Pharmacology and Experimental Therapeutics*, *270*(1), 414–423.

Shinkyo, R., & Guengerich, F. P. (2011). Inhibition of human cytochrome P450 3A4 by cholesterol. *The Journal of Biological Chemistry*, *286*(21), 18426–18433.

Silverman, R. B. (1995). Mechanism-based enzyme inactivators. *Methods in Enzymology*, *249*, 240–283.

Stark, K., Dostalek, M., & Guengerich, F. P. (2008). Expression and purification of orphan cytochrome P450 4X1 and oxidation of anandamide. *The FEBS Journal*, *275*(14), 3706–3717.

Stringer, R. A., Williams, G., Picard, F., Sohal, B., Kretz, O., McKenna, J., et al. (2014). Application of a deuterium replacement strategy to modulate the pharmacokinetics of 7-(3,5-dimethyl-1*H*-1,2,4-triazol-1-yl)3-(4-methoxy-2-methylphenyl)-2,6-*d* imethylpyrazolo 5,1-*b* oxazole, a novel CRF1 antagonist. *Drug Metabolism and Disposition*, *42*(5), 954–962.

Takakusa, H., Masumoto, H., Yukinaga, H., Makino, C., Nakayama, S., Okazaki, O., et al. (2008). Covalent binding and tissue distribution/retention assessment of drugs associated with idiosyncratic drug toxicity. *Drug Metabolism and Disposition*, *36*(9), 1770–1779.

Thomas, P. E., Bandiera, S., Maines, S. L., Ryan, D. E., & Levin, W. (1987). Regulation of cytochrome P-450_j, a high-affinity *N*-nitrosodimethylamine demethylase, in rat hepatic microsomes. *Biochemistry*, *26*, 2280–2289.

Thompson, R. A., Isin, E. M., Li, Y., Weidolf, L., Page, K., Wilson, I., et al. (2012). In vitro approach to assess the potential for risk of idiosyncratic adverse reactions caused by candidate drugs. *Chemical Research in Toxicology*, *25*(8), 1616–1632.

Thompson, D., & Oster, G. (1996). Use of terfenadine and contraindicated drugs. *Journal of the American Medical Association*, *275*, 1339–1341.

Tirona, R. G., Lee, W., Leake, B. F., Lan, L. B., Cline, C. B., Lamba, V., et al. (2003). The orphan nuclear receptor HNF4α determines PXR- and CAR-mediated xenobiotic induction of CYP3A4. *Nature Medicine*, *9*(2), 220–224.

Ueng, Y.-F., Shimada, T., Yamazaki, H., & Guengerich, F. P. (1995). Oxidation of aflatoxin B_1 by bacterial recombinant human cytochrome P450 enzymes. *Chemical Research in Toxicology*, *8*, 218–225.

Underhill, G. H., & Khetani, S. R. (2018). Advances in engineered human liver platforms for drug metabolism studies. *Drug Metabolism and Disposition*, *46*(11), 1626–1637.

Vineis, P., & Perera, F. (2007). Molecular epidemiology and biomarkers in etiologic cancer research: The new in light of the old. *Cancer Epidemiology, Biomarkers & Prevention*, *16*(10), 1954–1965.

Vogt, A. D., & Di Cera, E. (2012). Conformational selection or induced fit? A critical appraisal of the kinetic mechanism. *Biochemistry*, *51*(30), 5894–5902.

Vogt, A. D., Pozzi, N., Chen, Z., & Di Cera, E. (2014). Essential role of conformational selection in ligand binding. *Biophysical Chemistry*, *186*, 13–21.

Wang, C., Pallan, P. S., Zhang, W., Lei, L., Yoshimoto, F. K., Waterman, M. R., et al. (2017). Functional analysis of human cytochrome P450 21A2 variants involved in congenital adrenal hyperplasia. *The Journal of Biological Chemistry*, *292*(26), 10767–10778.

Waxman, D. J., Dannan, G. A., & Guengerich, F. P. (1985). Regulation of rat hepatic cytochrome P-450: Age-dependent expression, hormonal imprinting, and xenobiotic inducibility of sex-specific isoenzymes. *Biochemistry*, *24*(16), 4409–4417.

Waxman, D. J., & Holloway, M. G. (2009). Sex differences in the expression of hepatic drug metabolizing enzymes. *Molecular Pharmacology*, *76*(2), 215–228.

Wilbur, K., & Ensom, M. H. (2000). Pharmacokinetic drug interactions between oral contraceptives and second-generation anticonvulsants. *Clinical Pharmacokinetics*, *38*(4), 355–365.

Williams, P. A., Cosme, J., Sridhar, V., Johnson, E. F., & MeRee, D. E. (2000). Mammalian microsomal cytochrome P450 monooxygenase: Strutural adaptations for membrane binding and functional diversity. *Molecular Cell*, *5*, 121–131.

Wilson, A. G., White, A. C., & Mueller, R. A. (2003). Role of predictive metabolism and toxicity modeling in drug discovery—A summary of some recent advancements. *Current Opinion in Drug Discovery & Development*, *6*(1), 123–128.

Wiwi, C. A., & Waxman, D. J. (2005). Role of hepatocyte nuclear factors in transcriptional regulation of male-specific *CYP2A2*. *The Journal of Biological Chemistry*, *280*(5), 3259–3268.

Wolbold, R., Klein, K., Burk, O., Nussler, A. K., Neuhaus, P., Eichelbaum, M., et al. (2003). Sex is a major determinant of CYP3A4 expression in human liver. *Hepatology*, *38*(4), 978–988.

Xiong, G., Wu, Z., Yi, J., Fu, L., Yang, Z., Hsieh, C., et al. (2021). ADMETlab 2.0: an integrated online platform for accurate and comprehensive predictions of ADMET properties. *Nucleic Acids Research*, *49*(W1), W5–w14.

Yamazaki, H., Nakamura, M., Komatsu, T., Ohyama, K., Hatanaka, N., Asahi, S., et al. (2002). Roles of NADPH-P450 reductase and apo- and holo-cytochrome b_5 on xenobiotic oxidations catalyzed by 12 recombinant human cytochrome P450s expressed in membranes of *Escherichia coli*. *Protein Expression and Purification*, *24*(3), 329–337.
Yamazaki, H., Suemizu, H., Mitsui, M., Shimizu, M., & Guengerich, F. P. (2016). Combining chimeric mice with humanized liver, mass spectrometry, and physiologically-based pharmcokinetic modeling in toxicology. *Chemical Research in Toxicology*, *29*, 1903–1911.
Yang, X., Zhang, B., Molony, C., Chudin, E., Hao, K., Zhu, J., et al. (2010). Systematic genetic and genomic analysis of cytochrome P450 enzyme activities in human liver. *Genome Research*, *20*(8), 1020–1036.
Yano, J. K., Denton, T. T., Cerny, M. A., Zhang, X., Johnson, E. F., & Cashman, J. R. (2006). Synthetic inhibitors of cytochrome P-450 2A6: Inhibitory activity, difference spectra, mechanism of inhibition, and protein cocrystallization. *Journal of Medicinal Chemistry*, *49*(24), 6987–7001.
Yano, J. K., Wester, M. R., Schoch, G. A., Griffin, K. J., Stout, C. D., & Johnson, E. F. (2004). The structure of human microsomal cytochrome P450 3A4 determined by X-ray crystallography to 2.05 Å resolution. *The Journal of Biological Chemistry*, *279*, 38091–38094.
Yasuda, K., Nishikawa, M., Okamoto, K., Horibe, K., Mano, H., Yamaguchi, M., et al. (2021). Elucidation of metabolic pathways of 25-hydroxyvitamin D3 mediated by CYP24A1 and CYP3A using Cyp24a1 knockout rats generated by CRISPR/Cas9 system. *The Journal of Biological Chemistry*, *296*, 100668.
Yoshimoto, F. K., & Guengerich, F. P. (2014). Mechanism of the third oxidative step in the conversion of androgens to estrogens by cytochrome P450 19A1 steroid aromatase. *Journal of the American Chemical Society*, *136*(42), 15016–15025.
Yu, J. J., Zhou, Z., Tay-Sontheimer, J., Levy, R. H., & Ragueneau-Majlessi, I. (2018). Risk of clinically relevant pharmacokinetic-based drug-drug interactions with drugs approved by the US Food and Drug Administration between 2013 and 2016. *Drug Metabolism and Disposition*, *46*(6), 835–845.
Yun, C.-H., Kim, K. H., Calcutt, M. W., & Guengerich, F. P. (2005). Kinetic analysis of oxidation of coumarins by human cytochrome P450 2A6. *The Journal of Biological Chemistry*, *280*(13), 12279–12291.
Yun, C.-H., Okerholm, R. A., & Guengerich, F. P. (1993). Oxidation of the antihistaminic drug terfenadine in human liver microsomes. Role of cytochrome P-450 3A(4) in N-dealkylation and C-hydroxylation. *Drug Metabolism and Disposition*, *21*(3), 403–409.
Zhang, D., Flint, O., Wang, L., Gupta, A., Westhouse, R. A., Zhao, W., et al. (2012). Cytochrome P450 11A1 bioactivation of a kinase inhibitor in rats: Use of radioprofiling, modulation of metabolism, and adrenocortical cell lines to evaluate adrenal toxicity. *Chemical Research in Toxicology*, *25*(3), 556–571.
Zhang, Y., Klein, K., Sugathan, A., Nassery, N., Dombkowski, A., Zanger, U. M., et al. (2011). Transcriptional profiling of human liver identifies sex-biased genes associated with polygenic dyslipidemia and coronary artery disease. *PLoS One*, *6*(8), e23506.
Zimmerlin, A., Trunzer, M., & Faller, B. (2011). CYP3A time-dependent inhibition risk assessment validated with 400 reference drugs. *Drug Metabolism and Disposition*, *39*(6), 1039–1046.

CHAPTER TWO

Pharmacogenetics of the cytochromes P450: Selected pharmacological and toxicological aspects

Ann K. Daly*
Translational and Clinical Research Institute, Newcastle University, Newcastle Upon Tyne, United Kingdom
*Corresponding author: e-mail address: a.k.daly@ncl.ac.uk

Contents

Abstract

With the availability of detailed genomic data on all 57 human cytochrome P450 genes, it is clear that there is substantial variability in gene product activity with functionally significant polymorphisms reported across almost all isoforms. This article is concerned mainly with 13 P450 isoforms of particular relevance to xenobiotic metabolism. After brief review of the extent of polymorphism in each, the relevance of selected P450 isoforms to both adverse drug reaction and disease susceptibility is considered in detail. Bleeding due to warfarin and other coumarin anticoagulants is considered as an example of a type A reaction with idiosyncratic adverse drug reactions affecting the liver and skin as type B. It is clear that *CYP2C9* variants contribute significantly to warfarin dose requirement and also risk of bleeding, with a minor contribution from *CYP4F2*. In the

Advances in Pharmacology, Volume 95
ISSN 1054-3589
https://doi.org/10.1016/bs.apha.2022.05.001

case of idiosyncratic adverse drug reactions, *CYP2B6* variants appear relevant to both liver and skin reactions to several drugs with *CYP2C9* variants also relevant to phenytoin-related skin rash. The relevance of P450 genotype to disease susceptibility is also considered but detailed genetic studies now suggest that CYP2A6 is the only P450 relevant to risk of lung cancer with alleles associated with low or absent activity clearly protective against disease. Other cytochrome P450 genotypes are generally not predictors for risk of cancer or other complex disease development.

Abbreviations

cDNA copy DNA
CPIC Clinical Pharmacogenetics Implementation Group
DILI drug-induced liver injury
DOAC direct acting oral anticoagulant
GWAS genome-wide association study
HLA human leukocyte antigen
p-HPPH 5-parahydroxyphenyl-5-phenylhydantoin
INR international normalized ratio
NNK 4-(methylnitrosamino)-1-(3-pyridyl)-1-butanone
PharmVar pharmacogene variation consortium

1. Introduction

The cytochrome P450 genes are the most widely studied gene family in the area of pharmacogenetics. It was possible to understand phenotype-genotype relationships earlier for this gene family than for most other human genes. This situation arose by a mixture of chance observations but also from sustained work at the boundary of pharmacology, especially with respect to drug metabolism, and human genetics. Early approaches to pharmacogenetics involved population phenotyping studies where the ability of individuals to metabolize certain xenobiotics, particularly prescribed drugs, was studied. Often only the parent drug levels could be determined but sometimes levels of certain metabolites could also be detected chromatographically. Initially, the main well characterized pharmacogenetic polymorphism was that affecting acetylation. This reaction is not catalysed by P450 but variation in drug acetylation was well described during the late 1950s and early 1960s. Drug oxidation was subsequently shown to be subject to interindividual variation in pioneering studies, mainly on nortryptiline metabolism, from Sjoqvist and colleagues during the late 1960s and early 1970s (Alexanderson, Evans, & Sjoqvist, 1969; Sjöqvist & von Bahr, 1973). These involved both general population phenotyping and twin studies. However, at that time, the characteristic bimodality in population phenotype seen for acetylation was not reported for nortryptiline oxidation. Studies on oxidative metabolism of two other drugs, debrisoquine and sparteine, in the late 1970s by separate teams working in London and Stuttgart respectively resulted in finding bimodal distributions for metabolism and the first reports of "poor metabolizers" who lacked the ability to oxidize both these drugs (Eichelbaum, Spannbrucker, Steincke, & Dengler, 1979; Mahgoub, Idle, Dring, Lancaster, & Smith, 1977). It was subsequently confirmed that the same oxidation deficiency appeared to be responsible for the previously reported variable nortryptiline oxidation (Bertilsson, Dengler, Eichelbaum, & Schulz, 1980).

These early studies on interindividual variation in drug oxidation did not focus specifically on cytochromes P450 but, by the early 1980s, evidence emerged for cytochrome P450 involvement in debrisoquine oxidation (Kahn, Boobis, Murray, Brodie, & Davies, 1982; Meier, Mueller, Dick, & Meyer, 1983) with purification of the human enzyme now termed CYP2D6 achieved in 1985 (Distelrath et al., 1985), followed by cloning of the relevant cDNA in 1988 and identification of the first genetic variant responsible for CYP2D6-related poor metabolism by 1990 (Gonzalez et al., 1988; Gough et al., 1990; Hanioka, Kimura, Meyer, & Gonzalez, 1990).

During the acquisition of knowledge and understanding of the CYP2D6 polymorphism as a key pharmacogenetic example, studies on oxidative metabolism of a range of other drugs in humans proceeded in parallel. The most important of these drug examples in terms of current pharmacogenetic knowledge was *S*-mephenytoin for which a "new" pharmacogenetic polymorphism was reported in 1984 (Kupfer & Preisig, 1984). Though it was quickly established that this oxidation reaction was mediated by a cytochrome P450, cloning of the relevant cDNA (CYP2C19) and identification of two common sequence variants was not achieved until 1994 (de Morais, Wilkinson, Blaisdell, Meyer, et al., 1994; de Morais, Wilkinson, Blaisdell, Nakamura, et al., 1994), due both to the complexity of the CYP2C subfamily compared with CYP2D and the lower abundance of CYP2C19 compared with CYP2D6 and indeed other CYP2C family members. Other drug substrates providing evidence for existence of functionally significant genetic polymorphisms on the basis of variable population phenotypes included tolbutamide (CYP2C9) (Scott & Poffenbarger, 1978), coumarin (CYP2A6) (Fernandez-Salguero et al., 1995) and caffeine (CYP1A2) (Butler et al., 1992).

Now that complete genomic data are available for the 57 human cytochrome P450 genes, it is clear that many, especially those with roles mainly in xenobiotic metabolism, are subject to functionally significant genetic polymorphisms, though the extent of this varies. A recent article in this series has reviewed polymorphism in each individual isoform relevant to drug metabolism in detail, particularly pharmacokinetic effects (Tornio & Backman, 2018) but a summary of the current position about P450 polymorphism, with emphasis on those genes encoding proteins relevant to drug and xenobiotic metabolism, is provided in Table 1. Ongoing projects such as PharmVar have facilitated compilation of data on P450 polymorphisms and development of systematic and consistent nomenclature (Gaedigk, Casey, Whirl-Carrillo, Miller, & Klein, 2021). CYP2D6, CYP2C9, CYP2C19, CYP2A6, CYP2B6 and CYP3A4 show the largest number of variant alleles but the other P450 genes also listed in Table 1 show some relatively common polymorphisms. The current chapter is concerned with genetic polymorphisms that affect P450 expression and function directly. There is a recent report of a polymorphism in the transcription factor NFIB which affects CYP2D6 levels and activity (Lenk et al., 2022) and it seems likely that this type of polymorphism may also be relevant to expression of other CYP genes. Levels and activity of P450 proteins may also be affected by a range of non-genetic factors including induction and inhibition as discussed elsewhere (Tracy et al., 2016). For example, activity of the major drug metabolizing enzyme CYP3A4 is not greatly affected by genetic polymorphism within the coding gene but levels of activity show considerable interindividual variability with non-genetic factors accounting for much of this variation.

It is now clear that the knowledge gained to date on P450 polymorphisms is relevant to safe and effective prescription of a number of commonly used drugs but for a number of reasons progress on clinical implementation of this knowledge by introduction of pharmacogenetic tests to guide treatment has been slow. This will be discussed in detail below using the example of warfarin and CYP2C9 genotype, with other important and well studied examples of clinical implementation of pharmacogenetics discussed elsewhere in this volume (chapter "Cytochrome P450 polymorphism: From evolution to clinical use" by Ingelman-Sundberg). There is also continuing interest in the question of whether P450 genotypes can predict susceptibility to a range of adverse drug reactions. The relevance of P450 genotyping to susceptibility to idiosyncratic or type B adverse drug reactions will be illustrated by consideration of the examples of drug-induced liver injury and skin injury. A relatively large number of studies during the 1990s, following identification of the molecular basis of a number of

Table 1 Genetic polymorphisms in cytochrome P450 genes relevant to drug and xenobiotic metabolism.

Gene	Common variant allele examples	Overall relevance
CYP1A1	CYP1A1*2 to *13	Still relatively unclear despite large number of reports.
CYP1A2	CYP1A1*2 to *21; numerous CYP1A1*1 suballeles	Limited data on functional significance for most variants but CYP1A2*1F appears to be associated with higher levels of inducibility via the Ah receptor (Sim, 2013).
CYP2A6	CYP2A6*2 to *45; numerous CYP2A6*1 and *4 suballeles	CYP2A6*2 and *4 well established to be associated with absence of enzyme activity (Tanner & Tyndale, 2017). Other variants are associated with loss of or decreased activity.
CYP2A13	CYP2A13*2 to *10; range of CYP2A13*1 suballeles	Most variants appear to be associated with decreased activity. CYP2A13*4 may result in absence of activity (Vrzal, 2021).
CYP2B6	CYP2B6*2 to *38; some CYP2B6*1 suballeles	Complex pattern of variants summarized by PharmVar (Desta et al., 2021) but alleles associated with absence of activity are rare. Alleles with missense variant c.516G>T have been designated as either decreased clinical function (CYP2B6*6, *7, *9, *19, *20, *26, *34, and *36) or as no function due to the presence of other polymorphisms (CYP2B6*13, *37 and *38). At least one increased activity allele is known (CYP2B6*4). Some CYP2B6/CYP2B7 hybrid genes showing decreased or no activity have been reported (CYP2B6*29, *30). Some decreased function alleles may show substrate-dependent effects.
CYP2C8	CYP2C8*2 to *18; many CYP2C8*1 suballeles	The more common variants are associated with amino acid substitutions but functional relevance of these still not clear with some evidence for substrate-dependent effects (Tornio & Backman, 2018). A few rare frameshifts or truncated variants known.
CYP2C9	CYP2C9*2 to *75; many CYP2C9*1 suballeles	As reviewed recently (Sangkuhl et al., 2021), most known variants are missense but a few variants include frameshifts leading to no activity (e.g., CYP2C9*6). Missense variants are generally associated with decreased activity but level of effect varies with the possibility of some substrate-dependent effects.

Continued

Table 1 Genetic polymorphisms in cytochrome P450 genes relevant to drug and xenobiotic metabolism.—cont'd

Gene	Common variant allele examples	Overall relevance
CYP2C19	CYP2C19*2 to *39; many CYP2C19*1 and *2 suballeles	Several common null variants including CYP2C19*2 and *3. Decreased activity (e.g., CYP2C19*9) and increased activity variants (CYP2C19*17 and TG haplotype) also described resulting in a range of different phenotypes of poor, intermediate, extensive and ultrarapid metabolizers (Botton et al., 2021; Bråten et al., 2021).
CYP2D6	CYP2D6*2 to *149; many *1, *2, *4 and *10 suballeles	As discussed in detail elsewhere (Nofziger et al., 2020), a large number of null variants are known with some very common (e.g., CYP2D6*3 to *6). Decreased activity variants, some common, also exist (e.g., CYP2D6*10, *17). Increased activity variants due to gene duplication, including of the reference sequence, also common (e.g., CYP2D6*1 × 2). This results in a range of different phenotypes, namely poor, intermediate, extensive and ultrarapid.
CYP2E1	CYP2E1*2 to *7; some *1, *5 and *7 suballeles	A few rare missense variants are known with at least one of these, CYP2E1*2, associated with decreased activity (Hu et al., 1997). Other variants in non-coding regions may affect expression levels but data on these remains unclear.
CYP3A4	CYP3A4*1 to *35; several *1 suballeles	Information still limited on functional effects (Tornio & Backman, 2018). At least two rare variants CYP3A4*20 and *26 predicted to give rise to non-functional protein. Several missense variants may be associated with decreased enzyme activity. CYP3A4*22 affects splicing and may associate with decreased activity.
CYP3A5	CYP3A5*1 to *9; several *1 suballeles	The reference sequence (CYP3A5*1) is the minor form of this gene in many ethnic groups. The most common variant CYP3A5*3 affects splicing and codes for an inactive protein. Other variants including CYP3A5*5 to *7 are associated with splice defects or frameshifts and also encode inactive proteins.
CYP3A7	CYP3A7*1 to *3; several *1 suballeles	This gene is predominantly expressed in fetal tissue. However, at least one variant CYP3A7*1C (CYP3A7*1.003) is relatively common and associated with continued expression of the isoform in adults.

Data on variant alleles taken from PharmVar (https://www.pharmvar.org/).

common cytochrome P450 polymorphisms, concerned the possibility that these polymorphisms were relevant to cancer and other disease susceptibility due to the general role of the P450s in xenobiotic metabolism. This aspect will be considered in the final section of this chapter below.

2. Relevance of cytochrome P450 polymorphisms to warfarin dosing and bleeding risk

2.1 Historic aspects of warfarin metabolism in relation to the cytochromes P450

Since its initial therapeutic use in the 1950s, treatment with the anticoagulant warfarin has involved individualization of dosing based on patient response by measuring clotting rate (international normalized ratio (INR)). This clinical assay is very effective but means that the dose required by the individual patient cannot be calculated prior to start of therapy and there is a risk that some patients will suffer serious bleeding due to high warfarin levels during initiation of treatment. The important role of cytochromes P450 in warfarin metabolism was established by animal studies (Fasco, Vatsis, Kaminsky, & Coon, 1978), followed by human liver microsome studies (Kaminsky et al., 1984). Once cloning and expression of the main human P450 cDNAs had been achieved, it was demonstrated that 7-hydroxylation of S-warfarin was catalysed by CYP2C9 (Rettie et al., 1992). This was important because it was already known that the S-enantiomer accounted for the majority of anticoagulant activity and that oxidation by 7-hydroxylation was the major metabolic pathway (Rettie, Eddy, Heimark, Gibaldi, & Trager, 1989). In parallel with the studies showing a role for P450 in warfarin metabolism, population phenotyping studies suggested that metabolism of the antidiabetic drug tolbutamide showed a bimodal distribution for metabolism (Scott & Poffenbarger, 1978). When cDNA clones for CYP2C9 became available, a major role for this P450 in tolbutamide metabolism as well as S-warfarin 7-hydroxylation was confirmed and CYP2C9 became the third P450 known to be subject to a functionally significant polymorphism affecting metabolism of a range of different drugs (Furuya et al., 1995; Rettie, Wienkers, Gonzalez, Trager, & Korzekwa, 1994; Sullivan-Close et al., 1996). The nature of this polymorphism is slightly different to those common in CYP2D6 and CYP2C19 with the most common CYP2C9 variant alleles encoding amino acid substitutions that impair but don't completely abolish catalytic activity (reviewed by Daly, Rettie, Fowler, & Miners, 2017).

2.2 Warfarin dosing and relevance of P450 and other genotypes

The effect of CYP2C9 genotype on warfarin dose requirements and also on risk of bleeding with warfarin has been studied very extensively during the last 20–30 years. Similar studies on other coumarin anticoagulants which are related in structure to warfarin have also been performed and reached largely similar conclusions. Early studies showed an effect of the two common variant alleles *CYP2C9*2* and *CYP2C9*3* on warfarin dose requirements (Aithal, Day, Kesteven, & Daly, 1999; Furuya et al., 1995; Steward et al., 1997), with an increased risk of bleeding also demonstrated directly (Aithal et al., 1999). Several randomized clinical trials on the value of genotyping for common variants in both CYP2C9 and a second non-P450 gene VKORC1 which encodes the warfarin target enzyme to determine dosing prior to warfarin treatment have now been performed (for review, see Daly et al., 2017). Two clinical trials performed on European populations show clear benefit for genotyping in terms INR stability (Gage et al., 2017; Pirmohamed et al., 2013) but another on a mixed ethnicity population from the USA did not detect any advantage (Kimmel et al., 2013). This difference is likely to be due, at least in part, to the inclusion in the negative study of African-American patients for whom genetic factors affecting dose are still less clear. Study design and general clinical characteristics of the patients participating may have also contributed to the difference (Pirmohamed, Kamali, Daly, & Wadelius, 2015).

An additional cytochrome P450 CYP4F2 is also relevant to warfarin dosing due to a role in vitamin K metabolism. It was observed initially that a common variant in CYP4F2 giving rise to a valine to methionine substitution was associated with a higher warfarin dose requirement by genotyping patient samples with a drug metabolism gene chip which included a wide range of P450 polymorphisms (Caldwell et al., 2008). The basis for this observation was then discovered to relate to a role for CYP4F2 in vitamin K1 metabolism (McDonald, Rieder, Nakano, Hsia, & Rettie, 2009). The variant was associated with slower vitamin K metabolism resulting in higher circulating vitamin K levels and therefore a higher warfarin dose requirement. The clinical relevance of the variant was investigated in detail in a further study which showed no association with warfarin dose requirement but a significant relationship with time to therapeutic INR (Zhang et al., 2009). Though an interesting finding, most studies concluded that the contribution of CYP4F2 genotype to warfarin dose requirement was small and therefore of limited clinical relevance.

The pharmacogenetic observations concerning CYP2C9, VKORC1 and warfarin dose requirements feature in CPIC dosing guidelines (Johnson et al., 2017) but implementation to date worldwide has been very limited. This is likely to reflect the increasing prescription of direct-acting oral anticoagulants (DOACs) to patients requiring anticoagulant treatment who in the past would have been prescribed warfarin on grounds of both convenience together with lower risks for ischemic stroke or systemic embolism and major bleeding than in new users of warfarin (Dawwas et al., 2021).

2.3 CYP2C9 genotype relevance more broadly

In addition to warfarin and other coumarin anticoagulants, knowledge of CYP2C9 genotype may be relevant to safe prescribing of several other drugs, particularly phenytoin (Karnes et al., 2021). As described above, the common *CYP2C9*2* and **3* variants have been well characterized, especially in terms of effects on warfarin hydroxylation, but a large number of other variants, mostly rare with allele frequencies of less than 1%, are now known to occur (see Table 1). For example, in the gnomAD database (https://gnomad.broadinstitute.org/), 464 missense variants in addition to those within *CYP2C9*2* and **3* are listed (Amorosi et al., 2021). A recent study has investigated such variants using a systematic approach involving expression in a yeast-based system to determine both enzyme activity and protein abundance and found evidence for decreased activity in many cases (Amorosi et al., 2021).

3. Idiosyncratic adverse drug reactions and cytochrome P450 polymorphisms

There are numerous examples of contributions by cytochrome P450 polymorphisms to type A adverse drug reactions, including the serious bleeding that may occur due to warfarin overdosing discussed in Section 2. However, cytochrome P450 polymorphisms may also be relevant to the rarer type B idiosyncratic adverse drug reactions. These idiosyncratic adverse reactions are less dependent on drug concentration so the effect of P450 genotype may be more subtle. Some recent advances in this area on both idiosyncratic drug-induced liver injury and skin injury will be considered here.

3.1 Idiosyncratic liver injury and cytochrome P450 polymorphisms

For idiosyncratic drug-induced liver injury (DILI), a contribution by cytochrome P450 polymorphisms to risk has been proposed by a number of workers in the field (Corsini & Bortolini, 2013; Stachulski et al., 2013; Uetrecht, 2019; Yu et al., 2014). This seems reasonable since many of the drugs that cause idiosyncratic DILI undergo hepatic metabolism, sometimes to reactive metabolites. A reactive metabolite-mediated mechanism is well established to underly acetaminophen-induced liver injury in acetaminophen overdose which is a concentration-dependent adverse drug reaction (type A); whether this mechanism also underlies idiosyncratic DILI is less clear. As reviewed recently (Guengerich, 2020b), there are a number of mainly historic examples of drugs withdrawn from the market due to idiosyncratic hepatotoxicity where reactive metabolite formation, frequently involving cytochrome P450, appears to be the underlying toxicity mechanism. However, whether this is also the case for drugs that are still licensed but sometimes cause idiosyncratic DILI is less clear. There is increasing evidence that idiosyncratic DILI commonly involves inappropriate immune responses with certain HLA genotypes acting as strong susceptibility factors (Osanlou, Pirmohamed, & Daly, 2018; Urban, Daly, & Aithal, 2014). However, not all forms of idiosyncratic DILI show HLA associations. Where HLA associations occur, formation of reactive metabolites may contribute to an immune mechanism which is likely to involve inappropriate presentation of modified host peptides to T cells. Absent or low activity of the main P450 isoform involved in metabolism of a particular drug may result in other metabolic routes resulting in reactive metabolites not found via the normal metabolic route. This could lead to toxic effects including protein adduct formation and cellular stress or damage. On the other hand, if the normal metabolic route results in formation of a reactive metabolite, individuals with higher than normal levels of the metabolic enzyme could be at increased risk of toxicity. A few specific examples of licensed drugs known to cause idiosyncratic DILI where there is a possible contribution of P450 genotype to susceptibility are discussed below and summarized also in Table 2. The studies listed

Table 2 Reported contributions of cytochrome P450 polymorphisms to idiosyncratic drug-induced liver injury reactions involving currently licensed drugs.

Causative drug	P450 isoform	References
Ticlopidine	CYP2B6	Ariyoshi et al. (2010)
Efavirenz	CYP2B6	Yimer et al. (2012)
Diclofenac	CYP2C8	Daly et al. (2007)
Isoniazid	CYP2E1	Huang et al. (2003)

The above findings are from candidate gene studies.

here generally involve small numbers of patients and relatively small though statistically significant associations, with only limited replication achieved. This continues to be a problem in studying pharmacogenetic aspects of rare adverse drug reactions though global efforts to standardize phenotypic aspects of these reactions (Aithal et al., 2011; Hayashi et al., 2022; Pirmohamed et al., 2011) may help mitigate this limitation.

Diclofenac is a widely prescribed non-steroidal antiinflammatory drug which is a relatively common cause of DILI worldwide (Banks, Zimmerman, Ishak, & Harter, 1995; Bjornsson, Bergmann, Bjornsson, Kvaran, & Olafsson, 2013). Susceptibility to DILI due to this drug does not appear to be associated with particular HLA genotypes (Nicoletti et al., 2017; Urban et al., 2012). Diclofenac undergoes phase I metabolism by CYP2C9 and several other P450s including CYP2C8 and phase II metabolism by the UDP-glucuronosyltransferase UGT2B7. There is no evidence that the common CYP2C9 variant alleles are relevant to risk of DILI (Aithal, Day, Leathart, & Daly, 2000; Daly et al., 2007; Urban et al., 2012) but some evidence that CYP2C8 genotype might contribute, consistent with the role of this isoform in metabolism of diclofenac to 5-hydroxydiclofenac which may form an reactive imine metabolite (Daly et al., 2007; Lazarska, Dekker, Vermeulen, & Commandeur, 2018; Shen, Marchick, Davis, Doss, & Pohl, 1999). Both candidate gene and GWAS analysis indicate an additional role for polymorphic phase II metabolism and transporter polymorphisms in diclofenac-induced DILI, possibly linked to increased formation of reactive diclofenac acylglucuronide metabolites (Daly et al., 2007; Urban et al., 2012).

For DILI due to ticlopidine, an upstream SNP (rs7254579 which results in −2320T > C included in *CYP2B6*1.007*) that appears to be associated with increased CYP2B6 expression (Hesse et al., 2004) was significantly more common among cases (Ariyoshi et al., 2010). This variant might be associated with higher reactive metabolite levels resulting in an increased risk of DILI. In addition to the association with CYP2B6, there are replicated data showing that individuals positive for *HLA-A*33* alleles show an increased risk of ticlopidine DILI (Hirata et al., 2008; Nicoletti et al., 2017). Ticlopidine remains one of only a few currently licensed drugs associated with DILI where there is evidence that both HLA genotype and genotype for a drug-metabolizing enzyme contribute jointly to DILI risk.

CYP2B6 genotype may also be relevant to risk of DILI due to the anti-HIV drug efavirenz. The CYP2B6 variant rs3745274 (c.516G > T) appears to be more common in cases of DILI due to this drug (Yimer et al., 2012). This variant is associated with lower than normal CYP2B6 activity suggesting that for efavirenz, accumulation of the parent drug and not a metabolite might be an important factor in the toxicity mechanism. Limited independent replication of this CYP2B6 association has been reported (Elsharkawy et al., 2013; Manosuthi et al., 2014).

An association between certain CYP2E1 genotypes and isoniazid-related DILI has been suggested due to the role of CYP2E1 in metabolism of acetylhydrazine (Wang, Pradhan, Zhong, & Ma, 2016). A candidate gene study involving the *CYP2E1*5* variant (rs2031920) (detectable with the restriction enzyme *Rsa*I) reported a positive association (Huang et al., 2003) and other reports followed, some positive but others negative. However, recent GWAS analysis performed on East Asian, South Asian and European populations with isoniazid DILI did not detect any statistically significant signal in the area of CYP2E1 (Nicoletti et al., 2021; Suvichapanich et al., 2019). More specific investigation of CYP2E1 as a candidate gene in the same European population also yielded negative data (Nicoletti et al., 2021). It is possible that larger studies may show a small effect for CYP2E1 variants as risk factors for this form of DILI but any large effect seems unlikely. Compared with other P450 genes, the sequence of CYP2E1 is highly conserved (Harjumäki, Pridgeon, & Ingelman-Sundberg, 2021), making it less likely to contribute to a relatively common toxicity such as isoniazid-induced liver injury.

3.2 Idiosyncratic skin reactions and cytochrome P450 polymorphisms

Cytochrome P450 polymorphisms are also relevant to risk of idiosyncratic adverse drug reactions affecting the skin. Local metabolism by P450s expressed in skin tissue may be important in these reactions. The reactions vary considerably in severity ranging from severe blistering skin reactions such as Stevens-Johnson syndrome to a mild rash and can be induced by a number of prescribed drugs. The best studied pharmacogenomic examples are those induced by anticonvulsant drugs, including phenytoin and carbamazepine, and by anti-HIV drugs including nevirapine. Similar to DILI, HLA genes are the important risk factors for these reactions (Oussalah et al., 2020). However, the overall contribution by HLA genotype appears stronger for skin rash than for DILI whereas data on non-HLA genetic risk factors for drug-induced skin rash, especially polymorphisms affecting drug disposition including cytochromes P450, are more limited than for DILI.

CYP2C9 has a major role in phase I metabolism of phenytoin and common variants, especially *CYP2C9*2* and *CYP2C9*3*, have been shown to be associated with decreased rates of oxidative metabolism of this drug (Aynacioglu et al., 1999). Phenytoin is a well-established cause of skin injury and susceptibility to this type of toxicity has been shown to be association with *HLA B*15:02* which is also a major risk factor for carbamazepine-induced skin rash (Hung et al., 2010). When the effect size for *B*15:02* as a risk factor for carbamazepine versus phenytoin-induced toxicity is compared, the HLA-associated risk is much lower for phenytoin, suggesting that other genetic factors may contribute. Using GWAS, genetic factors for risk of skin injury with phenytoin were investigated in East Asians (Chung et al., 2014). A signal was detected on chromosome 10, with the strongest effect seen for the variant coding for the nonsynonymous polymorphism resulting in the base change I359L associated with the *CYP2C9*3* allele. The finding was replicated in additional cases from East Asia, and more recent studies from this geographic region confirm this CYP2C9 association (Hikino et al., 2020). The reason for the observed association with *CYP2C9*3* only is probably due to studies to date being based in East Asia where this allele is common but other variants such as *CYP2C9*2* are rarer. The basis for the toxicity may be due to the role of CYP2C9 in forming the metabolite p-HPPH which proceeds via a reactive arene oxide intermediate. It is possible that the low CYP2C9 activity seen in individuals carrying *CYP2C9*3* may result in higher levels of arene oxide formation leading to adduct formation which triggers the hypersensitivity reaction mediated by HLA. CYP2C9 variants common elsewhere in the world including that within the *CYP2C9*2* allele may also be relevant to risk of this toxicity. A recent small study based in the USA suggests that homozygosity for *CYP2C9*2* or any carriage of *CYP2C9*3* increases risk of skin reaction with phenytoin (Fohner et al., 2020).

The anti-HIV drug nevirapine causes skin rash quite commonly (Phillips et al., 2007). This drug is subject to P450-mediated metabolism by several isoforms with CYP2B6 showing a major role (Riska et al., 1999). The relationship between selected CYP2B6 variants and nevirapine skin rash has been investigated in several studies though, similar to the liver injury studies discussed in Section 3.1, the number of cases studied was small. The earliest of these studies on rs3745274 (c.516G>T) in CYP2B6 was worldwide. As discussed in Section 3.1, this decreased activity variant may also be associated with DILI linked to efavirenz. A significantly increased risk for development of nevirapine skin reactions with carriage of one or more CYP2B6 variant alleles, especially in cases of African ethnicity, was found (Yuan et al., 2011). In a smaller study also based in Africa on Stevens-Johnson syndrome and toxic epidermal necrolysis only, the same variant was investigated together with rs28399499 (c.983T>C)(*CYP2B6**18*), a variant associated with absence of activity (Ciccacci et al., 2013). The significant association of c.516G>T could not be confirmed, though a trend toward significance in the same direction as previously was reported. For c.983T>C, a highly statistically significant association was reported but this was based on small numbers. In a more recent and larger African study (Carr et al., 2014), carriage of c.983T>C was significantly more common in cases with Stevens-Johnson syndrome or toxic epidermal necrolysis but no effect was seen for c.516G>T. These studies together point to low CYP2B6 activity being a risk factor for nevirapine skin rash, possibly due to accumulation of the parent drug increasing risk of a HLA-mediated hypersensitivity reaction for which certain HLA-C alleles are risk factors (Pavlos et al., 2017).

4. Cytochrome P450 polymorphisms and disease susceptibility

4.1 Cancer

In addition to metabolism of prescribed drugs, cytochromes P450 contribute to metabolism of a range of other xenobiotics. A role for human cytochromes P450 in carcinogen activation is well established (Rendic & Guengerich, 2021). Since the first reports of P450 polymorphisms emerged in the 1970s, the possibility that interindividual variation in P450 levels could contribute to cancers relating to exposure to tobacco, alcohol and other xenobiotics together with oxidative stress more generally has received considerable attention. The availability of simple genotyping approaches to predict phenotype contributed to a large number of studies from the 1990s onward. This area has been reviewed in detail relatively recently (Daly, 2015), so the emphasis in this section is on the most recent advances. There are extensive reports in the literature, especially but not exclusively from prior to 2008 when the first GWAS analyses on disease susceptibility were published, that genotype for certain CYP1A1, CYP2D6 and, to a more limited extent, CYP2E1 and CYP2A6 polymorphisms predict risk of lung cancer. GWAS analyses on lung cancer now provide data on over 50 different susceptibility loci (reviewed by Bossé & Amos, 2018). The only P450 gene showing a positive association for risk of lung cancer development by GWAS is CYP2A6, with a protective effect for several polymorphisms that are associated with either low or absent CYP2A6 activity reported (McKay et al., 2017). The CYP2A6 association was detected in both adenocarcinoma and squamous cell carcinoma and likely relates to the role of CYP2A6 in nicotine metabolism with low activity resulting in altered smoking behaviour which may protect against exposure to carcinogens and procarcinogens in tobacco smoke (Murphy, 2021). CYP2A6 has a well established role in activation of nitrosamines such as NNK (4-(methylnitrosamino)-1-(3-pyridyl)-1-butanone) in addition to detoxicating nicotine so it is possible that the protective effect of low activity CYP2A6 variants against lung cancer may be due to lower levels of NNK activation together with lower smoking intensity (Yuan et al., 2017). CYP2A6 variants but no other P450 polymorphisms are included in a recently developed polygenic risk score for lung cancer (Hung et al., 2021).

It is possible that CYP2A6 genotype may contribute to susceptibility to other smoking-related cancers such as bladder cancer and pancreatic cancer but CYP2A6 data on these cancers are limited compared with lung cancer. This may be down to more data being available on lung cancer since it remains the leading cause of cancer mortality worldwide and the most common cancer diagnosed in many countries. In addition, while smoking contributes to risk of cancers affecting other organs in addition to the lung, the overall contribution is lower and any effect from CYP2A6 genotype therefore likely to be lower and more difficult to measure.

As well as CYP2A6, CYP2E1 remains a plausible candidate gene for a role in susceptibility to cancer. This reflects both its general substrate specificity which includes certain low molecular weight drugs, ethanol and procarcinogens such as NNK together with an ability to form reactive oxygen species during its catalytic cycle (Guengerich, 2020a). Despite a relatively large number of early reports of associations of CYP2E1 genotypes with cancer susceptibility, no associations have been detected in recent large GWAS on several cancers where this genotype for this P450 seemed of some potential relevance such as lung cancer (McKay et al., 2017), nasopharyngeal cancer (Cui et al., 2016) and various aerodigestive tract cancers (McKay et al., 2011). This may be due to the rarity of most functionally significant CYP2E1 polymorphisms as discussed in Section 3.1.

4.2 Other diseases

A role for P450 genotype in susceptibility to certain other common diseases where xenobiotic exposure is considered to contribute to pathogenesis has also been proposed. The role of cytochromes P450 in metabolism of endogenous compounds also raises the possibility that absence of activity could affect susceptibility to a range of common diseases. As with the cancer examples discussed above, GWAS have not confirmed associations. This is particularly the case for CYP2E1 where a contribution by this P450 to alcoholic liver disease and more recently to nonalcoholic liver disease development and progression has been proposed on the basis of ethanol as a substrate and the ability of the enzyme to generate reactive oxygen species (Harjumäki et al., 2021). Though CYP2E1 may well contribute to overall disease biology, there is no evidence from GWAS for a role for CYP2E1 genotype in either alcoholic liver disease or nonalcoholic fatty liver disease progression with instead genes that are more directly relevant to lipid metabolism key contributors (Anstee et al., 2020; Schwantes-An et al., 2021; Vujkovic et al., 2021). Elevation of CYP2E1 expression at the protein level in liver from steatosis and nonalcoholic steatohepatitis patients has been detected (Weltman, Farrell, Hall, Ingelman-Sundberg, & Liddle, 1998) but this was not confirmed at the mRNA level by sequencing (Govaere et al., 2020) so CYP2E1 genotype may not be relevant here.

5. Conclusion

Since the first reports on cytochrome P450 polymorphisms appeared more than 40 years ago, considerable progress has been made in understanding the underlying basis for variable levels of cytochrome P450-mediated metabolism. The overall extent of variability in P450 genes is now clear with functionally-significant polymorphisms reported across almost all isoforms. Genome sequencing has advanced this area considerably with large numbers of rare variants now reliably identified (Ingelman-Sundberg, Mkrtchian, Zhou, & Lauschke, 2018; chapter "Cytochrome P450 polymorphism: From evolution to clinical use" by Ingelman-Sundberg). The issue of functional significance of individual variants, especially when the effect may be substrate-dependent, is still not always clear, despite some recent advances (Amorosi et al., 2021), and further studies are needed. From the CPIC and other projects concerned with clinical implementation of pharmacogenetics, a large number of examples of drugs where genotyping for P450 polymorphisms (alongside other genes relevant to pharmacogenomics) prior to prescription is recommended have been described with detailed guidelines on how adjust prescribing to deal with genotype data now available. However, as discussed recently by selected experts in the field

(Chenoweth et al., 2020), challenges in implementing routine pharmacogenetic testing remain, despite well demonstrated advantages in having this knowledge available prior to prescription and successful implementation in some specialist centers. This chapter has focussed on some specific examples to illustrate the impact of P450 polymorphisms. Further examples are considered elsewhere in this volume (chapter "Cytochrome P450 polymorphism: From evolution to clinical use" by Ingelman-Sundberg).

Conflict of interest

The author has no conflicts of interest to declare.

References

Aithal, G. P., Day, C. P., Kesteven, P. J., & Daly, A. K. (1999). Association of polymorphisms in the cytochrome P450 CYP2C9 with warfarin dose requirement and risk of bleeding complications. *Lancet*, *353*(9154), 717–719. https://doi.org/10.1016/S0140-6736(98)04474-2.

Aithal, G. P., Day, C. P., Leathart, J. B. S., & Daly, A. K. (2000). Relationship of polymorphism in CYP2C9 to genetic susceptibility to diclofenac-induced hepatitis. *Pharmacogenetics*, *10*, 511–518.

Aithal, G. P., Watkins, P. B., Andrade, R. J., Larrey, D., Molokhia, M., Takikawa, H., et al. (2011). Case definition and phenotype standardization in drug-induced liver injury. *Clinical Pharmacology and Therapeutics*, *89*(6), 806–815. https://doi.org/10.1038/clpt.2011.58.

Alexanderson, B., Evans, D. A., & Sjoqvist, F. (1969). Steady-state plasma levels of nortriptyline in twins: Influence of genetic factors and drug therapy. *British Medical Journal*, *4*(5686), 764–768. https://doi.org/10.1136/bmj.4.5686.764.

Amorosi, C. J., Chiasson, M. A., McDonald, M. G., Wong, L. H., Sitko, K. A., Boyle, G., et al. (2021). Massively parallel characterization of CYP2C9 variant enzyme activity and abundance. *American Journal of Human Genetics*, *108*(9), 1735–1751. https://doi.org/10.1016/j.ajhg.2021.07.001.

Anstee, Q. M., Darlay, R., Cockell, S., Meroni, M., Govaere, O., Tiniakos, D., et al. (2020). Genome-wide association study of non-alcoholic fatty liver and steatohepatitis in a histologically characterised cohort. *Journal of Hepatology*, *73*(3), 505–515. https://doi.org/10.1016/j.jhep.2020.04.003.

Ariyoshi, N., Iga, Y., Hirata, K., Sato, Y., Miura, G., Ishii, I., et al. (2010). Enhanced susceptibility of HLA-mediated ticlopidine-induced idiosyncratic hepatotoxicity by CYP2B6 polymorphism in Japanese. *Drug Metabolism and Pharmacokinetics*, *25*(3), 298–306.

Aynacioglu, A. S., Brockmoller, J., Bauer, S., Sachse, C., Guzelbey, P., Ongen, Z., et al. (1999). Frequency of cytochrome P450 CYP2C9 variants in a Turkish population and functional relevance for phenytoin. *British Journal of Clinical Pharmacology*, *48*(3), 409–415.

Banks, A. T., Zimmerman, H. J., Ishak, K. G., & Harter, J. G. (1995). Diclofenac-associated hepatotoxicity—Analysis of 180 cases reported to the food-and-drug-administration as adverse reactions. *Hepatology*, *22*(3), 820–827.

Bertilsson, L., Dengler, H. J., Eichelbaum, M., & Schulz, H. U. (1980). Pharmacogenetic covariation of defective N-oxidation of sparteine and 4-hydroxylation of debrisoquine. *European Journal of Clinical Pharmacology*, *17*(2), 153–155.

Bjornsson, E. S., Bergmann, O. M., Bjornsson, H. K., Kvaran, R. B., & Olafsson, S. (2013). Incidence, presentation, and outcomes in patients with drug-induced liver injury in the general population of Iceland. *Gastroenterology*, *144*(7), 1419–1425. 1425 e1411-1413; quiz e1419-1420 https://doi.org/10.1053/j.gastro.2013.02.006.

Bossé, Y., & Amos, C. I. (2018). A decade of GWAS results in lung cancer. *Cancer Epidemiology, Biomarkers & Prevention*, *27*(4), 363–379. https://doi.org/10.1158/1055-9965.Epi-16-0794.

Botton, M. R., Whirl-Carrillo, M., Del Tredici, A. L., Sangkuhl, K., Cavallari, L. H., Agúndez, J. A. G., et al. (2021). PharmVar GeneFocus: CYP2C19. *Clinical Pharmacology and Therapeutics*, *109*(2), 352–366. https://doi.org/10.1002/cpt.1973.

Bråten, L. S., Haslemo, T., Jukic, M. M., Ivanov, M., Ingelman-Sundberg, M., Molden, E., et al. (2021). A novel CYP2C-haplotype associated with ultrarapid metabolism of escitalopram. *Clinical Pharmacology and Therapeutics*, *110*(3), 786–793. https://doi.org/10.1002/cpt.2233.

Butler, M. A., Lang, N. P., Young, J. F., Caporaso, N. E., Vineis, P., Hayes, R. B., et al. (1992). Determination of CYP1A2 and NAT2 phenotypes in human populations by analysis of caffeine urinary metabolites. *Pharmacogenetics*, *2*(3), 116–127. https://doi.org/10.1097/00008571-199206000-00003.

Caldwell, M. D., Awad, T., Johnson, J. A., Gage, B. F., Falkowski, M., Gardina, P., et al. (2008). CYP4F2 genetic variant alters required warfarin dose. *Blood*, *111*(8), 4106–4112. https://doi.org/10.1182/blood-2007-11-122010.

Carr, D. F., Chaponda, M., Cornejo Castro, E. M., Jorgensen, A. L., Khoo, S., Van Oosterhout, J. J., et al. (2014). CYP2B6 c.983T > C polymorphism is associated with nevirapine hypersensitivity in Malawian and Ugandan HIV populations. *The Journal of Antimicrobial Chemotherapy*, *69*(12), 3329–3334. https://doi.org/10.1093/jac/dku315.

Chenoweth, M. J., Giacomini, K. M., Pirmohamed, M., Hill, S. L., van Schaik, R. H. N., Schwab, M., et al. (2020). Global pharmacogenomics within precision medicine: Challenges and opportunities. *Clinical Pharmacology and Therapeutics*, *107*(1), 57–61. https://doi.org/10.1002/cpt.1664.

Chung, W. H., Chang, W. C., Lee, Y. S., Wu, Y. Y., Yang, C. H., Ho, H. C., et al. (2014). Genetic variants associated with phenytoin-related severe cutaneous adverse reactions. *JAMA*, *312*(5), 525–534. https://doi.org/10.1001/jama.2014.7859.

Ciccacci, C., Di Fusco, D., Marazzi, M. C., Zimba, I., Erba, F., Novelli, G., et al. (2013). Association between CYP2B6 polymorphisms and Nevirapine-induced SJS/TEN: A pharmacogenetics study. *European Journal of Clinical Pharmacology*, *69*(11), 1909–1916. https://doi.org/10.1007/s00228-013-1549-x.

Corsini, A., & Bortolini, M. (2013). Drug-induced liver injury: The role of drug metabolism and transport. *Journal of Clinical Pharmacology*, *53*(5), 463–474. https://doi.org/10.1002/jcph.23.

Cui, Q., Feng, Q. S., Mo, H. Y., Sun, J., Xia, Y. F., Zhang, H., et al. (2016). An extended genome-wide association study identifies novel susceptibility loci for nasopharyngeal carcinoma. *Human Molecular Genetics*, *25*(16), 3626–3634. https://doi.org/10.1093/hmg/ddw200.

Daly, A. K. (2015). Polymorphic variants of cytochrome P450: Relevance to cancer and other diseases. *Advances in Pharmacology*, *74*, 85–111. https://doi.org/10.1016/bs.apha.2015.03.001.

Daly, A. K., Aithal, G. P., Leathart, J. B., Swainsbury, R. A., Dang, T. S., & Day, C. P. (2007). Genetic susceptibility to diclofenac-induced hepatotoxicity: Contribution of UGT2B7, CYP2C8, and ABCC2 genotypes. *Gastroenterology*, *132*(1), 272–281.

Daly, A. K., Rettie, A. E., Fowler, D. M., & Miners, J. O. (2017). Pharmacogenomics of CYP2C9: Functional and clinical considerations. *Journal of Personalized Medicine*, *8*(1). https://doi.org/10.3390/jpm8010001.

Dawwas, G. K., Dietrich, E., Cuker, A., Barnes, G. D., Leonard, C. E., & Lewis, J. D. (2021). Effectiveness and safety of direct Oral anticoagulants versus warfarin in patients with valvular atrial fibrillation: A population-based cohort study. *Annals of Internal Medicine, 174*(7), 910–919. https://doi.org/10.7326/m20-6194.

de Morais, S. M. F., Wilkinson, G. R., Blaisdell, J., Meyer, U. A., Nakamura, K., & Goldstein, J. A. (1994). Identification of a new genetic defect responsible for the polymorphism of *(S)*-mephenytoin metabolism in Japanese. *Molecular Pharmacology, 46*, 594–598.

de Morais, S. M. F., Wilkinson, G. R., Blaisdell, J., Nakamura, K., Meyer, U. A., & Goldstein, J. A. (1994). The major genetic defect responsible for the polymorphism of *S*-mephenytoin metabolism in humans. *The Journal of Biological Chemistry, 269*, 15419–15422.

Desta, Z., El-Boraie, A., Gong, L., Somogyi, A. A., Lauschke, V. M., Dandara, C., et al. (2021). PharmVar GeneFocus: CYP2B6. *Clinical Pharmacology and Therapeutics, 110*(1), 82–97. https://doi.org/10.1002/cpt.2166.

Distelrath, L. M., Reilly, P. E. B., Martin, M. V., Davis, G. G., Wilkinson, G. R., & Guengerich, F. P. (1985). Purification and characterisation of the human liver cytochromes P450 involved in debrisoquine 4-hydroxylation and phenacetin O-deethylation, two prototypes for genetic polymorphism in oxidative drug metabolism. *The Journal of Biological Chemistry, 260*, 9057–9067.

Eichelbaum, M., Spannbrucker, N., Steincke, B., & Dengler, H. J. (1979). Defective N-oxidation of sparteine in man: A new pharmacogenetic defect. *European Journal of Clinical Pharmacology, 17*, 153–155.

Elsharkawy, A. M., Schwab, U., McCarron, B., Burt, A. D., Daly, A. K., Hudson, M., et al. (2013). Efavirenz induced acute liver failure requiring liver transplantation in a slow drug metaboliser. *Journal of Clinical Virology, 58*(1), 331–333. https://doi.org/10.1016/j.jcv.2013.05.003.

Fasco, M. J., Vatsis, K. P., Kaminsky, L. S., & Coon, M. J. (1978). Regioselective and stereoselective hydroxylation of R and S warfarin by different forms of purified cytochrome P-450 from rabbit liver. *The Journal of Biological Chemistry, 253*(21), 7813–7820.

Fernandez-Salguero, P., Hoffman, S. M. G., Cholerton, S., Mohrenweiser, H., Raunio, H., Pelkonen, O., et al. (1995). A genetic polymorphism in coumarin 7-hydroxylation: Sequence of the human *CYP2A* genes and identification of variant *CYP2A6* alleles. *American Journal of Human Genetics, 57*, 651–660.

Fohner, A. E., Rettie, A. E., Thai, K. K., Ranatunga, D. K., Lawson, B. L., Liu, V. X., et al. (2020). Associations of CYP2C9 and CYP2C19 pharmacogenetic variation with phenytoin-induced cutaneous adverse drug reactions. *Clinical and Translational Science*. https://doi.org/10.1111/cts.12787.

Furuya, H., FernandezSalguero, P., Gregory, W., Taber, H., Steward, A., Gonzalez, F. J., et al. (1995). Genetic polymorphism of CYP2C9 and its effect on warfarin maintenance dose requirement in patients undergoing anticoagulation therapy. *Pharmacogenetics, 5*(6), 389–392.

Gaedigk, A., Casey, S. T., Whirl-Carrillo, M., Miller, N. A., & Klein, T. E. (2021). Pharmacogene variation consortium: A global resource and repository for pharmacogene variation. *Clinical Pharmacology and Therapeutics, 110*(3), 542–545. https://doi.org/10.1002/cpt.2321.

Gage, B. F., Bass, A. R., Lin, H., Woller, S. C., Stevens, S. M., Al-Hammadi, N., et al. (2017). Effect of genotype-guided warfarin dosing on clinical events and anticoagulation control among patients undergoing hip or knee arthroplasty: The GIFT randomized clinical trial. *JAMA, 318*(12), 1115–1124. https://doi.org/10.1001/jama.2017.11469.

Gonzalez, F. J., Vilbois, F., Hardwick, J. P., McBride, O. W., Nebert, D. W., Gelboin, H. V., et al. (1988). Human debrisoquine 4-hydroxylase (P450IID1):

cDNA and deduced amino acid sequence and assignment of the CYP2D locus to chromosome 22. *Genomics, 2*, 174–179.

Gough, A. C., Miles, J. S., Spurr, N. K., Moss, J. E., Gaedigk, A., Eichelbaum, M., et al. (1990). Identification of the primary gene defect at the cytochrome P450 *CYP2D* locus. *Nature, 347*, 773–776.

Govaere, O., Cockell, S., Tiniakos, D., Queen, R., Younes, R., Vacca, M., et al. (2020). Transcriptomic profiling across the nonalcoholic fatty liver disease spectrum reveals gene signatures for steatohepatitis and fibrosis. *Science Translational Medicine, 12*(572). https://doi.org/10.1126/scitranslmed.aba4448.

Guengerich, F. P. (2020a). Cytochrome P450 2E1 and its roles in disease. *Chemico-Biological Interactions, 322*, 109056. https://doi.org/10.1016/j.cbi.2020.109056.

Guengerich, F. P. (2020b). A history of the roles of cytochrome P450 enzymes in the toxicity of drugs. *Toxicology Research, 37*(1), 1–23. https://doi.org/10.1007/s43188-020-00056-z.

Hanioka, N., Kimura, S., Meyer, U. A., & Gonzalez, F. J. (1990). The human *CYP2D* locus associated with a common genetic defect in drug oxidation: A G_{1934} to a base change in intron 3 of a mutant *CYP2D6* allele results in an aberrant 3′ splice recognition site. *American Journal of Human Genetics, 47*, 994–1001.

Harjumäki, R., Pridgeon, C. S., & Ingelman-Sundberg, M. (2021). CYP2E1 in alcoholic and non-alcoholic liver injury. Roles of ROS, reactive intermediates and lipid overload. *International Journal of Molecular Sciences, 22*(15). https://doi.org/10.3390/ijms22158221.

Hayashi, P. H., Lucena, M. I., Fontana, R. J., Bjornsson, E. S., Aithal, G. P., Barnhart, H., et al. (2022). A revised electronic version of RUCAM for the diagnosis of DILI. *Hepatology*. https://doi.org/10.1002/hep.32327.

Hesse, L. M., He, P., Krishnaswamy, S., Hao, Q., Hogan, K., von Moltke, L. L., et al. (2004). Pharmacogenetic determinants of interindividual variability in bupropion hydroxylation by cytochrome P450 2B6 in human liver microsomes. *Pharmacogenetics, 14*(4), 225–238. https://doi.org/10.1097/00008571-200404000-00002.

Hikino, K., Ozeki, T., Koido, M., Terao, C., Kamatani, Y., Mizukawa, Y., et al. (2020). HLA-B*51:01 and CYP2C9*3 are risk factors for phenytoin-induced eruption in the Japanese population: Analysis of data from the biobank Japan project. *Clinical Pharmacology and Therapeutics, 107*(5), 1170–1178. https://doi.org/10.1002/cpt.1706.

Hirata, K., Takagi, H., Yamamoto, M., Matsumoto, T., Nishiya, T., Mori, K., et al. (2008). Ticlopidine-induced hepatotoxicity is associated with specific human leukocyte antigen genomic subtypes in Japanese patients: A preliminary case-control study. *The Pharmacogenomics Journal, 8*(1), 29–33.

Hu, Y., Oscarson, M., Johansson, I., Yue, Q. Y., Dahl, M. L., Tabone, M., et al. (1997). Genetic polymorphism of human CYP2E1: Characterization of two variant alleles. *Molecular Pharmacology, 51*(3), 370–376.

Huang, Y. S., Chern, H. D., Su, W. J., Wu, J. C., Chang, S. C., Chiang, C. H., et al. (2003). Cytochrome P450 2E1 genotype and the susceptibility to antituberculosis drug-induced hepatitis. *Hepatology, 37*(4), 924–930. https://doi.org/10.1053/jhep.2003.50144.

Hung, S. I., Chung, W. H., Liu, Z. S., Chen, C. H., Hsih, M. S., Hui, R. C., et al. (2010). Common risk allele in aromatic antiepileptic-drug induced Stevens-Johnson syndrome and toxic epidermal necrolysis in Han Chinese. *Pharmacogenomics, 11*(3), 349–356. https://doi.org/10.2217/pgs.09.162.

Hung, R. J., Warkentin, M. T., Brhane, Y., Chatterjee, N., Christiani, D. C., Landi, M. T., et al. (2021). Assessing lung cancer absolute risk trajectory based on a polygenic risk model. *Cancer Research, 81*(6), 1607–1615. https://doi.org/10.1158/0008-5472.Can-20-1237.

Ingelman-Sundberg, M., Mkrtchian, S., Zhou, Y., & Lauschke, V. M. (2018). Integrating rare genetic variants into pharmacogenetic drug response predictions. *Human Genomics, 12*(1), 26. https://doi.org/10.1186/s40246-018-0157-3.

Johnson, J. A., Caudle, K. E., Gong, L., Whirl-Carrillo, M., Stein, C. M., Scott, S. A., et al. (2017). Clinical pharmacogenetics implementation consortium (CPIC) guideline for pharmacogenetics-guided warfarin dosing: 2017 update. *Clinical Pharmacology and Therapeutics*, *102*(3), 397–404. https://doi.org/10.1002/cpt.668.

Kahn, G. C., Boobis, A. R., Murray, S., Brodie, M. J., & Davies, D. S. (1982). Assay and characterisation of debrisoquine 4-hydroxylase activity of microsomal fractions of human liver. *British Journal of Clinical Pharmacology*, *13*(5), 637–645.

Kaminsky, L. S., Dunbar, D. A., Wang, P. P., Beaune, P., Larrey, D., Guengerich, F. P., et al. (1984). Human hepatic cytochrome P-450 composition as probed by in vitro microsomal metabolism of warfarin. *Drug Metabolism and Disposition*, *12*(4), 470–477.

Karnes, J. H., Rettie, A. E., Somogyi, A. A., Huddart, R., Fohner, A. E., Formea, C. M., et al. (2021). Clinical pharmacogenetics implementation consortium (CPIC) guideline for CYP2C9 and HLA-B genotypes and phenytoin dosing: 2020 update. *Clinical Pharmacology and Therapeutics*, *109*(2), 302–309. https://doi.org/10.1002/cpt.2008.

Kimmel, S. E., French, B., Kasner, S. E., Johnson, J. A., Anderson, J. L., Gage, B. F., et al. (2013). A pharmacogenetic versus a clinical algorithm for warfarin dosing. *The New England Journal of Medicine*, *369*(24), 2283–2293. https://doi.org/10.1056/NEJMoa1310669.

Kupfer, A., & Preisig, R. (1984). Pharmacogenetics of mephenytoin: A new drug hydroxylation polymorphism in man. *European Journal of Clinical Pharmacology*, *26*, 753–759.

Lazarska, K. E., Dekker, S. J., Vermeulen, N. P. E., & Commandeur, J. N. M. (2018). Effect of UGT2B7*2 and CYP2C8*4 polymorphisms on diclofenac metabolism. *Toxicology Letters*, *284*, 70–78. https://doi.org/10.1016/j.toxlet.2017.11.038.

Lenk, H., Klöditz, K., Johansson, I., Smith, R. L., Jukic, M., Molden, E., et al. (2022). The polymorphic nuclear factor NFIB regulates hepatic CYP2D6 expression and influences risperidone metabolism in psychiatric patients. *Clinical Pharmacology and Therapeutics*. https://doi.org/10.1002/cpt.2571.

Mahgoub, A., Idle, J. R., Dring, L. G., Lancaster, R., & Smith, R. L. (1977). Polymorphic hydroxylation of debrisoquine in man. *Lancet*, *ii*, 584–586.

Manosuthi, W., Sukasem, C., Lueangniyomkul, A., Mankatitham, W., Thongyen, S., Nilkamhang, S., et al. (2014). CYP2B6 haplotype and biological factors responsible for hepatotoxicity in HIV-infected patients receiving efavirenz-based antiretroviral therapy. *International Journal of Antimicrobial Agents*, *43*(3), 292–296. https://doi.org/10.1016/j.ijantimicag.2013.10.022.

McDonald, M. G., Rieder, M. J., Nakano, M., Hsia, C. K., & Rettie, A. E. (2009). CYP4F2 is a vitamin K1 oxidase: An explanation for altered warfarin dose in carriers of the V433M variant. *Molecular Pharmacology*, *75*(6), 1337–1346. https://doi.org/10.1124/mol.109.054833.

McKay, J. D., Hung, R. J., Han, Y., Zong, X., Carreras-Torres, R., Christiani, D. C., et al. (2017). Large-scale association analysis identifies new lung cancer susceptibility loci and heterogeneity in genetic susceptibility across histological subtypes. *Nature Genetics*, *49*(7), 1126–1132. https://doi.org/10.1038/ng.3892.

McKay, J. D., Truong, T., Gaborieau, V., Chabrier, A., Chuang, S. C., Byrnes, G., et al. (2011). A genome-wide association study of upper aerodigestive tract cancers conducted within the INHANCE consortium. *PLoS Genetics*, 7(3). https://doi.org/10.1371/journal.pgen.1001333, e1001333.

Meier, P. J., Mueller, H. K., Dick, B., & Meyer, U. A. (1983). Hepatic monooxygenase activities in subjects with a genetic defect in drug oxidation. *Gastroenterology*, *85*(3), 682–692.

Murphy, S. E. (2021). Biochemistry of nicotine metabolism and its relevance to lung cancer. *The Journal of Biological Chemistry*, *296*, 100722. https://doi.org/10.1016/j.jbc.2021.100722.

Nicoletti, P., Aithal, G. P., Bjornsson, E. S., Andrade, R. J., Sawle, A., Arrese, M., et al. (2017). Association of liver injury from specific drugs, or groups of drugs, with polymorphisms in HLA and other genes in a genome-wide association study. *Gastroenterology, 152*(5), 1078–1089. https://doi.org/10.1053/j.gastro.2016.12.016.

Nicoletti, P., Devarbhavi, H., Goel, A., Venkatesan, R., Eapen, C. E., Grove, J. I., et al. (2021). Genetic risk factors in drug-induced liver injury due to isoniazid-containing antituberculosis drug regimens. *Clinical Pharmacology and Therapeutics, 109*(4), 1125–1135. https://doi.org/10.1002/cpt.2100.

Nofziger, C., Turner, A. J., Sangkuhl, K., Whirl-Carrillo, M., Agúndez, J. A. G., Black, J. L., et al. (2020). PharmVar GeneFocus: CYP2D6. *Clinical Pharmacology and Therapeutics, 107*(1), 154–170. https://doi.org/10.1002/cpt.1643.

Osanlou, O., Pirmohamed, M., & Daly, A. K. (2018). Pharmacogenetics of adverse drug reactions. *Advances in Pharmacology, 83*, 155–190. https://doi.org/10.1016/bs.apha.2018.03.002.

Oussalah, A., Yip, V., Mayorga, C., Blanca, M., Barbaud, A., Nakonechna, A., et al. (2020). Genetic variants associated with T cell-mediated cutaneous adverse drug reactions: A PRISMA-compliant systematic review—An EAACI position paper. *Allergy, 75*(5), 1069–1098. https://doi.org/10.1111/all.14174.

Pavlos, R., McKinnon, E. J., Ostrov, D. A., Peters, B., Buus, S., Koelle, D., et al. (2017). Shared peptide binding of HLA class I and II alleles associate with cutaneous nevirapine hypersensitivity and identify novel risk alleles. *Scientific Reports*, 7(1), 8653. https://doi.org/10.1038/s41598-017-08876-0.

Phillips, E., Gutiérrez, S., Jahnke, N., Yip, B., Lima, V. D., Hogg, R. S., et al. (2007). Determinants of nevirapine hypersensitivity and its effect on the association between hepatitis C status and mortality in antiretroviral drug-naive HIV-positive patients. *AIDS, 21*(12), 1561–1568. https://doi.org/10.1097/QAD.0b013e3282170a9d.

Pirmohamed, M., Burnside, G., Eriksson, N., Jorgensen, A. L., Toh, C. H., Nicholson, T., et al. (2013). A randomized trial of genotype-guided dosing of warfarin. *The New England Journal of Medicine, 369*(24), 2294–2303. https://doi.org/10.1056/NEJMoa1311386.

Pirmohamed, M., Friedmann, P. S., Molokhia, M., Loke, Y. K., Smith, C., Phillips, E., et al. (2011). Phenotype standardization for immune-mediated drug-induced skin injury. *Clinical Pharmacology and Therapeutics, 89*(6), 896–901. https://doi.org/10.1038/clpt.2011.79.

Pirmohamed, M., Kamali, F., Daly, A. K., & Wadelius, M. (2015). Oral anticoagulation: A critique of recent advances and controversies. *Trends in Pharmacological Sciences, 36*(3), 153–163. https://doi.org/10.1016/j.tips.2015.01.003.

Rendic, S. P., & Guengerich, F. P. (2021). Human family 1-4 cytochrome P450 enzymes involved in the metabolic activation of xenobiotic and physiological chemicals: An update. *Archives of Toxicology, 95*(2), 395–472. https://doi.org/10.1007/s00204-020-02971-4.

Rettie, A. E., Eddy, A. C., Heimark, L. D., Gibaldi, M., & Trager, W. F. (1989). Characteristics of warfarin hydroxylation catalyzed by human liver microsomes. *Drug Metabolism and Disposition, 17*(3), 265–270.

Rettie, A. E., Korzekwa, K. R., Kunze, K. L., Lawrence, R. F., Eddy, A. C., Aoyama, T., et al. (1992). Hydroxylation of warfarin by human cDNA-expressed cytochrome P-450: A role for P-4502C9 in the etiology of (S)-warfarin-drug interactions. *Chemical Research in Toxicology, 5*(1), 54–59. https://doi.org/10.1021/tx00025a009.

Rettie, A. E., Wienkers, L. C., Gonzalez, F. J., Trager, W. F., & Korzekwa, K. R. (1994). Impaired *(S)*-warfarin metabolism catalysed by the R144C allelic variant of CYP2C9. *Pharmacogenetics, 4*, 39–42.

Riska, P., Lamson, M., MacGregor, T., Sabo, J., Hattox, S., Pav, J., et al. (1999). Disposition and biotransformation of the antiretroviral drug nevirapine in humans. *Drug Metabolism and Disposition, 27*(8), 895–901.

Sangkuhl, K., Claudio-Campos, K., Cavallari, L. H., Agundez, J. A. G., Whirl-Carrillo, M., Duconge, J., et al. (2021). PharmVar GeneFocus: CYP2C9. *Clinical Pharmacology and Therapeutics*, *110*(3), 662–676. https://doi.org/10.1002/cpt.2333.

Schwantes-An, T. H., Darlay, R., Mathurin, P., Masson, S., Liangpunsakul, S., Mueller, S., et al. (2021). Genome-wide association study and meta-analysis on alcohol-associated liver cirrhosis identifies genetic risk factors. *Hepatology*, *73*(5), 1920–1931. https://doi.org/10.1002/hep.31535.

Scott, J., & Poffenbarger, P. L. (1978). Pharmacogenetics of tolbutamide metabolism in humans. *Diabetes*, *28*, 41–51.

Shen, S., Marchick, M. R., Davis, M. R., Doss, G. A., & Pohl, L. R. (1999). Metabolic activation of diclofenac by human cytochrome P450 3A4: Role of 5-hydroxydiclofenac. *Chemical Research in Toxicology*, *12*(2), 214–222. https://doi.org/10.1021/tx9802365.

Sim, S. C. (2013). CYP1A2*1F [corrected] contains the -163C > A substitution and is highly inducible. *Pharmacogenetics and Genomics*, *23*(2), 104–105. https://doi.org/10.1097/FPC.0b013e32835ccc76.

Sjöqvist, F., & von Bahr, C. (1973). Interindividual differences in drug oxidation: clinical importance. *Drug Metabolism and Disposition*, *1*(1), 469–482.

Stachulski, A. V., Baillie, T. A., Park, B. K., Obach, R. S., Dalvie, D. K., Williams, D. P., et al. (2013). The generation, detection, and effects of reactive drug metabolites. *Medicinal Research Reviews*, *33*(5), 985–1080. https://doi.org/10.1002/med.21273.

Steward, D. J., Haining, R. L., Henne, K. R., Davis, G., Rushmore, T. H., Trager, W. F., et al. (1997). Genetic association between sensitivity to warfarin and expression of CYP2C9*3. *Pharmacogenetics*, 7(5), 361–367.

Sullivan-Close, T. H., Ghanayem, B. I., Bell, D. A., Zhang, Z.-Y., Kaminsky, L. S., Shenfield, G. M., et al. (1996). The role of the *CYP2C9*-Leu359 allelic variant in the tolbutamide polymorphism. *Pharmacogenetics*, *6*(4), 341–349.

Suvichapanich, S., Wattanapokayakit, S., Mushiroda, T., Yanai, H., Chuchottawon, C., Kantima, T., et al. (2019). Genomewide association study confirming the association of NAT2 with susceptibility to antituberculosis drug-induced liver injury in Thai patients. *Antimicrobial Agents and Chemotherapy*, *63*(8). https://doi.org/10.1128/aac.02692-18.

Tanner, J. A., & Tyndale, R. F. (2017). Variation in CYP2A6 activity and personalized medicine. *Journal of Personalized Medicine*, 7(4). https://doi.org/10.3390/jpm7040018.

Tornio, A., & Backman, J. T. (2018). Cytochrome P450 in pharmacogenetics: An update. *Advances in Pharmacology*, *83*, 3–32. https://doi.org/10.1016/bs.apha.2018.04.007.

Tracy, T. S., Chaudhry, A. S., Prasad, B., Thummel, K. E., Schuetz, E. G., Zhong, X. B., et al. (2016). Interindividual variability in cytochrome P450-mediated drug metabolism. *Drug Metabolism and Disposition*, *44*(3), 343–351. https://doi.org/10.1124/dmd.115.067900.

Uetrecht, J. (2019). Mechanisms of idiosyncratic drug-induced liver injury. *Advances in Pharmacology*, *85*, 133–163. https://doi.org/10.1016/bs.apha.2018.12.001.

Urban, T. J., Daly, A. K., & Aithal, G. P. (2014). Genetic basis of drug-induced liver injury: Present and future. *Seminars in Liver Disease*, *34*(2), 123–133. https://doi.org/10.1055/s-0034-1375954.

Urban, T. J., Shen, Y., Stolz, A., Chalasani, N., Fontana, R. J., Rochon, J., et al. (2012). Limited contribution of common genetic variants to risk for liver injury due to a variety of drugs. *Pharmacogenetics and Genomics*, *22*(11), 784–795. https://doi.org/10.1097/FPC.0b013e3283589a76.

Vrzal, R. (2021). Genetic and enzymatic characteristics of CYP2A13 in relation to lung damage. *International Journal of Molecular Sciences*, *22*(22). https://doi.org/10.3390/ijms222212306.

Vujkovic, M., Ramdas, S., Lorenz, K. M., Guo, X., Darlay, R., Cordell, H. J., et al. (2021). A trans-ancestry genome-wide association study of unexplained chronic ALT elevation as a proxy for nonalcoholic fatty liver disease with histological and radiological validation. *medRxiv*. https://doi.org/10.1101/2020.12.26.20248491. 2020.2012.2026. 20248491.

Wang, P., Pradhan, K., Zhong, X. B., & Ma, X. (2016). Isoniazid metabolism and hepatotoxicity. *Acta Pharmaceutica Sinica B*, *6*(5), 384–392. https://doi.org/10.1016/j.apsb.2016.07.014.

Weltman, M. D., Farrell, G. C., Hall, P., Ingelman-Sundberg, M., & Liddle, C. (1998). Hepatic cytochrome P450 2E1 is increased in patients with nonalcoholic steatohepatitis. *Hepatology*, *27*(1), 128–133. https://doi.org/10.1002/hep.510270121.

Yimer, G., Amogne, W., Habtewold, A., Makonnen, E., Ueda, N., Suda, A., et al. (2012). High plasma efavirenz level and CYP2B6*6 are associated with efavirenz-based HAART-induced liver injury in the treatment of naive HIV patients from Ethiopia: A prospective cohort study. *The Pharmacogenomics Journal*, *12*(6), 499–506. https://doi.org/10.1038/tpj.2011.34.

Yu, K., Geng, X., Chen, M., Zhang, J., Wang, B., Ilic, K., et al. (2014). High daily dose and being a substrate of cytochrome P450 enzymes are two important predictors of drug-induced liver injury. *Drug Metabolism and Disposition*, *42*(4), 744–750. https://doi.org/10.1124/dmd.113.056267.

Yuan, J., Guo, S., Hall, D., Cammett, A. M., Jayadev, S., Distel, M., et al. (2011). Toxicogenomics of nevirapine-associated cutaneous and hepatic adverse events among populations of African, Asian, and European descent. *AIDS*, *25*(10), 1271–1280.

Yuan, J. M., Nelson, H. H., Carmella, S. G., Wang, R., Kuriger-Laber, J., Jin, A., et al. (2017). CYP2A6 genetic polymorphisms and biomarkers of tobacco smoke constituents in relation to risk of lung cancer in the Singapore Chinese Health Study. *Carcinogenesis*, *38*(4), 411–418. https://doi.org/10.1093/carcin/bgx012.

Zhang, J. E., Jorgensen, A. L., Alfirevic, A., Williamson, P. R., Toh, C. H., Park, B. K., et al. (2009). Effects of CYP4F2 genetic polymorphisms and haplotypes on clinical outcomes in patients initiated on warfarin therapy. *Pharmacogenetics and Genomics*, *19*(10), 781–789. https://doi.org/10.1097/FPC.0b013e3283311347.

CHAPTER THREE

Cytochrome P450 enzymes and metabolism of drugs and neurotoxins within the mammalian brain

Marlaina R. Stocco[a] and Rachel F. Tyndale[b,c,d,*]
[a]Department of Psychological and Brain Sciences, University of California, Santa Barbara, Santa Barbara, CA, United States
[b]Department of Pharmacology and Toxicology, University of Toronto, Toronto, ON, Canada
[c]Campbell Family Mental Health Research Institute, CAMH, Toronto, ON, Canada
[d]Department of Psychiatry, University of Toronto, Toronto, ON, Canada
[*]Corresponding author: e-mail address: r.tyndale@utoronto.ca

Contents

Abstract

Cytochrome P450 enzymes (CYPs) that metabolize xenobiotics are expressed and active in the brain. These CYPs contribute to the metabolism of many centrally acting compounds, including clinically used drugs, drugs of abuse, and neurotoxins. Although CYP levels are lower in the brain than in the liver, they may influence central substrate and metabolite concentrations, which could alter resulting centrally-mediated responses to these compounds. Additionally, xenobiotic metabolizing CYPs are highly variable due to genetic polymorphisms and regulation by endogenous and xenobiotic molecules. In the brain, these CYPs are sensitive to xenobiotic induction. As a result, CYPs

Advances in Pharmacology, Volume 95
ISSN 1054-3589
https://doi.org/10.1016/bs.apha.2022.04.003

in the brain vary widely, including among humans, and this CYP variation may influence central metabolism and resulting response to centrally acting compounds. It has been demonstrated, using experimental manipulation of CYP activity *in vivo* selectively within the brain, that CYP metabolism in the brain alters central substrate and metabolite concentrations, as well as drug response and neurotoxic effects. This suggests that variability in xenobiotic metabolizing CYPs in the human brain may meaningfully contribute to individual differences in response to, and effects of, centrally acting drugs and neurotoxins. This chapter will provide an overview of CYP expression in the brain, endogenous- and xenobiotic-mediated CYP regulation, and the functional impact of CYP-mediated metabolism of drugs and neurotoxins in the brain, with a focus on experimental approaches in mice, rats, and non-human primates, and a discussion regarding the potential role of xenobiotic metabolizing CYPs in the human brain.

Abbreviations

AhR aryl hydrocarbon receptor
CAR constitutive androstane receptor
CNS central nervous system
CYP cytochrome P450
MPP^+ 1-methyl-4-phenylpyridinium
MPTP 1-methyl-4-phenyl-1,2,3,6-tetrahydropyridine
PPAR peroxisome proliferator-activated receptor
PXR pregnane X receptor

1. Introduction

1.1 Xenobiotic metabolizing CYPs in the brain

In addition to the liver, cytochrome P450 enzymes (CYPs), whose principal role is in drug metabolism, are expressed in extrahepatic tissues, where their activity can influence local xenobiotic metabolism and alter organ- and tissue-specific exposure to substrates and their metabolites (Choudhary, Jansson, Stoilov, Sarfarazi, & Schenkman, 2005; Ding & Kaminsky, 2003; Oesch, Fabian, Guth, & Landsiedel, 2014; Su et al., 2000; Thum & Borlak, 2000). CYPs are expressed and active in the brains of numerous mammalian species, including humans and other primates, rats, mice, and other rodents (Chung-Davidson, Rees, Wu, Yun, & Li, 2004; Martignoni, Groothuis, & de Kanter, 2006; Miksys & Tyndale, 2004; Renaud, Cui, Khan, & Klaassen, 2011; Sasame, Ames, & Nelson, 1977). Many CYPs located in the brain are involved predominantly in the metabolism of endogenous compounds, including neurotransmitters, hormones and other sterols, fatty acids, vitamins, and eicosanoids (Dutheil, Beaune, & Loriot, 2008; Haduch & Daniel, 2018; Petrov, Mast, Li, Denker, & Pikuleva, 2020). However, xenobiotic metabolizing CYPs, including members of the CYP1A, -2B, -2C, -2D, -2E, and -3A subfamilies, are also expressed in the brain (Table 1) (Bhamre, Anandatheerathavarada, Shankar, Boyd, & Ravindranath, 1993; Toselli et al., 2015). In addition to having endogenous substrates, these CYP subfamilies are responsible for the majority of known drug and toxin metabolism, including that of centrally active clinically used drugs, psychoactive drugs of abuse, and environmental neurotoxins (Anzenbacher & Anzenbacherova, 2001; Miksys & Tyndale, 2013; Shimada, Yamazaki, Mimura, Inui, & Guengerich, 1994; Stingl, Brockmoller, & Viviani, 2013). This chapter will focus on these subfamilies of CYPs specifically.

CYP expression in the brain is much lower than in the liver (<5%), suggesting that brain CYP activity is unlikely to impact circulating concentrations of xenobiotics and their metabolites (Hedlund, Gustafsson, & Warner, 2001; Renaud et al., 2011; Warner, Kohler, Hansson, & Gustafsson, 1988).

Table 1 Examples of CYPs expressed in the brain and their xenobiotic substrates.

	Centrally acting substrates	
Enzyme	**Drug**	**Neurotoxin**
CYP1A1	Caffeine[a]	Benzo[a]pyrene (toxification)[b]
CYP2B6	Nicotine[c]	Chlorpyrifos (toxification)[d]
CYP2C9/19	Fluoxetine[e]	Harmine, chlorpyrifos (detoxification)[d,f]
CYP2D6	Oxycodone, methamphetamine[g,h]	Harmine, MPTP (detoxification)[f,i]
CYP2E1	Caffeine[a]	Ethanol (toxification)[j]
CYP3A4	Oxycodone, alprazolam[g,k]	MPTP (detoxification)[i]

[a]Ha, Chen, Krahenbuhl, and Follath (1996)
[b]Esteves et al. (2021)
[c]Yamazaki et al. (1999)
[d]Tang et al. (2001)
[e]Liu et al. (2001)
[f]Yu et al. (2003)
[g]Lalovic et al. (2004)
[h]Lin et al. (1997)
[i]Coleman et al. (1996)
[j]Heit et al. (2013)
[k]Allqvist, Miura, Bertilsson, and Mirghani, 2007)

Nevertheless, CYP activity within the brain is sufficient to alter substrate metabolism in the central nervous system (CNS), yielding distinct substrate-metabolite concentration profiles in the brain versus the periphery, which could meaningfully influence the central effects of drugs and neurotoxins (Britto & Wedlund, 1992). Many xenobiotic metabolizing CYPs exhibit interindividual variation in expression and activity due to genetic polymorphisms and due to regulation (Honkakoski & Negishi, 2000; Ingelman-Sundberg, 1999; Ingelman-Sundberg, Sim, Gomez, & Rodriguez-Antona, 2007; Wang et al., 2011). Moreover, CYPs in the brain are sensitive to xenobiotic-mediated induction, which can regulate CYPs in a brain-specific manner (Bergh & Strobel, 1996; Hedlund et al., 1996; Miksys & Tyndale, 2004). Thus, variation in CYPs within the brain may yield variability in central xenobiotic metabolism, which in turn may contribute to individual differences in response to centrally acting drugs and neurotoxins (Dutheil et al., 2008; Toselli, Dodd, & Gillam, 2016).

1.2 Studying CYPs in the brain

CYP expression in the brain can be assessed at the mRNA level in whole brain or in discrete brain regions using PCR and Northern Blot approaches (Funae, Kishimoto, Cho, Niwa, & Hiroi, 2003; Hiroi, Imaoka, Chow, & Funae, 1998; Komori, 1993; Norris, Hardwick, & Emson, 1996). Hybridization techniques, such as fluorescence *in situ* hybridization can be used to investigate the distribution of CYP mRNA in tissues, cell types, and subcellular spaces within the brain (Chinta, Kommaddi, Turman, Strobel, & Ravindranath, 2005; Chinta, Pai, Upadhya, Boyd, & Ravindranath, 2002; Norris et al., 1996). Similarly, the presence of CYP protein within the brain can be assessed and quantified using Western Blot, while various *in situ* and *in cyto* labelling techniques are applied to visualize the spatial distribution of CYP proteins within brain regions, tissues, and cells (Cheng et al., 2013; Chinta et al., 2005; Miksys, Rao, Hoffmann, Mash, & Tyndale, 2002; Ravindranath, Anandatheerthavarada, & Shankar, 1989).

Assessing CYP metabolic activity in the brain is challenging due to low CYP protein levels overall and rapid degradation in brain tissue collected post-mortem (Sasame et al., 1977; Tyndale et al., 1999). Nevertheless, CYP enzymatic activity can be assessed *in vitro* in brain by quantifying enzymatic product formation following incubation of brain tissue with a CYP-selective substrate (Bhamre et al., 1993; Ravindranath et al., 1989; Tyndale et al., 1999). Alternatively, following substrate administration *in vivo*, concentrations of the substrate and its CYP-produced metabolites can be assessed in brain tissue or brain dialysate; brain analyte concentrations and metabolic ratios can serve as measures of *in vivo* substrate metabolism in the CNS (Arguelles, Miksys, & Tyndale, 2021; Tolledo, Stocco, Miksys, Gonzalez, & Tyndale, 2020).

To investigate the functional impact of CYPs in the brain and central CYP-catalyzed xenobiotic metabolism, the impact of selectively manipulating CYPs in the brain on CNS substrate concentrations and resulting responses to exogenously administered compounds is assessed (Fig. 1). CYPs within the brain can be manipulated via induction and/or inhibition, with or without affecting CYPs in the liver (Haduch, Rysz, Papp, & Daniel, 2018; Hedlund et al., 1996; Miksys & Tyndale, 2004). While certain inducers enhance CYP expression in the liver and in extrahepatic tissues, some inducers increase CYP expression selectively within the brain (Kuban & Daniel, 2021; Lee, Joshi, Yue, & Tyndale, 2006; Lee, Miksys, & Tyndale, 2006; Mann, Miksys, Lee, Mash, & Tyndale, 2008; Yue, Miksys, Hoffmann, & Tyndale, 2008). To inhibit CYPs specifically within the brain without affecting CYPs in the liver, low doses of pharmacological inhibitors can be administered intracerebrally; moreover,

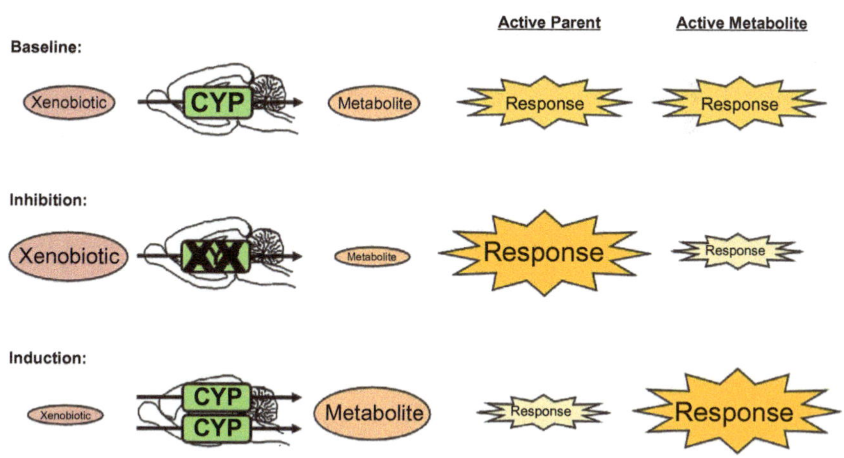

Fig. 1 The impact of manipulating CYPs selectively within the rodent brain via inhibition or induction, on resulting response depends on whether the xenobiotic parent versus metabolite is more pharmacologically active. Inhibiting CYP in the brain decreases metabolite production, increasing xenobiotic concentrations and xenobiotic-induced response. Inducing CYP in the brain enhances metabolite formation and metabolite-mediated response.

irreversible inhibitors can be used to selectively inactivate a specific CYP in the brain, allowing for a greater interval between intracerebral inhibitor pretreatment and subsequent substrate administration and behavioral testing (McMillan, El-Sherbeni, Richards, & Tyndale, 2020; McMillan & Tyndale, 2015; Miksys & Tyndale, 2009; Wang et al., 2015; Zhou, Khokhar, Zhao, & Tyndale, 2013).

2. CYP expression in the brain

Xenobiotic metabolizing CYP1A, -2B, -2C, -2D, -2E, and -3A are constitutively expressed in the mammalian brain (Dutheil et al., 2008; Renaud et al., 2011; Toselli et al., 2016). CYP mRNA, protein, and catalytic activity are detected broadly throughout different brain regions and exhibit a distinctly diffuse subcellular distribution in human, non-human primate, and rodent brains (Ghosh et al., 2016; Ravindranath, Anandatheerthavarada, & Shankar, 1990; Voirol et al., 2000). Brain CYPs are localized in the cell bodies of neurons and glia, in neuronal dendrites, axons, and synaptic terminals, as well as in glial processes (Miksys, Rao, et al., 2000; Toselli et al., 2016; Walther, Ghersi-Egea, Minn, & Siest, 1986). Moreover, protein and catalytic activity are detected in microsomal, mitochondrial, and plasma membrane fractions derived from primate and rodent brains (Ghersi-Egea et al., 1993; Neve & Ingelman-Sundberg, 2008; Walther et al., 1986). Individual CYP expression is heterogeneous in the mammalian brain, with mRNA, protein, and catalytic activity concentrated within specific brain structures, cell types, and subcellular compartments (Chinta et al., 2005; Chinta et al., 2002; Ferguson, Miksys, Palmour, & Tyndale, 2013; Woodland, Huang, Gryz, Bendayan, & Fawcett, 2008).

For instance, CYP1A1 is expressed broadly throughout human and rodent brains, and CYP1A1 protein is localized predominantly in neurons (Chinta et al., 2005). CYP1A1 protein is detected in cell bodies and apical dendrites of pyramidal neurons in the cerebral cortex and hippocampus, Purkinje and granule neurons in the cerebellum, and in midbrain reticular neurons (Chinta et al., 2005; Farin & Omiecinski, 1993; McFadyen, Melvin, & Murray, 1998). In rodents, CYP1A1 has also been identified in endothelial cells of the blood brain barrier and choroid plexus (Granberg, Ostergren, Brandt, & Brittebo, 2003). In humans, African green monkeys, and rats, CYP2E1 is also expressed predominantly in neurons, although CYP2E1 protein is detected almost exclusively in pyramidal neurons, with the highest levels in the frontal cortex, hippocampus, and cerebellum (Garcia-Suastegui et al., 2017; Lee, Joshi, et al., 2006).

Brain CYP2B expression exhibits species-specific differences. In African green monkeys, CYP2B6 is expressed constitutively in both neurons and astrocytes (Ferguson et al., 2013; Lee, Miksys, et al., 2006). CYP2B6 is also induced across several brain regions, including the frontal cortex, thalamus, hippocampus, caudate putamen, cerebellum, and brain stem (Ferguson et al., 2013; Lee, Miksys, et al., 2006). In contrast, constitutive expression of CYP2B6 is low in the human brain, with some protein detected in hippocampal neurons and in astrocytes of the frontal cortex and surrounding cerebral blood vessels (Miksys, Lerman, Shields, Mash, & Tyndale, 2003; Toselli et al., 2016). Human CYP2B6 is higher in the cerebellum, hippocampus, and caudate putamen of individuals who smoke and have alcohol use disorder, indicating CYP2B6 may be inducible in the human brain (Miksys et al., 2003). In rat brain, constitutive CYP2B1 expression is similarly low, with the exception of high CYP2B1 protein levels in astrocytes surrounding brain endothelium (Miksys, Hoffmann, & Tyndale, 2000). An inducible form of CYP2B1 is detected in the rat frontal cortex, brain stem, olfactory bulb, and substantia nigra (Miksys et al., 2000).

In contrast, CYP2C, -2D, and -3A are widely expressed within human, monkey, and rodent brains (Booth Depaz, Toselli, Wilce, & Gillam, 2015; Miksys, Cheung, Gonzalez, & Tyndale, 2005; Woodland et al., 2008). These CYPs are expressed in the cerebral cortex, hippocampus, amygdala, basal ganglia, and cerebellum (Booth Depaz et al., 2015; Miksys et al., 2005; Yadav, Johri, Dhawan, Seth, & Parmar, 2006); CYP2D and CYP3A are also detected in the olfactory bulbs, hypothalamus, thalamus, and brain stem (Miksys, Rao, et al., 2000; Miller, Miksys, Hoffmann, & Tyndale, 2014; Woodland et al., 2008; Yadav et al., 2006). These three CYP subfamilies are expressed in diverse cell types in the brain, including multiple neuronal subtypes, astrocytes and other glia, as well as endothelial cells (Booth Depaz et al., 2015; Ghosh et al., 2016; Miksys, Rao, et al., 2000; Norris et al., 1996). CYP2C, -2D, and -3A protein is localized in cell bodies and processes, and these have been detected in mitochondrial and plasma membrane fractions of neurons (Booth Depaz et al., 2015; Chinta et al., 2002; Ghersi-Egea et al., 1993; Neve & Ingelman-Sundberg, 2008).

3. Factors influencing CYPs in the brain

3.1 Endogenous factors

3.1.1 Genetics

Some CYP genes are highly genetically variable, and genetic polymorphisms can alter gene expression and influence the amount or function of CYP protein produced (Ingelman-Sundberg, 2004; Ingelman-Sundberg, Oscarson, & McLellan, 1999; Preissner et al., 2013). Genetic variation affecting CYP expression and/or activity yields altered metabolic phenotypes, including absent, reduced, normal, and increased catalytic activity (termed poor, intermediate, extensive, and ultra-rapid metabolism, respectively) (Ingelman-Sundberg, 1999; Ingelman-Sundberg et al., 2007). While genetic variation affects peripheral and central catalytic activity, the xenobiotic metabolizing human CYP2B6, -2C19, -2D6, and -3A4 are among the most highly genetically polymorphic, and these are expressed in the brain and have many centrally acting substrates; thus, genetic polymorphisms in these *CYPs* are likely to influence centrally mediated responses to their xenobiotic substrates (Dutheil et al., 2008; Haufroid & Hantson, 2015; Ingelman-Sundberg et al., 2007; Preissner et al., 2013; Stingl et al., 2013).

3.1.2 Hormones

Several xenobiotic metabolizing CYPs are sexually dimorphic in liver and extrahepatic tissues, due to being regulated by sex hormones. Estrogen-activated transcription factors bind to estrogen response elements in the promotor region of some CYP genes, such as *CYP1B1*, to regulate transcription (Tsuchiya, Nakajima, & Yokoi, 2005). Some transcription regulators are activated by other sex hormones, such as progesterone and testosterone, and these regulate expression of CYP2B, -2C, and -3A isoforms (Mikamo, Harada, Nishikawa, & Nishihara, 2003; Tsuchiya et al., 2005). Growth hormone regulates CYP gene transcription and contributes to sex differences in CYP expression (Dhir, Dworakowski, Thangavel, & Shapiro, 2006; Waxman & Holloway, 2009). Post-transcriptional regulation has also been demonstrated, with thyroid hormone (T3) inducing CYP2E1 expression *in vitro* by increasing the half-life of CYP2E1 mRNA, consistent with increased mRNA stability and/or decreased degradation (Peng & Coon, 1998).

Although the above examples occur in hepatic and extrahepatic tissues, some hormonal CYP regulation occurs in a brain-specific manner. CYP2D expression in the rat brain can be regulated by exogenous administration of sex hormones; testosterone increases CYP2D in the female rat brain and estrogen modestly increases CYP2D in the brain of ovariectomized female rats (Baum & Strobel, 1997; Bergh & Strobel, 1996). CYP2D-mediated drug metabolism is lower *in vivo* in the brain of female rats in diestrus compared to females in estrus and male rats (Arguelles et al., 2021; Arguelles, Richards, El-Sherbeni, Miksys, & Tyndale, 2022). Growth hormone induces CYP2D transcription *in vitro* in human neuron cultures and *in vivo* in mouse brain via regulation of peroxisome proliferator-activated receptor (PPAR) expression and binding to the CYP2D gene promotor region (Zhang et al., 2018).

3.2 Xenobiotics

3.2.1 Transcriptional regulation and induction

Xenobiotic exposure can increase or decrease *CYP* gene transcription through activation of transcription regulators; briefly, xenobiotics bind and activate intracellular receptors, which interact with other proteins to facilitate translocation to the nucleus, DNA binding, and initiation or repression of gene transcription (Honkakoski & Negishi, 2000). The aryl hydrocarbon receptor (AhR) is activated by toxins, such as methylcholanthrene, dioxin, and other polycyclic hydrocarbons, and its activation induces *CYP1A* gene transcription (Kapoor et al., 2006; Moscovitz et al., 2018; Terashima et al., 2018). In addition to the liver, AhR is highly expressed in the CNS, including in endothelial cells, neurons, and oligodendrocytes, and AhR activation induces CYP1A1 expression in the brain (Juricek & Coumoul, 2018).

The constitutive androstane receptor (CAR) and pregnane X receptor (PXR) are activated by xenobiotic ligands and can mediate the induction of CYP2B6, -2C8, -2C9, -2C19, and -3A4 (Klein & Zanger, 2013; Mikamo et al., 2003; Moscovitz et al., 2018; Zanger & Klein, 2013). CAR and PXR are activated by common drug inducers like rifampicin and phenobarbital, respectively (Zanger & Klein, 2013; Zanger & Schwab, 2013). CAR and PXR are highly expressed in the liver, although they are also present in the brain, where their activation can contribute to transcriptional regulation of *CYP2B*, *-2C*, and *-3A* (Gervot et al., 1999; Wang et al., 2019). Transcription induction by xenobiotics can substantially alter protein expression; for example, in African green monkeys, phenobarbital pretreatment increased CYP2B6 protein levels up to 150-fold in the frontal cortex (Lee, Miksys, et al., 2006).

PPARs comprise a family of ligand-activated transcriptional regulators that are mostly activated by endogenous compounds, but also by some drugs and environmental toxins (Honkakoski & Negishi, 2000). PPARs interact with the nuclear receptors retinoid X receptor (RXR), farsenoid X receptor (FXR), and hepatic nuclear factor 4 (HNF4), to regulate gene transcription in the liver and extrahepatic tissues (Hall, Quignodon, & Desvergne, 2008; Honkakoski & Negishi, 2000; Rakhshandehroo, Knoch, Muller, & Kersten, 2010). PPARs are expressed in the brain, in both neurons and glia (Hall et al., 2008; Warden et al., 2016). PPARs are implicated in regulating expression of brain CYPs with endogenous substrates, including CYP4A, -7A, and -8A (Honkakoski & Negishi, 2000; Rakhshandehroo et al., 2010). PPARs are also involved in transcriptional regulation of xenobiotic metabolizing CYPs in the brain, including CYP2C, -2D, and -2E (Cizkova, Konieczna, Erdosova, Lichnovska, & Ehrmann, 2012; Rakhshandehroo et al., 2010; Zhang et al., 2018).

3.2.2 Post-transcriptional induction

In contrast to transcriptional regulation, CYPs can be induced via post-transcriptional mechanisms, typically yielding higher CYP protein levels and catalytic activity regardless of changes in mRNA levels. Thus, some compounds induce CYP protein and catalytic activity in the absence of altered *CYP* gene expression. This could occur via several mechanisms, such as increased translational efficiency, protein stabilization, and reduced protein degradation (Tompkins & Wallace, 2007). Post-transcriptional induction can affect CYP2B, -2D, and -2E subfamily enzymes in the brain; nicotine and ethanol are commonly consumed inducers of these CYPs in the brain via these mechanisms (Miksys & Tyndale, 2004). While the exact mechanisms have not been identified for each inducer for each CYP, ethanol and nicotine have both been shown to alter expression of ubiquitination proteins, which could alter ubiquitin-mediated degradation of CYP proteins in the brain and/or periphery. The reduction of CYP2E1 ubiquitination in rat liver microsomes was implicated in ethanol-pretreatment-mediated CYP2E1 protein stabilization, and brain-specific changes in the expression of ubiquitination-related proteins in nicotine pretreated rats may contribute to a reduction in CYP2D degradation in the rat brain but not liver (Kane, Konu, Ma, & Li, 2004; Roberts, Song, Soh, Park, & Shoaf, 1995).

Induction of CYPs in the brain is, in some cases, also associated with CYP induction in the liver (Howard, Miksys, Hoffmann, Mash, & Tyndale, 2003; Yue, Khokhar, Miksys, & Tyndale, 2009). Daily nicotine pretreatments increase CYP2D and CYP2E1 protein, but not mRNA, in the rat brain; this is consistent with post-transcriptional induction (Howard et al., 2003; Yue et al., 2009). Of note, CYP2E1 is also induced in the liver, while CYP2D is not (Howard, Micu, Sellers, & Tyndale, 2001; Yue et al., 2008). Ethanol pretreatment also increases CYP2D and CYP2E1 protein in the rat brain, as well as inducing CYP2E1 in the rat liver (Upadhya, Tirumalai, Boyd, Mori, & Ravindranath, 2000; Warner & Gustafsson, 1994; Yue et al., 2009). CYP2B1 is induced by daily nicotine pretreatments in the rat brain and liver, although mRNA is also increased suggesting that transcriptional regulation may be involved (Miksys, Hoffmann, et al., 2000; Yue et al., 2009).

In African green monkeys, chronic nicotine administration and/or chronic ethanol intake increases CYP2B6, -2D, and -2E1 protein, but not mRNA, in the brain, consistent with post-transcriptional induction (Ferguson et al., 2013; Mann et al., 2008; Miller et al., 2014). In the liver, CYP2E1 is induced by both drugs, CYP2B6 is increased following chronic ethanol intake alone, and CYP2D is not affected; thus, CYP2D induction by nicotine and ethanol is brain-specific in African green monkeys (Ferguson, Miksys, Palmour, & Tyndale, 2011; Ferguson, Miksys, Palmour, & Tyndale, 2012; Miller et al., 2014). Interestingly, CYP2E1 is induced in the monkey brain, but not in the liver, by chronic phenobarbital pretreatments (Lee, Joshi, et al., 2006). Phenobarbital is a transcriptional inducer of other CYPs (i.e., CYP2C and CYP3A subfamily enzymes), and CYP2E1 is particularly susceptible to post-translational induction, suggesting that a non-transcriptional mechanism may mediate the phenobarbital-induced increase in brain CYP2E1 protein (Miksys & Tyndale, 2004; Ohno, Motojima, Okano, & Taniguchi, 2009).

Consistent with these data in rats and non-human primates, humans who smoked cigarettes or had alcohol use disorder had higher levels of CYP2B6, -2D6, and -2E1 protein in the brain post-mortem compared to controls (Howard et al., 2003; Mann et al., 2008; Miksys et al., 2003; Miksys et al., 2002). Moreover, smoking cigarettes and alcohol use disorder together have an additive effect on the association with higher protein levels of these CYPs in the human brain (Howard et al., 2003; Miksys et al., 2003; Miksys & Tyndale, 2004). While the mechanism of CYP2B6 induction in brain is somewhat unclear, alcohol use history was associated with increased CYP2B6 mRNA, protein, and catalytic activity in human liver microsomes, suggesting alcohol induces human hepatic CYP2B6 transcription (Hesse et al., 2004). Similarly, alcohol use history is associated with elevated human hepatic CYP2E1, consistent with CYP2E1 induction by alcohol; however, hepatic CYP2E1 can be induced with and without increased mRNA, consistent with multiple mechanisms of induction in the liver (Hukkanen, Jacob Iii, Peng, Dempsey, & Benowitz, 2010; Miksys & Tyndale, 2004; Tsutsumi, Lasker, Shimizu, Rosman, & Lieber, 1989). As in non-human primates, human CYP2D6 protein levels do not differ in the livers of humans who smoke cigarettes and/or have alcohol use disorder, compared to healthy controls, indicating that human CYP2D6 may be induced by both nicotine and alcohol via non-transcriptional mechanisms in the brain but not in the liver (Mann et al., 2008; S. Miksys et al., 2002).

3.2.3 Inhibition

Xenobiotics can interact directly with CYP enzymes to inhibit catalytic activity. Competitive inhibitors occupy the catalytic site of the enzyme and temporarily prevent substrate binding, which can cause drug-drug interactions (Bertz & Granneman, 1997; Fonne-Pfister & Meyer, 1988; Pelkonen et al., 2008). Some CYP substrates act as irreversible inhibitors (Bertz & Granneman, 1997; Zhou, Chan, Duan, Huang, & Chen, 2005). Among these are mechanism-based (also termed "suicide") inhibitors, which undergo CYP-mediated metabolism to a reactive intermediate that binds covalently to form a drug-enzyme complex; irreversible inhibition is long-lasting, due to inactivating the enzyme and requiring resynthesis of the enzyme for recovery of catalytic activity (Masubuchi, Narimatsu, Hosokawa, & Suzuki, 1994; Pelkonen et al., 2008; Sridar, Kenaan, & Hollenberg, 2012; Zhou et al., 2005). CYP inhibition by a systemically administered xenobiotic typically inhibits enzyme activity in all tissues reachable by the inhibitor and where the CYP is active; however, in some cases, an inhibitor may have organ-specific effects. For example, although propranolol is an irreversible inhibitor of human and rat CYP2D isoforms, propranolol acts as an irreversible inhibitor of CYP2D in the mouse liver and as a competitive inhibitor of CYP2D in the mouse brain (Masubuchi et al., 1994; Stocco et al., 2020; Tolledo et al., 2020). This could be due to the heterogeneous expression of mouse CYP2D isoforms between these two organs, with only the liver-expressed CYP2D isoforms being susceptible to irreversible inhibition by propranolol, leading to distinct forms of inhibition in the mouse brain versus liver (Tolledo et al., 2020).

4. Functional impact of brain CYP metabolism

4.1 Drugs

Response to centrally active drugs is often variable and does not always reflect circulating drug concentrations (Michels & Marzuk, 1993;

Sellers & Tyndale, 2000; Tauscher, Jones, Remington, Zipursky, & Kapur, 2002). This may be due, in part, to variable CYP-mediated drug metabolism in the brain yielding distinct drug and metabolite concentration profiles in the brain versus periphery. For example, CYP2B6 metabolizes the general anesthetic propofol (Court, Duan, Hesse, Venkatakrishnan, & Greenblatt, 2001). In rats, irreversible inhibition of CYP2B1 selectively in the brain increased central, but not peripheral, propofol concentrations, and this was associated with a prolonged sleep time, indicating enhanced drug effect (Khokhar & Tyndale, 2011). Conversely, inducing CYP2B1 selectively in the brain with daily nicotine pretreatments decreased brain propofol concentrations and reduced propofol-induced sleep duration (Khokhar, Miksys, & Tyndale, 2010; Khokhar & Tyndale, 2011). Thus, the sleep response in rats is dependent on brain propofol concentrations, which are impacted by central CYP2B1 activity (Khokhar & Tyndale, 2011). CYP2B6 variation in the human brain may similarly alter brain propofol concentrations and influence the depth of anesthetic response in clinical settings.

CYP2D metabolizes many opioids, including oxycodone, codeine, hydrocodone, and tramadol (Dayer, Desmeules, Leemann, & Striberni, 1988; Haufroid & Hantson, 2015; Lalovic, Phillips, Risler, Howald, & Shen, 2004). Selective manipulation of CYP2D in the rat brain *in vivo* alters drug and metabolite concentrations in the brain, as well as analgesic response following acute and repeated opioid administration (Li et al., 2015; McMillan, Miksys, & Tyndale, 2019; McMillan & Tyndale, 2015, 2017; Zhou et al., 2013). For example, rats with CYP2D inhibited in the brain have greater oxycodone-induced analgesia, which is associated with elevated brain, but not plasma, oxycodone concentrations (McMillan et al., 2019). In contrast, rats with brain CYP2D induced by daily nicotine pretreatments have lower brain, but not plasma, oxycodone concentrations and reduced oxycodone-induced analgesia (McMillan et al., 2019). Consistent with this, among humans undergoing post-operative treatment with oxycodone, those who smoked cigarettes required higher doses for effective pain management, consistent with potentially higher CYP2D6 in the brains of cigarette smokers metabolizing oxycodone more rapidly, reducing brain oxycodone concentrations and resulting analgesia (Kim et al., 2017; Mann et al., 2008).

In contrast with oxycodone, codeine requires CYP2D-mediated activation to morphine for its pharmacological effect (Dayer et al., 1988). Thus, inhibiting CYP2D in rat brain decreased acute codeine-induced analgesia, due to reduced CYP2D-mediated morphine production in the brain, and inducing CYP2D in the brain with daily nicotine pretreatments increased brain morphine concentrations and acute analgesia response (McMillan & Tyndale, 2015; Zhou et al., 2013). CYP2D in the rat brain also modulated the acquisition of analgesic tolerance to repeated codeine, which was associated with the impact of CYP2D in the brain on initial analgesia response; specifically, initial analgesic response was correlated with the rate of analgesic tolerance formation (McMillan & Tyndale, 2017). Thus, CYP2D induction in the rat brain increased acute codeine-induced analgesia, and this increase in acute analgesia was associated with a faster rate of tolerance to the analgesic effects upon subsequent daily codeine injections (McMillan & Tyndale, 2017). This indicates that CYP2D6 variation in the human brain may alter opioid response in acute clinical settings and during prolonged use.

Outcomes in psychiatric pharmacotherapy are highly variable, and therapeutic drug monitoring is often insufficient to predict treatment efficacy or the occurrence of adverse effects (Hiemke et al., 2018; Nierenberg et al., 2008; Volavka et al., 1992). Many drugs used in psychiatric medicine are metabolized by highly variable xenobiotic metabolizing CYPs, including CYP2C and CYP2D subfamily isoforms, which are expressed in the brain (Grasmader et al., 2004; Hiemke et al., 2018; Stingl et al., 2013). CYP2D6 contributes to the metabolism of many antipsychotic medications, including first- and second-generation drugs (Stingl et al., 2013). First-generation antipsychotics, such as haloperidol, produce extrapyramidal side effects, which can occur in both the acute and chronic treatment phases (Casey, 1991, 1994). CYP2D6-mediated haloperidol metabolism in the brain may influence the occurrence and severity of these acute and chronic extrapyramidal side effects. Inhibiting CYP2D in the rat brain increased CNS haloperidol concentrations and reduced acute haloperidol-induced catalepsy, while inducing CYP2D reduced brain haloperidol concentrations and exacerbated acute catalepsy response, which models acute extrapyramidal side effects (Castagne, Moser, & Porsolt, 2009; Miksys et al., 2017). Moreover, catalepsy response was positively correlated with CYP2D activity in the brain but not in the liver (Miksys et al., 2017). This suggests that brain CYP2D-mediated haloperidol metabolism contributes to acute catalepsy response, potentially through the production of a toxic catalepsy-causing metabolite in the brain. In a human CYP2D6-expressing transgenic mouse line, selective and irreversible inhibition of human CYP2D6 expressed in the transgenic mouse brain similarly reduced acute haloperidol-induced catalepsy, without changing peripheral haloperidol concentrations

(Tolledo et al., 2020). This provides further evidence for a role of CYP2D6 metabolism *in vivo* in the human brain enhancing risk of acute antipsychotic-induced extrapyramidal side effects.

In contrast, CYP2D metabolism in the brain is protective in animal models of chronic haloperidol-induced side effects. Irreversible inhibition of CYP2D in the rat brain increased CNS haloperidol concentrations and exacerbated chronic haloperidol-induced vacuous chewing motions, which model tardive dyskinesia, a debilitating side effect of first-generation antipsychotic treatment (Casey, 1991, 2000; Miksys et al., 2017). Conversely, using a different paradigm, chronic nicotine treatment reduced chronic haloperidol-induced vacuous chewing motions; this effect was not mediated via the nicotinic acetylcholine receptor, suggesting that this nicotine treatment may have induced CYP2D in the rat brain and decreased CNS haloperidol concentrations and vacuous chewing motions, although a specific role for CYP2D in the brain was not explored (Bordia, McIntosh, & Quik, 2012). Consistent with these data, cigarette smoking was associated with reduced chronic extrapyramidal side effects among humans undergoing chronic treatment with first-generation antipsychotics, despite historical antipsychotic dose being higher in smokers compared to non-smokers (Decina et al., 1990). Higher CYP2D6 in the human brain was associated with being a cigarette smoker versus non-smoker, and thus humans who smoke cigarettes would be expected to metabolize antipsychotics more rapidly within the brain (Mann et al., 2008). Having more CYP2D6 in the brain or liver may necessitate higher antipsychotic doses to attain sufficient CNS drug concentrations for therapeutic effect, while higher CYP2D6 in brain specifically may provide some protection against chronic extrapyramidal side effects.

In addition to clinically used drugs, xenobiotic metabolizing CYPs in the brain also metabolize drugs of abuse; thus, variation in brain CYP activity may meaningfully contribute to individual differences drug response, risk for addiction and relapse, and adverse outcomes of chronic use (Haufroid & Hantson, 2015; Sellers & Tyndale, 2000). In contrast to the liver where CYP2A6 is primarily responsible for nicotine metabolism, in the human brain, CYP2B6 may contribute more significantly to nicotine metabolism (Yamazaki, Inoue, Hashimoto, & Shimada, 1999). In rats, CYP2B1 in brain influences CNS nicotine concentrations and addiction-related behavioral responses; CYP2B1 induction in the brain reduces CNS nicotine concentrations, while inhibiting CYP2B1 in the brain increases CNS nicotine concentrations, both without affecting plasma drug concentrations

(Garcia, Coen, Miksys, Le, & Tyndale, 2015; Garcia, Le, & Tyndale, 2017). Inhibiting rat brain CYP2B1 also enhanced acquisition of nicotine self-administration at a lower dose, suggesting a leftward shift in nicotine abuse liability (Garcia et al., 2015). Moreover, rats with inhibited CYP2B1 in brain had higher breakpoints in a progressive ratio self-administration schedule, indicating greater motivation to acquire nicotine (Garcia et al., 2015). Consistent with this, in a smoking cessation trial, humans lacking CYP2B6, due to genetic polymorphisms, experienced more cravings and greater relapse rates while trying to remain abstinent (Lerman et al., 2002). Taken together, this suggests that CYP2B6 variation in the human brain may impact central nicotine metabolism, affecting psychological and behavioral aspects of nicotine addiction.

CYP2D6 metabolizes many psychostimulants, including catalyzing the p-hydroxylation of methamphetamine and amphetamine to p-hydroxymethamphetamine and p-hydroxyamphetamine, respectively (Law, Slawson, & Moody, 2000; Lin et al., 1997; Wu, Otton, Inaba, Kalow, & Sellers, 1997). Inhibiting CYP2D in rat brain increased brain methamphetamine concentrations, enhanced repeated methamphetamine-induced dopamine release in the dorsal striatum, and exacerbated both the acute behavioral response and repeated methamphetamine-induced behavioral sensitization (Stocco, El-Sherbeni, Zhao, Novalen, & Tyndale, 2021). This indicates that altered CYP2D in the brain can influence central and behavioral responses to acute and daily administration of psychostimulants like methamphetamine, independent of differences in hepatic metabolism and peripheral drug concentrations (Stocco et al., 2021). In humans, genetically poor (versus extensive) CYP2D6 metabolizers are more sensitive to changes in methamphetamine dose on subjective measures of methamphetamine-induced stimulation, euphoria, and good drug effect, despite there being no differences in peripheral methamphetamine concentrations (Sellers & Tyndale, 2000). This suggests that differences in brain CYP2D6 may influence CNS methamphetamine concentrations and resulting drug responses. Moreover, among humans who use methamphetamine, those who exhibit the highest nicotine dependence also use methamphetamine in larger amounts (Wang et al., 2014). This is consistent with higher CYP2D6 in the brains of cigarette smokers metabolizing methamphetamine more rapidly, decreasing methamphetamine concentrations in the brain, and in turn necessitating increased intake to achieve the desired central effects (Mann et al., 2008).

4.2 Neurotoxins

CYP1A1 contributes to the metabolism of various toxins and carcinogens, including polycyclic aromatic hydrocarbons, heterocyclic aromatic amines, and nitrosamines (Esteves, Rueff, & Kranendonk, 2021). CYP1A1 and related isoforms catalyze bioactivation of these compounds into reactive electrophilic intermediates, which form DNA adducts, leading to carcinogenesis (Esteves et al., 2021; Go, Hwang, & Choi, 2015). CYP1A-mediated production of reactive intermediates is implicated in the pathogenesis of cancers throughout the body, including in the liver, bladder, and brain (Go et al., 2015). In rodents administered polycyclic aromatic hydrocarbons, drug-DNA adducts were detected in the brain, colocalized in brain regions where CYP1A1 is expressed (Granberg et al., 2003). This suggests that CYP1A1 activity in the brain produces reactive intermediates, DNA adducts, and potentially eventually cancer. This is consistent with elevated levels of CYP1A1 in human brain glioma samples (Geng & Strobel, 1997; Go et al., 2015; Wahid, Mahjabeen, Baig, & Kayani, 2013). Thus, CYP1A1 variation in the brain may influence risk for environmental toxin-related brain cancers.

Similarly, CYP2E1 catalyzes the biotransformation of various toxic or carcinogenic compounds, including nitrosamines and alcohols (Esteves et al., 2021; Heit et al., 2013). CYP2E1-mediated metabolism generates reactive oxygen species, particularly superoxide and hydrogen peroxide (Garcia-Suastegui et al., 2017). CYP2E1 catalysis therefore exacerbates oxidative stress and can contribute to macromolecule adduct formation and damage, inflammation, and neurotoxicity in local tissues, including within the brain (Garcia-Suastegui et al., 2017; Gonzalez, 2005). Via these mechanisms, central CYP2E1-mediated alcohol metabolism is implicated in the hippocampal and cerebellar neurodegeneration typical of chronic alcohol use disorder (Garcia-Suastegui et al., 2017; Zhong et al., 2012). Therefore, variation in CYP2E1 in brain may influence risk for chronic xenobiotic exposure-induced oxidative stress and neurotoxicity (Novak & Woodcroft, 2000).

Chlorpyrifos is an organophosphate insecticide used broadly worldwide (Foong et al., 2020). Exposure can cause neurotoxicity, cognitive deficits, and other neurological effects (Steenland et al., 2000). Chlorpyrifos is a protoxin that is bioactivated by CYP2B6 to chlorpyrifos oxon (Tang et al., 2001). The chlorpyrifos oxon acts as an acetylcholinesterase inhibitor, causes cholinergic toxicity, and is primarily responsible for the neurotoxic effects of chlorpyrifos (Eyer et al., 2009; Kousba, Sultatos, Poet, & Timchalk, 2004). Inhibiting CYP2B1 in the rat brain reduced oxon production from chlorpyrifos in the brain but not in the periphery (Khokhar & Tyndale, 2012, 2014). The decrease in brain chlorpyrifos oxon concentrations was associated with reduced acetylcholinesterase inhibition in the brain (but not plasma) and less severe measures of behavioral neurotoxicity (Khokhar & Tyndale, 2012, 2014). This suggests that CYP2B6 variation in the human brain may influence susceptibility to chlorpyrifos oxon-induced neurotoxicity following exposure to chlorpyrifos.

Beta-carbolines are naturally occurring compounds that can be metabolically activated by *N*-methyltransferases to highly neurotoxic beta-carbolinium cations (Matsubara et al., 1993; Matsubara et al., 1998; Matsubara, Neafsey, & Collins, 1992). Elevated concentrations of these compounds are associated with Parkinson's disease and essential tremor, as well as with the severity of neurodegeneration in human patients (Kuhn, Muller, Grosse, & Rommelspacher, 1996; Louis et al., 2013; Louis, Zheng, Mao, & Shungu, 2007). CYP2C and CYP2D enzymes catalyze beta-carboline detoxification (Herraiz, Guillen, Aran, Idle, & Gonzalez, 2006; Yu, Idle, Krausz, Kupfer, & Gonzalez, 2003). Humanized CYP2D6-expressing transgenic mice metabolize beta-carbolines, such as harmine and harmaline, more rapidly compared to wild type mice and exhibit less severe beta-carboline-induced behavioral neurotoxicity, consistent with a protective effect of CYP2D6 metabolism (Cheng et al., 2013; Wu, Jiang, Shen, & Yu, 2009; Stocco et al., 2020; Yu et al., 2003). Consistent with this, genetic *CYP2D6* poor metabolizers have elevated risk for developing Parkinson's disease, and *CYP2C19* poor metabolizers have elevated risk for essential tremor (Alonso-Navarro et al., 2006; Anwarullah et al., 2017). Additionally, inhibiting human CYP2D6 expressed in the brain of humanized CYP2D6-expressing transgenic mice exacerbated measures of beta-carboline-induced behavioral neurotoxicity, consistent with a protective effect of CYP2D6 metabolism *in vivo* specifically within the brain (Fig. 2) (Stocco et al., 2020). Moreover, in humans, CYP2D6 protein was lower in the brains of individuals with Parkinson's disease compared to healthy controls, even when controlling for genotype (Mann et al., 2012). This suggests that CYP2C19 and CYP2D6 in the brain may confer protection against neurotoxicity and may reduce risk for neurodegenerative diseases.

The synthetic protoxin 1-methyl-4-phenyl-1,2,3,6-tetrahydropyridine (MPTP) also undergoes toxification to a potent neurotoxin, 1-methyl-4-phenylpyridinium (MPP^+), which induces parkinsonism through

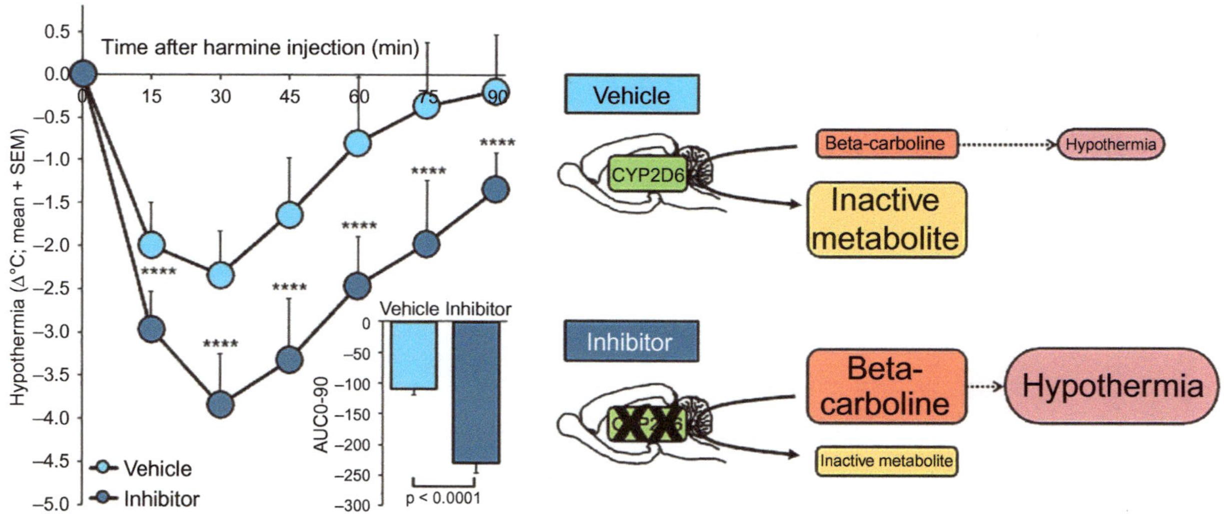

Fig. 2 Irreversible inhibition of human CYP2D6 expressed in the brain of humanized CYP2D6-expressing transgenic mice exacerbated hypothermia response induced by the peripheral administration of the beta-carboline harmine. Inhibiting the human CYP2D6, but not mouse CYP2D, expressed in the transgenic mouse brain may reduce central beta-carboline detoxification, increasing beta-carboline concentrations in the brain, and in turn enhancing centrally-mediated responses, including hypothermia. Data is graphed as mean and standard error of the mean (SEM). *Adapted from Stocco, M. R., Tolledo, C., Wadji, F. B., Gonzalez, F. J., Miksys, S., & Tyndale, R. F. (2020). Human CYP2D6 in the brain is protective against harmine-induced neurotoxicity: evidence from humanized CYP2D6 transgenic mice.* Molecular Neurobiology *doi:10.1007/s12035-020-02050-w.*

destruction of nigrostriatal dopamine neurons. CYP2D6 and CYP3A4 catalyze detoxification of MPTP (Coleman, Ellis, Martin, Lennard, & Tucker, 1996; Gilham et al., 1997; Mann & Tyndale, 2010; Modi et al., 1997). Inhibiting CYP2D6 or CYP3A4 *in vitro* in cultured neurons exacerbated MPP^{+}-induced toxicity (Mann & Tyndale, 2010). Inducing CYP2D in the mouse brain reduced striatal neurodegeneration *in vivo* in MPTP-treated mice (Singh et al., 2009). In humans, smoking cigarettes reduces risk for Parkinson's disease and essential tremor (Alves, Kurz, Lie, & Larsen, 2004; Benito-Leon, Louis, Bermejo-Pareja, & Neurological Disorders in Central Spain Study, 2008). Taken together, this suggests that the protective effect of smoking cigarettes may be due, at least in part, to the elevated CYP2D6 in the brains of smokers protecting against xenobiotic-induced neurotoxicity and eventual neurodegeneration underlying Parkinson's disease and essential tremor (Elbaz et al., 2004; Mann et al., 2008).

5. Conclusion

CYPs in the brain are a potentially important component of pharmacology, and insufficiently understood, particularly as it relates to centrally acting drugs and toxins. Xenobiotic metabolizing CYPs that are expressed in the brain, including CYP1A, -2B, -2C, -2D, -2E, and -3A subfamilies, are highly genetically variable, undergo various forms of regulation, and are sensitive to xenobiotic induction (Kuban & Daniel, 2021; Toselli et al., 2016; Zanger & Schwab, 2013). Moreover, many of these CYPs, particularly CYP2B, -2D, and -2E, are regulated to a greater extent in the brain versus the liver, or in a brain- versus liver-specific manner, suggesting that their activity may vary to a greater extent in the human brain than in the liver (Miksys & Tyndale, 2004). These CYPs have many substrates that are centrally active, including clinically used drugs, drugs of abuse, and neurotoxins (Britto & Wedlund, 1992; Dutheil et al., 2008). For many of these, dosage, exposure levels, and peripheral drug concentrations are poor predictors of drug response or central effects (Cherner et al., 2010; Eyer et al., 2009; Michels & Marzuk, 1993; Tauscher et al., 2002). The *in vivo* animal models described herein, including the humanized CYP2D6-expressing transgenic mice, have demonstrated that differences in CYPs within the brain, including human CYP2D6, can meaningfully alter central substrate and metabolite concentrations, and in turn influence central and behavioral responses. Thus, variation in CYPs in the human brain may alter central drug metabolism, thereby contributing to individual differences in drug response, therapeutic efficacy, and adverse effects, as well as neurotoxicity, neurodegeneration, and risk for neurodegenerative disease.

Acknowledgments

This work was undertaken, in part, thanks to funding from the Canada Research Chairs program (Dr. Tyndale, the Canada Research Chair in Pharmacogenomics), a Canadian Institutes of Health Research Foundation grant (FDN-154294), a R01 grant from the National Institutes of Health (DA043526), and the Centre for Addiction and Mental Health and the CAMH Foundation.

Conflict of interest

R.F.T has consulted for Quinn Emanuel and Ethismos Research Inc on unrelated topics. M.R.S has no conflicts to declare.

References

Allqvist, A., Miura, J., Bertilsson, L., & Mirghani, R. A. (2007). Inhibition of CYP3A4 and CYP3A5 catalyzed metabolism of alprazolam and quinine by ketoconazole as racemate and four different enantiomers. *European Journal of Clinical Pharmacology, 63*(2), 173–179. https://doi.org/10.1007/s00228-006-0230-z.

Alonso-Navarro, H., Martinez, C., Garcia-Martin, E., Benito-Leon, J., Garcia-Ferrer, I., Vazquez-Torres, P., et al. (2006). CYP2C19 polymorphism and risk for essential tremor. *European Neurology, 56*(2), 119–123. https://doi.org/10.1159/000095702.

Alves, G., Kurz, M., Lie, S. A., & Larsen, J. P. (2004). Cigarette smoking in Parkinson's disease: influence on disease progression. *Movement Disorders, 19*(9), 1087–1092. https://doi.org/10.1002/mds.20117.

Anwarullah, Aslam, M., Badshah, M., Abbasi, R., Sultan, A., Khan, K., et al. (2017). Further evidence for the association of CYP2D6*4 gene polymorphism with Parkinson's disease: a case control study. *Genes and Environment, 39*, 18. https://doi.org/10.1186/s41021-017-0078-8.

Anzenbacher, P., & Anzenbacherova, E. (2001). Cytochromes P450 and metabolism of xenobiotics. *Cellular and Molecular Life Sciences, 58*(5-6), 737–747. https://doi.org/10.1007/pl00000897.

Arguelles, N., Miksys, S., & Tyndale, R. F. (2021). Sex and Estrous Cycle Differences in Analgesia and Brain Oxycodone Levels. *Molecular Neurobiology, 58*(12), 6540–6551. https://doi.org/10.1007/s12035-021-02560-1.

Arguelles, N., Richards, J., El-Sherbeni, A. A., Miksys, S., & Tyndale, R. F. (2022). Sex, estrous cycle, and hormone regulation of CYP2D in the brain alters oxycodone metabolism and analgesia. *Biochemical Pharmacology, 198*, 114949. https://doi.org/10.1016/j.bcp.2022.114949.

Baum, L. O., & Strobel, H. W. (1997). Regulation of expression of cytochrome P-450 2D mRNA in rat brain with steroid hormones. *Brain Research, 765*(1), 67–73. https://doi.org/10.1016/s0006-8993(97)00428-9.

Benito-Leon, J., Louis, E. D., Bermejo-Pareja, F., & Neurological Disorders in Central Spain (NEDICES) Study Group. (2008). Population-based case-control study of cigarette smoking and essential tremor. *Movement Disorders, 23*(2), 246–252. https://doi.org/10.1002/mds.21810.

Bergh, A. F., & Strobel, H. W. (1996). Anatomical distribution of NADPH-cytochrome P450 reductase and cytochrome P4502D forms in rat brain: effects of xenobiotics and sex steroids. *Molecular and Cellular Biochemistry, 162*(1), 31–41. https://doi.org/10.1007/BF00250993.

Bertz, R. J., & Granneman, G. R. (1997). Use of in vitro and in vivo data to estimate the likelihood of metabolic pharmacokinetic interactions. *Clinical Pharmacokinetics, 32*(3), 210–258. https://doi.org/10.2165/00003088-199732030-00004.

Bhamre, S., Anandatheerathavarada, H. K., Shankar, S. K., Boyd, M. R., & Ravindranath, V. (1993). Purification of multiple forms of cytochrome P450 from a human brain and reconstitution of catalytic activities. *Archives of Biochemistry and Biophysics, 301*(2), 251–255. https://doi.org/10.1006/abbi.1993.1141.

Booth Depaz, I. M., Toselli, F., Wilce, P. A., & Gillam, E. M. (2015). Differential expression of cytochrome P450 enzymes from the CYP2C subfamily in the human brain. *Drug Metabolism and Disposition, 43*(3), 353–357. https://doi.org/10.1124/dmd.114.061242.

Bordia, T., McIntosh, J. M., & Quik, M. (2012). Nicotine reduces antipsychotic-induced orofacial dyskinesia in rats. *The Journal of Pharmacology and Experimental Therapeutics, 340*(3), 612–619. https://doi.org/10.1124/jpet.111.189100.

Britto, M. R., & Wedlund, P. J. (1992). Cytochrome P-450 in the brain. Potential evolutionary and therapeutic relevance of localization of drug-metabolizing enzymes. Drug Metabolism and Disposition, 20(3), 446-450. Retrieved from https://www.ncbi.nlm.nih.gov/pubmed/1355722.

Casey, D. E. (1991). Neuroleptic drug-induced extrapyramidal syndromes and tardive dyskinesia. *Schizophrenia Research, 4*(2), 109–120. https://doi.org/10.1016/0920-9964(91)90029-q.

Casey, D. E. (1994). Motor and mental aspects of acute extrapyramidal syndromes. *Acta Psychiatrica Scandinavica. Supplementum, 380*, 14–20. https://doi.org/10.1111/j.1600-0447.1994.tb05826.x.

Casey, D. E. (2000). Tardive dyskinesia: pathophysiology and animal models. *The Journal of Clinical Psychiatry, 61*(Suppl 4), 5–9. Retrieved from https://www.ncbi.nlm.nih.gov/pubmed/10739324.

Castagne, V., Moser, P. C., & Porsolt, R. D. (2009). Preclinical behavioral models for predicting antipsychotic activity. *Advances in Pharmacology, 57*, 381–418. https://doi.org/10.1016/S1054-3589(08)57010-4.

Cheng, J., Zhen, Y., Miksys, S., Beyoglu, D., Krausz, K. W., Tyndale, R. F., et al. (2013). Potential role of CYP2D6 in the central nervous system. *Xenobiotica, 43*(11), 973–984. https://doi.org/10.3109/00498254.2013.791410.

Cherner, M., Suarez, P., Casey, C., Deiss, R., Letendre, S., Marcotte, T., et al. (2010). Methamphetamine use parameters do not predict neuropsychological impairment in currently abstinent dependent adults. *Drug and Alcohol Dependence, 106*(2-3), 154–163. https://doi.org/10.1016/j.drugalcdep.2009.08.010.

Chinta, S. J., Kommaddi, R. P., Turman, C. M., Strobel, H. W., & Ravindranath, V. (2005). Constitutive expression and localization of cytochrome P-450 1A1 in rat and human brain: presence of a splice variant form in human brain. *Journal of Neurochemistry, 93*(3), 724–736. https://doi.org/10.1111/j.1471-4159.2005.03061.x.

Chinta, S. J., Pai, H. V., Upadhya, S. C., Boyd, M. R., & Ravindranath, V. (2002). Constitutive expression and localization of the major drug metabolizing enzyme, cytochrome P4502D in human brain. *Brain Research. Molecular Brain Research, 103*(1-2), 49–61. https://doi.org/10.1016/s0169-328x(02)00177-8.

Choudhary, D., Jansson, I., Stoilov, I., Sarfarazi, M., & Schenkman, J. B. (2005). Expression patterns of mouse and human CYP orthologs (families 1-4) during development and in different adult tissues. *Archives of Biochemistry and Biophysics, 436*(1), 50–61. https://doi.org/10.1016/j.abb.2005.02.001.

Chung-Davidson, Y. W., Rees, C. B., Wu, H., Yun, S. S., & Li, W. (2004). beta-naphthoflavone induction of CYP1A in brain of juvenile lake trout (Salvelinus namaycush Walbaum). *The Journal of Experimental Biology*, *207*(Pt 9), 1533–1542. https://doi.org/10.1242/jeb.00919.

Cizkova, K., Konieczna, A., Erdosova, B., Lichnovska, R., & Ehrmann, J. (2012). Peroxisome proliferator-activated receptors in regulation of cytochromes P450: new way to overcome multidrug resistance? *Journal of Biomedicine & Biotechnology*, *2012*, 656428. https://doi.org/10.1155/2012/656428.

Coleman, T., Ellis, S. W., Martin, I. J., Lennard, M. S., & Tucker, G. T. (1996). 1-Methyl-4-phenyl-1,2,3,6-tetrahydropyridine (MPTP) is N-demethylated by cytochromes P450 2D6, 1A2 and 3A4- -implications for susceptibility to Parkinson's disease. *The Journal of Pharmacology and Experimental Therapeutics*, *277*(2), 685–690. Retrieved from https://www.ncbi.nlm.nih.gov/pubmed/8627546.

Court, M. H., Duan, S. X., Hesse, L. M., Venkatakrishnan, K., & Greenblatt, D. J. (2001). Cytochrome P-450 2B6 is responsible for interindividual variability of propofol hydroxylation by human liver microsomes. *Anesthesiology*, *94*(1), 110–119. https://doi.org/10.1097/00000542-200101000-00021.

Dayer, P., Desmeules, J., Leemann, T., & Striberni, R. (1988). Bioactivation of the narcotic drug codeine in human liver is mediated by the polymorphic monooxygenase catalyzing debrisoquine 4-hydroxylation (cytochrome P-450 dbl/bufl). *Biochemical and Biophysical Research Communications*, *152*(1), 411–416. https://doi.org/10.1016/s0006-291x(88)80729-0.

Decina, P., Caracci, G., Sandik, R., Berman, W., Mukherjee, S., & Scapicchio, P. (1990). Cigarette smoking and neuroleptic-induced parkinsonism. *Biological Psychiatry*, *28*(6), 502–508. https://doi.org/10.1016/0006-3223(90)90483-i.

Dhir, R. N., Dworakowski, W., Thangavel, C., & Shapiro, B. H. (2006). Sexually dimorphic regulation of hepatic isoforms of human cytochrome p450 by growth hormone. *The Journal of Pharmacology and Experimental Therapeutics*, *316*(1), 87–94. https://doi.org/10.1124/jpet.105.093773.

Ding, X., & Kaminsky, L. S. (2003). Human extrahepatic cytochromes P450: function in xenobiotic metabolism and tissue-selective chemical toxicity in the respiratory and gastrointestinal tracts. *Annual Review of Pharmacology and Toxicology*, *43*, 149–173. https://doi.org/10.1146/annurev.pharmtox.43.100901.140251.

Dutheil, F., Beaune, P., & Loriot, M. A. (2008). Xenobiotic metabolizing enzymes in the central nervous syste contribution of cytochrome P450 enzymes in normal and pathological human brain. *Biochimie*, *90*(3), 426–436. https://doi.org/10.1016/j.biochi.2007.10.007.

Elbaz, A., Levecque, C., Clavel, J., Vidal, J. S., Richard, F., Amouyel, P., et al. (2004). CYP2D6 polymorphism, pesticide exposure, and Parkinson's disease. *Annals of Neurology*, *55*(3), 430–434. https://doi.org/10.1002/ana.20051.

Esteves, F., Rueff, J., & Kranendonk, M. (2021). The Central Role of Cytochrome P450 in Xenobiotic Metabolism-A Brief Review on a Fascinating Enzyme Family. *Journal of Xenobiotics*, *11*(3), 94–114. https://doi.org/10.3390/jox11030007.

Eyer, F., Roberts, D. M., Buckley, N. A., Eddleston, M., Thiermann, H., Worek, F., et al. (2009). Extreme variability in the formation of chlorpyrifos oxon (CPO) in patients poisoned by chlorpyrifos (CPF). *Biochemical Pharmacology*, *78*(5), 531–537. https://doi.org/10.1016/j.bcp.2009.05.004.

Farin, F. M., & Omiecinski, C. J. (1993). Regiospecific expression of cytochrome P-450s and microsomal epoxide hydrolase in human brain tissue. *Journal of Toxicology and Environmental Health*, *40*(2-3), 317–335. https://doi.org/10.1080/15287399309531797.

Ferguson, C. S., Miksys, S., Palmour, R., & Tyndale, R. F. (2011). Independent and combined effects of ethanol self-administration and nicotine treatment on hepatic CYP2E1 in African green monkeys. *Drug Metabolism and Disposition, 39*(12), 2233–2241. https://doi.org/10.1124/dmd.111.040378.

Ferguson, C. S., Miksys, S., Palmour, R. M., & Tyndale, R. F. (2012). Differential effects of nicotine treatment and ethanol self-administration on CYP2A6, CYP2B6 and nicotine pharmacokinetics in African green monkeys. *The Journal of Pharmacology and Experimental Therapeutics, 343*(3), 628–637. https://doi.org/10.1124/jpet.112.198564.

Ferguson, C. S., Miksys, S., Palmour, R. M., & Tyndale, R. F. (2013). Ethanol self-administration and nicotine treatment induce brain levels of CYP2B6 and CYP2E1 in African green monkeys. *Neuropharmacology, 72*, 74–81. https://doi.org/10.1016/j.neuropharm.2013.04.022.

Fonne-Pfister, R., & Meyer, U. A. (1988). Xenobiotic and endobiotic inhibitors of cytochrome P-450dbl function, the target of the debrisoquine/sparteine type polymorphism. *Biochemical Pharmacology, 37*(20), 3829–3835. https://doi.org/10.1016/0006-2952(88)90063-9.

Foong, S. Y., Ma, N. L., Lam, S. S., Peng, W., Low, F., Lee, B. H. K., et al. (2020). A recent global review of hazardous chlorpyrifos pesticide in fruit and vegetables: Prevalence, remediation and actions needed. *Journal of Hazardous Materials, 400*, 123006. https://doi.org/10.1016/j.jhazmat.2020.123006.

Funae, Y., Kishimoto, W., Cho, T., Niwa, T., & Hiroi, T. (2003). CYP2D in the brain. *Drug Metabolism and Pharmacokinetics, 18*(6), 337–349. https://doi.org/10.2133/dmpk.18.337.

Garcia, K. L., Coen, K., Miksys, S., Le, A. D., & Tyndale, R. F. (2015). Effect of Brain CYP2B Inhibition on Brain Nicotine Levels and Nicotine Self-Administration. *Neuropsychopharmacology, 40*(8), 1910–1918. https://doi.org/10.1038/npp.2015.40.

Garcia, K. L. P., Le, A. D., & Tyndale, R. F. (2017). Brain CYP2B induction can decrease nicotine levels in the brain. *Addiction Biology, 22*(5), 1257–1266. https://doi.org/10.1111/adb.12411.

Garcia-Suastegui, W. A., Ramos-Chavez, L. A., Rubio-Osornio, M., Calvillo-Velasco, M., Atzin-Mendez, J. A., Guevara, J., et al. (2017). The Role of CYP2E1 in the Drug Metabolism or Bioactivation in the Brain. *Oxidative Medicine and Cellular Longevity, 2017*, 4680732. https://doi.org/10.1155/2017/4680732.

Geng, J., & Strobel, H. W. (1997). Expression and induction of cytochrome P-450 1A1 and P-450 2D subfamily in the rat glioma C6 cell line. *Brain Research, 774*(1-2), 11–19. https://doi.org/10.1016/s0006-8993(97)81681-2.

Gervot, L., Rochat, B., Gautier, J. C., Bohnenstengel, F., Kroemer, H., de Berardinis, V., et al. (1999). Human CYP2B6: expression, inducibility and catalytic activities. *Pharmacogenetics, 9*(3), 295–306. Retrieved from https://www.ncbi.nlm.nih.gov/pubmed/10471061.

Ghersi-Egea, J. F., Perrin, R., Leininger-Muller, B., Grassiot, M. C., Jeandel, C., Floquet, J., et al. (1993). Subcellular localization of cytochrome P450, and activities of several enzymes responsible for drug metabolism in the human brain. *Biochemical Pharmacology, 45*(3), 647–658. https://doi.org/10.1016/0006-2952(93)90139-n.

Ghosh, C., Hossain, M., Solanki, J., Dadas, A., Marchi, N., & Janigro, D. (2016). Pathophysiological implications of neurovascular P450 in brain disorders. *Drug Discovery Today, 21*(10), 1609–1619. https://doi.org/10.1016/j.drudis.2016.06.004.

Gilham, D. E., Cairns, W., Paine, M. J., Modi, S., Poulsom, R., Roberts, G. C., et al. (1997). Metabolism of MPTP by cytochrome P4502D6 and the demonstration of 2D6 mRNA in human foetal and adult brain by in situ hybridization. *Xenobiotica, 27*(1), 111–125. https://doi.org/10.1080/004982597240802.

Go, R. E., Hwang, K. A., & Choi, K. C. (2015). Cytochrome P450 1 family and cancers. *The Journal of Steroid Biochemistry and Molecular Biology, 147*, 24–30. https://doi.org/10.1016/j.jsbmb.2014.11.003.

Gonzalez, F. J. (2005). Role of cytochromes P450 in chemical toxicity and oxidative stress: studies with CYP2E1. *Mutation Research*, *569*(1-2), 101–110. https://doi.org/10.1016/j.mrfmmm.2004.04.021.

Granberg, L., Ostergren, A., Brandt, I., & Brittebo, E. B. (2003). CYP1A1 and CYP1B1 in blood-brain interfaces: CYP1A1-dependent bioactivation of 7,12-dimethylbenz(a)anthracene in endothelial cells. *Drug Metabolism and Disposition*, *31*(3), 259–265. https://doi.org/10.1124/dmd.31.3.259.

Grasmader, K., Verwohlt, P. L., Rietschel, M., Dragicevic, A., Muller, M., Hiemke, C., et al. (2004). Impact of polymorphisms of cytochrome-P450 isoenzymes 2C9, 2C19 and 2D6 on plasma concentrations and clinical effects of antidepressants in a naturalistic clinical setting. *European Journal of Clinical Pharmacology*, *60*(5), 329–336. https://doi.org/10.1007/s00228-004-0766-8.

Ha, H. R., Chen, J., Krahenbuhl, S., & Follath, F. (1996). Biotransformation of caffeine by cDNA-expressed human cytochromes P-450. *European Journal of Clinical Pharmacology*, *49*(4), 309–315. https://doi.org/10.1007/BF00226333.

Haduch, A., & Daniel, W. A. (2018). The engagement of brain cytochrome P450 in the metabolism of endogenous neuroactive substrates: a possible role in mental disorders. *Drug Metabolism Reviews*, *50*(4), 415–429. https://doi.org/10.1080/03602532.2018.1554674.

Haduch, A., Rysz, M., Papp, M., & Daniel, W. A. (2018). The activity of brain and liver cytochrome P450 2D (CYP2D) is differently affected by antidepressants in the chronic mild stress (CMS) model of depression in the rat. *Biochemical Pharmacology*, *156*, 398–405. https://doi.org/10.1016/j.bcp.2018.09.005.

Hall, M. G., Quignodon, L., & Desvergne, B. (2008). Peroxisome Proliferator-Activated Receptor beta/delta in the Brain: Facts and Hypothesis. *PPAR Research*, *2008*, 780452. https://doi.org/10.1155/2008/780452.

Haufroid, V., & Hantson, P. (2015). CYP2D6 genetic polymorphisms and their relevance for poisoning due to amfetamines, opioid analgesics and antidepressants. *Clinical Toxicology (Philadelphia, Pa.)*, *53*(6), 501–510. https://doi.org/10.3109/15563650.2015.1049355.

Hedlund, E., Gustafsson, J. A., & Warner, M. (2001). Cytochrome P450 in the brain; a review. *Current Drug Metabolism*, *2*(3), 245–263. https://doi.org/10.2174/1389200013338513.

Hedlund, E., Wyss, A., Kainu, T., Backlund, M., Kohler, C., Pelto-Huikko, M., et al. (1996). Cytochrome P4502D4 in the brain: specific neuronal regulation by clozapine and toluene. *Molecular Pharmacology*, *50*(2), 342–350. Retrieved from https://www.ncbi.nlm.nih.gov/pubmed/8700142.

Heit, C., Dong, H., Chen, Y., Thompson, D. C., Deitrich, R. A., & Vasiliou, V. K. (2013). The role of CYP2E1 in alcohol metabolism and sensitivity in the central nervous system. *Sub-Cellular Biochemistry*, *67*, 235–247. https://doi.org/10.1007/978-94-007-5881-0_8.

Herraiz, T., Guillen, H., Aran, V. J., Idle, J. R., & Gonzalez, F. J. (2006). Comparative aromatic hydroxylation and N-demethylation of MPTP neurotoxin and its analogs, N-methylated beta-carboline and isoquinoline alkaloids, by human cytochrome P450 2D6. *Toxicology and Applied Pharmacology*, *216*(3), 387–398. https://doi.org/10.1016/j.taap.2006.06.003.

Hesse, L. M., He, P., Krishnaswamy, S., Hao, Q., Hogan, K., von Moltke, L. L., et al. (2004). Pharmacogenetic determinants of interindividual variability in bupropion hydroxylation by cytochrome P450 2B6 in human liver microsomes. *Pharmacogenetics*, *14*(4), 225–238. https://doi.org/10.1097/00008571-200404000-00002.

Hiemke, C., Bergemann, N., Clement, H. W., Conca, A., Deckert, J., Domschke, K., et al. (2018). Consensus Guidelines for Therapeutic Drug Monitoring in Neuropsychopharmacology: Update 2017. *Pharmacopsychiatry*, *51*(1-02), e1. https://doi.org/10.1055/s-0037-1600991.

Hiroi, T., Imaoka, S., Chow, T., & Funae, Y. (1998). Tissue distributions of CYP2D1, 2D2, 2D3 and 2D4 mRNA in rats detected by RT-PCR. *Biochimica et Biophysica Acta*, *1380*(3), 305–312. https://doi.org/10.1016/s0304-4165(97)00157-8.

Honkakoski, P., & Negishi, M. (2000). Regulation of cytochrome P450 (CYP) genes by nuclear receptors. *The Biochemical Journal*, *347*(Pt 2), 321–337. https://doi.org/10.1042/0264-6021:3470321.

Howard, L. A., Micu, A. L., Sellers, E. M., & Tyndale, R. F. (2001). Low doses of nicotine and ethanol induce CYP2E1 and chlorzoxazone metabolism in rat liver. *The Journal of Pharmacology and Experimental Therapeutics*, *299*(2), 542–550. Retrieved from https://www.ncbi.nlm.nih.gov/pubmed/11602665.

Howard, L. A., Miksys, S., Hoffmann, E., Mash, D., & Tyndale, R. F. (2003). Brain CYP2E1 is induced by nicotine and ethanol in rat and is higher in smokers and alcoholics. *British Journal of Pharmacology*, *138*(7), 1376–1386. https://doi.org/10.1038/sj.bjp.0705146.

Hukkanen, J., Jacob Iii, P., Peng, M., Dempsey, D., & Benowitz, N. L. (2010). Effects of nicotine on cytochrome P450 2A6 and 2E1 activities. *British Journal of Clinical Pharmacology*, *69*(2), 152–159. https://doi.org/10.1111/j.1365-2125.2009.03568.x.

Ingelman-Sundberg, M. (1999). Duplication, multiduplication, and amplification of genes encoding drug-metabolizing enzymes: evolutionary, toxicological, and clinical pharmacological aspects. *Drug Metabolism Reviews*, *31*(2), 449–459. https://doi.org/10.1081/dmr-100101930.

Ingelman-Sundberg, M. (2004). Pharmacogenetics of cytochrome P450 and its applications in drug therapy: the past, present and future. *Trends in Pharmacological Sciences*, *25*(4), 193–200. https://doi.org/10.1016/j.tips.2004.02.007.

Ingelman-Sundberg, M., Oscarson, M., & McLellan, R. A. (1999). Polymorphic human cytochrome P450 enzymes: an opportunity for individualized drug treatment. *Trends in Pharmacological Sciences*, *20*(8), 342–349. https://doi.org/10.1016/s0165-6147(99)01363-2.

Ingelman-Sundberg, M., Sim, S. C., Gomez, A., & Rodriguez-Antona, C. (2007). Influence of cytochrome P450 polymorphisms on drug therapies: pharmacogenetic, pharmacoepigenetic and clinical aspects. *Pharmacology & Therapeutics*, *116*(3), 496–526. https://doi.org/10.1016/j.pharmthera.2007.09.004.

Juricek, L., & Coumoul, X. (2018). The Aryl Hydrocarbon Receptor and the Nervous System. *International Journal of Molecular Sciences*, *19*(9). https://doi.org/10.3390/ijms19092504.

Kane, J. K., Konu, O., Ma, J. Z., & Li, M. D. (2004). Nicotine coregulates multiple pathways involved in protein modification/degradation in rat brain. *Brain Research. Molecular Brain Research*, *132*(2), 181–191. https://doi.org/10.1016/j.molbrainres.2004.09.010.

Kapoor, N., Pant, A. B., Dhawan, A., Dwievedi, U. N., Seth, P. K., & Parmar, D. (2006). Cytochrome P450 1A isoenzymes in brain cells: Expression and inducibility in cultured rat brain neuronal and glial cells. *Life Sciences*, *79*(25), 2387–2394. https://doi.org/10.1016/j.lfs.2006.08.002.

Khokhar, J. Y., Miksys, S. L., & Tyndale, R. F. (2010). Rat brain CYP2B induction by nicotine is persistent and does not involve nicotinic acetylcholine receptors. *Brain Research*, *1348*, 1–9. https://doi.org/10.1016/j.brainres.2010.06.035.

Khokhar, J. Y., & Tyndale, R. F. (2011). Drug metabolism within the brain changes drug response: selective manipulation of brain CYP2B alters propofol effects. *Neuropsychopharmacology*, *36*(3), 692–700. https://doi.org/10.1038/npp.2010.202.

Khokhar, J. Y., & Tyndale, R. F. (2012). Rat brain CYP2B-enzymatic activation of chlorpyrifos to the oxon mediates cholinergic neurotoxicity. *Toxicological Sciences*, *126*(2), 325–335. https://doi.org/10.1093/toxsci/kfs029.

Khokhar, J. Y., & Tyndale, R. F. (2014). Intracerebroventricularly and systemically delivered inhibitor of brain CYP2B (C8-Xanthate), even following chlorpyrifos exposure, reduces chlorpyrifos activation and toxicity in male rats. *Toxicological Sciences*, *140*(1), 49–60. https://doi.org/10.1093/toxsci/kfu075.

Kim, D. H., Park, J. Y., Karm, M. H., Bae, H. Y., Lee, J. Y., Soo Ahn, H., et al. (2017). Smoking may increase postoperative opioid consumption in patients who underwent distal gastrectomy with gastroduodenostomy for early stomach cancer: a retrospective analysis. *The Clinical Journal of Pain*, *33*(10), 905–911. https://doi.org/10.1097/AJP.0000000000000472.

Klein, K., & Zanger, U. M. (2013). Pharmacogenomics of Cytochrome P450 3A4: Recent Progress Toward the "Missing Heritability" Problem. *Frontiers in Genetics*, *4*, 12. https://doi.org/10.3389/fgene.2013.00012.

Komori, M. (1993). A novel P450 expressed at the high level in rat brain. *Biochemical and Biophysical Research Communications*, *196*(2), 721–728. https://doi.org/10.1006/bbrc.1993.2309.

Kousba, A. A., Sultatos, L. G., Poet, T. S., & Timchalk, C. (2004). Comparison of chlorpyrifos-oxon and paraoxon acetylcholinesterase inhibition dynamics: potential role of a peripheral binding site. *Toxicological Sciences*, *80*(2), 239–248. https://doi.org/10.1093/toxsci/kfh163.

Kuban, W., & Daniel, W. A. (2021). Cytochrome P450 expression and regulation in the brain. *Drug Metabolism Reviews*, *53*(1), 1–29. https://doi.org/10.1080/03602532.2020.1858856.

Kuhn, W., Muller, T., Grosse, H., & Rommelspacher, H. (1996). Elevated levels of harman and norharman in cerebrospinal fluid of parkinsonian patients. *Journal of Neural Transmission (Vienna)*, *103*(12), 1435–1440. https://doi.org/10.1007/BF01271257.

Lalovic, B., Phillips, B., Risler, L. L., Howald, W., & Shen, D. D. (2004). Quantitative contribution of CYP2D6 and CYP3A to oxycodone metabolism in human liver and intestinal microsomes. *Drug Metabolism and Disposition*, *32*(4), 447–454. https://doi.org/10.1124/dmd.32.4.447.

Law, M. Y., Slawson, M. H., & Moody, D. E. (2000). Selective involvement of cytochrome P450 2D subfamily in in vivo 4-hydroxylation of amphetamine in rat. *Drug Metabolism and Disposition*, *28*(3), 348–353. Retrieved from https://www.ncbi.nlm.nih.gov/pubmed/10681381.

Lee, A. M., Joshi, M., Yue, J., & Tyndale, R. F. (2006). Phenobarbital induces monkey brain CYP2E1 protein but not hepatic CYP2E1, in vitro or in vivo chlorzoxazone metabolism. *European Journal of Pharmacology*, *552*(1-3), 151–158. https://doi.org/10.1016/j.ejphar.2006.09.006.

Lee, A. M., Miksys, S., & Tyndale, R. F. (2006). Phenobarbital increases monkey in vivo nicotine disposition and induces liver and brain CYP2B6 protein. *British Journal of Pharmacology*, *148*(6), 786–794. https://doi.org/10.1038/sj.bjp.0706787.

Lerman, C., Shields, P. G., Wileyto, E. P., Audrain, J., Pinto, A., Hawk, L., et al. (2002). Pharmacogenetic investigation of smoking cessation treatment. *Pharmacogenetics*, *12*(8), 627–634. https://doi.org/10.1097/00008571-200211000-00007.

Li, J., Xie, M., Wang, X., Ouyang, X., Wan, Y., Dong, G., et al. (2015). Sex hormones regulate cerebral drug metabolism via brain miRNAs: down-regulation of brain CYP2D by androgens reduces the analgesic effects of tramadol. *British Journal of Pharmacology*, *172*(19), 4639–4654. https://doi.org/10.1111/bph.13206.

Lin, L. Y., Di Stefano, E. W., Schmitz, D. A., Hsu, L., Ellis, S. W., Lennard, M. S., et al. (1997). Oxidation of methamphetamine and methylenedioxymethamphetamine by CYP2D6. *Drug Metabolism and Disposition*, *25*(9), 1059–1064. Retrieved from https://www.ncbi.nlm.nih.gov/pubmed/9311621.

Liu, Z. Q., Shu, Y., Huang, S. L., Wang, L. S., He, N., & Zhou, H. H. (2001). Effects of CYP2C19 genotype and CYP2C9 on fluoxetine N-demethylation in human liver microsomes. *Acta Pharmacologica Sinica*, *22*(1), 85–90. Retrieved from https://www.ncbi.nlm.nih.gov/pubmed/11730569.

Louis, E. D., Factor-Litvak, P., Liu, X., Vonsattel, J. P., Galecki, M., Jiang, W., et al. (2013). Elevated brain harmane (1-methyl-9H-pyrido[3,4-b]indole) in essential tremor cases vs. controls. *Neurotoxicology*, *38*, 131–135. https://doi.org/10.1016/j.neuro.2013.07.002.

Louis, E. D., Zheng, W., Mao, X., & Shungu, D. C. (2007). Blood harmane is correlated with cerebellar metabolism in essential tremor: a pilot study. *Neurology*, *69*(6), 515–520. https://doi.org/10.1212/01.wnl.0000266663.27398.9f.

Mann, A., Miksys, S. L., Gaedigk, A., Kish, S. J., Mash, D. C., & Tyndale, R. F. (2012). The neuroprotective enzyme CYP2D6 increases in the brain with age and is lower in Parkinson's disease patients. *Neurobiology of Aging*, *33*(9), 2160–2171. https://doi.org/10.1016/j.neurobiolaging.2011.08.014.

Mann, A., Miksys, S., Lee, A., Mash, D. C., & Tyndale, R. F. (2008). Induction of the drug metabolizing enzyme CYP2D in monkey brain by chronic nicotine treatment. *Neuropharmacology*, *55*(7), 1147–1155. https://doi.org/10.1016/j.neuropharm.2008.07.017.

Mann, A., & Tyndale, R. F. (2010). Cytochrome P450 2D6 enzyme neuroprotects against 1-methyl-4-phenylpyridinium toxicity in SH-SY5Y neuronal cells. *The European Journal of Neuroscience*, *31*(7), 1185–1193. https://doi.org/10.1111/j.1460-9568.2010.07142.x.

Martignoni, M., Groothuis, G. M., & de Kanter, R. (2006). Species differences between mouse, rat, dog, monkey and human CYP-mediated drug metabolism, inhibition and induction. *Expert Opinion on Drug Metabolism & Toxicology*, *2*(6), 875–894. https://doi.org/10.1517/17425255.2.6.875.

Masubuchi, Y., Narimatsu, S., Hosokawa, S., & Suzuki, T. (1994). Role of the CYP2D subfamily in metabolism-dependent covalent binding of propranolol to liver microsomal protein in rats. *Biochemical Pharmacology*, *48*(10), 1891–1898. https://doi.org/10.1016/0006-2952(94)90587-8.

Matsubara, K., Collins, M. A., Akane, A., Ikebuchi, J., Neafsey, E. J., Kagawa, M., et al. (1993). Potential bioactivated neurotoxicants, N-methylated beta-carbolinium ions, are present in human brain. *Brain Research*, *610*(1), 90–96. https://doi.org/10.1016/0006-8993(93)91221-d.

Matsubara, K., Gonda, T., Sawada, H., Uezono, T., Kobayashi, Y., Kawamura, T., et al. (1998). Endogenously occurring beta-carboline induces parkinsonism in nonprimate animals: a possible causative protoxin in idiopathic Parkinson's disease. *Journal of Neurochemistry*, *70*(2), 727–735. https://doi.org/10.1046/j.1471-4159.1998.70020727.x.

Matsubara, K., Neafsey, E. J., & Collins, M. A. (1992). Novel S-adenosylmethionine-dependent indole-N-methylation of beta-carbolines in brain particulate fractions. *Journal of Neurochemistry*, *59*(2), 511–518. https://doi.org/10.1111/j.1471-4159.1992.tb09400.x.

McFadyen, M. C. E., Melvin, W. T., & Murray, G. I. (1998). Regional distribution of individual forms of cytochrome P450 mRNA in normal adult human brain. *Biochemical Pharmacology*, *55*(6), 825–830. https://doi.org/10.1016/s0006-2952(97)00516-9.

McMillan, D. M., El-Sherbeni, A. A., Richards, J., & Tyndale, R. F. (2020). Centrally administered CYP2D inhibitors increase oral tramadol analgesia in rats. *Brain Research Bulletin*, *164*, 400–406. https://doi.org/10.1016/j.brainresbull.2020.09.001.

McMillan, D. M., Miksys, S., & Tyndale, R. F. (2019). Rat brain CYP2D activity alters in vivo central oxycodone metabolism, levels and resulting analgesia. *Addiction Biology*, *24*(2), 228–238. https://doi.org/10.1111/adb.12590.

McMillan, D. M., & Tyndale, R. F. (2015). Nicotine increases codeine analgesia through the induction of brain CYP2D and central activation of codeine to morphine. *Neuropsychopharmacology*, *40*(7), 1804–1812. https://doi.org/10.1038/npp.2015.32.

McMillan, D. M., & Tyndale, R. F. (2017). Inducing rat brain CYP2D with nicotine increases the rate of codeine tolerance; predicting the rate of tolerance from acute analgesic response. *Biochemical Pharmacology*, *145*, 158–168. https://doi.org/10.1016/j.bcp.2017.08.015.

Michels, R., & Marzuk, P. M. (1993). Progress in psychiatry (1). *The New England Journal of Medicine*, *329*(8), 552–560. https://doi.org/10.1056/NEJM199308193290808.

Mikamo, E., Harada, S., Nishikawa, J., & Nishihara, T. (2003). Endocrine disruptors induce cytochrome P450 by affecting transcriptional regulation via pregnane X receptor. *Toxicology and Applied Pharmacology*, *193*(1), 66–72. https://doi.org/10.1016/j.taap.2003.08.001.

Miksys, S. L., Cheung, C., Gonzalez, F. J., & Tyndale, R. F. (2005). Human CYP2D6 and mouse CYP2Ds: organ distribution in a humanized mouse model. *Drug Metabolism and Disposition*, *33*(10), 1495–1502. https://doi.org/10.1124/dmd.105.005488.

Miksys, S., Hoffmann, E., & Tyndale, R. F. (2000). Regional and cellular induction of nicotine-metabolizing CYP2B1 in rat brain by chronic nicotine treatment. *Biochemical Pharmacology*, *59*(12), 1501–1511. https://doi.org/10.1016/s0006-2952(00)00281-1.

Miksys, S., Lerman, C., Shields, P. G., Mash, D. C., & Tyndale, R. F. (2003). Smoking, alcoholism and genetic polymorphisms alter CYP2B6 levels in human brain. *Neuropharmacology*, *45*(1), 122–132. https://doi.org/10.1016/s0028-3908(03)00136-9.

Miksys, S., Rao, Y., Hoffmann, E., Mash, D. C., & Tyndale, R. F. (2002). Regional and cellular expression of CYP2D6 in human brain: higher levels in alcoholics. *Journal of Neurochemistry*, *82*(6), 1376–1387. https://doi.org/10.1046/j.1471-4159.2002.01069.x.

Miksys, S., Rao, Y., Sellers, E. M., Kwan, M., Mendis, D., & Tyndale, R. F. (2000). Regional and cellular distribution of CYP2D subfamily members in rat brain. *Xenobiotica*, *30*(6), 547–564. https://doi.org/10.1080/004982500406390.

Miksys, S., & Tyndale, R. F. (2004). The unique regulation of brain cytochrome P450 2 (CYP2) family enzymes by drugs and genetics. *Drug Metabolism Reviews*, *36*(2), 313–333. https://doi.org/10.1081/dmr-120034149.

Miksys, S., & Tyndale, R. F. (2009). Brain drug-metabolizing cytochrome P450 enzymes are active in vivo, demonstrated by mechanism-based enzyme inhibition. *Neuropsychopharmacology*, *34*(3), 634–640. https://doi.org/10.1038/npp.2008.110.

Miksys, S., & Tyndale, R. F. (2013). Cytochrome P450-mediated drug metabolism in the brain. *Journal of Psychiatry & Neuroscience*, *38*(3), 152–163.

Miksys, S., Wadji, F. B., Tolledo, E. C., Remington, G., Nobrega, J. N., & Tyndale, R. F. (2017). Rat brain CYP2D enzymatic metabolism alters acute and chronic haloperidol side-effects by different mechanisms. *Progress in Neuro-Psychopharmacology & Biological Psychiatry*, *78*, 140–148. https://doi.org/10.1016/j.pnpbp.2017.04.030.

Miller, R. T., Miksys, S., Hoffmann, E., & Tyndale, R. F. (2014). Ethanol self-administration and nicotine treatment increase brain levels of CYP2D in African green monkeys. *British Journal of Pharmacology*, *171*(12), 3077–3088. https://doi.org/10.1111/bph.12652.

Modi, S., Gilham, D. E., Sutcliffe, M. J., Lian, L. Y., Primrose, W. U., Wolf, C. R., et al. (1997). 1-methyl-4-phenyl-1,2,3,6-tetrahydropyridine as a substrate of cytochrome P450 2D6: allosteric effects of NADPH-cytochrome P450 reductase. *Biochemistry*, *36*(15), 4461–4470. https://doi.org/10.1021/bi962633p.

Moscovitz, J. E., Kalgutkar, A. S., Nulick, K., Johnson, N., Lin, Z., Goosen, T. C., et al. (2018). Establishing transcriptional signatures to differentiate PXR-, CAR-, and AhR-mediated regulation of drug metabolism and transport genes in cryopreserved human hepatocytes. *The Journal of Pharmacology and Experimental Therapeutics*, *365*(2), 262–271. https://doi.org/10.1124/jpet.117.247296.

Neve, E. P., & Ingelman-Sundberg, M. (2008). Intracellular transport and localization of microsomal cytochrome P450. *Analytical and Bioanalytical Chemistry*, *392*(6), 1075–1084. https://doi.org/10.1007/s00216-008-2200-z.

Nierenberg, A. A., Ostacher, M. J., Huffman, J. C., Ametrano, R. M., Fava, M., & Perlis, R. H. (2008). A brief review of antidepressant efficacy, effectiveness, indications, and usage for major depressive disorder. *Journal of Occupational and Environmental Medicine, 50*(4), 428–436. https://doi.org/10.1097/JOM.0b013e31816b5034.

Norris, P. J., Hardwick, J. P., & Emson, P. C. (1996). Regional distribution of cytochrome P450 2D1 in the rat central nervous system. *The Journal of Comparative Neurology, 366*(2), 244–258. https://doi.org/10.1002/(SICI)1096-9861(19960304)366:2<244::AID-CNE5>3.0.CO;2-5.

Novak, R. F., & Woodcroft, K. J. (2000). The alcohol-inducible form of cytochrome P450 (CYP 2E1): role in toxicology and regulation of expression. *Archives of Pharmacal Research, 23*(4), 267–282. https://doi.org/10.1007/BF02975435.

Oesch, F., Fabian, E., Guth, K., & Landsiedel, R. (2014). Xenobiotic-metabolizing enzymes in the skin of rat, mouse, pig, guinea pig, man, and in human skin models. *Archives of Toxicology, 88*(12), 2135–2190. https://doi.org/10.1007/s00204-014-1382-8.

Ohno, M., Motojima, K., Okano, T., & Taniguchi, A. (2009). Induction of drug-metabolizing enzymes by phenobarbital in layered co-culture of a human liver cell line and endothelial cells. *Biological & Pharmaceutical Bulletin, 32*(5), 813–817. https://doi.org/10.1248/bpb.32.813.

Pelkonen, O., Turpeinen, M., Hakkola, J., Honkakoski, P., Hukkanen, J., & Raunio, H. (2008). Inhibition and induction of human cytochrome P450 enzymes: current status. *Archives of Toxicology, 82*(10), 667–715. https://doi.org/10.1007/s00204-008-0332-8.

Peng, H. M., & Coon, M. J. (1998). Regulation of rabbit cytochrome P450 2E1 expression in HepG2 cells by insulin and thyroid hormone. *Molecular Pharmacology, 54*(4), 740–747. Retrieved from https://www.ncbi.nlm.nih.gov/pubmed/9765518.

Petrov, A. M., Mast, N., Li, Y., Denker, J., & Pikuleva, I. A. (2020). Brain sterol flux mediated by cytochrome P450 46A1 affects membrane properties and membrane-dependent processes. *Brain Communications, 2*(1). https://doi.org/10.1093/braincomms/fcaa043.

Preissner, S. C., Hoffmann, M. F., Preissner, R., Dunkel, M., Gewiess, A., & Preissner, S. (2013). Polymorphic cytochrome P450 enzymes (CYPs) and their role in personalized therapy. *PLoS One, 8*(12), e82562. https://doi.org/10.1371/journal.pone.0082562.

Rakhshandehroo, M., Knoch, B., Muller, M., & Kersten, S. (2010). Peroxisome proliferator-activated receptor alpha target genes. *PPAR Research, 2010.* https://doi.org/10.1155/2010/612089.

Ravindranath, V., Anandatheerthavarada, H. K., & Shankar, S. K. (1989). Xenobiotic metabolism in human brain- -presence of cytochrome P-450 and associated mono-oxygenases. *Brain Research, 496*(1-2), 331–335. https://doi.org/10.1016/0006-8993(89)91083-4.

Ravindranath, V., Anandatheerthavarada, H. K., & Shankar, S. K. (1990). NADPH cytochrome P-450 reductase in rat, mouse and human brain. *Biochemical Pharmacology, 39*(6), 1013–1018. https://doi.org/10.1016/0006-2952(90)90279-t.

Renaud, H. J., Cui, J. Y., Khan, M., & Klaassen, C. D. (2011). Tissue distribution and gender-divergent expression of 78 cytochrome P450 mRNAs in mice. *Toxicological Sciences, 124*(2), 261–277. https://doi.org/10.1093/toxsci/kfr240.

Roberts, B. J., Song, B. J., Soh, Y., Park, S. S., & Shoaf, S. E. (1995). Ethanol induces CYP2E1 by protein stabilization. Role of ubiquitin conjugation in the rapid degradation of CYP2E1. *The Journal of Biological Chemistry, 270*(50), 29632–29635. https://doi.org/10.1074/jbc.270.50.29632.

Sasame, H. A., Ames, M. M., & Nelson, S. D. (1977). Cytochrome P-450 and NADPH cytochrome c reductase in rat brain: formation of catechols and reactive catechol metabolites. *Biochemical and Biophysical Research Communications, 78*(3), 919–926. https://doi.org/10.1016/0006-291x(77)90510-1.

Sellers, E. M., & Tyndale, R. F. (2000). Mimicking gene defects to treat drug dependence. *Annals of the New York Academy of Sciences*, *909*, 233–246. https://doi.org/10.1111/j.1749-6632.2000.tb06685.x.

Shimada, T., Yamazaki, H., Mimura, M., Inui, Y., & Guengerich, F. P. (1994). Interindividual variations in human liver cytochrome P-450 enzymes involved in the oxidation of drugs, carcinogens and toxic chemicals: studies with liver microsomes of 30 Japanese and 30 Caucasians. *The Journal of Pharmacology and Experimental Therapeutics*, *270*(1), 414–423. Retrieved from https://www.ncbi.nlm.nih.gov/pubmed/8035341.

Singh, S., Singh, K., Patel, D. K., Singh, C., Nath, C., Singh, V. K., et al. (2009). The expression of CYP2D22, an ortholog of human CYP2D6, in mouse striatum and its modulation in 1-methyl 4-phenyl-1,2,3,6-tetrahydropyridine-induced Parkinson's disease phenotype and nicotine-mediated neuroprotection. *Rejuvenation Research*, *12*(3), 185–197. https://doi.org/10.1089/rej.2009.0850.

Sridar, C., Kenaan, C., & Hollenberg, P. F. (2012). Inhibition of bupropion metabolism by selegiline: mechanism-based inactivation of human CYP2B6 and characterization of glutathione and peptide adducts. *Drug Metabolism and Disposition*, *40*(12), 2256–2266. https://doi.org/10.1124/dmd.112.046979.

Steenland, K., Dick, R. B., Howell, R. J., Chrislip, D. W., Hines, C. J., Reid, T. M., et al. (2000). Neurologic function among termiticide applicators exposed to chlorpyrifos. *Environmental Health Perspectives*, *108*(4), 293–300. https://doi.org/10.1289/ehp.00108293.

Stingl, J. C., Brockmoller, J., & Viviani, R. (2013). Genetic variability of drug-metabolizing enzymes: the dual impact on psychiatric therapy and regulation of brain function. *Molecular Psychiatry*, *18*(3), 273–287. https://doi.org/10.1038/mp.2012.42.

Stocco, M. R., El-Sherbeni, A. A., Zhao, B., Novalen, M., & Tyndale, R. F. (2021). The role of CYP2D in rat brain in methamphetamine-induced striatal dopamine and serotonin release and behavioral sensitization. *Psychopharmacology*, *238*(7), 1791–1804. https://doi.org/10.1007/s00213-021-05808-9.

Stocco, M. R., Tolledo, C., Wadji, F. B., Gonzalez, F. J., Miksys, S., & Tyndale, R. F. (2020). Human CYP2D6 in the brain is protective against harmine-induced neurotoxicity: evidence from humanized CYP2D6 transgenic mice. *Molecular Neurobiology*. https://doi.org/10.1007/s12035-020-02050-w.

Su, T., Bao, Z., Zhang, Q. Y., Smith, T. J., Hong, J. Y., & Ding, X. (2000). Human cytochrome P450 CYP2A13: predominant expression in the respiratory tract and its high efficiency metabolic activation of a tobacco-specific carcinogen, 4-(methylnitrosamino)-1-(3-pyridyl)-1-butanone. *Cancer Research*, *60*(18), 5074–5079. Retrieved from https://www.ncbi.nlm.nih.gov/pubmed/11016631.

Tang, J., Cao, Y., Rose, R. L., Brimfield, A. A., Dai, D., Goldstein, J. A., et al. (2001). Metabolism of chlorpyrifos by human cytochrome P450 isoforms and human, mouse, and rat liver microsomes. *Drug Metabolism and Disposition*, *29*(9), 1201–1204. Retrieved from https://www.ncbi.nlm.nih.gov/pubmed/11502728.

Tauscher, J., Jones, C., Remington, G., Zipursky, R. B., & Kapur, S. (2002). Significant dissociation of brain and plasma kinetics with antipsychotics. *Molecular Psychiatry*, *7*(3), 317–321. https://doi.org/10.1038/sj.mp.4001009.

Terashima, J., Jimma, Y., Jimma, K., Hakata, S., Yachi, M., Habano, W., et al. (2018). The regulation mechanism of AhR activated by benzo[a]pyrene for CYP expression are different between 2D and 3D culture of human lung cancer cells. *Drug Metabolism and Pharmacokinetics*, *33*(4), 211–214. https://doi.org/10.1016/j.dmpk.2018.04.002.

Thum, T., & Borlak, J. (2000). Gene expression in distinct regions of the heart. *Lancet*, *355*(9208), 979–983. https://doi.org/10.1016/S0140-6736(00)99016-0.

Tolledo, C., Stocco, M. R., Miksys, S., Gonzalez, F. J., & Tyndale, R. F. (2020). Human CYP2D6 Is functional in brain in vivo: evidence from humanized CYP2D6 transgenic mice. *Molecular Neurobiology*, *57*(6), 2509–2520. https://doi.org/10.1007/s12035-020-01896-4.

Tompkins, L. M., & Wallace, A. D. (2007). Mechanisms of cytochrome P450 induction. *Journal of Biochemical and Molecular Toxicology*, *21*(4), 176–181. https://doi.org/10.1002/jbt.20180.

Toselli, F., de Waziers, I., Dutheil, M., Vincent, M., Wilce, P. A., Dodd, P. R., et al. (2015). Gene expression profiling of cytochromes P450, ABC transporters and their principal transcription factors in the amygdala and prefrontal cortex of alcoholics, smokers and drug-free controls by qRT-PCR. *Xenobiotica*, *45*(12), 1129–1137. https://doi.org/10.3109/00498254.2015.1040102.

Toselli, F., Dodd, P. R., & Gillam, E. M. (2016). Emerging roles for brain drug-metabolizing cytochrome P450 enzymes in neuropsychiatric conditions and responses to drugs. *Drug Metabolism Reviews*, *48*(3), 379–404. https://doi.org/10.1080/03602532.2016.1221960.

Tsuchiya, Y., Nakajima, M., & Yokoi, T. (2005). Cytochrome P450-mediated metabolism of estrogens and its regulation in human. *Cancer Letters*, *227*(2), 115–124. https://doi.org/10.1016/j.canlet.2004.10.007.

Tsutsumi, M., Lasker, J. M., Shimizu, M., Rosman, A. S., & Lieber, C. S. (1989). The intralobular distribution of ethanol-inducible P450IIE1 in rat and human liver. *Hepatology*, *10*(4), 437–446. https://doi.org/10.1002/hep.1840100407.

Tyndale, R. F., Li, Y., Li, N. Y., Messina, E., Miksys, S., & Sellers, E. M. (1999). Characterization of cytochrome P-450 2D1 activity in rat brain: high-affinity kinetics for dextromethorphan. *Drug Metabolism and Disposition*, *27*(8), 924–930. Retrieved from https://www.ncbi.nlm.nih.gov/pubmed/10421620.

Upadhya, S. C., Tirumalai, P. S., Boyd, M. R., Mori, T., & Ravindranath, V. (2000). Cytochrome P4502E (CYP2E) in brain: constitutive expression, induction by ethanol and localization by fluorescence in situ hybridization. *Archives of Biochemistry and Biophysics*, *373*(1), 23–34. https://doi.org/10.1006/abbi.1999.1477.

Voirol, P., Jonzier-Perey, M., Porchet, F., Reymond, M. J., Janzer, R. C., Bouras, C., et al. (2000). Cytochrome P-450 activities in human and rat brain microsomes. *Brain Research*, *855*(2), 235–243. https://doi.org/10.1016/s0006-8993(99)02354-9.

Volavka, J., Cooper, T., Czobor, P., Bitter, I., Meisner, M., Laska, E., et al. (1992). Haloperidol blood levels and clinical effects. *Archives of General Psychiatry*, *49*(5), 354–361. https://doi.org/10.1001/archpsyc.1992.01820050018002.

Wahid, M., Mahjabeen, I., Baig, R. M., & Kayani, M. A. (2013). Expression of CYP1A1 and GSTP1 in human brain tumor tissues in Pakistan. *Asian Pacific Journal of Cancer Prevention*, *14*(12), 7187–7191. https://doi.org/10.7314/apjcp.2013.14.12.7187.

Walther, B., Ghersi-Egea, J. F., Minn, A., & Siest, G. (1986). Subcellular distribution of cytochrome P-450 in the brain. *Brain Research*, *375*(2), 338–344. https://doi.org/10.1016/0006-8993(86)90754-7.

Wang, Z., Bao, Y., Yan, S., Lian, Z., Jia, Z., & Liu, Z. (2014). An investigation of cigarettes smoking behavior and nicotine dependence among Chinese methamphetamine users in two provinces. *BioMed Research International*, *2014*, 175205. https://doi.org/10.1155/2014/175205.

Wang, Q., Han, X., Li, J., Gao, X., Wang, Y., Liu, M., et al. (2015). Regulation of cerebral CYP2D alters tramadol metabolism in the brain: interactions of tramadol with propranolol and nicotine. *Xenobiotica*, *45*(4), 335–344. https://doi.org/10.3109/00498254.2014.981609.

Wang, D., Jiang, Z., Shen, Z., Wang, H., Wang, B., Shou, W., et al. (2011). Functional evaluation of genetic and environmental regulators of p450 mRNA levels. *PLoS One*, *6*(10), e24900. https://doi.org/10.1371/journal.pone.0024900.

Wang, Y., Tang, H., Xu, M., Luo, J., Zhao, L., Shi, F., et al. (2019). Effect of copper nanoparticles on brain cytochrome P450 enzymes in rats. *Molecular Medicine Reports*, *20*(1), 771–778. https://doi.org/10.3892/mmr.2019.10302.

Warden, A., Truitt, J., Merriman, M., Ponomareva, O., Jameson, K., Ferguson, L. B., et al. (2016). Localization of PPAR isotypes in the adult mouse and human brain. *Scientific Reports*, *6*, 27618. https://doi.org/10.1038/srep27618.

Warner, M., & Gustafsson, J. A. (1994). Effect of ethanol on cytochrome P450 in the rat brain. *Proceedings of the National Academy of Sciences of the United States of America*, *91*(3), 1019–1023. https://doi.org/10.1073/pnas.91.3.1019.

Warner, M., Kohler, C., Hansson, T., & Gustafsson, J. A. (1988). Regional distribution of cytochrome P-450 in the rat brain: spectral quantitation and contribution of P-450b,e, and P-450c,d. *Journal of Neurochemistry*, *50*(4), 1057–1065. https://doi.org/10.1111/j.1471-4159.1988.tb10573.x.

Waxman, D. J., & Holloway, M. G. (2009). Sex differences in the expression of hepatic drug metabolizing enzymes. *Molecular Pharmacology*, *76*(2), 215–228. https://doi.org/10.1124/mol.109.056705.

Woodland, C., Huang, T. T., Gryz, E., Bendayan, R., & Fawcett, J. P. (2008). Expression, activity and regulation of CYP3A in human and rodent brain. *Drug Metabolism Reviews*, *40*(1), 149–168. https://doi.org/10.1080/03602530701836712.

Wu, C., Jiang, X. L., Shen, H. W., & Yu, A. M. (2009). Effects of CYP2D6 status on harmaline metabolism, pharmacokinetics and pharmacodynamics, and a pharmacogenetics-based pharmacokinetic model. *Biochemical Pharmacology*, *78*(6), 617–624. https://doi.org/10.1016/j.bcp.2009.05.011.

Wu, D., Otton, S. V., Inaba, T., Kalow, W., & Sellers, E. M. (1997). Interactions of amphetamine analogs with human liver CYP2D6. *Biochemical Pharmacology*, *53*(11), 1605–1612. https://doi.org/10.1016/s0006-2952(97)00014-2.

Yadav, S., Johri, A., Dhawan, A., Seth, P. K., & Parmar, D. (2006). Regional specificity in deltamethrin induced cytochrome P450 expression in rat brain. *Toxicology and Applied Pharmacology*, *217*(1), 15–24. https://doi.org/10.1016/j.taap.2006.07.008.

Yamazaki, H., Inoue, K., Hashimoto, M., & Shimada, T. (1999). Roles of CYP2A6 and CYP2B6 in nicotine C-oxidation by human liver microsomes. *Archives of Toxicology*, *73*(2), 65–70. https://doi.org/10.1007/s002040050588.

Yu, A. M., Idle, J. R., Krausz, K. W., Kupfer, A., & Gonzalez, F. J. (2003). Contribution of individual cytochrome P450 isozymes to the O-demethylation of the psychotropic beta-carboline alkaloids harmaline and harmine. *The Journal of Pharmacology and Experimental Therapeutics*, *305*(1), 315–322. https://doi.org/10.1124/jpet.102.047050.

Yue, J., Khokhar, J., Miksys, S., & Tyndale, R. F. (2009). Differential induction of ethanol-metabolizing CYP2E1 and nicotine-metabolizing CYP2B1/2 in rat liver by chronic nicotine treatment and voluntary ethanol intake. *European Journal of Pharmacology*, *609*(1-3), 88–95. https://doi.org/10.1016/j.ejphar.2009.03.015.

Yue, J., Miksys, S., Hoffmann, E., & Tyndale, R. F. (2008). Chronic nicotine treatment induces rat CYP2D in the brain but not in the liver: an investigation of induction and time course. *Journal of Psychiatry & Neuroscience*, *33*(1), 54–63. Retrieved from https://www.ncbi.nlm.nih.gov/pubmed/18197273.

Zanger, U. M., & Klein, K. (2013). Pharmacogenetics of cytochrome P450 2B6 (CYP2B6): advances on polymorphisms, mechanisms, and clinical relevance. *Frontiers in Genetics*, *4*, 24. https://doi.org/10.3389/fgene.2013.00024.

Zanger, U. M., & Schwab, M. (2013). Cytochrome P450 enzymes in drug metabolis regulation of gene expression, enzyme activities, and impact of genetic variation. *Pharmacology & Therapeutics*, *138*(1), 103–141. https://doi.org/10.1016/j.pharmthera.2012.12.007.

Zhang, F., Li, J., Na, S., Wu, J., Yang, Z., Xie, X., et al. (2018). The involvement of PPARs in the selective regulation of brain CYP2D by growth hormone. *Neuroscience*, *379*, 115–125. https://doi.org/10.1016/j.neuroscience.2018.03.009.

Zhong, Y., Dong, G., Luo, H., Cao, J., Wang, C., Wu, J., et al. (2012). Induction of brain CYP2E1 by chronic ethanol treatment and related oxidative stress in hippocampus, cerebellum, and brainstem. *Toxicology*, *302*(2-3), 275–284. https://doi.org/10.1016/j.tox.2012.08.009.

Zhou, S., Chan, E., Duan, W., Huang, M., & Chen, Y. Z. (2005). Drug bioactivation, covalent binding to target proteins and toxicity relevance. *Drug Metabolism Reviews*, *37*(1), 41–213. https://doi.org/10.1081/dmr-200028812.

Zhou, K., Khokhar, J. Y., Zhao, B., & Tyndale, R. F. (2013). First demonstration that brain CYP2D-mediated opiate metabolic activation alters analgesia in vivo. *Biochemical Pharmacology*, *85*(12), 1848–1855. https://doi.org/10.1016/j.bcp.2013.04.014.

CHAPTER FOUR

Mammalian cytochrome P450 biodiversity: Physiological importance, function, and protein and genomic structures of cytochromes P4502B in multiple species of woodrats with different dietary preferences

Michele M. Skopec[a], James R. Halpert[b,*], and M. Denise Dearing[c,*]
[a]Department of Zoology, Weber State University, Ogden, UT, United States
[b]Department of Pharmacology and Toxicology, College of Pharmacy, University of Arizona, Tucson, AZ, United States
[c]School of Biological Sciences, University of Utah, Salt Lake City, UT, United States
*Corresponding authors: e-mail address: jhalpert1@arizona.edu; denise.dearing@utah.edu

Contents

Advances in Pharmacology, Volume 95
ISSN 1054-3589
https://doi.org/10.1016/bs.apha.2022.05.002

Abstract

The vast diversity of cytochrome P450 enzymes in mammals has been proposed to result in large measure from plant-animal warfare, whereby evolution of chemical defenses such as phenolics and terpenoids in plants led to duplication and divergence of P450 genes in herbivores. Over evolutionary time, natural selection is predicted to have produced P450s with high affinity and enhanced metabolism of substrates that are ingested regularly by herbivores. Interestingly, however, almost all knowledge of the interactions of mammalian P450 enzymes with substrates stems from studies of the metabolism of drugs and model compounds rather than studies on wild mammalian herbivores and their respective PSMs. A question of particular interest centers on the role of individual P450 enzymes in the ability of certain herbivores to specialize on plants that are lethal to most other species, including those from the same genus as the specialists. We tackled this intricate problem using a tractable natural system (herbivorous woodrats, genus *Neotoma*) focusing on comparisons of the specialist *N. stephensi*, the facultative specialist *N. lepida*, and the generalist *N. albigula*, and employing a cross-disciplinary approach involving ecology, biochemistry, pharmacology, structural biology, and genomics. Based on multiple findings suggesting the importance of CYP2B enzymes for ingestion of juniper and a major constituent, α-pinene, we characterized the structure, function and activity of several CYP2B enzymes in woodrats with different dietary habits. Results to date suggest that differences in CYP2B gene copy number may contribute to differential tolerance of PSMs among woodrat species, although additional work is warranted to firmly link gene copy number to juniper tolerance.

Abbreviations

ABT	1-aminobenzotriazole
BROD	benzyloxyresorufin-O-dealkylation
GST	glutathione S-transferase
NDGA	nordihydroguaiaretic acid
PSM	plant secondary metabolite
SRS	substrate recognition sites
245-HCB	2,2′,4,4′,5′5′-hexachlorobiphenyl
4-CPI	4-(4-chlorophenyl)imidazole
7-BR	7-benzyloxyresorufin
7-EFC	7-ethoxy-4-(trifluoromethyl)coumarin
7-MFC	7-methoxy-4-(trifluoromethyl)coumarin

1. Introduction

The diversity of mammalian P450 enzymes has been attributed in part to the co-evolutionary arms race between plants and herbivores (Nebert & Dieter, 2000; Nelson, 2003, 2011). As plants evolved chemical defenses such as phenolics and terpenoids, P450 genes in herbivores are proposed to have evolved through duplication and divergence to metabolize plant secondary metabolites (PSMs) that can be toxic (Ehrlich & Raven, 1964; Schuler, 2011). Over evolutionary time, natural selection is predicted to produce P450s with high affinity and enhanced metabolism of substrates that are ingested regularly by herbivores. This evolutionary process has resulted in a stunning diversity of functional P450 enzymes that remain an exciting and active area of investigation.

In the early days of elucidation of function of individual P450 enzymes, ecologists Freeland and Janzen proposed that "detoxification" enzymes mediated the interactions between mammalian herbivores and the plants on which they feed, and that there were fundamental physiological constraints in the biotransformation systems of mammals restricting their ability to feed on plants that produce high levels of PSMs (Freeland & Janzen, 1974). The generalist feeding strategy observed in the majority of mammalian herbivores (thousands of species) was surmised to result from limitations in the hepatic detoxification system that had evolved to process a wide range of substrates with low catalytic activity toward any particular substrate. The dozen or so mammalian species capable of specializing on plants with high levels of PSMs were predicted to have evolved biotransformation (detoxification) enzymes with enhanced function to facilitate efficient catalysis of the more restricted set of PSMs in their diet. Specialization was predicted to result in a reduction in the ability to transform novel compounds that differ chemically from those typically found in the diet (Sorensen, McLister, & Dearing, 2005a; Torregrossa, Azzara, & Dearing, 2012). This idea that enzymatic biochemical tradeoffs govern the diet breadth of herbivores has become entrenched in the field of plant-animal interactions despite limited empirical studies (Marsh, Wallis, Andrew, & Foley, 2006).

In this chapter, we review our research to test the biochemical trade-offs hypothesis. We tackled this intricate problem using a tractable natural system (herbivorous woodrats, *Neotoma* species) in a cross-disciplinary approach involving ecology, biochemistry, pharmacology, and structural biology. Woodrats, genus *Neotoma*, are an exceptional natural system for comparative studies on P450 enzymes (Fig. 1). All of 20 or so species of woodrats in *Neotoma* are herbivorous. This genus is unparalleled by any other mammalian genus with respect to the variety of generalist and specialist species, thereby enabling comparisons among species/populations with similar morphologies and ecologies (Weinstein et al., 2021).

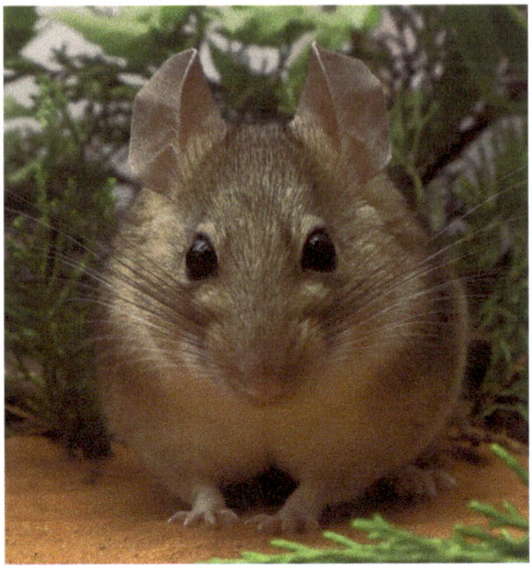

Fig. 1 Woodrat (genus *Neotoma)* and juniper. *Neotoma lepida* is one of a very few mammalian herbivores that is able to specialize on a plant, juniper, that is high in plant secondary metabolites (PSMs). Juniper produces a variety of terpenes with α-pinene being a dominant one.

Woodrats (120–600 g) are easily kept under laboratory conditions, and their relationship to laboratory rats (25-million-year divergence time) is recent enough that molecular reagents designed for pharmacological studies on laboratory rats work on woodrats (Haley, Lamb, Franklin, Constance, & Denise Dearing, 2007; Lamb, Sorensen, & Dearing, 2001; Skopec, Haley, & Dearing, 2007). Genomic tools now exist for some species of woodrats (Greenhalgh et al., 2022) and more are in the works. In addition, woodrats consume a wide range of PSMs (e.g., terpenes, alkaloids, aromatic hydrocarbons) in differing amounts (Weinstein et al., 2021).

For this chapter, we focus on three woodrat species in particular that vary in dietary specialization and their ingestion of juniper and its terpenes, which are potent inducers and inhibitors of CYP2B1 in laboratory rats (De-Oliveira, Ribeiro-Pinto, & Paumgartten, 1997; Hiroi, Miyazaki, Kobayashi, Imaoka, & Funae, 1995; Lamb, Marick, Sorensen, Haley, & Dearing, 2004). *Neotoma stephensi* is an obligate specialist that consumes almost exclusively juniper foliage *(Juniperus monosperma)* year round (Dial, 1988; Skopec, Kohl, Schramm, Halpert, & Dearing, 2015; Vaughn, 1982). The dose of terpenes that *N. stephensi* ingests daily in its juniper diet would be lethal to other mammalian species. *Neotoma stephensi* is sympatric (shares the same habitat) with a generalist, *N. albigula,* that consumes far less juniper in nature

(18–34%; Dial, 1988; Weinstein et al., 2021). In feeding trials, *N. albigula* also consumes less juniper and a major juniper component, α-pinene (Torregrossa & Dearing, 2009b). Indeed, the generalist tends to store food until the terpenes have volatilized (Torregrossa & Dearing, 2009a). These two woodrat species permit an interspecies comparison of a specialist and generalist that occur in sympatry.

In addition, we investigated CYP2B enzymes in two populations of *N. lepida*. This comparison is an intraspecies one between a population that regularly consumes high levels of juniper (*Juniperus osteosperma*: 40–90%) in the Great Basin desert and another population in the Mojave desert that currently does not consume juniper or terpene-rich plants but has historically done so (Mangione, Dearing, & Karasov, 2000; Skopec et al., 2015). The Mojave desert population switched from a diet containing juniper to one of creosote bush (*Larrea tridentata*) ca.18,000 years ago when juniper was extirpated and creosote bush invaded as a result of natural climatic changes in the desert southwest. Evidence from fossilized woodrat middens (homes and food storage structures) from the Mojave desert indicates that woodrats stopped collecting juniper and started collecting creosote bush at this time (Van Devender, 1977). Creosote bush and juniper produce very different suites of PSMs. Terpenes are the primary PSMs in juniper (Adams, Beauchamp, Dev, & Dutz, 2007), whereas creosote bush produces a phenolic-rich resin that can comprise 10–25% of the dry mass of leaves (Mabry, Difeo, Sakakibara, Bohnstedt, & Seigler, 1977). The majority of this resin is composed of nordihydroguaiaretic acid (NDGA), a phenolic compound that causes kidney cysts in lab rats (Goodman, Grice, Becking, & Salem, 1970). The switch from a diet of juniper (terpenes) to creosote (phenolic resin) are predicted to have resulted in new biotransformation challenges for *N. lepida* that could have favored different forms of CYP2B enzymes.

The fact that *N. stephensi* and *N. lepida* specialize on two different species of juniper creates another interesting aspect of the interspecies comparison. *N. stephensi* consumes *J. monosperma* or one-seeded juniper, which is less chemically diverse than *J. osteosperma* or Utah juniper. One-seeded juniper has a lower overall terpene content (~4.5% dry weight), and α-pinene is the predominant terpene at 61.8% of the overall terpene content, whereas Utah juniper has a higher overall terpene content (~9% dry weight) and a larger diversity of terpenes, including α-pinene, sabinene, and bornyl acetate (Skopec et al., 2015). *N. stephensi's* long history with a less chemically diverse juniper may have allowed it to become more specialized, as evidenced by a

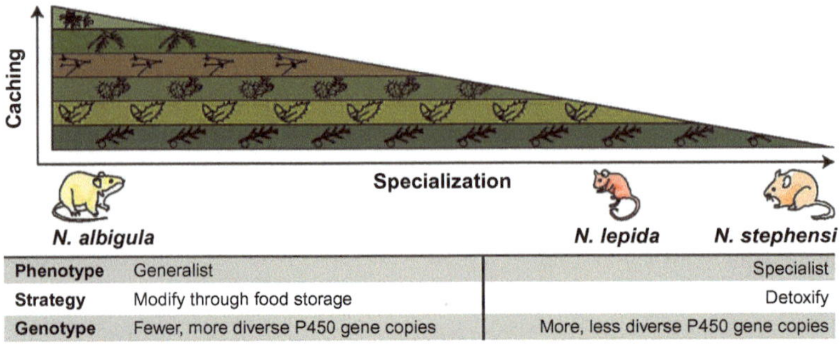

Fig. 2 Three species of woodrats and their likely evolutionary pathways to being able to consume juniper. *Neotoma albigula* is a dietary generalist that is only able to consume a diet of ~30% juniper and relies on behavioral strategies to deal with the terpenes present in juniper. The two specialists, *N. lepida* and *N. stephensi,* can consume a diet of >70% juniper and rely on biotransformation pathways to detoxify the terpenes present in juniper.

preference for one-seeded juniper over Utah juniper and for consumption of one-seeded juniper rather than caching, which would otherwise allow the terpenes to volatilize (Skopec, Adams, & Muir, 2019; Skopec et al., 2015). *Neotoma lepida,* on the other hand, shows no preference for its native Utah juniper compared with one-seeded juniper and chooses to cache more than consume relative to *N. stephensi* (Skopec et al., 2019, 2015). The caching behavior and intake of diverse PSMs exhibited by *N. lepida* may have allowed it to adapt to new diets such as creosote. Studying these three species that span the generalist to specialist spectrum has led us to propose a new paradigm for understanding how woodrats deal with plants high in PSMs. Generalists modify their food before consuming it to decrease their exposure to PSMs, while specialists will rely on specialized biotransformation pathways to detoxify the high doses of PSM. In short, specialists detoxify, and generalists modify (Fig. 2).

2. Results

2.1 Early work implicating CYP2B in dietary specialization

Our initial foray (early to late 2000s) in understanding the role of CYP2B in dietary specialization in woodrats leveraged experimental approaches available at that time. In the juniper specialist *N. stephensi*, we found much higher total P450 content and messenger RNA expression of CYP2B (and also CYP3A) compared with Sprague-Dawley rats including those induced with α-pinene (Lamb et al., 2004). CYP2B activity levels utilizing benzyloxyresorufin-O-dealkylation (BROD) did not differ between *N. stephensi* and *N. albigula* feeding on low doses of juniper, but doubled in the specialist on high doses of juniper (Haley et al., 2007). Studies using the early microarray technology designed for laboratory rats further supported the role of CYP2B in enabling juniper specialization in *N. stephensi*, which exhibited >fourfold expression of CYP2B compared with *N. albigula* on both the control and low juniper diet (25%). In addition, CYP2B expression in *N. stephensi* fed the high juniper diet (70%) was 5 × greater than when it was fed on the low juniper diet (25%; Skopec et al., 2007).

A series of parallel studies of the juniper and creosote bush feeding populations of *N. lepida*, also pointed to the importance of CYP2B with respect to PSMs. Counter to our expectations, BROD was higher in the creosote than juniper feeding population on both control (PSM free) and creosote containing diets suggesting that CYP2B may be an important pathway for metabolizing the phenolics present in creosote (Haley, Lamb, Franklin, Constance, & Dearing, 2008). However, woodrats of both populations showed increased expression of five CYP2B isoforms when ingesting 50% juniper compared with creosote in experiments using the laboratory rat microarray, suggesting that CYP2B may have a larger role in metabolizing the terpenes in juniper than the phenolics in creosote (Magnanou, Malenke, & Dearing, 2009).

2.2 Functional assays implicating the role of P450s and of CYP2B in juniper ingestion by woodrats

Administration of the suicide P450 inhibitor (1-aminobenzotriazole; ABT) to *N. lepida* reduced intake of a juniper diet by 35%; this reduction was greater than that observed with a non-PSM control diet (Skopec, Malenke, Halpert, & Dearing, 2013). In *N. stephensi,* ABT administration resulted in a 47% reduction in intake of a juniper diet (unpublished). Although ABT is not a specific CYP2B inhibitor, the results clearly show the importance of P450s for juniper intake by both species. In addition, ABT increases the clearance time of hexobarbital (a known CYP2B substrate in laboratory rats) three- to fourfold (Lewis & Lake, 1997; Skopec et al., 2013; Sorensen, Skopec, & Dearing, 2006).

In addition, we found species differences in hexobarbital clearance times (determined with hypnotic state assays) that correlate with voluntary levels of juniper consumption in *N. albigula* and *N. stephensi*. The generalist *N. albigula* had longer clearance times and lower voluntary juniper consumption,

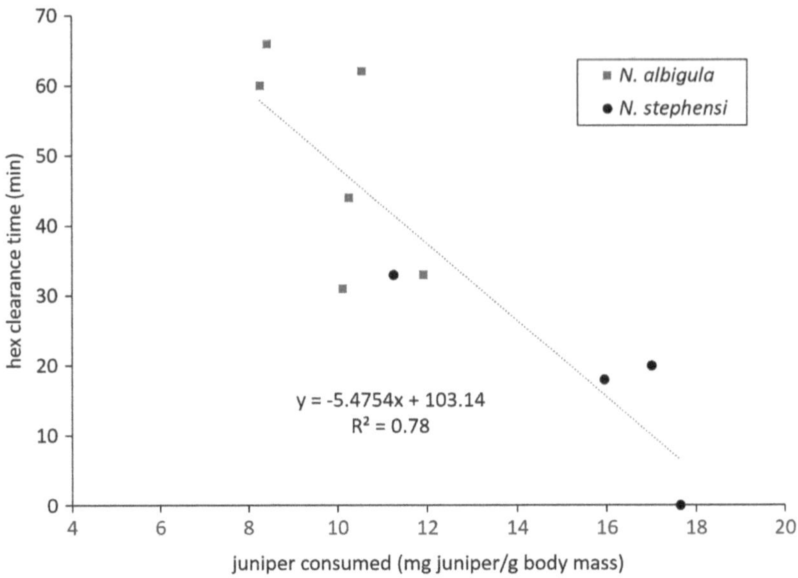

Fig. 3 Correlation between hexobarbital (hex) clearance times and juniper consumption. Juniper consumed (mg juniper/g body mass) was calculated based on dry matter intake over 3 days when the generalist, *N. albigula* ($n = 6$) and specialist, *N. stephensi* ($n = 4$) were fed a 25% juniper diet. Hex clearance times were measured on animals given intraperitoneal injections of hex (100 mg/kg) dose of hex after eating 25% juniper for 3 days. Hex clearance times were measured as time from loss of righting reflex to time righting reflex was regained (Skopec et al., 2013). There was a significant correlation between juniper intake and hex clearance times ($R^2 = 0.78$, $P = 0.014$).

whereas the specialist *N. stephensi* had shorter clearance times and higher voluntary juniper consumption (Fig. 3). These experiments were accompanied by more detailed efforts to understand the role of specific woodrat CYP2B isoforms in juniper feeding and to characterize their structure and function.

2.3 Enormous diversity of CYP2B isoforms in woodrats

Early in 2010, we began cloning and sequencing CYP2B in woodrats using primers designed from the limited information in Genbank for the isoforms present in *Rattus norvegicus* and *Mus muscuslus*. Ironically, if we had any inkling at the time of the tremendous CYP2B diversity present in woodrats, we likely would have abandoned this effort and waited for the development of more efficient approaches. Our initial study contained a total 11 *N. lepida* woodrats distributed relatively evenly between the juniper and creosote feeders. From these animals, we generated 87 CYP2B clones consisting of 62 unique CYP2B nucleotide sequences that translated into 53 unique amino acid sequences. These amino acid sequences were further reduced into a dozen unique combinations of important residues at substrate recognition sites (SRSs). The variability observed likely represents a combination of allelic variation at individual loci as well as a sampling of multiple CYP2B isoforms. Indeed, analysis of CYP2B copy number by Southern blot and quantitative PCR methods revealed multiple copies of CYP2B, ranging from two to eight. The diversity of CYP2B amino acid sequences in *N. lepida* indicated a connection between particular CYP2B isoforms and particular diets and populations. Our evolutionary analysis of the CYP2B SRS variants suggested that CYP2B genes in *N. lepida* initially evolved in response to dietary terpenes and were later modified in populations that switched to creosote (Malenke, Magnanou, Thomas, & Dearing, 2012). We have since characterized the structure and function of three of these isoforms: CYP2B35, 36 and 37 (Wilderman et al., 2014), as described in more detail below.

In addition to *N. lepida*, we also evaluated CYP2B variation and copy number in *N. stephensi* and *N. albigula*. Based on quantitative PCR and sequencing, we found that the specialist possessed five more CYP2B gene copies on average than the generalist; however, the specialist's CYP2B sequences were far less diverse. The greater abundance of unique CYP2B nucleotide sequences in the generalist is consistent with the hypothesis that these genes likely evolved via neofunctionalization, a process in which duplicated genes mutate and assume new function, such as altered substrate specificity (Hahn, 2009).

Identifying and characterizing the diversity of CYP2B isoforms demands high quality and annotated reference genomes; however, unlike model species, these resources were lacking for woodrats. In 2016, we generated the first draft genome for *Neotoma* (Campbell, Oakeson, Yandell, Halpert, & Dearing, 2016). Due to the limitations of short-read sequencing, we were unable to resolve the P450 region of this genome, and the assembly as a whole was quite fragmented (scaffold N50 length of 151 kb). Recently, using a novel approach (trio-binning), we generated high quality genomes (97% complete) for two species of *Neotoma*: *N. lepida* and its sister species, *N. bryanti*. Most importantly, we were able to resolve the CYP2B region along with other duplicated P450 regions for both woodrat species. Although *CYP2B* genes in many species (e.g., humans and other primates; *Mus musculus*) are typically found only between *CYP2G* and *CYP2S* genes in the CYP2ABFGST gene array (Hu et al., 2008), New World rodents such as *Neotoma* vary in their arrangement of *CYP2B* genes within this array. Within *Neotoma*, we found a novel gene island outside the bounds of the typical array, comprised solely of variable numbers of duplicated *CYP2B* genes most similar to CYP2B37, a woodrat specific CYP2B gene (Greenhalgh et al., 2022; Wilderman et al., 2014). The other known woodrat specific CYP2B genes (*CYP2B35*, *CYP2B36)* appear to be contained within the bounds of standard CYP2ABFGST gene array. Our analyses of these genomes are consistent with our earlier findings of multiple gene copies of CYP2B in *Neotoma*, with a spectacular expansion evident in *N. lepida* consisting of a total of 15 apparently functional CYP2B genes and a number of pseudogenes, indicating high turnover of these genes.

2.4 Background to biochemical and structural studies of woodrat CYP2B enzymes

For P450s in species such as the human, rat and rabbit, site-directed mutagenesis, molecular modeling, and crystal structures underscore the importance of single amino acid substitutions not only within the active site of the CYP2B enzymes but also at other residues (Jang, Davydov, Lee, Yun, & Halpert, 2014; Shah, Liu, Zhang, Stout, & Halpert, 2017; Wilderman & Halpert, 2012). We hypothesized that studies of woodrat CYP2B enzymes with their natural substrates might yield new insights into P450 structure-function relationships. In addition, we sought to explore whether structural differences among woodrat CYP2B enzymes played a role in the inter- and intraspecies differences in woodrat dietary preferences. The paradigm followed in this work was our previous studies of the metabolism of 2,2′,4,4′,5′5′-hexachlorobiphenyl (245-HCB) by dog liver microsomes and dog CYP2B11 (Duignan, Sipes, Ciaccio, & Halpert, 1988; Duignan, Sipes, Leonard, & Halpert, 1987; Graves, Elhag, Ciaccio, Bourque, & Halpert, 1990; Hasler et al., 1994). In those studies, we demonstrated that the unusual ability of dogs to metabolize and eliminate certain polychlorinated biphenyls including 245-HCB compared with rats results from: (1) high constitutive expression of CYP2B11 and (2) 20-fold greater turnover of 245-HCB by CYP2B11 than rat CYP2B1. Furthermore, site-directed mutagenesis showed that three substrate recognition site residues (V114, D290, and L363) in CYP2B11 that differ from CYP2B1 are essential for 2-hydroxylation of 245-HCB and important for 3-hydroxylation. Thus, small differences in a few amino acids in CYP2B enzymes indeed result in a major species difference in handling of an important synthetic environmental contaminant.

One caveat, however, in terms of relevance for the woodrat studies of natural dietary constituents is that absolute turnover of 245-HCB by CYP2B11 (0.2 nmol/min/nmol) is very low.

2.5 Studies of woodrat CYP2B enzymes and of monoterpene binding to human CYP2B6

As a first step toward functional and structural characterization of woodrat CYP2B enzymes, we selected two variant clones from three major clades identified in *N. lepida* (Malenke et al., 2012). They were termed CYP2B35v1 or v2 (Clade A), CYP2B36v1 or v2 (Clade F), and CYP2B37v1 or v2 (Clade H) (Wilderman et al., 2014). Based on expression levels in *E. coli*, ease of purification, and enzyme activity, we focused in this and subsequent studies on CYP2B35v1, CYP 2B36v1, and CYP 2B37v2. For simplicity, they are referred to as CYP2B35, CYP2B36, and CYP2B37 in this chapter. CYP2B36 and CYP2B37, showed dealkylation activity with the model substrates 7-ethoxy-4-(trifluoromethyl)coumarin (7-EFC) and 7-benzyloxyresorufin (7-BR), whereas CYP2B35 was inactive. Binding of the monoterpene (+)-α-pinene produced a Type I shift in the absorbance spectrum of each enzyme with K_S values ~1 μM, similar to CYP2B1. Modest differences in functional profiles between CYP2B36 and CYP2B37 were partially explained by changes in substrate recognition site residues 114 and 480. The most intriguing finding was the lack of activity of 2B35 toward 7-EFC and 7-BR, which are dealkylated by most if not all other CYP2B enzymes.

In parallel with these nascent studies of woodrat CYP2B enzymes, we added monoterpenes to our long-standing research on the lone CYP2B in humans, namely CYP2B6. After four painstaking years, we had finally figured out how to crystallize the enzyme (Gay et al., 2010), and subsequent structural studies documented the remarkable plasticity of CYP2B6 previously shown with rabbit CYP2B4 (Shah et al., 2012). In addition to demonstrating tight binding of (+)-α-pinene to CYP2B6 by spectral titrations, thermodynamics of ligand binding was explored using isothermal titration calorimetry (Wilderman, Shah, Jang, Stout, & Halpert, 2013). Comparison was made to CYP2A6, which is much less flexible than CYP2B6 based on comparison of multiple X-ray crystal structures. Consistent with expectation, entropy was the major driving force for hydrocarbon binding to CYP2A6, whereas formation of the CYP2B6-(+)-α-pinene complex had a significant enthalpic component. A 2.0 Å resolution crystal structure of this enzyme ligand complex was solved

(Wilderman et al., 2013). Comparison with prior structures confirmed that CYP2B6 is highly plastic and suggested that the specific components of enthalpic contribution to ligand binding are closely tied to the degree of enzyme flexibility.

To explore this question further, we solved X-ray crystal structures of complexes of CYP2B6 and CYP2A6 with another monoterpene, namely sabinene (Shah et al., 2015). In CYP2B6, sabinene positioned itself with the putative oxidation site located closer to the heme iron (Fig. 4A). In contrast, sabinene was found in an alternate conformation in the more compact CYP2A6, where the larger hydrophobic side chains resulted in a significantly reduced active-site cavity. Furthermore, results from isothermal titration calorimetry indicated a much more substantial contribution of favorable enthalpy to sabinene binding to CYP2B6 as opposed to CYP2A6, consistent with the previous observations with (+)-α-pinene. Structural analysis of CYP2B6 complexes with sabinene and the structurally similar (3)-carene,

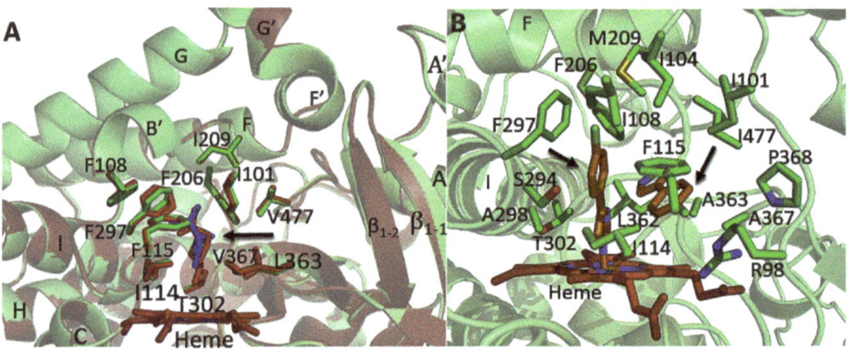

Fig. 4 (A) Overlay of CYP2B6-sabinene (green) and CYP2B6-(+)-3-carene (red) structures in a cartoon representation showing active-site residues in sticks within a 5 Å radius of the ligand. Heme is shown in red sticks. The arrow points to the ligands. Sabinene is shown in blue and (+)-3-carene in red sticks. (B) Active site of the CYP2B35 structure showing residues located within 5 Å from either molecule of 4-(4-chlorophenyl)imidazole (arrows). A total of 19 residues that include A363 and A367 are shown, constituting the active site of CYP2B35. *Panel (A) from Shah, M. B., Wilderman, P. R., Liu, J., Jang, H. H., Zhang, Q., Stout, C. D., & Halpert, J. R. (2015). Structural and biophysical characterization of human cytochromes P450 2B6 and 2A6 bound to volatile hydrocarbons: Analysis and comparison.* Molecular Pharmacology, *87(4), 649–659. (25585967). https://doi.org/10.1124/mol.114.097014 with permission from publisher. Panel (B) from Shah, M. B., Liu, J., Huo, L., Zhang, Q., Dearing, M. D., Wilderman, P. R., … Halpert, J. R. (2016). Structure-function analysis of mammalian CYP2B enzymes using 7-substituted coumarin derivatives as probes: Utility of crystal structures and molecular modeling in understanding xenobiotic metabolism.* Molecular Pharmacology, *89(4), 435–445. (26826176). https://doi.org/10.1124/mol.115.102111 with permission from publisher.*

and comparison with previously solved structures revealed how the movement of the F206 side chain facilitates monoterpene binding. The overall inference was that CYP2B6 (and presumably rat and rabbit CYP2B enzymes) are almost tailor-made to bind monoterpenes with high affinity even though any dietary pressure to detoxify such compounds must have preceded the species divergence.

After several years of effort, crystal structures of CYP2B35 and CYP2B37 were solved in complex with 4-(4-chlorophenyl)imidazole (4-CPI) (Shah et al., 2016). Similar efforts with monoterpenes and with CYP2B36 were unsuccessful. The closed conformation of CYP2B35 contained two molecules of 4-CPI within the active site (Fig. 4B), whereas the CYP2B37 structure demonstrated an open conformation with three 4-CPI molecules, one within the active site and the other two in the substrate access channel. To probe structure-function relationships of CYP2B35, CYP2B36, and CYP2B37, we tested the *O*-dealkylation of 7-alkoxycoumarins and 7-alkoxy-4-(trifluoromethyl)coumarins (Fig. 5) with a C1–C7 side chain. CYP2B35 showed the highest catalytic efficiency (k_{cat}/K_M) with 7-heptoxycoumarin as a substrate, followed by 7-hexoxycoumarin. In contrast, CYP2B37 showed the highest catalytic efficiency with 7-ethoxy-4-(trifluoromethyl)coumarin (7-EFC), followed by 7-methoxy-4-(trifluoromethyl)coumarin (7-MFC). CYP2B35 had no dealkylation activity with 7-MFC or 7-EFC. Furthermore, the new 4-CPI–bound structures were used as templates for docking the 7-substituted coumarin derivatives, which revealed orientations consistent with the functional studies. In particular, the A363-A367 motif in CYP2B35 appeared to be responsible for the larger active site and ability to accommodate larger substrates.

In a subsequent mutagenesis study, CYP2B35 A367V showed maximal activity with 7-butoxycoumarin as opposed to 7-heptoxycoumarin in the parental enzyme, and CYP2B35 A363I/A367V produced an activity profile like that generated by CYP2B37 (Huo et al., 2017). CYP2B35 A363I/A367V/I477F showed 7-ethoxycoumarin and 7-EFC O-dealkylation rates similar to those of CYP2B37 and higher than those of the double mutant. A CYP2B35 sextuple mutant with the corresponding CYP2B37 residue at positions 104, 114, 209, 363, 367, and 477 produced an activity profile that

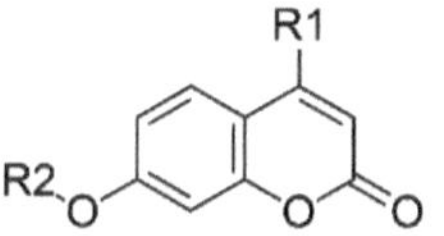

Fig. 5 Chemical structure of 4-substituted 7-alkoxycoumarins. R1 = —H or —CF_3. R2 = methyl to heptyl.

was a hybrid of that of CYP2B35 and CYP2B37, which could be explained by docking of 7-substituted coumarin derivatives into a model based on the crystal structure of the 4-CPI bound CYP2B37. Intriguingly, after literally decades of site-directed mutagenesis studies on CYP2B enzymes in our laboratory, this was the first example of a such a hybrid function mutant.

Returning to studies of monoterpenes, we compared liver microsomal metabolism in *N. stephensi* and *N. albigula* (Orr et al., 2020). In both species, a 30% juniper diet increased the total CYP2B concentration in microsomes two- to threefold and microsomal α-pinene metabolism fourfold. In *N. stephensi*, higher levels of dietary juniper (60% and 100%) further induced CYP2B and increased microsomal turnover of α-pinene. Rates of α-pinene turnover by microsomes from both species ranged from 10 to 19 nmol/min/nmol P450. Similar rates were observed with CYP2B1, CYP2B35, and CYP2B37 (12–14 nmol/min/nmol). The results do not suggest higher turnover by specialist CYP2B enzymes as being responsible for the ability of *N. stephensi* to tolerate high levels of juniper in the diet. Rather, the CYP2B enzymes from multiple species are very well adapted to bind and turn over α-pinene, and calorimetric and spectral titrations show much tighter binding of monoterpenes to CYP2B6 than to CYP2A6 due to a greater enthalpic component. Thus, in contrast to our initial paradigm of unique 245-HCB turnover by dog CYP2B11 compared with other CYP2B enzymes, CYP2B enzymes as a sub-family appear to have evolved to handle monoterpenes. This is certainly consistent with the ancient nature of the monoterpenes as opposed to the very recent synthetic PCBs. In support of this hypothesis is the observation that maximal activity of CYP2B enzymes toward α-pinene is >50-fold higher than turnover of 245-HCB by CYP2B11. Accordingly, subsequent studies are warranted to investigate other possible mechanisms underlying dietary specialization such as differential inducibility of P450s and other biotransformation enzymes by juniper, as well as differences in Phase 3 or gut microbiome metabolism.

2.6 Role of enzyme induction in species differences

To determine whether the generalist *N. albigula* is limited by the ability to up-regulate CYP2B, we recently designed a study where the generalist and specialist were fed either juniper to induce the expression of CYP2B (diet induction) or injected with phenobarbital a potent inducer of CYP2B (pharmacological induction; Waxman & Azaroff, 1992) and then fed a high juniper diet (60%). *N. albigula* consumed a similar amount of juniper and had a similar amount of CYP2B enzyme as *N. stephensi* after the diet treatment but not after the pharmacological treatment (Fig. 6A). However,

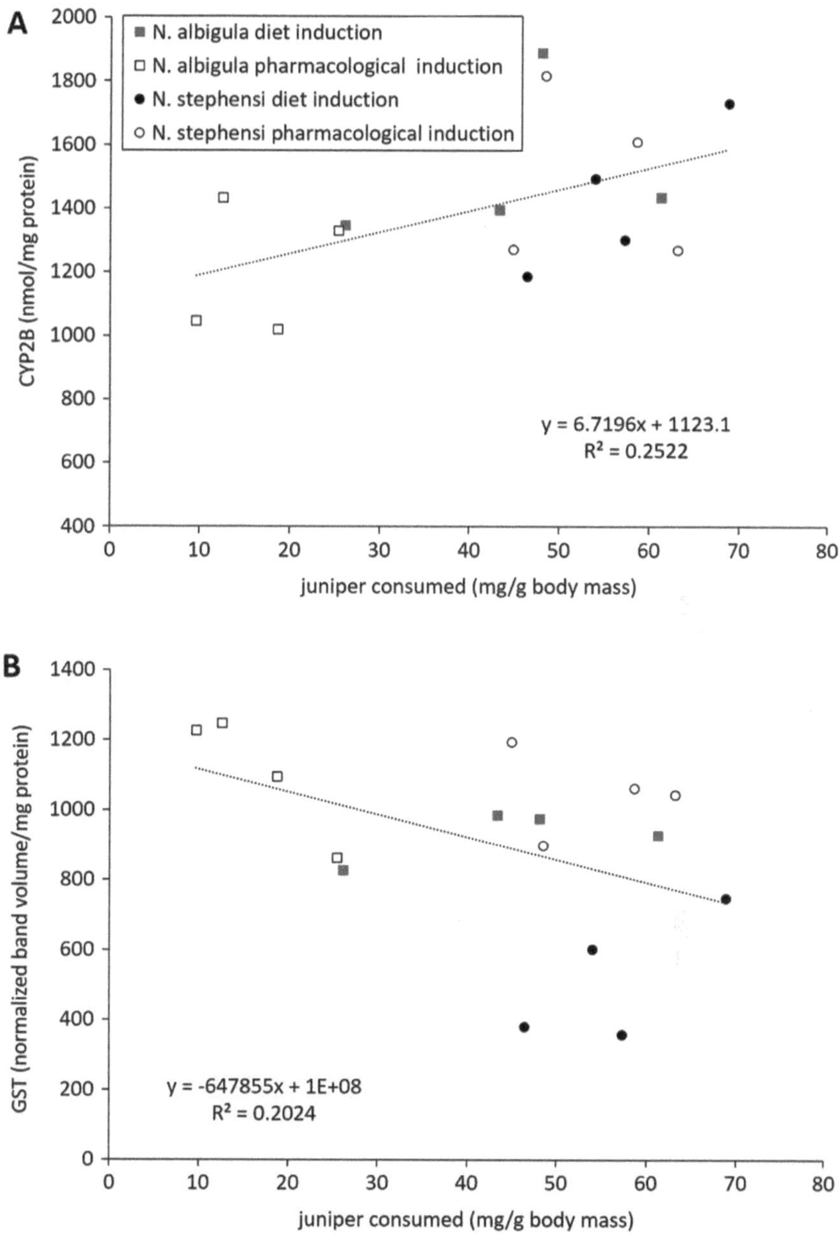

Fig. 6 Correlation between juniper consumption and protein content of CYP2B or GST in liver of woodrats. The generalist, *N. albigula* (squares, $n = 4$ each treatment) and specialist, *N. stephensi* (circles, $n = 4$ each treatment) were either fed increasing amounts of juniper for 4 days (10% juniper for 2 days and 30% juniper for 2 days, diet induction, filled symbols) or given intraperitoneal injections of phenobarbital (80 mg/kg) for 4 days (pharmacological induction, open symbols) to induce the production of CYP2B. Juniper consumed (mg juniper/g body mass) was calculated based on 3 days dry matter intakes of a 60% juniper diet. (A) CYP2B protein content in the liver of the woodrats (as measured by Western blot) is positively correlated with juniper consumption ($R^2 = 0.25$, $P = 0.039$). (B) cytosolic GST Ya protein content in the liver of woodrats (as measured by Western blot) is negatively correlated with juniper consumption ($R^2 = 0.20$, $P = 0.043$).

N. albigula was unable to maintain body mass on the 60% juniper diet, and therefore in nature would only be able to consume such a high level of juniper for a few days. We found, in addition to increased expression of CYP2B on high juniper diets, *N. stephensi* also shows lower expression of the cytosolic phase II glutathione S-transferases (GSTs) compared to *N. abigula* (Fig. 6B; Haley et al., 2007; Skopec et al., 2007).

3. Conclusion

3.1 Summary of main results

As hoped, the genus *Neotoma* has proved to be an outstanding system for studying the role of P450 enzymes, especially CYP2B, in the normal physiology of mammalian herbivores. Based on the biochemical tradeoff hypothesis (Freeland & Janzen, 1974) that provided the initial impetus for the work, we expected that the obligate specialist *N. stephensi* and facultative specialist *N. lepida* would have evolved P450 enzymes with enhanced function to facilitate efficient catalysis of the major monoterpenes present in juniper, including α-pinene. Moreover, we expected a reduction in the ability to transform novel compounds—those that differ chemically from compounds typically found in the specialist's diet—based on previous work documenting signs of toxicosis in the specialist, *N. stephensi,* fed novel diets containing resin from creosote bush (Sorensen, McLister, & Dearing, 2005a, 2005b; (Torregrossa et al., 2012)). Experimentally, we found little difference in liver microsomal α-pinene turnover between specialists and generalists but higher levels of total CYP2B enzymes in the specialist on a control or 30% juniper diet.

By employing technologies that were not even imaginable in 1974, we found some remarkable differences in gene copy number and genomic structures of CYP2B in specialist vs generalist woodrats. The greater gene copy number coupled with less sequence variation in the specialist is consistent with specialization to a narrow range of PSMs and may underpin the ability of the specialist to express higher quantities of CYP2B enzyme when feeding on high quantities of juniper. CYP2B in the generalist appears to be under selection for differentiation, likely as a result of its highly varied diet. Short-term feeding trials with >30% juniper suggest that the generalist *N. albigula* is not limited by its ability to up-regulate CYP2B, but rather that some physiological change occurs leading to failure to continue to consume the diet.

Our current working hypothesis is that some of the CYP2B enzymes in *N. stephensi* produce non-toxic metabolites that do not need to be conjugated by GST. The P450 enzymes of other specialist herbivores (e.g., koalas, ringtail possum) polyoxygenate terpenes to a greater extent than generalist mammals and with negligible conjugation (reviewed in Dearing, Foley, & McLean, 2005). The extra CYP2B gene copies of specialist woodrats may enable such extensive oxidation without much need for conjugation, and may explain why *N. stephensi* excretes half as much glucuronic acid as does *N. albigula* on the same amount of juniper (Sorensen et al., 2005b). Duplication of CYP2B genes in the specialist would then mimic the well-studied CYP2D6 duplications in humans, where gene copy number correlates with and predicts the ability to metabolize drugs, and is postulated to have resulted from selection pressure to detoxify plant alkaloids in the diet (Ingelman-Sundberg, 2005). These results highlight the importance of further study into the different isoforms of CYP2B produced by woodrats.

3.2 Reflections

It is more than 40 years since one of us (JRH) first started studying rat CYP2B1. During those four decades, my research group performed in depth studies of the structure and function of CYP2B enzymes in rats, rabbits, dogs, and humans. After solving over 30 X-ray crystal structures and publishing more than 100 peer-reviewed articles on the above CYP2B enzymes, I would have thought that nothing about the sub-family would surprise me. I was very wrong!

I embarked on the collaborative studies with Denise Dearing in 2011 with the mindset that there might be a handful of CYP2B enzymes in woodrats, and that through the same basic approaches that had been successful until then, we would be able to decipher the reason why some woodrat species and/or populations could specialize on juniper with its high content of monoterpenes. In retrospect, I am grateful that we completely under-estimated the number of woodrat CYP2B genes. Otherwise, we would have never started to characterize only three of the enzymes from *N. lepida*. Fortuitously, one of them in particular, namely CYP2B35, turned out to be highly unusual in its substrate specificity, largely due to the unique presence of the small Ala residues at SRS positions 363 and 367. In addition, reciprocal mutagenesis studies of CYP2B35 and CYP2B37 yielded our first ever multiple CYP2B mutant with enhanced activity toward substrates of both parental enzymes. Equally fortuitously, the novel CYP2B gene island in *N. lepida* is comprised solely of variable numbers of duplicated genes most similar to CYP2B37. Very interesting to me after decades of studying human CYP2B6 was that these studies on a novel species—the woodrat—prompted us to explore monoterpene interactions with the human enzyme. Because of the extremely high affinity of CYP2B enzymes, including CYP2B6, for monoterpenes, they yielded high resolution crystals and were very amenable to thermodynamic studies. Through such studies, we were able to obtain our first evidence that the conformational plasticity of CYP2B enzyme that we had identified with model inhibitors had real significance for the thermodynamics of binding of these small, pure hydrocarbons. Furthermore, the high affinity of CYP2B enzymes for terpenes observed across a wide range of species is suggestive of an ancient relationship between CYP2B and terpenes, and that terpenes may have been one of the original substrates shaping the evolution of this sub-family. Thus, the basic science conducted on woodrat P450s served to inform our understanding of drug metabolism in humans.

The most unexpected finding for me came from Dr. Dearing studies of the *N. lepida* and *N. bryanti* genomes. Although there were preliminary indications of much higher CYP2B gene copy number in woodrat specialists than in other woodrat species, only the most recent genomic *structures* could provide definitive information. The expansion of the CYP2B sub-family presented above, as well as of the CYP2A and CYP3A subfamilies, and evolution of multiple novel gene islands within the CYP2B and CYP3A subfamilies is a remarkable discovery that opens up a multitude of avenues for new research.

3.3 Future directions

One promising direction for the future is an examination of the metabolites generated from monoterpenes by different woodrat CYP2B enzymes. Very early work in Dr. Dearing's laboratory in the late 1990s revealed an overall difference in the types of metabolites produced by *N. stephensi* and *N. albigula* fed α-pinene. Unfortunately, the metabolite libraries at the time did not facilitate identification of these metabolites aside from myrtenic acid. However, current analytical approaches could examine this hypothesis in engineered woodrat CYP2B enzymes. We hope this chapter spurs interest along these lines! Additionally, whole organism studies could examine through standard measurements of transaminases in the blood whether *N. albigula* incurs liver damage when forced to feed on juniper diets for long periods of time. The application of new gene editing techniques such as

CRISPR (Doudna & Charpentier, 2014) may enable alteration of P450 genes either in woodrats (which would take more development) or by inserting woodrat P450s into model species such as *M. musculus* to further explore the function of woodrat P450 enzymes. Additionally, the use of liver organoids (Harrison et al., 2021) may facilitate high-throughput and multi-substrate studies to understand the standing variation observed in woodrat CYP2B genes across individuals and the functional nature of this diversity.

Dr. Dearing and Dr. Skopec's research groups are currently applying genomic approaches to understand the genetic mechanisms enabling woodrats to feed on plants high in PSMs. The high copy number of detoxification enzymes discovered in the genomes of *N. lepida* and *N. bryanti* underscores the need for more high-quality genomes for the species-rich and diet-diverse genus *Neotoma*, particularly that of the specialist, *N. stephensi* and generalist, *N. albigula*, to fully understand the evolution of detoxification enzymes with respect to diet breadth. Moreover, newer longer read sequencing and genomic techniques should permit us to determine which CYP2B isoforms the generalist and specialist species up-regulate in response to juniper consumption—this would be a tremendous advancement from the early days of cloning and sequencing CYP2B. Finally, preliminary results from over 200 woodrat genomes (low coverage) implicate P450s other than CYP2B in the ability of woodrats to feed on creosote and its rich complement of PSMs such as phenolics.

In closing, the evolutionary arms race between woodrats and PSMs has in essence resulted in natural P450 mutagenesis screens, honed over the millennia, for different enzyme function and across a wide range of substrates (terpenes, phenolics, alkaloids). As such, mammalian herbivores in general offer myriad P450 diversity and an opportunity to understand P450s in context with the substrates that have shaped enzyme structure and function. Woodrats, with >20 species that feed on different PSMs and are easily kept in captivity, offer a superlative system for these studies of mammalian P450 biodiversity. We hope this work will spur the interest of current trainees to pursue future studies of P450 enzymes in woodrats.

Acknowledgments

We are grateful to the many creative members of research teams and our funding agencies for support of this work. M.D.D. thanks the National Science Foundation for multiple awards (0079865, 0236402, 0817527, 1256383, 1656497) and the University of Utah. J.R.H. thanks the NSF (1256480). We thank Dr. Sara Weinstein and Dylan Klure for the image of Meliodas, the woodrat in Fig. 1 and Dr. Robert Greenhalgh for creating Fig. 2.

Conflict of interest statement

The authors have no conflicts of interest to declare.

References

Adams, R. P., Beauchamp, P. S., Dev, V., & Dutz, S. M. (2007). New natural products isolated from one-seeded *Juniperus* of the southwestern United States: Isolation and occurrence of 2-ethenyl-3-methyl phenol and its derivatives. *Journal of Essential Oil Research, 19*, 146–152.

Campbell, M., Oakeson, K. F., Yandell, M., Halpert, J. R., & Dearing, D. (2016). The draft genome sequence and annotation of the desert woodrat *Neotoma lepida*. *Genome Data, 9*, 58–59. 27408812. https://doi.org/10.1016/j.gdata.2016.06.008.

Dearing, M. D., Foley, W. J., & McLean, S. (2005). The influence of plant secondary metabolites on the nutritional ecology of herbivorous terrestrial vertebrates. *Annual Review of Ecology Evolution and Systematics, 36*, 169–189. ISI:000234684900008.

De-Oliveira, A. C. A. X. F., Ribeiro-Pinto, L., & Paumgartten, F. J. R. (1997). *In vitro* inhibition of CYP2B1 monooxygenase by β-myrcene and other monoterpenoid compounds. *Toxicology Letters, 92*(1), 39–46. https://doi.org/10.1016/s0378-4274(97)00034-9.

Dial, K. P. (1988). Three sympatric species of *Neotoma*: Dietary specialization and coexisitence. *Oecologia, 76*, 531–537. https://doi.org/10.1007/BF00397865.

Doudna, J. A., & Charpentier, E. (2014). The new frontier of genome engineering with CRISPR-Cas9. *Science, 346*(6213), 1258096. https://doi.org/10.1126/science.1258096.

Duignan, D. B., Sipes, I. G., Ciaccio, P. J., & Halpert, J. R. (1988). The metabolism of xenobiotics and endogenous compounds by the constitutive dog liver cytochrome P450 PBD-2. *Archives of Biochemistry and Biophysics, 267*(1), 294–304. https://doi.org/10.1016/0003-9861(88)90035-5.

Duignan, D. B., Sipes, I. G., Leonard, T. B., & Halpert, J. R. (1987). Purification and characterization of the dog hepatic cytochrome P-450 isozyme responsible for the metabolism of 2,2′,4,4′,5,5′-hexachlorobiphenyl. *Archives of Biochemistry and Biophysics, 255*(2), 290–303. https://doi.org/10.1016/0003-9861(87)90396-1.

Ehrlich, P. R., & Raven, P. (1964). Butterflies and plants: A study in coevolution. *Evolution, 18*, 586–608.

Freeland, W. J., & Janzen, D. H. (1974). Strategies in herbivory by mammals: The role of plant secondary compounds. *The American Naturalist, 108*(961), 269–289.

Gay, S. C., Shah, M. B., Talakad, J. C., Maekawa, K., Roberts, A. G., Wilderman, P. R., et al. (2010). Crystal structure of a cytochrome P450 2B6 genetic variant in complex with the inhibitor 4-(4-Chlorophenyl)imidazole at 2.0-Å resolution. *Molecular Pharmacology*, 77(4), 529–538. https://doi.org/10.1124/mol.109.062570.

Goodman, T., Grice, H. C., Becking, G. C., & Salem, F. A. (1970). A cystic nephropathy induced by nordihydroguaiaretic acid in the rat. Light and electron microscopic investigations. *Laboratory Investigation, 23*(1), 93–107 (5431225).

Graves, P. E., Elhag, G. A., Ciaccio, P. J., Bourque, D. P., & Halpert, J. R. (1990). cDNA and deduced amino acid sequences of a dog hepatic cytochrome P450IIB responsible for the metabolism of 2,2′,4,4′,5,5′-hexachlorobiphenyl. *Archives of Biochemistry and Biophysics, 281*(1), 106–115. https://doi.org/10.1016/0003-9861(90)90419-Y.

Greenhalgh, R., Holding, M. L., Orr, T. J., Henderson, J. B., Parchman, T. L., Matocq, M. D., et al. (2022). Trio-binned genomes of the woodrats *Neotoma bryanti* and *N. lepida* reveal novel gene islands and rapid copy number evolution of xenobiotic metabolizing cytochrome p450 genes. *Molecular Ecology Resources*, In press. https://doi.org/10.1111/1755-0998.13650.

Hahn, M. W. (2009). Distinguishing among evolutionary models for the maintenance of gene duplicates. *Journal of Heredity, 100*(5), 605–617. https://doi.org/10.1093/jhered/esp047.

Haley, S. L., Lamb, J. G., Franklin, M. R., Constance, J. E., & Dearing, M. D. (2008). Pharm-ecology of diet shifting: Biotransformation of plant secondary compounds in creosote (*Larrea tridentata*) by a woodrat herbivore, *Neotoma lepida. Physiological Biochemistry and Zoology, 81*, 584–593. https://doi.org/10.1086/589951.

Haley, S. L., Lamb, J. G., Franklin, M. R., Constance, J. E., & Denise Dearing, M. (2007). Xenobiotic metabolism of plant secondary compounds in juniper (*Juniperus monosperma*) by specialist and generalist woodrat herbivores, genus *Neotoma. Comparative Biochemistry and Physiology C Toxicology and Pharmacology, 146*(4), 552–560. 17681888 https://doi.org/10.1016/j.cbpc.2007.06.007.

Harrison, S. P., Baumgarten, S. F., Verma, R., Lunov, O., Dejneka, A., & Sullivan, G. J. (2021). Liver organoids: Recent developments, limitations and potential. *Frontiers in Medicine, 8*, 574047. https://doi.org/10.3389/fmed.2021.574047.

Hasler, J. A., Harlow, G. R., Szklarz, G. D., John, G. H., Kedzie, K. M., Burnett, V. L., et al. (1994). Site-directed mutagenesis of putative substrate recognition sites in cytochrome P450 2B11: Importance of amino acid residues 114, 290, and 363 for substrate specificity. *Molecular Pharmacology, 46*(2), 338–345, (8078495).

Hiroi, T., Miyazaki, Y., Kobayashi, Y., Imaoka, S., & Funae, Y. (1995). Induction of hepatic P450s in rat by essential wood and leaf oils. *Xenobiotica, 25*(5), 457–467. (7571719) https://doi.org/10.3109/00498259509061865.

Hu, S., Wang, H., Knisely, A. A., Reddy, S., Kovacevic, D., Liu, Z., et al. (2008). Evolution of the CYP2ABFGST gene cluster in rat, and a fine-scale comparison among rodent and primate species. *Genetica, 133*(2), 215–226, (17876710). https://doi.org/10.1007/s10709-007-9206-x.

Huo, L., Liu, J., Dearing, M. D., Szklarz, G. D., Halpert, J. R., & Wilderman, P. R. (2017). Rational re-engineering of the O-dealkylation of 7-alkoxycoumarin derivatives by cytochromes P450 2B from the desert woodrat *Neotoma lepida. Biochemistry, 56*(16), 2238–2246, (28375626). https://doi.org/10.1021/acs.biochem.7b00097.

Ingelman-Sundberg, M. (2005). Genetic polymorphisms of cytochrome P450 2D6 (CYP2D6): Clinical consequences, evolutionary aspects and functional diversity. *The Pharmacogenomics Journal, 5*(1), 6–13. https://doi.org/10.1038/sj.tpj.6500285.

Jang, H.-H., Davydov, D. R., Lee, G.-Y., Yun, C.-H., & Halpert, J. R. (2014). The role of cytochrome P450 2B6 and 2B4 substrate access channel residues predicted based on crystal structures of the amlodipine complexes. *Archives of Biochemistry and Biophysics, 545*, 100–107. https://doi.org/10.1016/j.abb.2014.01.008.

Lamb, J. G., Marick, P., Sorensen, J., Haley, S., & Dearing, M. D. (2004). Liver biotransforming enzymes in woodrats *Neotoma stephensi* (Muridae). *Comparative Biochemistry and Physiology, Part C, 138*(2), 195–201, (15450867). https://doi.org/10.1016/j.cca.2004.07.003.

Lamb, J. G., Sorensen, J. S., & Dearing, M. D. (2001). Comparison of detoxification enzyme mRNAs in woodrats (*Neotoma lepida*) and laboratory rats. *Journal of Chemical Ecology, 27*(4), 845–857, (11446304). https://doi.org/10.1023/a:1010366322299.

Lewis, D. F. V., & Lake, B. G. (1997). Molecular modelling of mammalian CYP2B isoforms and their interaction with substrates, inhibitors and redox partners. *Xenobiotica, 27*(5), 443–478. https://doi.org/10.1080/004982597240433.

Mabry, T. J., Difeo, D. R. J., Sakakibara, M., Bohnstedt, C. F. J., & Seigler, D. (1977). The natural products chemistry of *Larrea*. In T. J. H. H. Mabry, & J. R. D. R. Difeo (Eds.), *Creosote Bush. Biology and Chemistry of Larrea in New World Deserts. Xvi + 284p. Illus. Maps: Vol. 6. Us/Ibp (International Biological Program) Synthesis Series* (pp. 115–134). Stroudsburg, PA., USA: Dowden, Hutchinson and Ross, Inc. (Dist. By Academic Press: New York,

N.Y., USA; London, Encland). Isbn 0-87933-282-4. 1977. (PREV197815053986 Copyright BIOSIS 2003.).

Magnanou, E., Malenke, J. R., & Dearing, M. D. (2009). Expression of biotransformation genes in woodrat (*Neotoma*) herbivores on novel and ancestral diets: Identification of candidate genes responsible for dietary shifts. *Molecular Ecology*, *18*(11), 2401–2414, (19389177). https://doi.org/10.1111/j.1365-294X.2009.04171.x.

Malenke, J. R., Magnanou, E., Thomas, K., & Dearing, M. D. (2012). Cytochrome P450 2B diversity and dietary novelty in the herbivorous, desert woodrat (*Neotoma lepida*). *PLoS One*, 7(8), e41410. https://doi.org/10.1371/journal.pone.0041510.

Mangione, A. M., Dearing, M. D., & Karasov, W. H. (2000). Interpopulation differences in tolerance to creosote bush resin in desert woodrats (*Neotoma lepida*). *Ecology*, *81*(8), 2067–2076, (ISI:000088888900002).

Marsh, K. J., Wallis, I. R., Andrew, R. L., & Foley, W. J. (2006). The detoxification limitation hypothesis: Where did it come from and where is it going? *Journal of Chemical Ecology*, *32*(6), 1247–1266, (16770716). https://doi.org/10.1007/s10886-006-9082-3.

Nebert, D. W., & Dieter, M. Z. (2000). The evolution of drug metabolism. *Pharmacology*, *61*, 124–135.

Nelson, D. R. (2003). Comparison of P450s from human and fugu: 420 million years of vertebrate P450 evolution. *Archives of Biochemistry and Biophysics*, *409*(1), 18–24, (12464240).

Nelson, D. R. (2011). Progress in tracing the evolutionary paths of cytochrome P450. *Biochimica et Biophysica Acta*, *1814*(1), 14–18.

Orr, T. J., Kitanovic, S., Schramm, K. M., Skopec, M. M., Wilderman, P. R., Halpert, J. R., et al. (2020). Strategies in herbivory by mammals revisited: The role of liver metabolism in a juniper specialist (*Neotoma stephensi*) and a generalist (*Neotoma albigula*). *Molecular Ecology*, *29*(9), 1674–1683. https://doi.org/10.1111/mec.15431.

Schuler, M. A. (2011). P450s in plant-insect interactions. *Biochimica et Biophysica Acta*, *1814*(1), 36–45 (20883828) https://doi.org/10.1016/j.bbapap.2010.09.012.

Shah, M. B., Liu, J., Huo, L., Zhang, Q., Dearing, M. D., Wilderman, P. R., et al. (2016). Structure-function analysis of mammalian CYP2B enzymes using 7-substituted coumarin derivatives as probes: Utility of crystal structures and molecular modeling in understanding xenobiotic metabolism. *Molecular Pharmacology*, *89*(4), 435–445 (26826176) https://doi.org/10.1124/mol.115.102111.

Shah, M. B., Liu, J., Zhang, Q., Stout, C. D., & Halpert, J. R. (2017). Halogen−π interactions in the cytochrome P450 active site: Structural insights into human CYP2B6 substrate selectivity. *American Chemical Society Chemical Biology*, *12*(5), 1204–1210. https://doi.org/10.1021/acschembio.7b00056.

Shah, M. B., Wilderman, P. R., Liu, J., Jang, H. H., Zhang, Q., Stout, C. D., et al. (2015). Structural and biophysical characterization of human cytochromes P450 2B6 and 2A6 bound to volatile hydrocarbons: Analysis and comparison. *Molecular Pharmacology*, *87*(4), 649–659, (25585967). https://doi.org/10.1124/mol.114.097014.

Shah, M. B., Wilderman, P. R., Pascual, J., Zhang, Q., Stout, C. D., & Halpert, J. R. (2012). Conformational adaptation of human cytochrome P450 2B6 and rabbit cytochrome P450 2B4 revealed upon binding multiple amlodipine molecules. *Biochemistry*, *51*(37), 7225–7238. https://doi.org/10.1021/bi300894z.

Skopec, M. M., Adams, R. P., & Muir, J. P. (2019). Terpenes may serve as feeding deterrents and foraging cues for mammalian herbivores. *Journal of Chemical Ecology*, *45*(11−12), 993–1003 (31755019) https://doi.org/10.1007/s10886-019-01117-w.

Skopec, M. M., Haley, S., & Dearing, M. D. (2007). Differential hepatic gene expression of a dietary specialist (*Neotoma stephensi*) and generalist (*Neotoma albigula*) in response to juniper (*Juniperus monosperma*) ingestion. *Comparative Biochemistry and Physiology Part D Genomics Proteomics*, *2*(1), 34–43, (20483276). https://doi.org/10.1016/j.cbd.2006.11.001.

Skopec, M. M., Kohl, K. D., Schramm, K., Halpert, J. R., & Dearing, M. D. (2015). Using the specialization framework to determine degree of dietary specialization in a herbivorous woodrat. *Journal of Chemical Ecology*, *41*(12), 1059–1068. https://doi.org/10.1007/s10886-015-0654-y.

Skopec, M. M., Malenke, J. R., Halpert, J. R., & Dearing, M. D. (2013). An in vivo assay for elucidating the importance of cytochromes P450 for the ability of a wild mammalian herbivore (*Neotoma lepida*) to consume toxic plants. *Physiological and Biochemical Zoology*, *86*(5), 595–601. https://doi.org/10.1086/672212.

Sorensen, J. S., McLister, J. D., & Dearing, M. D. (2005a). Novel plant secondary metabolites impact dietary specialists more than generalists. *Ecology*, *86*(1), 140–154. https://doi.org/10.1890/03-0669.

Sorensen, J. S., McLister, J. D., & Dearing, M. D. (2005b). Plant secondary metabolites compromise the energy budgets of specialist and generalist mammalian herbivores. *Ecology*, *86*(1), 125–139. https://doi.org/10.1890/03-0627.

Sorensen, J. S., Skopec, M. M., & Dearing, M. D. (2006). Application of pharmacological approaches to plant-mammal interactions. *Journal of Chemical Ecology*, *32*(6), 1229–1246, (16770715). https://doi.org/10.1007/s10886-006-9086-z.

Torregrossa, A-M., Azzara, A. V., & Dearing, M. D. (2012). Testing the diet-breadth trade-off hypothesis: Differential regulation of novel plant secondary compounds by a specialist and a generalist herbivore. *Oecologia*, *168*, 711–718. https://doi.org/10.1007/s00442-011-2121-y.

Torregrossa, A.-M., & Dearing, M. D. (2009b). Nutritional toxicology of mammals: Regulated intake of plant secondary compounds. *Functional Ecology*, *23*(1), 48–56. https://doi.org/10.1111/j.1365-2435.2008.01523.x.

Torregrossa, A-M., & Dearing, M. D. (2009a). Caching as a behavioral mechanism to reduce toxin intake. *Journal of Mammalogy*, *904*(4), 803–810. https://doi.org/10.1644/08-MAMM-A-261.1.

Van Devender, T. R. (1977). Holocene woodlands in the southwestern deserts. *Science*, *198*, 189–192.

Vaughn, T. A. (1982). Stephen's woodrat, a dietary specialist. *Journal of Mammalogy*, *63*, 53–62. https://doi.org/10.2307/1380671.

Waxman, D. J., & Azaroff, L. (1992). Phenobarbital induction of cytochrome *P*-450 gene expression. *Biochemical Journal*, *281*(3), 577–592. https://doi.org/10.1042/bj2810577.

Weinstein, S. B., Martínez-Mota, R., Stapleton, T. E., Klure, D. M., Greenhalgh, R., Orr, T. J., et al. (2021). Microbiome stability and structure is governed by host phylogeny over diet and geography in woodrats (*Neotoma* spp.). *Proceedings of the National Academy of Science of the United States of America*, *118*(47), e2108787118. https://doi.org/10.1073/pnas.2108787118.

Wilderman, P. R., & Halpert, J. R. (2012). Plasticity of CYP2B enzymes: Structural and solution biophysical methods. *Current Drug Metabolism*, *13*(2), 167–176.

Wilderman, P. R., Jang, H. H., Malenke, J. R., Salib, M., Angermeier, E., Lamime, S., et al. (2014). Functional characterization of cytochromes P450 2B from the desert woodrat *Neotoma lepida*. *Toxicology and Applied Pharmacology*, *274*(3), 393–401 (24361551) https://doi.org/10.1016/j.taap.2013.12.005.

Wilderman, P. R, Shah, M. B., Jang, H-H., Stout, D., & Halpert, J. R. (2013). Structural and thermodynamic basis of (+)-α-pinene binding to human cytochrome P450 2B6. *Journal of the American Chemical Society*, *135*, 10433–10440. https://doi.org/10.1021/ja403042k.

CHAPTER FIVE

Atypical kinetics of cytochrome P450 enzymes in pharmacology and toxicology

Jacqueline Wen Hui Leow, Lloyd Wei Tat Tang, and Eric Chun Yong Chan*

Department of Pharmacy, Faculty of Science, National University of Singapore, Singapore, Singapore
*Corresponding author: e-mail address: phaccye@nus.edu.sg

Contents

Abstract

Atypical kinetics are observed in metabolic reactions catalyzed by cytochrome P450 enzymes (P450). Yet, this phenomenon is regarded as experimental artifacts in some instances despite increasing evidence challenging the assumptions of typical Michaelis-Menten kinetics. As P450 play a major role in the metabolism of a wide range of substrates including drugs and endogenous compounds, it becomes critical to consider the impact of atypical kinetics on the accuracy of estimated kinetic and inhibitory parameters which could affect extrapolation of pharmacological and toxicological implications. The first half of this book chapter will focus on atypical non-Michaelis-Menten kinetics (*e.g.* substrate inhibition, biphasic and sigmoidal kinetics) as well as proposed underlying mechanisms supported by recent insights in mechanistic enzymology. In particular, substrate inhibition kinetics in P450 as well as concurrent drug inhibition of P450 in the presence of substrate inhibition will be further discussed.

Advances in Pharmacology, Volume 95
ISSN 1054-3589
https://doi.org/10.1016/bs.apha.2022.05.003

Moreover, mounting evidence has revealed that despite the high degree of sequence homology between CYP3A isoforms (*i.e.* CYP3A4 and CYP3A5), they have the propensities to exhibit vastly different susceptibilities and potencies of mechanism-based inactivation (MBI) with a common drug inhibitor. These experimental observations pertaining to the presence of these atypical isoform- and probe substrate-specific complexities in CYP3A isoforms by several clinically-relevant drugs will therefore be expounded and elaborated upon in the second half of this book chapter.

Abbreviations

CPR	Cytochrome P450 reductase
HLM	Human liver microsomes
IVIVE	*In vitro* to *in vivo* extrapolation
k_{inact}	maximum inactivation rate constant
K_i	inhibition constant
K_I	concentration of inactivator at half-maximum inactivation rate constant
K_m	substrate concentration at half maximal velocity
K_s	substrate inhibition constant
MBI	mechanism-based inactivation
NADPH	nicotinamide adenine dinucleotide phosphate
P450	Cytochrome P450 enzyme
RI	reversible inhibition
$[S]$	substrate concentration
V_{max}	maximal velocity
v	velocity

1. Introduction

The kinetic profiling of cytochrome P450 enzyme (P450)-mediated drug metabolism and interactions continue to be extensively studied (Guengerich, 2019) and relevant in many areas of pharmacology and toxicology including academia, drug discovery and regulatory domains (Guengerich, 2021). Primarily, the quantitation of the rate and extent of drug metabolism by P450 aids in the prediction of its systemic clearance and detoxication of drugs from the human body (Emoto, Murayama, Rostami-Hodjegan, & Yamazaki, 2010). In certain scenarios whereby P450-mediated metabolism of a drug forms an active metabolite which possesses pharmacological or toxic effects, the characterization of metabolite formation kinetics is additionally essential in the determination of its exposure. The experimental derivation of *in vitro* inhibitory parameters also aids in defining the degree of perpetrator drug inhibition or inactivation of P450 involved in victim drug disposition for an accurate extrapolation of the likelihood of significant drug-drug interaction (DDI) and exposure-dependent toxicity.

On another note, there has also been rising interest in the physiological and pathological functions of P450 involved in the metabolism of endogenous substances comprising hormones and fatty acids as substrates (Pikuleva & Waterman, 2013; Rendic & Guengerich, 2021). These endogenous substrates and their P450-derived metabolites have been shown to possess diverse biological activities and functions such as cardiac effects associated with eicosanoids (Jamieson, Endo, Darwesh, Samokhvalov, & Seubert, 2017). Moreover, P450 have also been implicated in the pathogenesis and progression of diseases such as diabetes (Elfaki, Mir, Almutairi, & Abu Duhier, 2018) and liver disorders (Shoieb, El-Ghiaty, Alqahtani, & El-Kadi, 2020). In particular, CYP19A1 and CYP17A1 are implicated in estrogen receptor-positive breast cancer (Friesenhengst, Pribitzer-Winner, Miedl, Pröstling, & Schreiber, 2018) and prostate cancer (Giatromanolaki et al., 2019), respectively, and have become drug targets for the management of these conditions (Guengerich, 2017). Hence, the accurate understanding of the metabolic and inhibitory kinetics of P450 associated with both drugs and endogenous substrates becomes important in drug discovery, pathophysiology, pharmacology and toxicology research.

The cornerstone of modern enzymatic kinetic analysis has remained largely unchanged since 1913 when the work of Leonor Michaelis and Maud Menten led to the inception and widespread applications of the Michaelis-Menten equation (Michaelis & Menten, 1913; Michaelis, Menten, Johnson, & Goody, 2011). The Michaelis-Menten equation and associated assumptions also set the foundation for the development and application of enzyme inhibition kinetic equations for reversible inhibition (RI) and mechanism-based inactivation (MBI). Hence, the almost habitual practice of assuming Michaelis-Menten kinetics, for all enzymatic reactions including P450-mediated reactions, continues to persist in the scientific community despite reports of atypical enzymatic kinetics associated with both drugs and endogenous substances. The frequent dismissal of atypical kinetics could be due to its perception as an *in vitro* artifact or lack of translation to *in vivo* consequences which further encourages forceful fitting and analysis of experimental data using the Michaelis-Menten equation. Therefore, increasing the mechanistic understanding of non-Michaelis-Menten atypical kinetics becomes vital in order to change the current narrative and investigate their significance.

Notably, the pharmacological implications of atypical kinetics should not be disregarded. For instance, the lack of consideration of underlying atypical kinetics could potentially affect the accuracy and performance of *in vitro* to *in vivo* extrapolation (IVIVE) of kinetic or inhibition parameters, which are scaled and integrated to derive physiologically-relevant parameters (*e.g.* hepatic clearance) for the prediction of *in vivo* outcomes (Chao, Uss, & Cheng, 2010). This could have major downstream consequences given the increasing adoption of physiologically-based pharmacokinetic and quantitative systems pharmacology modeling by pharmaceutical companies and regulatory authorities (Hariparsad et al., 2021). The successful development and validation of these models *via* bottom-up or middle-out approaches depend heavily on the assimilation of accurate mechanistic *in vitro* data before it can be applied and translated into real-world decisions (*e.g.* dose determination for first-in-human trials and waivers for clinical DDI studies) (Jamei, 2016; Tsamandouras, Rostami-Hodjegan, & Aarons, 2015). In the case of drug inhibitors targeting P450 as a mechanism of action, it is equally critical to consider atypical kinetics of specific substrates involved in the disease of interest, to obtain accurate estimations of drug inhibitor potencies and prediction of pharmacotherapeutic effect. Furthermore, it is plausible that toxicological implications of atypical kinetics could surface given that P450 is also involved in the formation of toxic metabolites from drugs (Guengerich, 2021). Off-target inhibition of P450 by drugs may also perturb endogenous metabolism and physiological levels of bioactive metabolites and culminate in adverse events. These scenarios collectively highlight the importance of accurately defining atypical Michaelis-Menten kinetics to address the pharmacological and toxicological implications.

This chapter will attempt to discuss current proposed mechanisms and supporting evidence of atypical Michaelis-Menten kinetics from recent advances in mechanistic enzymology research. A focus on substrate inhibition kinetics of the interactions between drugs and endogenous substrates implicating P450 will be explored. Furthermore, atypical complexities in MBI of P450 with a focus on probe substrate- and isoform-dependent inactivation of CYP3A enzymes will be discussed.

2. Atypical Michaelis-Menten kinetics and proposed mechanisms

It is well established that an enzymatic reaction adheres to typical Michaelis-Menten kinetics when the velocity (v) of the reaction plotted

Table 1 Graphical representations and steady-state empirical mathematical equations for typical and atypical Michaelis-Menten kinetics.

Kinetic profile	Graphical representation of *v* against [S][a]	Eadie-Hofstee plot of *v* against *v*/[S]	Steady-state empirical equation
Typical			
Michaelis-Menten kinetics	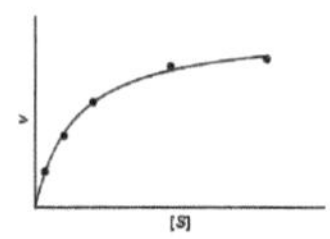	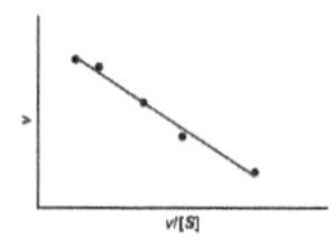	$v = \frac{V_{max}[S]}{K_m + [S]}$
Atypical			
Biphasic kinetics	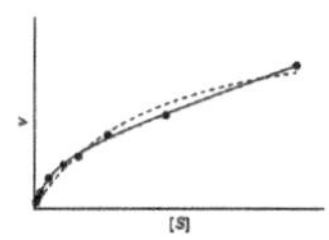	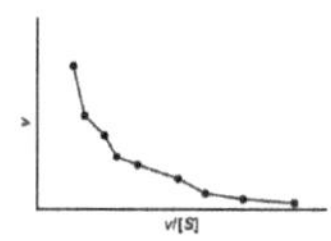	$v = \frac{V_{max(1)}[S] + \frac{V_{max(2)}}{K_{m(2)}}[S]^2}{K_{m(1)} + [S]}$
Substrate inhibition kinetics			
Partial	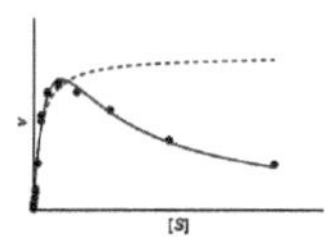	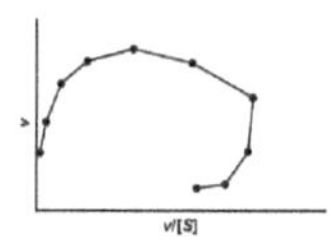	$v = \frac{V_{max}[S]}{K_m + [S]\left(1 + \frac{[S]}{K_s}\right)}$
Complete	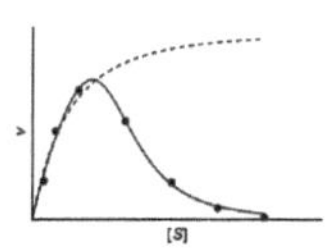	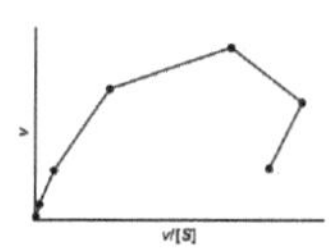	$v = \frac{V_{max}[S]}{K_m + [S]\left(1 + \frac{[S]^n}{K_s^n}\right)}$
Positive cooperative (sigmoidal) kinetics	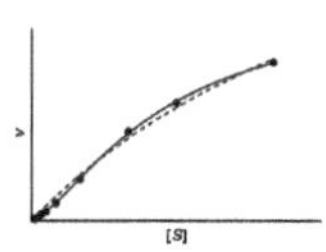	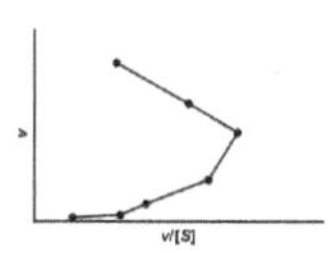	$v = \frac{V_{max}[S]^n}{K'^n + [S]^n}$

[a]Dotted lines for atypical kinetic profiles represent the fitted Michaelis-Menten relationships.
v = velocity; [S] = substrate concentration; V_{max} = maximal velocity; K_m = substrate concentration at half maximal velocity; K_s = substrate inhibition constant; n = Hill's coefficient; K′ = an associated parameter to K_m comprising additional interaction factors involved.

against increasing substrate concentrations ([*S*]) gives rise to a hyperbolic saturable curve approaching zero-order kinetics. In contrast, atypical kinetics such as biphasic, substrate inhibition (partial and complete) and positive cooperative kinetics have differing graphical profiles as outlined in Table 1. Briefly, both biphasic and substrate inhibition kinetics generally demonstrate an initial hyperbolic curve at low [*S*]. However, saturation does not occur at higher [*S*] and a linear increase in *v* proportional to increasing [*S*] is observed in the former compared to a decline in *v* beyond a certain [*S*] in the latter. For positive cooperative kinetics, a characteristic sigmoidal saturation profile is obtained instead. It has also been demonstrated that more than one feature of atypical kinetics could occur simultaneously such as in the case of both initial sigmoidal characteristics at low [*S*] and substrate inhibition at high [*S*] being observed (Muller et al., 2015; Wang, Neiner, & Kharasch, 2019).

The accurate identification of atypical kinetics solely *via* visual interpretation of *v* against [*S*] graphs might be tricky, considering that the assessment would be highly dependent on the selection and range of [*S*] values used in the *in vitro* enzymatic incubations. While adopting a full [*S*] range consisting of both low and high values is generally a good practice for enzyme-based assays to determine *v* against [*S*], strategic sampling at low [*S*] may be necessary to unveil a sigmoidal saturation profile although this could be limited by analytical sensitivity to product formation. Conversely, strategic sampling of higher [*S*] would be more essential for the definition of both biphasic and substrate inhibition profiles which may be constrained by aqueous insolubility and cost issues. Hence, consideration regarding suitable sampling of [*S*] within a range of low to high values surrounding the estimated Michaelis-Menten constant or [*S*] at half maximal *v* (K_m), to be adopted in an *in vitro* enzymatic assay is critical to avoid the false impression of Michaelis-Menten kinetics whereby underlying atypical kinetics may be obfuscated. Beyond *v* against [*S*] graphs, the use of secondary transformed plots can also be a useful tool to supplement the diagnosis of the presence or absence of atypical kinetics. A common example is the Eadie-Hofstee plot which is a linear representation of typical Michaelis-Menten kinetics where *v* is expressed as a function of the ratio *v*/[*S*]. A deviation from linearity in the form of a characteristic hook in the upper corner of the Eadie-Hofstee plot is commonly used to identify substrate inhibition (Table 1). Other characteristic Eadie-Hofstee plots for biphasic and positive cooperative kinetics are also shown in Table 1.

Importantly, even in the presence of graphical representations of atypical kinetics, there also lies a need to determine if any potential artefactual contributions have been excluded which would otherwise obfuscate the conclusions. Namely, this pertains to any controllable experimental factor that could disrupt Michaelis-Menten assumptions of free ligand and steady state approximations such as excessive substrate depletion greater than 10%

at each [*S*] that affects apparent free [*S*], sequential metabolism in both homogenous (*e.g.*, recombinant enzymes) and heterogenous *in vitro* enzyme systems (*e.g.*, human liver microsomes (HLMs)) and saturable non-productive non-specific protein binding that leads to false positive conclusions of atypical kinetics (Leow & Chan, 2019). Therefore, it is imperative that atypical profiles should be reproducible across multiple *in vitro* enzyme concentrations to establish its kinetic validity. In the case of endogenous substrates such as polyunsaturated fatty acids, substrate-substrate interactions in the form of micelle formation due to its inherent amphiphilic characteristics could also lead to a reduction in apparent free [*S*] at concentrations above the critical micellar concentration. Hence, interpretation of v against [*S*] plots with reference to the known critical micellar concentration of the fatty acid substrate would help avoid inaccurate deductions of atypical kinetics. Atypical kinetics arising from the use of cell-based systems such as primary human hepatocytes and immortalized hepatocellular cell lines could also be confounded by the presence of active transporters which would lead to a disconnect between intracellular and medium [*S*]. These factors, among others discussed in literature (Leow & Chan, 2019; Tracy, 2006), should be determined to be non-confounders before experimental data can be investigated as possible atypical kinetics.

In addition, it becomes more ambiguous in the determination of artefactual atypical kinetics when contrasting profiles for the same enzyme-substrate reaction are derived from different *in vitro* enzymatic systems. For instance, CYP3A4 metabolism of midazolam to 1′-hydroxymidazolam in microsomes prepared from transfected human liver epithelial cells was shown to demonstrate typical Michaelis-Menten kinetics which contrasted against partial substrate inhibition kinetics observed with microsomes prepared from baculovirus-infected insect cells with or without co-expressed cytochrome b_5 (Christensen, Mathiesen, Postvoll, Winther, & Molden, 2009). This difference in metabolism kinetics despite near identical incubation conditions was suggested to be due to differences in membrane lipid compositions of *in vitro* enzymatic systems (Gibson, Wang, Varkhede, & Ma, 2021). Similar enzyme source effects were also observed for other P450 such as CYP2C9 metabolism of diclofenac (Kumar, Rock, Warren, Tracy, & Wahlstrom, 2006) as well as in other forms of atypical kinetics such as positive cooperativity in CYP3A4 (Z. Zhang et al., 2004). It was also noted by Christensen et al. that the absence of cytochrome b_5 led to a more pronounced substrate inhibition effect compared to the presence of cytochrome b_5. Subsequently, the same research group established that insect microsomes co-expressing similar levels of human CYP3A5 but with a 12-fold difference range in cytochrome P450 reductase (CPR) activity displayed Michaelis-Menten kinetics for the same reaction when CPR activity was lowest and substrate inhibition kinetics when CPR activity was intermediate to high (Christensen, Hestad, Molden, & Mathiesen, 2011). The mechanism of how varying levels of accessory proteins contribute to atypical kinetics remain unclear given that research is still ongoing to understand the implications of CPR and cytochrome b_5 on overall P450 activity (Heintze, Klein, Hofmann, & Zanger, 2021; Henderson, McLaughlin, & Wolf, 2013; Schulz, Kammerer, & Küpper, 2019). Moreover, limited data is available regarding physiological levels of these accessory proteins in normal human livers. For instance, existing studies report large interindividual variations in CPR and cytochrome b_5 protein expression levels of up to 12.8- and 19-fold differences, respectively, across HLM samples obtained from Chinese populations (Zhang et al., 2015, 2016). Taken together, more work needs to be performed to understand the physiological relevance of enzyme source effects including membrane lipid compositions and the roles and abundances of accessory proteins before conclusions can be made regarding the validity of atypical or typical Michaelis-Menten kinetics observed under different experimental conditions.

Steady-state equations have been developed to describe atypical kinetics as compiled in Table 1. While these equations have limited mechanistic molecular insights, they are conventionally applied to characterize atypical kinetics based on the Occam's razor principle. More mechanistic equations for the various atypical kinetics as well as corresponding kinetic schemes have also been developed and discussed extensively in existing literature, which are not the focus of this chapter (Houston & Galetin, 2005; Korzekwa, 2021; Leow & Chan, 2019; Shou et al., 2001; Wu, 2011). For example, two-site mathematical models have been established for substrate inhibition based on the assumption of two substrate-binding sites whereby one is reactive and the other is inhibitory (Wu, 2011). The identification and interrogation of reactive and inhibitory substrate-binding sites can potentially be performed *via* the use of complementary experimental techniques including *in silico* methods such as molecular dynamics (MD) simulations and *in vitro* methods such as site-directed mutagenesis and enzymatic assays (Denisov et al., 2019; Denisov, Grinkova, Camp, McLean, & Sligar, 2021; Muller et al., 2015; Tracy et al., 2002).

For substrates of CYP3A4 namely midazolam, ticlopidine and diazepam which displayed non-Michaelis-Menten kinetics, it has been demonstrated that multi-substrate binding models provided better fitting to *in vitro* metabolism data and marked improvement in *in vivo* clearance predictions compared to the use of the Michaelis-Menten equation (Paragas, Wang, Korzekwa, & Nagar, 2021). The use of numerical methods in solving ordinary or partial differential equations describing complex enzyme kinetics has also been proposed alternatively as a solution to overcome limitations of explicit equations when Michaelis-Menten assumptions do not hold (Yadav, Korzekwa, & Nagar, 2021). Additionally, this method could be useful in statistically distinguishing the presence of atypical kinetics from artefactual contributions. The use of such mechanistic equations in data analysis and discussion may be useful in supporting the generation of hypotheses regarding underlying mechanisms of atypical kinetics. However, as all hypothesized mechanisms have not been definitively proven, one should avoid confirming the underlying molecular mechanisms simply based on the premise that an ideal goodness-of-fit has been achieved using these mechanistic equations.

Various mechanisms for atypical kinetics have thus far been proposed which challenge the validity of the assumptions undertaken for typical Michaelis-Menten kinetics (Fig. 1). One key assumption is the existence and involvement of only one catalytic binding site for each subunit of enzyme. In contrast, the most popular proposed mechanism for various forms of atypical kinetics, as briefly mentioned in the previous paragraph, revolves around the possibility of multiple substrate binding within the active site or access channel of each subunit of enzyme. In the case of biphasic kinetics, it was suggested that two catalytically active binding sites could exist whereby the semi-hyperbolic pattern at lower $[S]$ is due to substrate binding to the low K_m and low maximal velocity (V_{max}) site while the linear phase at higher $[S]$ is due to substrate binding to the high K_m and high $V_{\max}$ site of the enzyme (Leow & Chan, 2019). Similarly, this can also be used to explain positive cooperativity or sigmoidal kinetics with different K_m and $V_{\max}$ values for individual binding sites. On the other hand, the presence of one catalytic and one inhibitory site has been proposed to lead to substrate inhibition. However, it is prudent to note that multiple substrate binding may not necessarily lead to the observation of atypical kinetics in all cases. In the event whereby the K_m and $V_{\max}$ of substrate binding at both binding sites are similar, this can culminate in typical Michaelis-Menten kinetics in an enzyme kinetics assay.

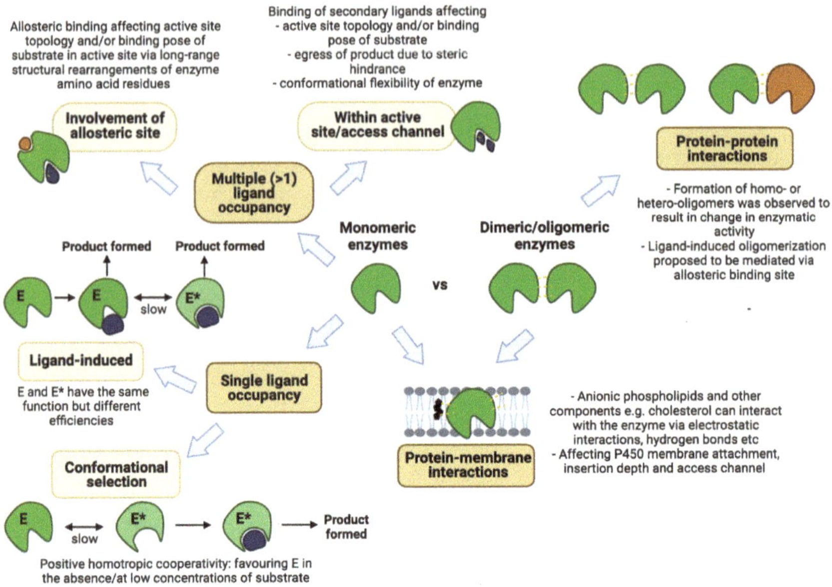

Fig. 1 Proposed mechanisms of atypical Michaelis-Menten kinetics including multiple substrate binding in active site, allosteric binding, protein-protein/protein-membrane interactions and ligand-induced or ligand-independent slow conformational change in enzyme.

Notably, X-ray crystallographic evidence is present for multiple ligand binding within the active sites of several P450 including CYP3A4 (Ekroos & Sjögren, 2006a), CYP2D6 (A. Wang, Stout, Zhang, & Johnson, 2015) and CYP21A2 (Zhao et al., 2012) for a diverse range of both drug-like and endogenous substrates. For example, CYP2C8 was co-crystallized with two 9-*cis*-retinoic acid moieties which were stacked upon each other within its large T- or Y-shaped active site (Fig. 2A and B) (Schoch et al., 2008). Despite such structural evidence, kinetic evidence of atypical kinetics has not been demonstrated for this reaction. Only one study reported kinetic parameters fitted to the Michaelis-Menten equation for this reaction but without the accompaniment of graphical data (Marill, Capron, Idres, & Chabot, 2002). On the other hand, although it was reported that biphasic kinetics appear to be observed for thioridazine S-oxidation by CYP2D6 along with X-ray crystallographic evidence of two thioridazine molecules co-crystallized with CYP2D6 (Wang et al., 2015), the authors still proceeded to fit the kinetic data to the Michaelis-Menten equation instead (Obach & Reed-Hagen, 2002).

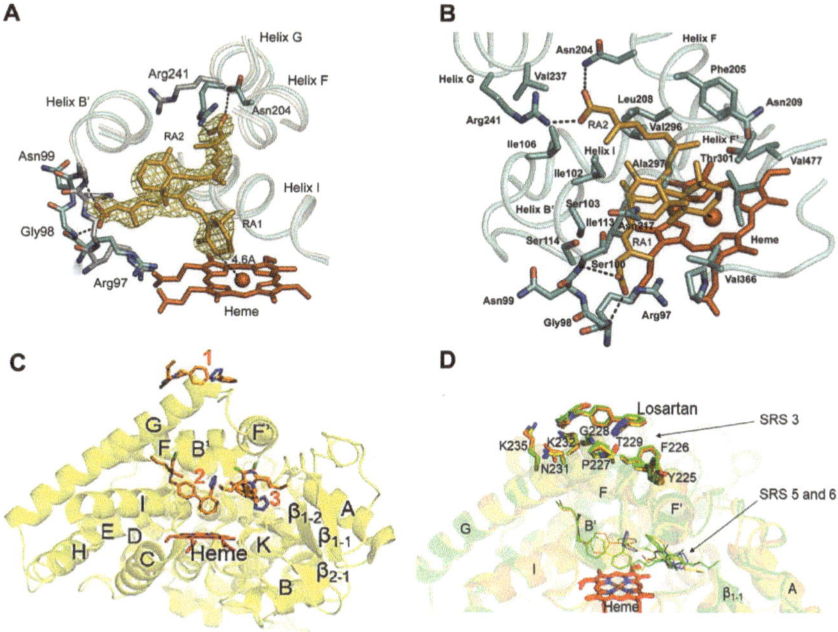

Fig. 2 Examples of X-ray crystallographic evidence of multiple ligand occupancy in cytochrome P450 enzymes either occurring within the active site or involving a distal allosteric site. (A and B) Ligand-binding site of cytochrome P450 2C8 illustrating interactions of two molecules 9-*cis*-retinoic acid within the active site of the protein. The substrates are depicted as stick figures with carbon atoms colored orange. Other atoms are colored red for oxygen. The proximal molecule of retinoic acid is designated as RA1, and the distal molecule is labeled as RA2. A gold mesh is used to render $2|Fo| - |Fc|\sigma$A-weighted ligand omit maps contoured at 1σ around the ligands. The heme prosthetic group is rendered as a red stick figure, with the central iron atom shown as a sphere. Portions of the secondary structure of the protein are rendered as a cyan ribbon, with side chains shown as stick figures with carbons colored cyan. In some cases, portions of the substrate-free structure (Protein Data Bank code 1pq2) are shown as a gray ribbon, with side chains shown as stick figures with carbons colored gray. The nitrogen, carbon, and oxygen atoms of the backbone are shown in some cases to illustrate hydrogen bonding interactions (black dashed lines). The distance between RA1 land the heme iron is indicated by black dashed lines. The views differ between panels to clearly depict different features of the structures. (C) Structure of wild-type cytochrome P450 2C9 WT (yellow) complexed with three molecules of losartan (orange sticks). Heme is shown as red sticks. The location of each losartan is represented by red numbers: 1, peripheral site; 2, active site; and 3,access channel. Correspondingly, (D) shows the structural overlay of CYP2C9–losartan complexes representing interactions of peripheral losartan (SRS3) with the amino acid residue side chains located within 5 Å. *Panels (A and B) Data are from Schoch, G. A., Yano, J. K., Sansen, S., Dansette, P. M., Stout, C. D., & Johnson, E. F. (2008). Determinants of Cytochrome P450 2C8 substrate binding: structures of complexes with montelukast, troglitazone, felodipine and 9-cis-retinoic acid.* Journal of Biological Chemistry, 283*(25), 17227–17237; Panel (D) Data are adapted from Maekawa, K., Adachi, M., Matsuzawa, Y., Zhang, Q., Kuroki, R., Saito, Y., & Shah, M. B. (2017). Structural basis of single-nucleotide polymorphisms in cytochrome P450 2C9.* Biochemistry, 56*(41), 5476–5480 with permission of the publisher.*

While X-ray crystallography is currently regarded as the gold standard in defining structural determinants of P450, the co-crystallization of multiple substrates has sometimes been regarded as a crystallographic artifact due to the high and non-physiological concentrations of ligands used in the process.

Beyond X-ray crystallography, other *in silico* modeling techniques such as molecular docking and MD simulations have also been commonly utilized to investigate the hypothesis of multiple ligand occupancy in P450 (Siu, Hao, Dixit, & Lai, 2018). For instance, substrate inhibition kinetics was observed in CYP2J2 metabolism of arachidonic acid (AA) and a homology model of CYP2J2 was developed to investigate the stepwise sequential binding of one AA substrate firstly to the catalytic or orthosteric binding site (OBS) prior to the binding of a second AA to a predicted secondary binding site (SBS) within the active site of CYP2J2 (Fig. 3A) (Leow, Verma, Lim, Fan, & Chan, 2021). The results revealed the novel possibility of two AA substrates binding concomitantly and stably to the OBS and SBS (Fig. 3B–F). Additionally, the distance between ω6 double bond of OBS-bound AA to the heme-iron, where epoxidation is favored to produce 14,15-epoxyeicosatrienoic acid (EET), was found to be significantly greater when two AA substrates are simultaneously bound to both OBS and SBS compared to when one AA was only bound to OBS. This suggests that the second AA binding at SBS could reduce the reaction potential of AA at OBS which aligns with the proposed mechanism of substrate inhibition. Alternatively, other theories of substrate inhibition kinetics due to multiple substrate binding includes the prevention of the egress of product formed due to direct blockage *via* steric hindrance, restriction in conformational flexibility of the enzyme or stabilization of a non-productive binding pose of the substrate in access to the heme iron which thus presents as an observed apparent decline in v (Kokkonen et al., 2021). Interestingly, the abovementioned points are comprehensively demonstrated in a study whereby kinetic analysis of wild-type CYP3A4 and other active site mutants revealed concurrent positive cooperativity and substrate inhibition kinetics in the epoxidation of carbamazepine and the underlying mechanisms were probed *via* MD simulations as well (Muller et al., 2015). While the simulated binding of a second carbamazepine molecule appears to stabilize the first carbamazepine molecule in a putative catalytic pose which may hence explain the observed positive cooperativity, the additional binding of more substrates was observed to lead to the prevention of complete egress of ligand from the catalytic site.

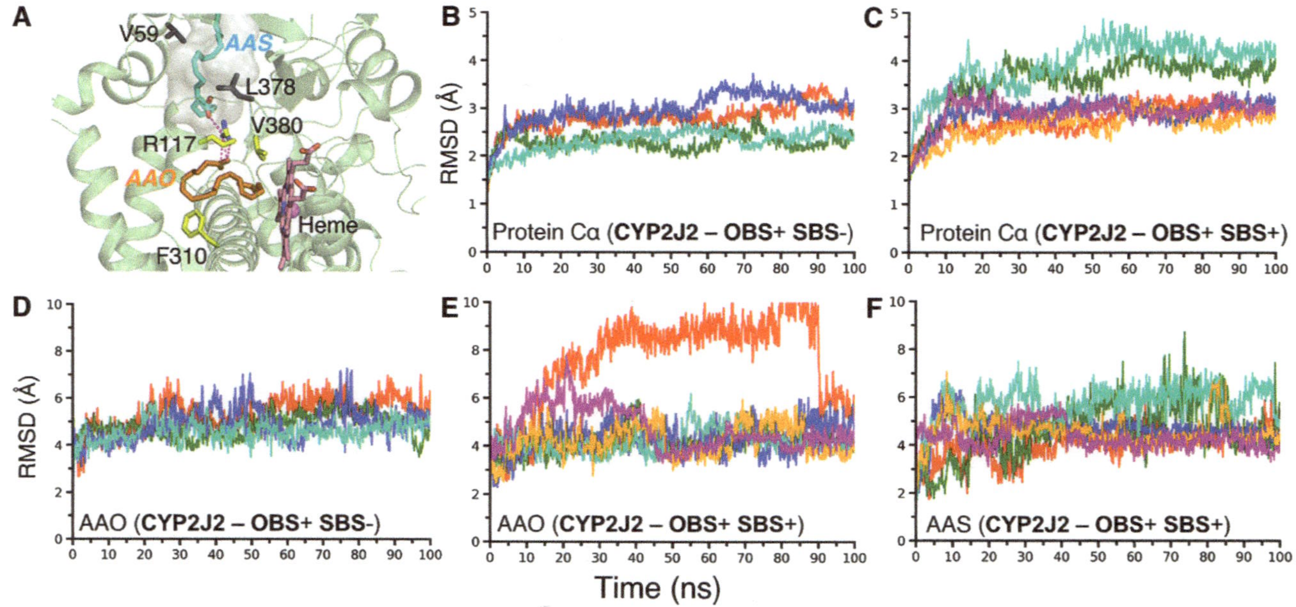

Fig. 3 (A) Docking of arachidonic acid (AA) to 3-dimensional homology model of cytochrome P450 2J2 (CYP2J2). AA could occupy both orthosteric (OBS) and secondary binding sites (SBS) in CYP2J2. OBS bound AA (AAO) and SBS bound AA (AAS) are as labeled in the figure. The location of SBS in CYP2J2 is shown in gray surface representation. Examples of AA binding residues in OBS and SBS observed in MD trajectories are R117, V380 and F310 as well as R117, V59 and L378 respectively as labeled. Salt-bridge interactions with R117 are shown by dashed lines. (B and C) Protein Cα atom RMSD in "CYP2J2—OBS+ SBS−" and "CYP2J2—OBS+ SBS+". (D and E*) AAO heavy atom RMSD in "CYP2J2—OBS+ SBS−" and "CYP2J2—OBS+ SBS+". (F) AAS heavy atom RMSD in "CYP2J2—OBS+ SBS+." *Some data points were omitted to reduce the y-axis for (E) which does not affect the interpretation of data. *Data are from Leow, J. W. H., Verma, R. K., Lim, A. B. H., Fan, H., & Chan, E. C. Y. (2021). Atypical kinetics of cytochrome P450 2J2: Epoxidation of arachidonic acid and reversible inhibition by xenobiotic inhibitors.* European Journal of Pharmaceutical Sciences, 164, *105889.*

A different opinion on the mechanics of multiple substrate binding involves the occurrence of allosteric binding at a secondary non-active site instead, which is defined for the purposes of this discussion as a site distant from the active site or access channel to the heme-iron. It has been postulated that allosteric binding could result in long-range structural rearrangements and changes in the conformation of amino acid side chains which eventually alters the positioning of the productive substrate and its metabolism at the active site. Reports of X-ray crystal structures of substrates present in allosteric binding sites are present in literature albeit lesser than reported for multiple substrates in the active site (Schoch et al., 2004; Williams et al., 2004). In one study, the crystal structure of CYP2C9 was derived with three losartan molecules co-crystallized which occupied the active site, access channel as well as a peripheral binding site (Fig. 2C and D) (Maekawa et al., 2017). A biphasic Eadie-Hofstee plot was also demonstrated with regards to the kinetics of CYP2C9 metabolism of losartan in HLM which hints at the potential involvement of allosteric modulation (Yasar et al., 2001). However, the lack of functional studies makes it difficult to identify the relative contribution of multiple substrate binding within the active site and access channel in comparison to allosteric effects in mediating the observed kinetic profile. In contrast, functional studies were performed to investigate the interactions of CYP3A4 and testosterone, a well-known substrate which exhibits sigmoidal kinetics with this P450 isoform (Denisov et al., 2016). Synthetic testosterone dimers were created to serve as active site binding ligands which were established in titration experiments to exhibit simple single-site binding. Interestingly, to probe for the effect of substrate binding at a peripheral allosteric site observed in X-ray crystallography (Sevrioukova & Poulos, 2015; Williams et al., 2004), titration with a mixture of monomeric and dimeric testosterone was performed (1:4 ratio). The results indicated a 2-fold higher apparent affinity and significant shift of spin equilibrium toward a high-spin configuration at saturation compared to titration with the dimeric molecule alone, which was attributed to allosteric site modulation by monomeric testosterone.

Other alternative hypotheses for the mechanisms underlying atypical Michaelis-Menten kinetics include protein-protein and protein-membrane interactions which are also phenomenon unaccounted for in typical Michaelis-Menten kinetics and assumptions. Currently, there are multiple structural and functional studies validating the physiological relevance of P450–P450 aggregation including the breakthrough use of cryogenic electron microscopy in characterizing the full-length dynamic and functional conformations of homodimeric CYP102A1 (Su, Chakraborty, Osawa, & Zhang, 2020) as well as the demonstration of a concentration-dependent equilibrium between monomeric and hetero-oligomeric states of CYP3A4, CYP3A5 and CYP2E1 with activation of CYP2E1 associated with oligomerization *via* luminescence resonance energy transfer technology (Davydov, Davydova, Sineva, & Halpert, 2015). Furthermore, protein-membrane interactions could also play a critical role in contributing to atypical kinetics especially in the case of mammalian P450 which are membrane-bound in nature and mostly co-localized in the endoplasmic reticulum (Seliskar & Rozman, 2007). Membrane bilayers of the endoplasmic reticulum are usually composed of a wide variety of neutral and charged phospholipids as well as other components such as cholesterol (Šrejber et al., 2018). It has been demonstrated that varying levels of these components could affect P450 activity by altering P450 membrane attachment patterns and orientations *via* forces such as hydrogen bonding and electrostatic interactions. However, while existing reviews and research articles in literature focus extensively on the mechanisms of these interactions, advances in experimental techniques and outcomes on enzymatic activity (Lampe, 2017; Reed & Backes, 2012), limited studies relate it to atypicalities in kinetic outcomes. Similarly, although it was also proposed that conformational selection or ligand-induced slow conformational change of monomeric enzymes could cause atypical kinetics (Porter & Miller, 2012; Redhair & Atkins, 2021), the relevance of these hypotheses with regards to experimental data of non-Michaelis Menten kinetics has yet to be established.

With respect to atypical Michaelis-Menten kinetics in P450 specifically, the frequency and prevalence observed across different isoforms remain largely unclear due to limited studies available in literature. While CYP3A4 appears to have the highest number of reported cases of atypical kinetics which is commonly hypothesized to be due to its large active site (1385 Å) being able to accommodate multiple substrate binding, other P450 with small and narrow active sites such as CYP1A2 (375 Å) have also been reported to display atypical kinetics (Lin et al., 2001a; Wang et al., 2009). While atypical kinetics associated with CYP2C9 was observed in 18% of 500 diverse drug-like compounds that were screened, less than 2% was observed for CYP2D6 (McMasters et al., 2007). The *in vivo* implications of various forms of atypical kinetics in P450 including sigmoidal kinetics have also been explored (Sakamoto, Itoh, & Fujiwara, 2013;

Witherow & Houston, 1999) which could be further complicated by concurrent DDIs (inhibition/activation) (Egnell, Houston, & Boyer, 2003, 2005; Mast, Verwilst, Wilkey, Guengerich, & Pikuleva, 2020). In the following subsections, a focus on P450 substrate inhibition in the absence and presence of drug inhibitors will be discussed.

2.1 Substrate inhibition kinetics in P450

Substrate inhibition kinetics have been estimated to occur in approximately 20% of known enzymes, presenting itself as likely the most common form of atypical kinetics observed in literature (Reed, Lieb, & Nijhout, 2010). In a single study, the metabolism kinetics of 13 P450 marker substrates including both drugs and endogenous substances were investigated with 10 recombinant P450 (Lin et al., 2001a). Six of the substrates screened exhibited partial substrate inhibition whereby v declines to a non-zero asymptote (see Table 1 for example). Furthermore, more than one unique substrate was screened for some P450. While ethoxyresorufin demonstrated substrate inhibition when metabolized by CYP1A2, other CYP1A2 substrates estrone and phenacetin revealed typical Michaelis-Menten behavior instead (Lin et al., 2001b). The same substrate may also exhibit differing kinetics when metabolized by different P450 isoforms. For example, bufotalin 5β-hydroxylation *via* CYP3A4 exhibited biphasic kinetics while the same reaction mediated by CYP3A5 displayed substrate inhibition kinetics (Dai et al., 2019). Even in the event of a specific substrate and enzyme pairing, differences in kinetic profiles for the formation of different metabolites could also occur such as in the case of 4-hydroxymidazolam formation by CYP3A4 which is commonly established to follow typical Michaelis-Menten kinetics compared to 1′-hydroxymidazolam whereby substrate inhibition is more commonly reported (Yang, Atkins, Isoherranen, Paine, & Thummel, 2012). Certain genetic variants of CYP2D6 were also found to contribute to substrate inhibition kinetics in the *in vitro* metabolism of nebivolol compared to typical Michaelis-Menten kinetics observed for wild-type CYP2D6, highlighting that atypical kinetics could precipitate due to genetic polymorphism (Hu et al., 2016). Taken together, this highlights how varied the presentation of substrate inhibition can be, alongside other forms of atypical kinetics. The specificity of this phenomenon for a particular enzyme-substrate interaction and formation of a particular metabolite emphasizes the need for evaluation on a case-by-case basis.

In alignment with Lin et al., a survey of existing literature also revealed that partial substrate inhibition is widely observed in contrast to only a few cases reported for complete substrate inhibition where product formation is fully inhibited by excess substrate, resulting in v decreasing to zero at high $[S]$ (see example in Table 1). However, this trend could be confounded by aqueous solubility constraints when performing *in vitro* enzymatic assays. Of note, complete substrate inhibition by a drug substrate was reported for *S*-efavirenz 8-hydroxylation by wild-type CYP2B6.1 and variants (Wang et al., 2019). Moreover, an oral selective estrogen receptor degrader, AZD9496, developed previously for the treatment of estrogen receptor-positive breast cancer also exhibited complete substrate inhibition in HLM, CYP2C8 and hepatocytes (Bapiro et al., 2018). For endogenous substrates, the phenomenon of complete substrate inhibition was also evident for AA when metabolized by CYP2J2 (Leow et al., 2021). The maximum v observed prior to the declining trend occurred at 20 to 30 μM AA which falls below its critical micellar concentration of 73 μM. Hence, while the formation of micelles is unlikely to confound the decline in v of AA metabolism by CYP2J2, it is unknown if it could have contributed partially to the substrate inhibition observed at the highest AA concentration of 80 μM adopted in the study. Regardless, complete substrate inhibition has been reported by AA at lower concentrations up to 50 μM when metabolized by non-P450 such as a mouse homolog of human 15-lipoxygenase-2 (Bender, Schexnaydre, Murphy, Uhlson, & Newcomer, 2016) and a mutant of mammalian 8*R*-lipoxygenase (Neau et al., 2014) which ascertains the validity of this phenomenon.

Given that one of the primary applications for conducting *in vitro* P450 metabolism studies is to predict *in vivo* disposition and systemic clearance using estimated kinetic parameters, it becomes critical to determine if the inaccurate fitting of substrate inhibition data to the Michaelis-Menten equation can result in significantly different kinetic parameters translating to inaccurate IVIVE. Several reviews have attempted to discuss this and the general consensus remains that an underestimation of V_{max} would be expected and accompanied by a poor estimation of K_m (Galetin, Ito, Hallifax, & Houston, 2005; Tracy, 2006). Conventionally, *in vitro* intrinsic clearance (CL_{int}) is heavily relied upon as a surrogate marker by regulatory authorities and pharmaceutical companies to predict *in vivo* clearance. CL_{int} is derived experimentally either *via* substrate depletion methods or calculation of the ratio of V_{max} to K_m. However, the use of *in vitro* CL_{int} inherently adopts the assumptions of non-saturable metabolism, first-order elimination and constant clearance. In the example of fitting data representing CYP2C9 hydroxylation of piroxicam which demonstrates substrate inhibition to both the empirical substrate inhibition model and Michaelis-Menten model, both K_m and V_{max} were underestimated by approximately 2-fold and 1.3-fold respectively when the latter model was incorrectly utilized which led to a 1.7-fold overestimation in *in vitro* CL_{int} (Tracy, 2003). Similarly, a 1.1- to 1.8-fold underestimation of V_{max} was also reported in another study investigating a range of different P450 and corresponding substrates exhibiting substrate inhibition when the data were fitted to the Michaelis-Menten equation instead (Lin et al., 2001b). The extent of deviation of the predicted *in vivo* clearance due to model misspecification as compared to the actual observed *in vivo* clearance could vary and be subjected to influence by the inclusion or exclusion of data points at high $[S]$ representing substrate inhibition in the process of analysis and regression.

It is commonly argued with respect to drug substrates exhibiting substrate inhibition that significant *in vivo* implications are improbable as the phenomenon only occurs at high $[S]$ which would be unlikely to fall within physiological limits. However, this assumption can be problematic especially if no effort is taken to evaluate and compare on a case-by-case basis if the systemic or intrahepatic concentrations of the drug of interest and its kinetic parameters of substrate inhibition could fall within the same range. This could be possible in the case of high-affinity drugs with corresponding high systemic and hepatic exposures whereby even in the case of substrates with typical Michaelis-Menten kinetics, adopting CL_{int} for IVIVE to estimate hepatic clearance would lead to inaccuracies (Back, Yun, Kim, & Kim, 2020). Using a previously mentioned example, a greater than dose-proportional increase in area under curve (AUC) and maximum plasma concentration (C_{max}) after a single dose administration of 600 mg AZD9496 in phase I clinical trials was observed (Hamilton et al., 2018). The absence of MBI of CYP2C8, which was determined to be the key P450 isoform responsible for the metabolism of this drug candidate, was demonstrated which would otherwise be a potential cause for nonlinear pharmacokinetics (Bapiro et al., 2018). Notably, it was estimated that the maximum unbound liver inlet concentration of AZD9496 was 1 μM for a single 600 mg dose which is higher than its K_m of 0.4 μM in HLM attributed to CYP2C8 based on reaction phenotyping for the formation of its major metabolite (Bapiro et al., 2018). Hence, it is reasonable to suggest that the metabolism of AZD9496 by CYP2C8 occurring at this level of systemic exposure is likely affected by substrate inhibition and leading to a reduction in v although the extent of this effect is unclear. It is also currently unknown whether AZD9496 is a substrate of hepatic uptake transporters which if demonstrated could imply that its intrahepatic concentration may be significantly higher than 1 μM and closer to its substrate inhibition constant (K_s) of 12 μM, increasing the *in vivo* relevance of substrate inhibition in potentially contributing to the apparent dose nonlinearity. The *in vivo* relevance of substrate inhibition occurring for drug substrates could also be increased in disease conditions such as renal or hepatic impairment as this could lead to increased systemic exposure in the event that significant renal excretion or hepatic metabolism is implicated in the elimination of these drugs from the body. However, in general it should be noted that observed *in vivo* outcomes of non-linear pharmacokinetics is likely a result of the complex interplay of multiple factors, in which it would be difficult to tease out the key contributing role of atypical kinetics without having a holistic understanding of other mechanisms that could also be implicated.

In addition, given that intestinal luminal concentrations of orally administered drugs are typically higher than corresponding systemic or intrahepatic concentrations, the *in vivo* implications of substrate inhibition could be considerable if the implicated enzymes are significantly expressed in the intestine and play a role in drug pharmacokinetics (*e.g.*, intestinal metabolism and first pass, bioactivation of prodrugs). Currently, limited evidence of atypical kinetics occurring with the use of human intestinal microsomes (HIMs) or other *in vitro* models of human intestinal metabolism have been reported in contrast to HLMs (Oda & Kharasch, 2001a, 2001b). Substrate inhibition kinetics has been reported for metabolite formation from indinavir oxidation in permeabilized enterocytes (Davies et al., 2020) although it is unknown if this atypical kinetics was correspondingly observed in indinavir oxidation in HLMs as only kinetic parameters K_m and V_{max} were reported without corresponding graphical representations (Chiba, Hensleigh, & Lin, 1997). With reference to a previous example on wild-type CYP2B6.1 metabolism of *S*-efavirenz which demonstrates complete substrate inhibition, CYP2B6 is significantly expressed in human intestine (relative P450 expression in jejunum of 4.9–7.8% and highest mean percentage contribution of colon P450 expression to intestinal P450 expression) (Fritz et al., 2019) and contributes significantly to the elimination of efavirenz with an estimated fraction metabolized of 62% (Ke, Barter, Rowland-Yeo, & Almond, 2016). The kinetic parameters for 8-hydroxyefavirenz formation from *S*-efavirenz metabolism by wild-type CYP2B6.1 revealed a K_m and K_s of 17 and 47 μM respectively

(Wang et al., 2019) which is significantly lower than the estimated intestinal luminal efavirenz concentration of 5 mM after a dose of 400 mg (Oswald et al., 2012) and also falls in a similar range to the reported therapeutic plasma concentration of up to 13 μM for the dose of 600 mg (Bednasz et al., 2017). Furthermore, CYP2B6 also exhibits genetic polymorphism whereby various degrees of substrate inhibition ranging from partial to complete was observed among the different CYP2B6 variants. CYP2B6.19 exhibited least substrate inhibition while 8-hydroxyefavirenz formation was reduced drastically to 4% of V_{max} for CYP2B6.1 and CYP2B6.4 at 100 μM *S*-efavirenz (Wang et al., 2019), adding another layer of complexity to our understanding of the *in vivo* implications of substrate inhibition on drug pharmacokinetics.

On the other hand, when *in vitro* substrate inhibition occurs for a P450 and an endogenous substrate, it is commonly proposed to be an *in vivo* homeostatic mechanism whereby negative feedback may be necessary. CYP2J2 metabolism of AA is important in the formation of regioisomeric EETs which possess a diverse range of biological activities including vasodilation, anti-inflammation and ion channel binding (Campbell, Imig, Schmitz, & Falck, 2017; Elinder & Liin, 2017; Xu, Zhang, & Wang, 2011). Hence, it is logical to assume that some form of regulatory mechanism may be required to maintain steady-state levels of such bioactive endogenous metabolites in the body. In particular, the biological significance of substrate inhibition has also been discussed extensively in non-P450, highlighting the various different biological functions that substrate inhibition can modulate in different contexts (Reed et al., 2010). Another relevant example of substrate inhibition kinetics being implicated in the metabolism of endogenous substrates includes the hydroxylation of 25-hydroxyvitamin D3 by CYP27B1 to produce its active metabolite (Tang, Voo, Nguyen, & Tuckey, 2010). Furthermore, physiological concentrations of endogenous substrates have a greater potential to be within the higher micromolar range as compared to drug substrates. As discussed for the case of CYP2J2 metabolism of AA by Leow et al., free AA plasma levels ranges from 0.1 to 50 μM in healthy humans but could increase to levels up to 500 μM under pathophysiological conditions (Abdelmagid et al., 2015; Pompeia, Lima, & Curi, 2003). Therefore, considering that the respective K_m and K_s values of 45 and 31 μM (Leow et al., 2021) fall within the physiological concentration range of AA, the *in vitro* substrate inhibition phenomenon has a reasonable potential to be implicated in metabolic regulation and may even be enhanced in disease conditions.

2.2 Drug inhibition of P450 in the presence of substrate inhibition

Being cognizant of how drug inhibition of P450 may be different in the presence of concurrent substrate inhibition becomes imperative as *in vitro* DDI assays such as RI are commonly performed using single surrogate probe substrates recommended by the regulatory authorities such as the United States Food and Drug Administration (FDA). Historically, this practice could be attributed to resource constraint reasons and the push for an accelerated timeline of drug to market even starting from early drug discovery processes. However, the success of this method of probe substrate surrogacy depends heavily on the assumption that the potency and mode of drug inhibition is unaffected by the probe substrate such that the results can be accurately extrapolated to other substrates for a particular enzyme. This assumption is now increasingly challenged even in cases whereby atypical kinetics are not implicated as various studies report substrate-dependent effects on the inhibitory constants (K_i) being observed for the same inhibitors (Jagdish et al., 2003; Stresser et al., 2000). With regards to the additional dimension of atypical kinetics in substrate-dependency, significantly less P450 inhibition studies have been conducted on this topic.

An earlier comprehensive study investigating interaction profiles between various CYP3A4 substrates and inhibitors displaying a mix of typical and atypical Michaelis-Menten kinetics revealed an 80-fold difference in K_i values (Galetin, Clarke, & Houston, 2003). A relatively more recent study also attempted to test the assumption of substrate independence on the potency of inhibitors *in vivo* for a set of eight victim drugs and eight inhibitors of CYP3A4 (Loue & Tod, 2014). Although the study reported that limited evidence of substrate-dependency exists for most of drugs screened, two substrate outliers nifedipine and cyclosporine were determined to exhibit significant substrate-dependent effect on the potency of inhibitors. Two out of eight inhibitors of CYP3A4 metabolism of cyclosporine and two out of three inhibitors of CYP3A4 metabolism of nifedipine showed significant variability in the estimated inhibition ratio value, a measure related to *in vitro* K_i, compared to when other substrates were used. Interestingly, both nifedipine (Galetin et al., 2003) and cyclosporine (Dai et al., 2004) have been reported to exhibit substrate inhibition when metabolized by CYP3A4. Although it was concluded by the authors in their discussion that strong and weak inhibitors were often accurately predicted independent of substrate utilized, this suggests that intermediate inhibitors might therefore be more likely to produce greater variability in K_i and the impact of this on victim drug disposition and pharmacokinetics should not be overlooked.

Further studies were also performed on the *in vitro* metabolism of AA by CYP2J2 which demonstrated substrate inhibition as discussed in the previous section, whereby the reaction was then subjected to a panel of nine drug inhibitors (Leow et al., 2021). The same panel of drug inhibitors were also tested when astemizole was substituted as a probe substrate yielding typical Michaelis-Menten behavior instead. It was revealed that drug inhibition of CYP2J2 metabolism of AA produced K_i values that differed from the inhibition of CYP2J2 metabolism of astemizole (Fig. 4A). A greater than 2-fold difference between K_i values was observed for six drugs, out of which four had a greater than 5-fold difference ranging from 5.02- to 10.1-fold. Differing modes of RI were also observed for almost half of the panel of drug inhibitors screened although no distinct correlation could be made between

A

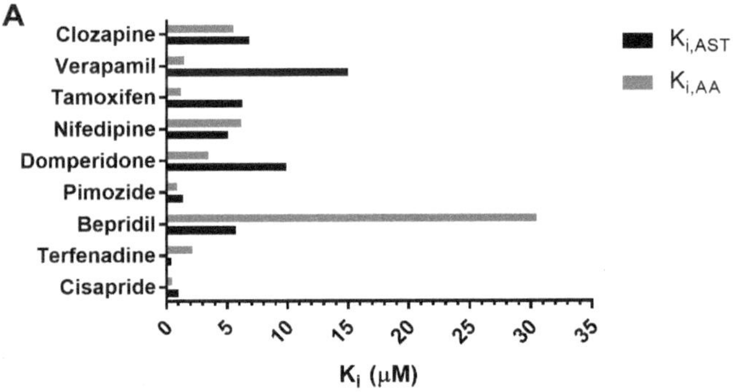

B

		$K_{i,AA}$	
		Competitive	**Mixed mode**
$K_{i,AST}$	**Competitive**	• Cisapride • Pimozide	• Terfenadine • Tamoxifen
	Mixed mode	• Nifedipine • Verapamil • Bepridil	• Domperidone • Clozapine

Fig. 4 (A) Inhibition constants of various drugs ($n = 9$) screened against CYP2J2-mediated arachidonic acid metabolism ($K_{i,\ AA}$) and against CYP2J2-mediated astemizole metabolism ($K_{i,\ AST}$), as well as (B) their corresponding modes of inhibition. *Data are modified and redrawn from Leow, J. W. H., Verma, R. K., Lim, A. B. H., Fan, H., & Chan, E. C. Y. (2021). Atypical kinetics of cytochrome P450 2J2: Epoxidation of arachidonic acid and reversible inhibition by xenobiotic inhibitors.* European Journal of Pharmaceutical Sciences, 164, *105889.*

the mode of inhibition and potency of CYP2J2 inhibition for both substrates AA and astemizole (Fig. 4B). The results also contrasted with majority of the existing literature in the context where kinetic profiles become more hyperbolic and progressively Michaelis-Menten-like with increasing inhibitor concentrations (Yang et al., 2012) (Fig. 5A and B). This has been postulated to be due to the growing dominance of a non-productive enzyme-substrate-inhibitor complex formed instead with the assumption of two binding sites present within the enzyme active site (Galetin et al., 2003). Interestingly, Leow et al. reported the persistence of substrate inhibition kinetics despite increasing concentrations of drug inhibitors against CYP2J2 metabolism of AA (Fig. 5C and D) which was also demonstrated in another study reporting carbamazepine inhibition of CYP3A4-mediated progesterone hydroxylation (Denisov et al., 2019). This observation of sustained substrate inhibition profile despite increasing inhibitor concentrations was hypothesized to be due to reasons such as the binding of three or more ligands preventing the egress of product, or the continued effect of allosteric binding by substrate or inhibitor that modulates metabolism at the active site at high substrate and inhibitor concentrations (Leow et al., 2021).

It is noteworthy that the K_i values determined for drug inhibition against CYP2J2 metabolism of AA were obtained using mathematical derivation of an equation utilizing Hill's coefficient (Leow et al., 2021), which is a quantitative but not mechanistic method of improving data fitting (Goutelle et al., 2008). Currently, only a few mechanistic equations and corresponding kinetic schemes have been developed to explain this interaction which are strongly based on the two-site model hypothesis that can also account for the simultaneous binding of multiple inhibitors (Wu, 2011). The lack of a standardized approach to selecting the appropriate equation as well as lack of coherence between mechanistic and empirical equations makes the comparison and understanding of K_i values and relevant caveats across different studies challenging. Hence, a deeper understanding of the underlying mechanisms of substrate inhibition as well as drug inhibition in the presence of substrate inhibition would be necessary for the development of more mechanistic and representative equations which will increase confidence in the accuracy of K_i values determined. In addition, it becomes difficult to assess solely the impact of atypical kinetics in affecting K_i given that the contributing roles of substrate-dependency which could not be delineated in current studies. It would be an ideal scenario if structural analogues or substrates that have similar physicochemical

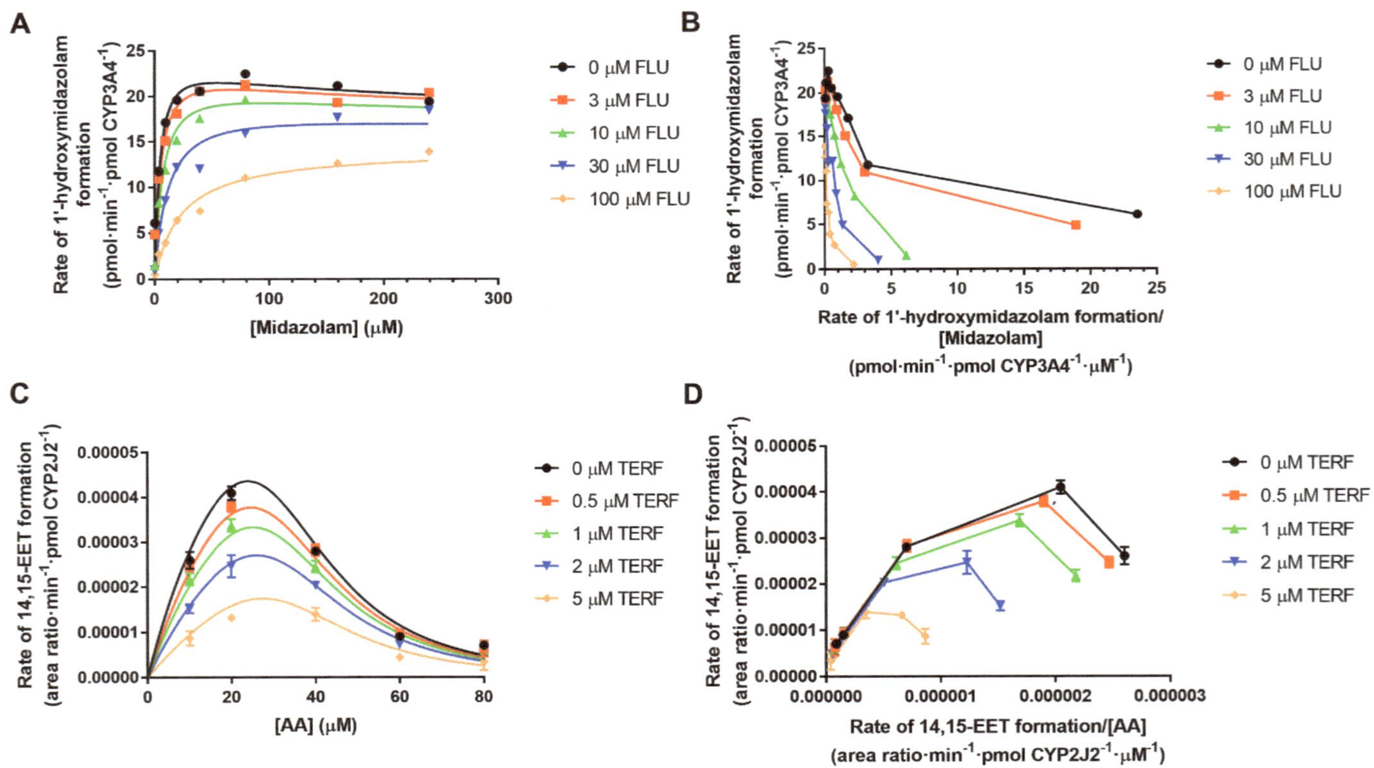

Fig. 5 See figure legend on opposite page.

properties but exhibit differing typical and atypical kinetics when metabolized by the same enzyme are utilized for a comparison study.

The *in vivo* implications of drug inhibition in the presence of substrate inhibition could also be more difficult to ascertain compared to substrate inhibition alone as discussed in the previous section due to the complexity of factors involved including additional considerations for perpetrator drug pharmacokinetics at different doses and dosage regimens. Another point of relevance could arise in the form of IVIVE of *in vitro* K_i to predicting changes in systemic exposure of victim drugs which might be inaccurate if USFDA-recommended probe substrates were used, as well as in the event that substrate inhibition kinetics of the victim drug is disregarded in the mathematical derivation of K_i. More research needs to be performed to determine if unaccounted substrate inhibition of the victim drug in *in vitro* DDI studies could affect the accuracy of IVIVE and caution should be taken especially for interactions between intermediate potency inhibitors and substrates that are known to exhibit substrate inhibition. Given that existing data suggests that intermediate potency inhibitors may have increased variability across substrates with atypical kinetics, it would be prudent to perform *in vitro* DDI studies using the specific inhibitor-substrate pairing of interest as well as escalating to clinical DDI studies for this category of inhibitors instead of only focusing on high

Fig. 5 *In vitro* substrate inhibition kinetics in the presence of a drug inhibitor. (A) Inhibitory effect of fluconazole (FLU) on substrate inhibition kinetics of recombinant human cytochrome P450 3A4 (CYP3A4) metabolism of midazolam to 1′-hydroxymidazolam. With increasing FLU concentrations (0–100 μM), the graph changes into a hyperbolic curve due to the increasing contribution of a non-productive enzyme-substrate-inhibitor complex. The corresponding Eadie-Hofstee plot (B) shows the representative change in the shape of the profile from a hook in the upper corner to an increasingly linear plot with increasing FLU concentrations. (C) Inhibitory effect of terfenadine (TERF) on substrate inhibition kinetics of recombinant human cytochrome P450 2J2 (CYP2J2) metabolism of arachidonic acid (AA) to 14,15-epoxysicosatrienoic acid (EET). The effect of substrate inhibition continued even at high concentrations of TERF (0–5 μM). Correspondingly, the Eadie-Hofstee plot (D) revealed the persistence of non-linearity which is characteristic for substrate inhibition. *(Panel B) Data are adapted and redrawn from Yang, J., Atkins, W. M., Isoherranen, N., Paine, M. F., & Thummel, K. E. (2012). Evidence of CYP3A allosterism in vivo: Analysis of fluconazole and midazolam interaction.* Clinical Pharmacology and Therapeutics, 91*(3), 442; (Panel D) Data are from Leow, J. W. H., Verma, R. K., Lim, A. B. H., Fan, H., & Chan, E. C. Y. (2021). Atypical kinetics of cytochrome P450 2J2: Epoxidation of arachidonic acid and reversible inhibition by xenobiotic inhibitors.* European Journal of Pharmaceutical Sciences, 164, *105889.*

potency inhibitors. This is because victim drug toxicodynamics also come into the equation and an intermediate potency inhibitor could potentially still cause significant adverse effects should the therapeutic window of victim drug be narrow, leading to observed toxicity even with small to moderate increases in systemic exposure.

3. Atypicalities in mechanism-based inactivation of cytochrome P450

As previously mentioned, P450 serve as one of the major driving forces of xenobiotic metabolism in the human body (Guengerich, 2001). It is estimated that the metabolism of >80% of all marketed drugs can be ascribed to just six P450 isoforms (Zanger & Schwab, 2013), thereby entrenching their significance in drug disposition. However, due to their wide substrate and catalytic promiscuity, there is broad consensus that the P450 may also inadvertently perpetrate metabolic activation of drugs (Guengerich, 2001). Also termed as bioactivation, they result in the generation of electrophilic, chemically reactive intermediates that could covalently adduct to the P450 apoprotein and/or prosthetic heme or coordinate with the heme ferrous and engender time-dependent inhibition of its catalytic activity *via* MBI (Ho, Chan, Hardy, & Chan, 2015). In contrast to the previous instances of enzymatic inhibition covered in the earlier sections of this chapter, the loss of enzymatic activity incited by MBI is irreversible and is only restored upon *de novo* synthesis of the implicated enzyme. Consequently, the extent of pharmacokinetic DDI tends to be more profound than with a direct reversible inhibitor and could also lead to autoinhibition of hepatic elimination, time-dependent and/or nonlinear pharmacokinetics (Bjornsson et al., 2003). Finally, covalent modification of the P450 protein may constitute neoantigens and trigger adaptive immune responses which can culminate in immune-mediated toxicities (Masubuchi & Horie, 2007). Due to its manifold ramifications in pharmacology and toxicology, it is clinically important to discern if a drug elicits MBI of P450.

More importantly, it is increasingly being recognized that MBI of P450 are also amenable to atypical kinetics and exhibits many complex phenomena such as multiple substrate binding, partial inactivation, quasi-irreversible inactivation and sequential metabolism which may hinder accurate parameterization of *in vitro* MBI kinetic parameters and subsequent prediction of DDI. This has been recently reviewed in-detail by Yadav et al. and the reader is referred to that publication for a more comprehensive overview (Yadav, Paragas, Korzekwa, & Nagar, 2020). Consequently, this second half of this chapter will focus on two intriguing emerging atypical complexities that are commonly observed in MBI of CYP3A by drugs which may affect extrapolation of pharmacological and toxicological implications.

3.1 Complexities in the mechanism-based inactivation of CYP3A

CYP3A4 is the most abundantly expressed hepatic P450 and is responsible for the metabolism of more than half of all marketed drugs (Wilkinson, 1996; Wrighton, VandenBranden, & Ring, 1996). Consequently, its inactivation *via* MBI is expected to have deep clinical significance. This is best exemplified by the calcium-channel blocker mibefradil which was pulled from the market 10 months following its FDA-approval due to the potential for harmful DDIs (*i.e.*, rhabdomyolysis, renal failure or bradycardia) with other co-administered drugs (Li Wan Po & Zhang, 1998). Following its withdrawal, it was revealed that mibefradil was a potent MBI of CYP3A4 and could markedly augment the plasma concentrations of several sensitive CYP3A substrates such as simvastatin and tacrolimus (Prueksaritanont et al., 1999; Zhou, Chan, Li, & Huang, 2005). Recently, CYP3A5—its highly homologous counterpart, has also gained prominence in the sphere of drug metabolism. Interestingly, multiple lines of evidence have revealed that CYP3A enzymes have the propensities to exhibit vastly disparate inactivation profiles with several clinically-relevant drugs depending on the probe substrate utilized (Guo et al., 2019; Okada et al., 2009; Sugiyama et al., 2011). These atypical observations appear to go against the conventional principles of enzyme inhibition and constitute an emerging paradigm in complex P450 kinetics whereby the inhibitory behavior exhibited by a particular compound is contingent on the identity of the probe substate employed in the *in vitro* assay (Tracy, 2006).

In contrast to the other instances of atypical P450 kinetics that have been expounded upon in the first half of this chapter, the implications of such probe substrate-dependent inhibition/inactivation lie more upstream in the drug development continuum and are closely entwined with its clinical efficacy and safety. For instance, the presence of such probe substrate-dependencies could confound IVIVE and result in gross underpredictions or overestimations of its potential DDI liabilities. Concordant with these previous reports, some rather interesting probe substrate-dependent experimental observations in CYP3A isoforms by several clinically-relevant drugs have recently been unraveled. These examples will be highlighted in this following section. Moreover, this section will also discuss and propose another dimension of complexity arising from the differential inactivation kinetic profiles between the highly homologous CYP3A isoforms (*i.e.*, CYP3A4 and CYP3A5).

3.2 Probe substrate-dependent inactivation in CYP3A

In vitro P450 inactivation assays conducted for a particular drug typically relies on a P450 isoform-selective probe substrate which functions as a surrogate marker of the residual enzyme activity. From these assays, two kinetic constants namely its K_I (inactivation concentration at half-maximum inactivation rate constant) and k_{inact} (maximal inactivation rate constant)—which are analogous to K_m and V_{max} in the Michaelis-Menten equation—can be obtained. From a drug discovery perspective, inactivators that possess a larger k_{inact} and smaller K_i generally have a greater propensity to elicit DDI *in vivo*. While these inactivation kinetic constants were traditionally regarded as intrinsic features of the inactivator and were thought to be *independent* of the probe substrate, it is now recognized that such assumptions are overly reductionistic and are only valid when both the probe substrate and inactivator are competing for access to the same catalytic binding site. In that regard, X-ray crystallographic structures of CYP3A have revealed that the active site of this P450 subfamily possesses considerable bulk and plasticity which may help mechanistically explain its substrate promiscuity (Ekroos & Sjögren, 2006b; Williams et al., 2004). More importantly, these pioneering studies also revealed the existence of multiple binding sites and the possibility for the simultaneous binding of more than one molecule of the substrate in different orientations within the active site. Taken together, the unique topology of the enzymatic active site of CYP3A facilitates different dynamic orientations of the inactivator in a probe-substrate dependent manner. Consequently, the biochemical interactions observed with one CYP3A probe substrate are not reflective of those obtained with another (Galetin et al., 2005; Kenworthy, Bloomer, Clarke, & Houston, 1999).

Indeed, it has been previously demonstrated that the inactivation potency (k_{inact}/K_i) of the benzofuran antiarrhythmic agent dronedarone and its major pharmacologically-active metabolite N-desbutyldronedarone was markedly greater when rivaroxaban was utilized as the probe substrate (*i.e.*, 185 and 53.7 min^{-1} mM^{-1}) in place of testosterone (*i.e.*, 44.8

and 15.9 min^{-1} mM^{-1}) (Cheong et al., 2017; Hong et al., 2016). Similarly, in a more recent study involving the fibroblast growth factor receptor inhibitors erdafitinib, infigratinib and pemigatinib, salient difference in their inactivation potencies against CYP3A4 were also observed when rivaroxaban was utilized in place of the FDA-recommended probes (*i.e.*, testosterone and/or midazolam) (Tang, Teng, Koh, et al., 2021; Tang, Teng, Verma, et al., 2021; Tang et al., 2022). Specifically, in the case of infigratinib, the k_{inact}/K_I ratio obtained with rivaroxaban was found to be ~2.0- and ~1.7-fold higher than that obtained with testosterone and midazolam respectively, thereby suggesting that the inactivation of CYP3A4-mediated rivaroxaban hydroxylation is expected to be more potent as compared with its FDA-recommended prototypical substrates. This trend is further substantiated by the plots of k_{obs} *vs* $[I]$ (infigratinib) and the resultant Kitz-Wilson plots against the three structurally-distinct substrates (Fig. 6). As rivaroxaban is routinely utilized in tandem with dronedarone for secondary stroke prophylaxis in the setting of atrial fibrillation (Hindricks et al., 2021) and is increasingly being adopted as the anticoagulation of choice in cancer-associated venous thromboembolism (Short & Connors, 2014), these probe substrate-dependent inactivation profiles reiterate the importance of utilizing a clinically-relevant substrate to derive accurate inactivation kinetic constants for pharmacokinetic DDI studies.

Apart from probe substrate-dependent effects in inactivation potency, there are also compelling reasons to believe that the choice of probe substrate employed in the assay could affect its susceptibility toward inactivation. This phenomenon is exemplified by the MBI of CYP3A5 by the dual epidermal growth factor receptor/human epidermal growth factor receptor 2 inhibitor lapatinib (Chan et al., 2012). Remarkably, it was discovered that lapatinib was metabolically activated by CYP3A5 to a quinoneimine reactive metabolite that covalently inactivated CYP3A5-mediated testosterone 6β hydroxylation but not midazolam 1′-hydroxylation in a time- and concentration-manner (Fig. 7). This is not surprising and is consistent with the notion of multiple binding sites within the active site of CYP3A enzymes. In fact, it may be rationalized that this probe substrate-dependent inactivation of lapatinib by CYP3A5 could have arisen from the covalent adduction of the lapatinib quinoneimine species to a specific region within the active site such that it impedes the productive binding of testosterone but not midazolam, thereby preserving its metabolism. From a pragmatic standpoint, this atypical finding is consequential as it suggests that any

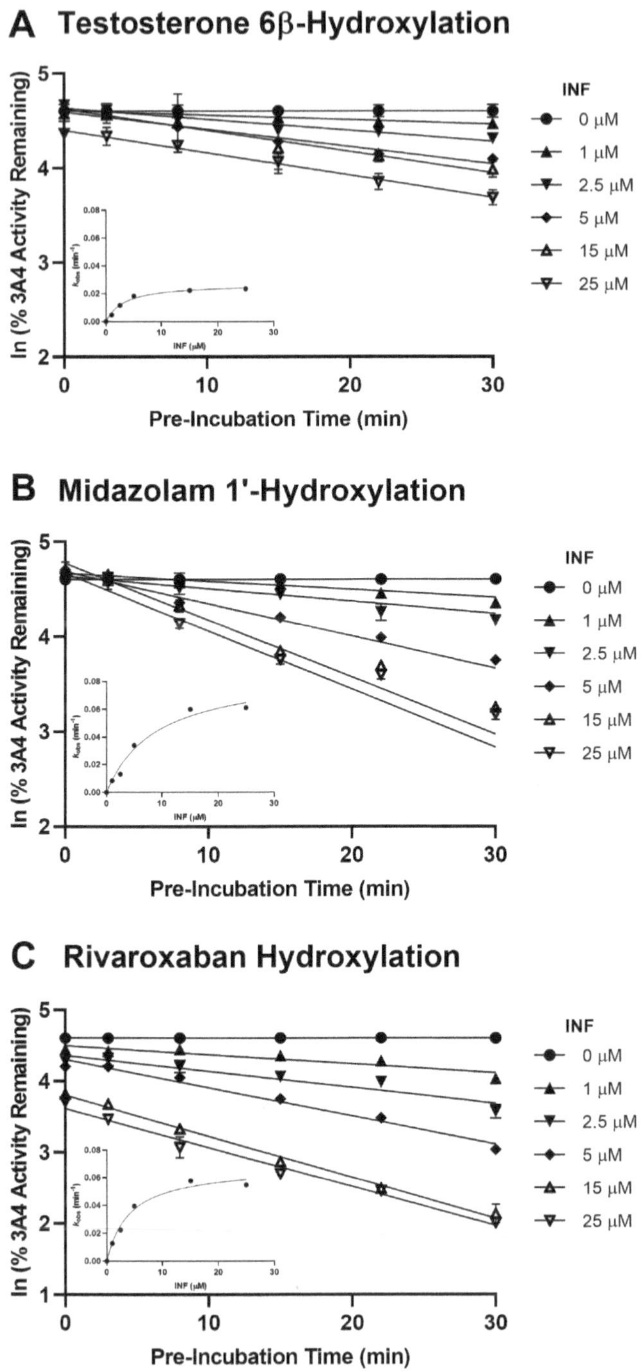

Fig. 6 See figure legend on opposite page.

potential clinical DDI arising from the inactivation of CYP3A5 by lapatinib would be substrate-specific. Therefore, in order for *in vitro* CYP3A inactivation assays to provide accurate quantitative insights into the potential and magnitude of clinically-significant DDI, it should be routinely advocated that such assays are conducted using the 'victim' drug of interest as the probe substrate.

3.3 Isoform-dependent inactivation in CYP3A

On one hand, as CYP3A5 shares ~85% sequence similarity with CYP3A4, they are known to possess overlapping substrate specificities. However, unlike CYP3A4, the expression levels of CYP3A5 can vary considerably between ethnic populations due to the occurrence of the defective *3 allele which encodes for a truncated and non-functional protein. Notably, the frequency of possessing at least one *3 allele ranges from as low as 10–30% in Caucasians to as high as 50–70% in African-Americans (Kuehl et al., 2001). Conversely, in wild-type *1 carriers, the hepatic protein expression of CYP3A5 may be on par with, or even surpass that of CYP3A4 in some individuals (Lamba, Lin, Schuetz, & Thummel, 2002; Lin et al., 2002). Consequently, CYP3A5 may further augment CYP3A-mediated drug metabolism and may be a significant contributor of interindividual variability in drug disposition (Kamdem et al., 2005). Importantly, mounting evidence has revealed that despite the high degree of sequence homology and substrate specificities between both CYP3A isoforms, these enzymes have the propensities to exhibit vastly different inactivation profiles with a common substrate. Although the exact mechanistic basis for these atypical experimental observations remains an area of

Fig. 6 Time- and concentration-dependent inactivation of CYP3A4 by the fibroblast growth factor receptor inhibitor infigratinib using (A) testosterone, (B) midazolam, and (C) rivaroxaban as probe substrates. Nonlinear regression of kobs *versus* INF concentration (inset plots) yielded KI and kinact values of $3.26 \pm 0.61\,\mu M$ and $0.027 \pm 0.002\,min^{-1}$ when testosterone was used as the probe substrate, $9.03 \pm 2.85\,\mu M$ and $0.088 \pm 0.011\,min^{-1}$ when midazolam was harnessed as the probe substrate, and $4.17 \pm 0.93\,\mu M$ and $0.068 \pm 0.005\,min^{-1}$ when rivaroxaban was employed as probe substrates respectively. *Data are modified and redrawn from Tang, L. W. T., Teng, J. W., Verma, R. K., Koh, S. K., Zhou, L., Go, M. L., … Chan, E. C. Y. (2021). Infigratinib is a reversible inhibitor and mechanism-based inactivator of Cytochrome P450 3A4.* Drug Metabolism and Disposition, 49*(9), 856–868.*

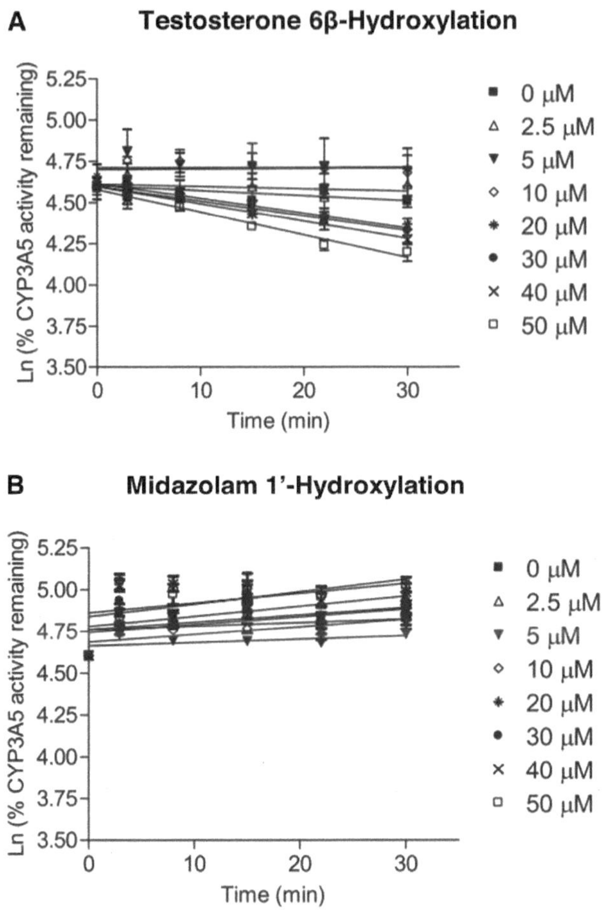

Fig. 7 (A) Time- and concentration-dependent inactivation of CYP3A5 by the dual epidermal growth factor receptor/human epidermal growth factor receptor 2 inhibitor lapatinib using testosterone as probe substrate. (B) Conversely, a lack of time- and concentration-dependent inactivation of CYP3A5 by lapatinib was observed when midazolam as utilized as the probe substrate. *Data are modified and redrawn from Chan, E. C. Y., New, L. S., Chua, T. B., Yap, C. W., Ho, H. K., & Nelson, S. D. (2012). Interaction of lapatinib with cytochrome P450 3A5.* Drug Metabolism and Disposition, *40(7), 1414–1422.*

ongoing research, there are compelling reasons to believe that it may be ascribed to the subtle yet importance nuances in the active site architecture of CYP3A4 and CYP3A5.

The covalent MBI of CYP3A4 by uricosuric agent benzbromarone (Tang, Verma, Fan, & Chan, 2021) was recently established. Utilizing a unique covalent docking methodology, the authors proposed that the mechanism of inactivation stemmed from the covalent adduction of epoxide-derived reactive intermediates of benzbromarone to an accessible cysteine residue in position 239 which lies vicinal to the F-F′ loop of CYP3A4—a region of the protein oriented directly above the active site which is known to play an instrumental role in regulating substrate access. Intriguingly, a follow-up study involving three structurally distinct probe substrates of CYP3A consistently demonstrated that such MBI was not elicited in CYP3A5 (Fig. 8) (Tang, Verma, Yong, et al., 2021). This was

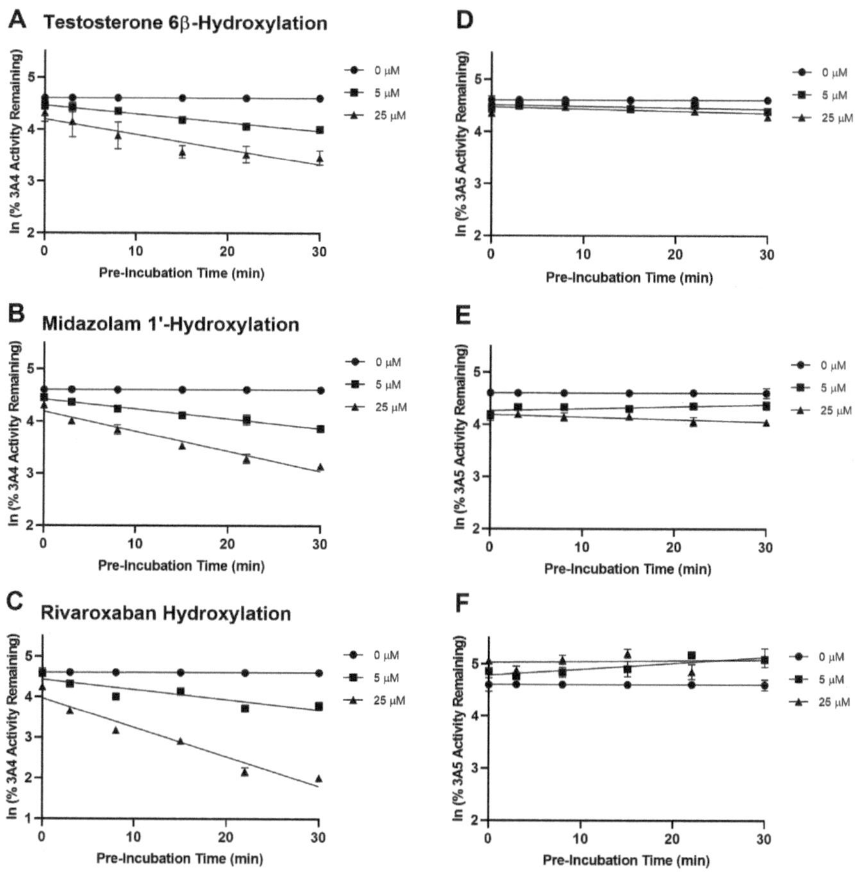

Fig. 8 (A–C) Time- and concentration-dependent inactivation of CYP3A4 by the uricosuric agent benzbromarone is confirmed by three structurally disparate probe substrates of CYP3A. (D–F) In contrast, no apparent time-dependent decrease in CYP3A5 activity elicited by BBR is observed with the same three probe substrates. *Data are modified and redrawn from Tang, L. W. T., Verma, R. K., Yong, R. P., Li, X., Wang, L., Lin, Q., … Chan, E. C. Y. (2021). Differential reversible and irreversible interactions between benzbromarone and human Cytochrome P450s 3A4 and 3A5.* Molecular Pharmacology, 100*(3), 224–236.*

rather peculiar as it was previously reported that benzbromarone could be bioactivated to its epoxide intermediates by both CYP3A4 and CYP3A5 (Wang et al., 2017), thereby implying that the salient differences in susceptibilities toward inactivation did not stem from a metabolic pathway that was unique to CYP3A4. This prompted the authors to delve further into the structural and molecular determinants underpinning this atypical isoform-specific inactivation. Juxtaposing the docked poses of benzbromarone to crystal structures of CYP3A4 to centroid frames of CYP3A5 generated *via* MD simulations, it was discovered that both CYP3A isoforms bear similar propensities to form adducts with benzbromarone despite the substitution of a cysteine residue to a serine in position 239 of CYP3A5. However, unlike in CYP3A4, the F-F′ loop of CYP3A5 possessed greater structural flexibility which allowed for the subsequent stabilization of an alternate 'open' conformation whereby the entrance to the active site is preserved (Fig. 9). Moreover, by generating *in silico* mutants of CYP3A5, it facilitated the verification of the biochemical basis for the increased

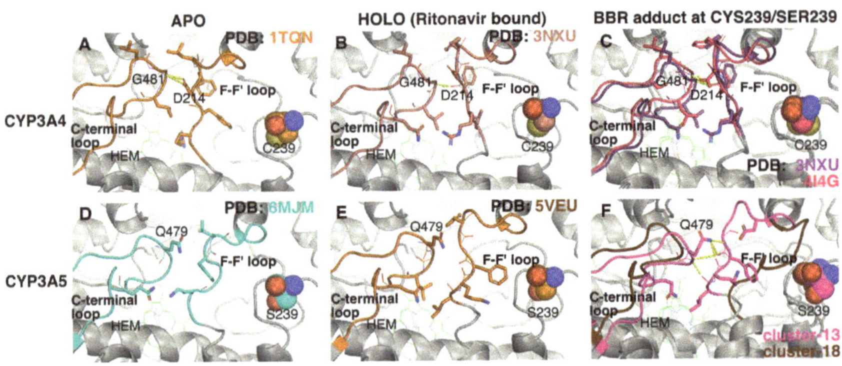

Fig. 9 F-F′ loop conformations of CYP3A4 and CYP3A5 in their apo-, holo-(ritonavir-bound) and BBR adduct forms. (A) "Closed" F-F′ loop conformation of apo CYP3A4 (PDB:1TQN). (B) "Closed" F-F′ loop conformation of ritonavir-bound CYP3A4 (PDB:3NXU). (C) "Closed" F-F′ loop conformation of BBR-adducted CYP3A4 (PDB:3NXU and 4I4G). (D) "Closed" F-F′ loop conformation of apo CYP3A5 (PDB:6MJM). (E) "Closed" F-F′ loop conformation of ritonavir-bound CYP3A5 (PDB:5VEU). (F) "Open" (cluster-18) or "closed" (cluster-13) F-F′ loop conformation of BBR-adducted CYP3A5. The F-F′ and C-terminal residues within 5 Å of each other are shown in sticks. Shade of the F-F′ and C-terminal loops corresponds to the respective PDB/Cluster ID code. *Data are from Tang, L. W. T., Verma, R. K., Yong, R. P., Li, X., Wang, L., Lin, Q., … Chan, E. C. Y. (2021). Differential reversible and irreversible interactions between benzbromarone and human cytochrome P450s 3A4 and 3A5.* Molecular Pharmacology, 100*(3), 224–236.*

flexibility in the F-F′ loop of CYP3A5—which arose from a D214G substitution that negated the formation of appreciable interactions with a glycine residue on the opposing C-terminal loop. Taken together it was postulated that the greater inherent flexibility coupled with the maintenance of an "open" F-F′ loop conformation may have preserved substrate accessibility to the active site and translated to a lack of MBI elicited by benzbromarone in CYP3A5. This proposed hypothesis is also corroborated by a study by Pearson et al. which underscored the key role of Cys239/Ser239 in the isoform-specific inactivation of CYP3A by raloxifene (Pearson et al., 2007). Overall, these findings reinforce the importance of discerning between the interactions of a common substate with both CYP3A4 and CYP3A5 due to their ability to exhibit isoform-specific inactivation.

3.4 In vivo implications of atypicalities and complexities in mechanism-based inactivation

Although *in vivo* observations of atypical kinetics stemming from TDI have been noted, their effects have been rather modest as compared to what was reported *in vitro* and, in most cases, did not produce a discernible or pronounced pharmacokinetic effect. This is likely due to the greater biological complexity and the associated increase in confounding elements as one transitions from a simpler human-relevant *in vitro* system (*i.e.*, single recombinant P450 systems, human tissue fractions or primary hepatic cultures) to the human *in vivo* situation (Tracy, 2006). Some notable examples of these extenuating factors include the presence of other drug metabolizing enzymes, involvement of non-P450 metabolic pathways and extensive protein binding to plasma proteins. Consequently, it is plausible that atypicalities in TDI may not precipitate *in vivo* due to the reduction of the effector concentration to a level below its necessary threshold or the compensation of substrate clearance by other competing metabolic routes.

However, one caveat associated with many of these earlier reports are that these data are analyzed using the conventional graphing method which is unable to accommodate atypicalities in P450 TDI kinetics. In that regard, numerical approaches using ordinary differential equation of the kinetic schemes may circumvent this limitation and yield more representative *in vitro* kinetic parameters (Yadav et al., 2020). Furthermore, the utilization of dynamic physiologically-based pharmacokinetic modeling approaches over static modeling methodologies may further facilitate more accurate predictions of prospective DDI.

4. Conclusion

In conclusion, atypical Michaelis-Menten kinetics are observed *in vitro* in many forms which have the potential to translate to significant *in vivo* consequences. Hence, the presence of atypical kinetics should be evaluated on a case-by-case basis while being cognizant of potential confounders in experimental design instead of being dismissed as experimental artifacts. Multiple mechanisms underlying atypical kinetics have been proposed although well-rounded evidence consisting of multiple biophysical methods that can establish both structural and functional features as well as corresponding enzyme kinetic analysis can be lacking in several instances, making it difficult thus far to ascertain the validity of these hypotheses. However, the current plethora of evidence does suggest a high likelihood that these mechanisms may not be mutually exclusive. In particular, substrate inhibition kinetics appear to be the most common form of atypical kinetics present in the P450 metabolism of both drugs and endogenous compounds. Notably, this can result in both pharmacological and toxicological implications due to the wide-ranging roles of P450 in drug metabolism, bioactivation, homeostasis and disease pathogenesis. In addition, atypical complexities in MBI were discussed such as probe substrate- and isoform-dependent inactivation of CYP3A enzymes that could hinder the successful extrapolation of *in vitro* CYP3A inhibition parameters to the prediction of *in vivo* DDI potential. Although the current understanding on their exact biochemical basis is still nascent, ongoing molecular modeling efforts and mechanistic studies are expected to shed more insights into these atypical phenomena.

Acknowledgments

This work was supported by the National University Heart Centre Singapore (NUHCS) Cardiovascular Research Institute (CVRI) - Core Fund [Grant NUHSRO/2019/082/Core] and the A*STAR Industry Alignment Fund—Pre-Positioning (IAF-PP) [Grant H18/01/a0/C14].

Conflict of interest

The authors declare no conflicts of interest. All data reported in the present review are from the public scientific literature.

References

Abdelmagid, S. A., Clarke, S. E., Nielsen, D. E., Badawi, A., El-Sohemy, A., Mutch, D. M., et al. (2015). Comprehensive profiling of plasma fatty acid concentrations in young healthy Canadian adults. *PLoS One*, *10*(2), e0116195. https://doi.org/10.1371/journal.pone.0116195.

Back, H., Yun, H., Kim, S. K., & Kim, J. K. (2020). Beyond the Michaelis-Menten: Accurate prediction of in vivo hepatic clearance for drugs with low K M. *Clinical and Translational Science*, *13*(6), 1199. https://doi.org/10.1111/CTS.12804.

Bapiro, T. E., Sykes, A., Martin, S., Davies, M., Yates, J. W. T., Hoch, M., et al. (2018). Complete substrate inhibition of cytochrome P450 2C8 by AZD9496, an oral selective estrogen receptor degrader. *Drug Metabolism and Disposition*, *46*(9), 1268–1276. https://doi.org/10.1124/dmd.118.081539.

Bednasz, C. J., Venuto, C. S., Ma, Q., Daar, E. S., Sax, P. E., Fischl, M. A., et al. (2017). Efavirenz therapeutic range in HIV-1 treatment Naïve participants HHS public access. *Therapeutic Drug Monitoring*, *39*(6), 596–603. https://doi.org/10.1097/FTD.0000000000000443.

Bender, G., Schexnaydre, E. E., Murphy, R. C., Uhlson, C., & Newcomer, M. E. (2016). Membrane-dependent activities of human 15-LOX-2 and its murine counterpart: Implications for murine models of atherosclerosis*. *The Journal of Biological Chemistry*, *291*(37), 19413. https://doi.org/10.1074/JBC.M116.741454.

Bjornsson, T. D., Callaghan, J. T., Einolf, H. J., Fischer, V., Gan, L., Grimm, S., et al. (2003). The conduct of in vitro and in vivo drug-drug interaction studies: A Pharmaceutical Research and Manufacturers of America (PhRMA) perspective. *Drug Metabolism and Disposition*, *31*(7), 815–832. https://doi.org/10.1124/dmd.31.7.815.

Campbell, W. B., Imig, J. D., Schmitz, J. M., & Falck, J. R. (2017). Orally active epoxyeicosatrienoic acid analogs. *Journal of Cardiovascular Pharmacology*, *70*(4), 211–224. https://doi.org/10.1097/FJC.0000000000000523.

Chan, E. C. Y., New, L. S., Chua, T. B., Yap, C. W., Ho, H. K., & Nelson, S. D. (2012). Interaction of lapatinib with cytochrome P450 3A5. *Drug Metabolism and Disposition*, *40*(7), 1414–1422. https://doi.org/10.1124/dmd.112.044958.

Chao, P., Uss, A. S., & Cheng, K. (2010). Use of intrinsic clearance for prediction of human hepatic clearance. *Expert Opinion on Drug Metabolism & Toxicology*, *6*(2), 189–198. https://doi.org/10.1517/17425250903405622.

Cheong, E. J. Y., Goh, J. J. N., Hong, Y., Venkatesan, G., Liu, Y., Chiu, G. N. C., et al. (2017). Application of static modeling in the prediction of in vivo drug-drug interactions between rivaroxaban and antiarrhythmic agents based on in vitro inhibition studies. *Drug Metabolism and Disposition*, *45*(3), 260–268. https://doi.org/10.1124/dmd.116.073890.

Chiba, M., Hensleigh, M., & Lin, J. H. (1997). Hepatic and intestinal metabolism of indinavir, an HIV protease inhibitor, in rat and human microsomes. Major role of CYP3A. *Biochemical Pharmacology*, *53*(8), 1187–1195. https://doi.org/10.1016/S0006-2952(97)00100-7.

Christensen, H., Hestad, A. L., Molden, E., & Mathiesen, L. (2011). CYP3A5-mediated metabolism of midazolam in recombinant systems is highly sensitive to NADPH-cytochrome P450 reductase activity. *Xenobiotica*, *41*(1), 1–5. https://doi.org/10.3109/00498254.2010.523734.

Christensen, H., Mathiesen, L., Postvoll, L. W., Winther, B., & Molden, E. (2009). Different enzyme kinetics of midazolam in recombinant CYP3A4 microsomes from human and insect sources. *Drug Metabolism and Pharmacokinetics*, *24*(3), 261–268. https://doi.org/10.2133/DMPK.24.261.

Dai, Y., Iwanaga, K., Lin, Y. S., Hebert, M. F., Davis, C. L., Huang, W., et al. (2004). In vitro metabolism of cyclosporine A by human kidney CYP3A5. *Biochemical Pharmacology*, *68*(9), 1889–1902. https://doi.org/10.1016/J.BCP.2004.07.012.

Dai, Z. R., Ning, J., Sun, G. B., Wang, P., Zhang, F., Ma, H. Y., et al. (2019). Cytochrome P450 3A enzymes are key contributors for hepatic metabolism of bufotalin, a natural constitute in Chinese medicine Chansu. *Frontiers in Pharmacology*, *10*(FEB), 52. https://doi.org/10.3389/fphar.2019.00052.

Davies, M., Peramuhendige, P., King, L., Golding, M., Kotian, A., Penney, M., et al. (2020). Evaluation of in vitro models for assessment of human intestinal metabolism in drug discovery. *Drug Metabolism and Disposition, 48*(11), 1169–1182. https://doi.org/10.1124/DMD.120.000111.

Davydov, D. R., Davydova, N. Y., Sineva, E. V., & Halpert, J. R. (2015). Interactions among cytochromes P450 in microsomal membranes: Oligomerization of cytochromes P450 3A4, 3A5, AND 2E1 and its functional consequences*. *Journal of Biological Chemistry, 290*(6), 3850–3864. https://doi.org/10.1074/jbc.M114.615443.

Denisov, I. G., Grinkova, Y. V., Camp, T., McLean, M. A., & Sligar, S. G. (2021). Midazolam as a probe for drug-drug interactions mediated by CYP3A4: homotropic allosteric mechanism of site-specific hydroxylation. *Biochemistry, 60*(21), 1670–1681. https://doi.org/10.1021/ACS.BIOCHEM.1C00161/SUPPL_FILE/BI1C00161_SI_001.PDF.

Denisov, I. G., Grinkova, Y. V., Nandigrami, P., Shekhar, M., Tajkhorshid, E., & Sligar, S. G. (2019). Allosteric interactions in human cytochrome P450 CYP3A4: the role of phenylalanine 213. *Biochemistry, 58*(10), 1411–1422. https://doi.org/10.1021/acs.biochem.8b01268.

Denisov, I. G., Mak, P. J., Grinkova, Y. V., Bastien, D., Bérubé, G., Sligar, S. G., et al. (2016). The use of isomeric testosterone dimers to explore allosteric effects in substrate binding to cytochrome P450 CYP3A4. *Journal of Inorganic Biochemistry, 158*, 77. https://doi.org/10.1016/J.JINORGBIO.2015.12.019.

Egnell, A. C., Houston, B., & Boyer, S. (2003). In vivo CYP3A4 heteroactivation is a possible mechanism for the drug interaction between felbamate and carbamazepine. *Journal of Pharmacology and Experimental Therapeutics, 305*(3), 1251–1262. https://doi.org/10.1124/JPET.102.047530.

Egnell, A. C., Houston, J. B., & Boyer, C. S. (2005). Predictive models of CYP3A4 heteroactivation: In vitro-in vivo scaling and pharmacophore modeling. *Journal of Pharmacology and Experimental Therapeutics, 312*(3), 926–937. https://doi.org/10.1124/JPET.104.078519.

Ekroos, M., & Sjögren, T. (2006a). Structural basis for ligand promiscuity in cytochrome P450 3A4. *Proceedings of the National Academy of Sciences of the United States of America, 103*(37), 13682–13687. https://doi.org/10.1073/pnas.0603236103.

Ekroos, M., & Sjögren, T. (2006b). Structural basis for ligand promiscuity in cytochrome P450 3A4. *Proceedings of the National Academy of Sciences of the United States of America, 103*(37), 13682–13687. https://doi.org/10.1073/pnas.0603236103.

Elfaki, I., Mir, R., Almutairi, F. M., & Abu Duhier, F. M. (2018). Cytochrome P450: Polymorphisms and roles in cancer, diabetes and atherosclerosis. *Asian Pacific Journal of Cancer Prevention: APJCP, 19*(8), 2057–2070. https://doi.org/10.22034/APJCP.2018.19.8.2057.

Elinder, F., & Liin, S. I. (2017). Actions and mechanisms of polyunsaturated fatty acids on voltage-gated ion channels. *Frontiers in Physiology, 8*, 43. https://doi.org/10.3389/fphys.2017.00043.

Emoto, C., Murayama, N., Rostami-Hodjegan, A., & Yamazaki, H. (2010). Methodologies for investigating drug metabolism at the early drug discovery stage: Prediction of hepatic drug clearance and P450 contribution. *Current Drug Metabolism, 11*(8), 678–685. https://doi.org/10.2174/138920010794233503.

Friesenhengst, A., Pribitzer-Winner, T., Miedl, H., Pröstling, K., & Schreiber, M. (2018). Elevated aromatase (CYP19A1) expression is associated with a poor survival of patients with estrogen receptor positive breast cancer. *Hormones & Cancer, 9*(2), 128. https://doi.org/10.1007/S12672-017-0317-2.

Fritz, A., Busch, D., Lapczuk, J., Ostrowski, M., Drozdzik, M., & Oswald, S. (2019). Expression of clinically relevant drug-metabolizing enzymes along the human intestine and their correlation to drug transporters and nuclear receptors: An intra-subject analysis. *Basic & Clinical Pharmacology & Toxicology, 124*(3), 245–255. https://doi.org/10.1111/BCPT.13137.

Galetin, A., Clarke, S. E., & Houston, J. B. (2003). Multisite kinetic analysis of interactions between prototypical CYP3A4 subgroup substrates: Midazolam, testosterone, and nifedipine. *Drug Metabolism and Disposition*, *31*(9), 1108–1116. https://doi.org/10.1124/dmd.31.9.1108.

Galetin, A., Ito, K., Hallifax, D., & Houston, J. B. (2005). CYP3A4 substrate selection and substitution in the prediction of potential drug-drug interactions. *Journal of Pharmacology and Experimental Therapeutics*, *314*(1), 180–190. https://doi.org/10.1124/jpet.104.082826.

Giatromanolaki, A., Fasoulaki, V., Kalamida, D., Mitrakas, A., Kakouratos, C., Lialiaris, T., et al. (2019). CYP17A1 and androgen-receptor expression in prostate carcinoma tissues and cancer cell lines. *Current Urology*, *13*(3), 157. https://doi.org/10.1159/000499276.

Gibson, C. R., Wang, Y. H., Varkhede, N., & Ma, B. (2021). Variability in human in vitro enzyme kinetics. In S. Nagar, U. A. Argikar, & D. Tweedie (Eds.), *Vol. 2342. Enzyme kinetics in drug metabolism. Methods in molecular biology* (pp. 443–479). New York, NY: Humana. https://doi.org/10.1007/978-1-0716-1554-6_16.

Goutelle, S., Maurin, M., Rougier, F., Barbaut, X., Bourguignon, L., Ducher, M., et al. (2008). The Hill equation: A review of its capabilities in pharmacological modelling. *Fundamental & Clinical Pharmacology*, *22*(6), 633–648. https://doi.org/10.1111/j.1472-8206.2008.00633.x.

Guengerich, F. P. (2001). Common and uncommon cytochrome P450 reactions related to metabolism and chemical toxicity. *Chemical Research in Toxicology*, *14*(6), 611–650, American Chemical Society. https://doi.org/10.1021/tx0002583.

Guengerich, F. P. (2017). Intersection of roles of cytochrome P450 enzymes with xenobiotic and endogenous substrates. Relevance to toxicity and drug interactions. *Chemical Research in Toxicology*, *30*(1), 2. https://doi.org/10.1021/ACS.CHEMRESTOX.6B00226.

Guengerich, F. P. (2019). Kinetic modeling of steady-state situations in cytochrome P450 enzyme reactions. *Drug Metabolism and Disposition*, *47*(11), 1232–1239. https://doi.org/10.1124/dmd.119.088732.

Guengerich, F. P. (2021). A history of the roles of cytochrome P450 enzymes in the toxicity of drugs. *Toxicological Research*, *37*(1), 1–23. https://doi.org/10.1007/s43188-020-00056-z.

Guo, X., Li, W., Li, Q., Chen, Y., Zhao, G., Peng, Y., et al. (2019). Tofacitinib is a mechanism-based inactivator of cytochrome P450 3A4. *Chemical Research in Toxicology*, *32*(9), 1791–1800. https://doi.org/10.1021/acs.chemrestox.9b00141.

Hamilton, E. P., Patel, M. R., Armstrong, A. C., Baird, R. D., Jhaveri, K., Hoch, M., et al. (2018). A first-in-human study of the new oral selective estrogen receptor degrader AZD9496 for ER+/HER2− advanced breast cancer. *Clinical Cancer Research*, *24*(15), 3510–3518. https://doi.org/10.1158/1078-0432.CCR-17-3102.

Hariparsad, N., Ramsden, D., Taskar, K., Badée, J., Venkatakrishnan, K., Reddy, M. B., et al. (2021). Current practices, gap analysis and proposed workflows for PBPK modeling of cytochrome P450 induction: An industry perspective. *Clinical Pharmacology and Therapeutics*. https://doi.org/10.1002/CPT.2503.

Heintze, T., Klein, K., Hofmann, U., & Zanger, U. M. (2021). Differential effects on human cytochromes P450 by CRISPR/Cas9-induced genetic knockout of cytochrome P450 reductase and cytochrome b5 in HepaRG cells. *Scientific Reports*, *11*(1), 1–14. https://doi.org/10.1038/s41598-020-79952-1.

Henderson, C. J., McLaughlin, L. A., & Wolf, C. R. (2013). Evidence that cytochrome b5 and cytochrome b5 reductase can act as sole electron donors to the hepatic cytochrome P450 system. *Molecular Pharmacology*, *83*(6), 1209–1217. https://doi.org/10.1124/MOL.112.084616.

Hindricks, G., Potpara, T., Dagres, N., Arbelo, E., Bax, J. J., Blomström-Lundqvist, C., et al. (2021). 2020 ESC Guidelines for the diagnosis and management of atrial fibrillation developed in collaboration with the European Association for Cardio-Thoracic Surgery (EACTS). *European Heart Journal*, *42*(5), 373–498. https://doi.org/10.1093/eurheartj/ehaa612.

Ho, H. K., Chan, J. C. Y., Hardy, K. D., & Chan, E. C. Y. (2015). Mechanism-based inactivation of CYP450 enzymes: A case study of lapatinib. *Drug Metabolism Reviews*, *47*(1), 21–28. https://doi.org/10.3109/03602532.2014.1003648.

Hong, Y., Chia, Y. M. F., Yeo, R. H., Venkatesan, G., Koh, S. K., Chai, C. L. L., et al. (2016). Inactivation of human cytochrome P450 3A4 and 3A5 by dronedarone and n-desbutyl dronedarone. *Molecular Pharmacology*, *89*(1), 1–13. https://doi.org/10.1124/mol.115.100891.

Houston, J. B., & Galetin, A. (2005). Modelling atypical CYP3A4 kinetics: Principles and pragmatism. *Archives of Biochemistry and Biophysics*, *433*(2), 351–360. https://doi.org/10.1016/j.abb.2004.09.010.

Hu, X., Lan, T., Dai, D., Xu, R. A., Yuan, L., Zhou, Q., et al. (2016). Evaluation of 24 CYP2D6 variants on the metabolism of nebivolol in vitro. *Drug Metabolism and Disposition: The Biological Fate of Chemicals*, *44*(11), 1828–1831. https://doi.org/10.1124/DMD.116.071811.

Jagdish, K. R., Zhao, S. Z., Olejnik, N., Moore, D., Satoh, H., Warner, N., et al. (2003). Substrate dependent inhibition profiles of fourteen drugs on CYP3A4 activity measured by a high throughput LCMS/MS method with four probe drugs, midazolam, testosterone, nifedipine and terfenadine. *Drug Metabolism and Pharmacokinetics*, *18*(2), 128–138. https://doi.org/10.2133/DMPK.18.128.

Jamei, M. (2016). Recent advances in development and application of physiologically-based pharmacokinetic (PBPK) models: A transition from academic curiosity to regulatory acceptance. *Current Pharmacology Reports*, *2*, 161–169. https://doi.org/10.1007/s40495-016-0059-9.

Jamieson, K. L., Endo, T., Darwesh, A. M., Samokhvalov, V., & Seubert, J. M. (2017). Cytochrome P450-derived eicosanoids and heart function. *Pharmacology & Therapeutics*, *179*, 47–83. https://doi.org/10.1016/j.pharmthera.2017.05.005.

Kamdem, L. K., Streit, F., Zanger, U. M., Brockmöller, J., Oellerich, M., Armstrong, V. W., et al. (2005). Contribution of CYP3A5 to the in vitro hepatic clearance of tacrolimus. *Clinical Chemistry*, *51*(8), 1374–1381. https://doi.org/10.1373/clinchem.2005.050047.

Ke, A., Barter, Z., Rowland-Yeo, K., & Almond, L. (2016). Towards a best practice approach in PBPK modeling: Case example of developing a unified efavirenz model accounting for induction of CYPs 3A4 and 2B6. *CPT: Pharmacometrics & Systems Pharmacology*, *5*(7), 367. https://doi.org/10.1002/PSP4.12088.

Kenworthy, K. E., Bloomer, J. C., Clarke, S. E., & Houston, J. B. (1999). CYP3A4 drug interactions: Correlation of 10 in vitro probe substrates. *British Journal of Clinical Pharmacology*, *48*(5), 716–727. https://doi.org/10.1046/j.1365-2125.1999.00073.x.

Kokkonen, P., Beier, A., Mazurenko, S., Damborsky, J., Bednar, D., & Prokop, Z. (2021). Substrate inhibition by the blockage of product release and its control by tunnel engineering. *RSC Chemical Biology*, *2*(2), 645–655. https://doi.org/10.1039/D0CB00171F.

Korzekwa, K. (2021). Enzyme kinetics of oxidative metabolism-cytochromes P450. In S. Nagar, U. A. Argikar, & D. Tweedie (Eds.), *Vol. 2342. Enzyme kinetics in drug metabolism. Methods in molecular biology* (pp. 237–256). New York, NY: Humana. https://doi.org/10.1007/978-1-0716-1554-6_9.

Kuehl, P., Zhang, J., Lin, Y., Lamba, J., Assem, M., Schuetz, J., et al. (2001). Sequence diversity in CYP3A promoters and characterization of the genetic basis of polymorphic CYP3A5 expression. *Nature Genetics*, *27*(4), 383–391. https://doi.org/10.1038/86882.

Kumar, V., Rock, D. A., Warren, C. J., Tracy, T. S., & Wahlstrom, J. L. (2006). Enzyme source effects on CYP2C9 kinetics and inhibition. *Drug Metabolism and Disposition: The Biological Fate of Chemicals*, *34*(11), 1903. https://doi.org/10.1124/DMD.106.010249.

Lamba, J. K., Lin, Y. S., Schuetz, E. G., & Thummel, K. E. (2002). Genetic contribution to variable human CYP3A-mediated metabolism. *Advanced Drug Delivery Reviews*, *54*(10), 1271–1294. https://doi.org/10.1016/S0169-409X(02)00066-2.

Lampe, J. N. (2017). Advances in the understanding of protein-protein interactions in drug metabolizing enzymes through the use of biophysical techniques. *Frontiers in Pharmacology*, *8*, 521. https://doi.org/10.3389/FPHAR.2017.00521.

Leow, J. W. H., & Chan, E. C. Y. (2019). Atypical Michaelis-Menten kinetics in cytochrome P450 enzymes: A focus on substrate inhibition. *Biochemical Pharmacology*, *169*, 113615. https://doi.org/10.1016/j.bcp.2019.08.017.

Leow, J. W. H., Verma, R. K., Lim, A. B. H., Fan, H., & Chan, E. C. Y. (2021). Atypical kinetics of cytochrome P450 2J2: Epoxidation of arachidonic acid and reversible inhibition by xenobiotic inhibitors. *European Journal of Pharmaceutical Sciences*, *164*, 105889. https://doi.org/10.1016/J.EJPS.2021.105889.

Li Wan Po, A., & Zhang, W. Y. (1998). What lessons can be learnt from withdrawal of mibefradil from the market? *The Lancet*, *351*(9119), 1829–1830. https://doi.org/10.1016/S0140-6736(05)78800-0.

Lin, Y. S., Dowling, A. L. S., Quigley, S. D., Farin, F. M., Zhang, J., Lamba, J., et al. (2002). Co-regulation of CYP3A4 and CYP3A5 and contribution to hepatic and intestinal midazolam metabolism. *Molecular Pharmacology*, *62*(1), 162–172. https://doi.org/10.1124/mol.62.1.162.

Lin, Y., Lu, P., Tang, C., Mei, Q., Rodrigues, A. D., Rushmore, T. H., et al. (2001a). Substrate inhibition kinetics for cytochrome P450-catalyzed reactions. *Drug Metabolism and Disposition*, *29*(4), 368–374.

Lin, Y., Lu, P., Tang, C., Mei, Q., Sandig, G., Rodrigues, A. D., et al. (2001b). Substrate inhibition kinetics for cytochrome P450-catalyzed reactions. *Drug Metabolism and Disposition*, *29*(4 Pt 1), 368–374.

Loue, C., & Tod, M. (2014). Reliability and extension of quantitative prediction of CYP3A4-mediated drug interactions based on clinical data. *The AAPS Journal*, *16*(6), 1309. https://doi.org/10.1208/S12248-014-9663-Y.

Maekawa, K., Adachi, M., Matsuzawa, Y., Zhang, Q., Kuroki, R., Saito, Y., et al. (2017). Structural basis of single-nucleotide polymorphisms in cytochrome P450 2C9. *Biochemistry*, *56*(41), 5476–5480. https://doi.org/10.1021/ACS.BIOCHEM.7B00795/SUPPL_FILE/BI7B00795_SI_001.PDF.

Marill, J., Capron, C. C., Idres, N., & Chabot, G. G. (2002). Human cytochrome P450s involved in the metabolism of 9-cis- and 13-cis-retinoic acids. *Biochemical Pharmacology*, *63*(5), 933–943. https://doi.org/10.1016/S0006-2952(01)00925-X.

Mast, N., Verwilst, P., Wilkey, C. J., Guengerich, F. P., & Pikuleva, I. A. (2020). In vitro activation of cytochrome P450 46A1 (CYP46A1) by efavirenz-related compounds. *Journal of Medicinal Chemistry*, *63*(12), 6477–6488. https://doi.org/10.1021/ACS.JMEDCHEM.9B01383/SUPPL_FILE/JM9B01383_SI_002.CSV.

Masubuchi, Y., & Horie, T. (2007). Toxicological significance of mechanism-based inactivation of cytochrome P450 enzymes by drugs. *Critical Reviews in Toxicology*, *37*(5), 389–412, Taylor & Francis. https://doi.org/10.1080/10408440701215233.

McMasters, D. R., Torres, R. A., Crathern, S. J., Dooney, D. L., Nachbar, R. B., Sheridan, R. P., et al. (2007). Inhibition of recombinant cytochrome P450 isoforms 2D6 and 2C9 by diverse drug-like molecules. *Journal of Medicinal Chemistry*, *50*(14), 3205. https://doi.org/10.1021/JM0700060.

Michaelis, L., & Menten, M. L. (1913). The kenetics of the inversion effect. *Biochemische Zeitschrift*, *49*, 333–369.

Michaelis, L., Menten, M. L., Johnson, K. A., & Goody, R. S. (2011). The original Michaelis constant: Translation of the 1913 Michaelis-Menten paper. *Biochemistry*, *50*(39), 8264–8269. https://doi.org/10.1021/bi201284u.

Muller, C. S., Knehans, T., Davydov, D. R., Bounds, P. L., von Mandach, U., Halpert, J. R., et al. (2015). Concurrent cooperativity and substrate inhibition in the epoxidation of carbamazepine by cytochrome P450 3A4 active site mutants inspired by molecular dynamics simulations. *Biochemistry*, *54*(3), 711–721. https://doi.org/10.1021/bi5011656.

Neau, D. B., Bender, G., Boeglin, W. E., Bartlett, S. G., Brash, A. R., & Newcomer, M. E. (2014). Crystal structure of a lipoxygenase in complex with substrate. *Journal of Biological Chemistry*, *289*(46), 31905–31913. https://doi.org/10.1074/JBC.M114.599662.

Obach, R. S., & Reed-Hagen, A. E. (2002). Measurement of Michaelis constants for cytochrome P450-mediated biotransformation reactions using a substrate depletion approach. *Drug Metabolism and Disposition*, *30*(7), 831–837. https://doi.org/10.1124/DMD.30.7.831.

Oda, Y., & Kharasch, E. D. (2001a). Metabolism of levo-α-acetylmethadol (LAAM) by human liver cytochrome P450: Involvement of CYP3A4 characterized by atypical kinetics with two binding sites. *Journal of Pharmacology and Experimental Therapeutics*, *297*(1), 410–422.

Oda, Y., & Kharasch, E. D. (2001b). Metabolism of methadone and levo-acetylmethadol (LAAM) by human intestinal cytochrome P450 3A4 (CYP3A4): Potential contribution of intestinal metabolism to presystemic clearance and bioactivation. *Journal of Pharmacology and Experimental Therapeutics*, *298*(3), 1021–1032.

Okada, Y., Murayama, N., Yanagida, C., Shimizu, M., Guengerich, F. P., & Yamazaki, H. (2009). Drug interactions of thalidomide with midazolam and cyclosporine a: heterotropic cooperativity of human cytochrome P450 3A5. *Drug Metabolism and Disposition*, *37*(1), 18–23. https://doi.org/10.1124/dmd.108.024679.

Oswald, S., Meyer Zu Schwabedissen, H. E., Nassif, A., Modess, C., Desta, Z., Ogburn, E. T., et al. (2012). Impact of efavirenz on intestinal metabolism and transport: Insights from an interaction study with ezetimibe in healthy volunteers. *Clinical Pharmacology and Therapeutics*, *91*(3), 506. https://doi.org/10.1038/CLPT.2011.255.

Paragas, E. M., Wang, Z., Korzekwa, K., & Nagar, S. (2021). Complex cytochrome P450 kinetics due to multisubstrate binding and sequential metabolism. Part 2. Modeling of experimental data. *Drug Metabolism and Disposition*, *49*(12), 1100–1108. https://doi.org/10.1124/DMD.121.000554.

Pearson, J. T., Wahlstrom, J. L., Dickmann, L. J., Kumar, S., Halpert, J. R., Wienkers, L. C., et al. (2007). Differential time-dependent inactivation of P450 3A4 and P450 3A5 by raloxifene: A key role for C239 in quenching reactive intermediates. *Chemical Research in Toxicology*, *20*(12), 1778–1786. https://doi.org/10.1021/tx700207u.

Pikuleva, I. A., & Waterman, M. R. (2013). Cytochromes P450: Roles in diseases. *The Journal of Biological Chemistry*, *288*(24), 17091. https://doi.org/10.1074/JBC.R112.431916.

Pompeia, C., Lima, T., & Curi, R. (2003). Arachidonic acid cytotoxicity: Can arachidonic acid be a physiological mediator of cell death? *Cell Biochemistry and Function*, *21*(2), 97–104. https://doi.org/10.1002/cbf.1012.

Porter, C. M., & Miller, B. G. (2012). Cooperativity in monomeric enzymes with single ligand-binding sites. *Bioorganic Chemistry*, *43*, 44–50. https://doi.org/10.1016/J.BIOORG.2011.11.001.

Prueksaritanont, T., Ma, B., Tang, C., Meng, Y., Assang, C., Lu, P., et al. (1999). Metabolic interactions between mibefradil and HMG-CoA reductase inhibitors: An in vitro investigation with human liver preparations. *British Journal of Clinical Pharmacology*, *47*(3), 291–298. https://doi.org/10.1046/J.1365-2125.1999.00903.X.

Redhair, M., & Atkins, W. M. (2021). Analytical and functional aspects of protein-ligand interactions: Beyond induced fit and conformational selection. *Archives of Biochemistry and Biophysics*, *714*, 109064. https://doi.org/10.1016/J.ABB.2021.109064.

Reed, J. R., & Backes, W. L. (2012). Formation of P450•P450 complexes and their effect on P450 function. *Pharmacology & Therapeutics*, *133*(3), 299–310. https://doi.org/10.1016/j.pharmthera.2011.11.009.

Reed, M. C., Lieb, A., & Nijhout, H. F. (2010). The biological significance of substrate inhibition: A mechanism with diverse functions. *BioEssays*, *32*(5), 422–429. https://doi.org/10.1002/BIES.200900167.

Rendic, S. P., & Guengerich, F. P. (2021). Human family 1-4 cytochrome P450 enzymes involved in the metabolic activation of xenobiotic and physiological chemicals: An update. *Archives of Toxicology*, *95*(2), 395–472. https://doi.org/10.1007/S00204-020-02971-4.

Sakamoto, M., Itoh, T., & Fujiwara, R. (2013). Prediction of in vivo carbamazepine 10,11-epoxidation from in vitro metabolic studies with human liver microsomes: Importance of its sigmoidal kinetics. *Biological & Pharmaceutical Bulletin*, *36*(12), 1959–1963. https://doi.org/10.1248/BPB.B13-00569.

Schoch, G. A., Yano, J. K., Sansen, S., Dansette, P. M., David, C., & Johnson, E. F. (2008). Determinants of cytochrome P450 2C8 substrate binding structures of complexes with montelukast, troglitazone, felodipine, and 9-cis-retinoic acid. *The Journal of Biological Chemistry*, *283*(25), 17227–17237. https://doi.org/10.1074/jbc.M802180200.

Schoch, G. A., Yano, J. K., Wester, M. R., Griffin, K. J., Stout, C. D., & Johnson, E. F. (2004). Structure of human microsomal cytochrome P450 2C8: Evidence for a peripheral fatty acid binding site. *Journal of Biological Chemistry*, *279*(10), 9497–9503. https://doi.org/10.1074/JBC.M312516200.

Schulz, C., Kammerer, S., & Küpper, J. H. (2019). NADPH-cytochrome P450 reductase expression and enzymatic activity in primary-like human hepatocytes and HepG2 cells for in vitro biotransformation studies. *Clinical Hemorheology and Microcirculation*, *73*(1), 249–260. https://doi.org/10.3233/CH-199226.

Seliskar, M., & Rozman, D. (2007). Mammalian cytochromes P450—Importance of tissue specificity. *Biochimica et Biophysica Acta*, *1770*(3), 458–466. https://doi.org/10.1016/J.BBAGEN.2006.09.016.

Sevrioukova, I. F., & Poulos, T. L. (2015). Anion-dependent stimulation of CYP3A4 monooxygenase. *Biochemistry*, *54*(26), 4083–4096. https://doi.org/10.1021/acs.biochem.5b00510.

Shoieb, S. M., El-Ghiaty, M. A., Alqahtani, M. A., & El-Kadi, A. O. S. (2020). Cytochrome P450-derived eicosanoids and inflammation in liver diseases. *Prostaglandins & Other Lipid Mediators*, *147*, 106400. https://doi.org/10.1016/J.PROSTAGLANDINS.2019.106400.

Short, N. J., & Connors, J. M. (2014). New oral anticoagulants and the cancer patient. *The Oncologist*, *19*(1), 82–93. https://doi.org/10.1634/theoncologist.2013-0239.

Shou, M., Lin, Y., Lu, P., Tang, C., Mei, Q., Cui, D., et al. (2001). Enzyme kinetics of cytochrome P450-mediated reactions. *Current Drug Metabolism*, *2*(1), 17–36.

Siu, Y. A., Hao, M. H., Dixit, V., & Lai, W. G. (2018). Celecoxib is a substrate of CYP2D6: Impact on celecoxib metabolism in individuals with CYP2C9*3 variants. *Drug Metabolism and Pharmacokinetics*, *33*(5), 219–227. https://doi.org/10.1016/J.DMPK.2018.06.001.

Šrejber, M., Navrátilová, V., Paloncýová, M., Bazgier, V., Berka, K., Anzenbacher, P., et al. (2018). Membrane-attached mammalian cytochromes P450: An overview of the membrane's effects on structure, drug binding, and interactions with redox partners. *Journal of Inorganic Biochemistry*, *183*, 117–136. https://doi.org/10.1016/J.JINORGBIO.2018.03.002.

Stresser, D. M., Blanchard, A. P., Turner, S. D., Erve, J. C. L., Dandeneau, A. A., Miller, V. P., et al. (2000). Substrate-dependent modulation of CYP3A4 catalytic activity: Analysis of 27 test compounds with four fluorometric substrates. *Drug Metabolism and Disposition*, *28*(12), 1440–1448.

Su, M., Chakraborty, S., Osawa, Y., & Zhang, H. (2020). Cryo-EM reveals the architecture of the dimeric cytochrome P450 CYP102A1 enzyme and conformational changes required for redox partner recognition. *The Journal of Biological Chemistry*, *295*(6), 1637–1645. https://doi.org/10.1074/JBC.RA119.011305.

Sugiyama, M., Fujita, K., Murayama, N., Akiyama, Y., Yamazaki, H., & Sasaki, Y. (2011). Sorafenib and sunitinib, two anticancer drugs, inhibit CYP3A4-mediated and activate CY3A5-mediated midazolam 1′-hydroxylation. *Drug Metabolism and Disposition*, *39*(5), 757–762. https://doi.org/10.1124/dmd.110.037853.

Tang, L. W. T., Teng, J. W., Koh, S. K., Zhou, L., Go, M. L., & Chan, E. C. Y. (2021). Mechanism-based inactivation of cytochrome P450 3A4 and 3A5 by the fibroblast growth factor receptor inhibitor erdafitinib. *Chemical Research in Toxicology*, *34*(7), 1800–1813. https://doi.org/10.1021/acs.chemrestox.1c00178.

Tang, L. W. T., Teng, J. W., Verma, R. K., Koh, S. K., Zhou, L., Go, M. L., et al. (2021). Infigratinib is a reversible inhibitor and mechanism-based inactivator of cytochrome P450 3A4. *Drug Metabolism and Disposition*, *49*(9), 856–868. https://doi.org/10.1124/dmd.121.000508.

Tang, L. W. T., Verma, R. K., Fan, H., & Chan, E. C. Y. (2021). Mechanism-based inactivation of cytochrome P450 3A4 by benzbromarone. *Molecular Pharmacology*, *99*(4), 266–276. https://doi.org/10.1124/molpharm.120.000086.

Tang, L. W. T., Verma, R. K., Yong, R. P., Li, X., Wang, L., Lin, Q., et al. (2021). Differential reversible and irreversible interactions between benzbromarone and human cytochrome P450s 3A4 and 3A5. *Molecular Pharmacology*, *100*(3), 224–236. https://doi.org/10.1124/molpharm.121.000256.

Tang, E. K., Voo, K. J., Nguyen, M. N., & Tuckey, R. C. (2010). Metabolism of substrates incorporated into phospholipid vesicles by mouse 25-hydroxyvitamin D3 1alpha-hydroxylase (CYP27B1). *The Journal of Steroid Biochemistry and Molecular Biology*, *119*(3–5), 171–179. https://doi.org/10.1016/j.jsbmb.2010.02.022.

Tang, L. W. T., Wei, W., Verma, R. K., Koh, S. K., Zhou, L., Fan, H., et al. (2022). Direct and sequential bioactivation of pemigatinib to reactive iminium ion intermediates culminate in mechanism-based inactivation of cytochrome P450 3A. *Drug Metabolism and Disposition*, *50*(5), 529–540. https://doi.org/10.1124/dmd.121.000804. DMD-AR-2021-000804.

Tracy, T. S. (2003). Atypical enzyme kinetics: their effect on in vitro-in vivo pharmacokinetic predictions and drug interactions. *Current Drug Metabolism*, *4*(5), 341–346.

Tracy, T. S. (2006). Atypical cytochrome p450 kinetics: implications for drug discovery. *Drugs in R&D*, 7(6), 349–363. https://doi.org/10.2165/00126839-200607060-00004.

Tracy, T. S., Hutzler, J. M., Haining, R. L., Rettie, A. E., Hummel, M. A., & Dickmann, L. J. (2002). Polymorphic variants (CYP2C9*3 and CYP2C9*5) and the F114L active site mutation of CYP2C9: Effect on atypical kinetic metabolism profiles. *Drug Metabolism and Disposition*, *30*(4), 385–390.

Tsamandouras, N., Rostami-Hodjegan, A., & Aarons, L. (2015). Combining the "bottom up" and "top down" approaches in pharmacokinetic modelling: Fitting PBPK models to observed clinical data. *British Journal of Clinical Pharmacology*, *79*(1), 48–55. https://doi.org/10.1111/BCP.12234.

Wang, P. F., Neiner, A., & Kharasch, E. D. (2019). Efavirenz metabolism: Influence of polymorphic CYP2B6 variants and stereochemistry. *Drug Metabolism and Disposition*, *47*(10), 1195–1205. https://doi.org/10.1124/dmd.119.086348.

Wang, H., Peng, Y., Zhang, T., Lan, Q., Zhao, H., Wang, W., et al. (2017). Metabolic epoxidation is a critical step for the development of benzbromarone-induced hepatotoxicity. *Drug Metabolism and Disposition*, *45*(12), 1354–1363. https://doi.org/10.1124/dmd.117.077818.

Wang, A., Stout, C. D., Zhang, Q., & Johnson, E. F. (2015). Contributions of Ionic interactions and protein dynamics to cytochrome P450 2D6 (CYP2D6) substrate and inhibitor binding. *Journal of Biological Chemistry, 290*(8), 5092–5104. https://doi.org/10.1074/JBC.M114.627661.

Wang, B., Yang, L. P., Zhang, X. Z., Huang, S. Q., Bartlam, M., & Zhou, S. F. (2009). New insights into the structural characteristics and functional relevance of the human cytochrome P450 2D6 enzyme. *Drug Metabolism Reviews, 41*(4), 573–643. https://doi.org/10.1080/03602530903118729.

Wilkinson, G. R. (1996). Cytochrome P4503A (CYP3A) metabolism: Prediction of in vivo activity in humans. *Journal of Pharmacokinetics and Biopharmaceutics, 24*(5), 475–490. https://doi.org/10.1007/BF02353475.

Williams, P. A., Cosme, J., Matak Vinković, D., Ward, A., Angove, H. C., Day, P. J., et al. (2004). Crystal structures of human cytochrome P450 3A4 bound to metyrapone and progesterone. *Science, 305*(5684), 683–686. https://doi.org/10.1126/science.1099736.

Witherow, L. E., & Houston, J. B. (1999). Sigmoidal kinetics of CYP3A substrates: An approach for scaling dextromethorphan metabolism in hepatic microsomes and isolated hepatocytes to predict in vivo clearance in rat. *Journal of Pharmacology and Experimental Therapeutics, 290*(1), 58–65.

Wrighton, S. A., VandenBranden, M., & Ring, B. J. (1996). The human drug metabolizing cytochromes P450. *Journal of Pharmacokinetics and Biopharmaceutics, 24*(5), 461–473. https://doi.org/10.1007/BF02353474.

Wu, B. (2011). Substrate inhibition kinetics in drug metabolism reactions. *Drug Metabolism Reviews, 43*(4), 440–456. https://doi.org/10.3109/03602532.2011.615320.

Xu, X., Zhang, X. A., & Wang, D. W. (2011). The roles of CYP450 epoxygenases and metabolites, epoxyeicosatrienoic acids, in cardiovascular and malignant diseases. *Advanced Drug Delivery Reviews, 63*(8), 597–609. https://doi.org/10.1016/j.addr.2011.03.006.

Yadav, J., Korzekwa, K., & Nagar, S. (2021). Numerical methods for modeling enzyme kinetics. *Methods in Molecular Biology (Clifton, N.J.), 2342*, 147–168. https://doi.org/10.1007/978-1-0716-1554-6_6.

Yadav, J., Paragas, E., Korzekwa, K., & Nagar, S. (2020). Time-dependent enzyme inactivation: Numerical analyses of in vitro data and prediction of drug-drug interactions. *Pharmacology & therapeutics, 206*, 107449. https://doi.org/10.1016/J.PHARMTHERA.2019.107449.

Yang, J., Atkins, W. M., Isoherranen, N., Paine, M. F., & Thummel, K. E. (2012). Evidence of CYP3A allosterism in vivo: Analysis of fluconazole and midazolam interaction. *Clinical Pharmacology and Therapeutics, 91*(3), 442. https://doi.org/10.1038/CLPT.2011.178.

Yasar, Ü., Tybring, G., Hidestrand, M., Oscarson, M., Ingelman-Sundberg, M., Dahl, M.-L., et al. (2001). Role of CYP2C9 polymorphism in losartan oxidation. *Drug Metabolism and Disposition, 29*(7), 1051–1056.

Zanger, U. M., & Schwab, M. (2013). Cytochrome P450 enzymes in drug metabolism: Regulation of gene expression, enzyme activities, and impact of genetic variation. *Pharmacology and Therapeutics, 138*(1), 103–141. https://doi.org/10.1016/j.pharmthera.2012.12.007. Pergamon.

Zhang, H., Gao, N., Liu, T., Fang, Y., Qi, B., Wen, Q., et al. (2015). Effect of cytochrome b5 content on the activity of polymorphic CYP1A2, 2B6, and 2E1 in human liver microsomes. *PLoS One, 10*(6), e0128547. https://doi.org/10.1371/JOURNAL.PONE.0128547.

Zhang, H. F., Li, Z. H., Liu, J. Y., Liu, T. T., Wang, P., Fang, Y., et al. (2016). Correlation of cytochrome P450 oxidoreductase expression with the expression of 10 isoforms of cytochrome P450 in human liver. *Drug Metabolism and Disposition, 44*(8), 1193–1200. https://doi.org/10.1124/DMD.116.069849/-/DC1.

Zhang, Z., Li, Y., Shou, M., Zhang, Y., Ngui, J. S., Stearns, R. A., et al. (2004). Influence of different recombinant systems on the cooperativity exhibited by cytochrome P4503A4. *Xenobiotica; The Fate of Foreign Compounds in Biological Systems*, *34*(5), 473–486. https://doi.org/10.1080/00498250410001691271.

Zhao, B., Lei, L., Kagawa, N., Sundaramoorthy, M., Banerjee, S., Nagy, L. D., et al. (2012). Three-dimensional structure of steroid 21-hydroxylase (cytochrome P450 21A2) with two substrates reveals locations of disease-associated variants. *The Journal of Biological Chemistry*, *287*(13), 10613–10622. https://doi.org/10.1074/JBC.M111.323501.

Zhou, S., Chan, E., Li, X., & Huang, M. (2005). Clinical outcomes and management of mechanism-based inhibition of cytochrome P450 3A4. *Therapeutics and Clinical Risk Management*, *1*(1), 3–13. https://doi.org/10.2147/TCRM.1.1.3.53600.

CHAPTER SIX

Biosynthesis using cytochrome P450 enzymes: Focus on synthesis of drug metabolites

W. Griffith Humphreys*
Aranmore Pharma Consulting, Lawrenceville, NJ, United States
*Corresponding author: e-mail address: wghumphreys@gmail.com

Contents

Abstract

While modern synthetic chemistry provides the ability to synthesize an incredible variety of new structures, the natural world provides unmatched chemical diversity. This diversity can be employed in the drug discovery process either through isolation of an organic molecule from a biological source as a drug candidate, usually referred to as natural product chemistry, or by providing enzymes that are capable to performing chemistry not available through synthetic chemistry approaches. Natural or engineered enzymes can be used in candidate discovery to generate chemical diversity in conjunction with synthetic efforts. As a candidate progresses into develop there is often a need to characterize metabolites, thus a need for metabolite standard synthesis. Metabolite synthesis is best accomplished with a flexible application of both chemical and biosynthetic approaches. This overview of the use of biosynthesis to aid in the drug discovery and development process will cover multiple methodologies with a focus on the use of microbes as a flexible and cost-effective resource.

Advances in Pharmacology, Volume 95
ISSN 1054-3589
https://doi.org/10.1016/bs.apha.2022.05.007

Abbreviations

ADME	absorption, disposition, metabolism and excretion
CYP	cytochrome P450
iPSC	induced pluripotent stem cells
LC-MS/MS	liquid chromatography-tandem mass spectrometry
MIST	metabolites in safety testing
NADP(H)	reduced nicotinamide adenine dinucleotide phosphate

1. Introduction

A full understanding of the pharmacology and toxicology of a new drug must account for the activities not just of the new drug molecule but of all metabolites as well. An obvious key activity along the way to characterizing the contribution of metabolites to the pharmacology and toxicology is to understand the structure, abundance and activity of key metabolites. Metabolite profiling involves multiple steps, beginning with simple determination of metabolite molecular weight all the way to full structural identification along with measurement of molecular properties (e.g., metabolite levels in plasma across species, determination of on- and off-target pharmacology). The process of characterization of the metabolite activity often requires metabolite standard syntheses, which can be accomplished through multiple methods using synthetic or biosynthetic approaches (Cusack et al., 2013).

Many metabolites can be synthesized with relatively small changes to the synthetic scheme used for the parent. This is often the case with metabolites formed from alterations of side chains that have simple points of attachment, e.g., N- or O-dealkylations or side-chain oxidation reactions. In these cases, chemical synthesis of the metabolite will likely be the most cost-effective method. For more complex metabolite structures, chemical synthesis may involve the full synthetic route used for parent or may even require a new synthetic scheme. In these cases, methods that directly convert parent into metabolite of interest will likely be very competitive in total resource costs and timelines. These methods include electrochemistry, use of chemical reagents such as synthetic porphyrins and biosynthetic methods (Cusack et al., 2013). Of these, biosynthesis offers a much wider applicability to access the full range of typical metabolic transformations.

There are many options for the process of metabolite biosynthesis metabolite production and isolation and include: (1) isolation from animal or human in vitro systems or urine/feces samples (Cusack et al., 2013; Dalvie et al., 2009; Walker et al., 2014), (2) isolation from systems expressing native or mutated P450 enzymes (Garrigós-Martínez et al., 2021; Hausjell, Halbwirth, & Spadiut, 2018; Sawayama et al., 2009; Schroer, Kittelmann, & Lütz, 2010; Vail, Homann, Hanna, & Zaks, 2005), and (3) isolation from incubations with bacteria or fungi (Griffiths, Best, & Jezequel, 1991; Li, Josephs, Skiles, & Humphreys, 2008; Li, Zhang, & Li, 2016; Murphy, 2015; Piska, Żelaszczyk, Jamrozik, Kubowicz-Kwaśny, & Pękala, 2016; Rosazza & Smith, 1979; Rosazza, Stocklinski, Gustafson, Adrian, & Smith, 1975; Salter et al., 2019; Smith, Humphrey, Engel, & Rosazza, 1976; Smith & Rosazza, 1974; Venisetty & Ciddi, 2003; Yousuf, Jamil, & Mammadova, 2019). The important factors to consider when selecting a method for metabolite synthesis are quantity of metabolite required, overall resource cost, timing of delivery that meets project needs, and quality of final product.

Biosynthesis can employ natural or engineered enzymes and can be used in candidate discovery and development during multiple stages, such as: (1) to generate chemical diversity in conjunction with synthetic efforts (Brodney, Sharma, Lazzaro, Walker, & Obach, 2018; Fessner, 2019; Masood et al., 2012; Obach et al., 2018; Zhang, Huang, & Arnold, 2019) (2) to provide metabolite standards during candidate characterization, or (3) to scale-up synthesis of a drug candidate molecule. Because they perform chemistry on an incredibly wide range of substrates and generate products with interesting pharmacology, the predominant enzymes appropriate for these activities are from the cytochrome P450 family.

The most common use of biosynthetic tools by ADME scientists is probably for targeted metabolite synthesis. This process begins with the identification of a metabolite of interest during an in vitro or in vivo experiment with a drug candidate. The initial system used for identification may provide sufficient quantities of the metabolite for structure identification and other characterization. However, this is often not the case and there is a need for larger quantities of the metabolites of interest for characterization purposes. This is especially true of the metabolite is present in quantities in human plasma that qualify it as a major metabolite according to the Metabolites in Safety Testing Guidance (FDA Guidance, 2016), i.e., it is present in quantities in human plasma at greater than 10% of the total drug-related material.

There have been many interesting new developments in engineered CYP proteins that may be useful for these applications (Gumulya & Gillam, 2017; Zhang et al., 2019). The engineered proteins described in these new studies have properties such as improved thermal stability or new functional capabilities. These systems are covered in a subsequent chapter of this book.

Another potential source of enzymatic activity useful for metabolite synthesis is microbial cultures. Bacteria and fungi synthesize many natural compounds that have drug-like properties. Indeed, the majority of antibiotics have been isolated from these sources. Since the initial publications on directed metabolite synthesis using microbes (Rosazza et al., 1975; Smith et al., 1976) this methodology has held promise as a key partner to stand alongside of chemical synthesis. However, routine microbial screening has not become routine with ADME groups in the pharmaceutical industry. This is likely the result of the challenges of incorporating the resources necessary for microbial culture, screening and scale-up into a typical ADME group. Also, it is cumbersome to screen multiple microbial strains for targeted activity if conducted with traditional shake flask cultures. One solution to this problem is to use methods that allow multiple strains to be simultaneously screened using multiwell plates to streamline the process (Li et al., 2008; Quinn, Dempsey, Casey, Kane, & Murphy, 2015; Salter et al., 2019).

While meeting the requirements of the MIST guidance is a very important goal, there are other potential benefits of metabolite characterization. In select cases, the metabolite may retain the potent pharmacology of the parent compound, and if found early enough in the discovery and development process, can become the lead compound (Fura et al., 2004). Furthermore, the process of complete characterization of metabolite structure and properties can be important regarding intellectual property. Metabolite characterization will continue to be an important part of drug development and can be accomplished by a multipronged and ever-evolving approach, including both synthetic and biosynthetic techniques.

This chapter will discuss metabolite synthesis and characterization methodology and the impacts of metabolite information on the drug discovery and development process.

2. Utility of metabolite biosynthesis

Biosynthesis methodology, predominately via CYP enzymes, can provide a valuable tool alongside of medicinal chemistry and synthesis efforts. Through directed or undirected biotransformation, these methods can be applied at multiple stages of the drug discovery and development process (Fig. 1).

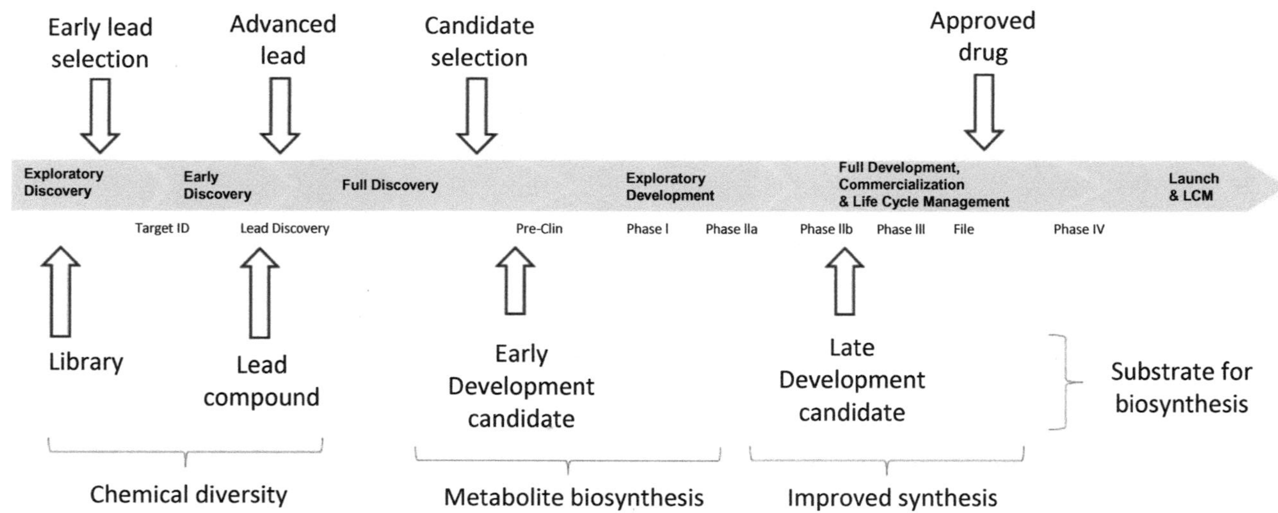

Fig. 1 Application of biosynthesis in drug discovery and development.

2.1 Discovery applications: Chemical diversity

The same diversity of enzymatic reactions that produces natural products can be tapped for the diversification of lead compounds or libraries. Although this technique is not often employed, there has been some published studies on lead diversification through enzymatic transformation, with an excellent example being a study by Arnold and coworkers that describes a small library being modified by a panel of mutated bacterial CYP BM-3 enzymes (Sawayama et al., 2009). This approach can be used to produce a modified library covering a significantly wider range of chemical space than synthetic libraries alone. It does, however, necessitate a more complex screening protocol with a deconvolution step to discriminate the activity of mixtures. Another approach is to use lead compounds as the starting point for enzymatic diversification (Brodney et al., 2018; Fessner, 2019; Masood et al., 2012; Obach et al., 2018). The incorporation of metabolism information into medicinal chemistry optimization efforts may lead to compounds that have dramatically improved ADME properties and provide important design elements for advanced lead compounds (Fura et al., 2004; Augeri et al., 2005.

Another interesting method to generate chemical diversity is to a multistep process to add a fluorine to a lead molecule. The first step is to use enzyme sources to form hydroxy derivatives of the lead. The hydroxylated compounds can then be converted to a fluoro derivative with the use of fluorinating agent such as diethylaminosulfur trifluoride (DAST) (Obach, Walker, & Brodney, 2016; Rentmeister, Arnold, & Fasan, 2009).

2.2 Early development: Meeting MIST requirements

The need to better characterize a metabolite can occur at multiple points during the late discovery or early development stages. Early metabolite identification via LC-MS/MS profiling analysis of in vitro or in vivo samples (from efficacy or PK studies) gives early information on metabolite structure but often assignments are as Markush structures, i.e., where exact structure is still unknown (e.g., the exact point of attachment of a hydroxyl group). Also, there is often only quantitative estimates based on mass spectrometry response factors (comparison of the mass spectrometer signal strength for two analytes) generated. More in-depth characterization often occurs after candidate nomination or upon receipt of samples from first-in human trials but still may not include full structural determination or any quantitative characterization data. The human ADME study conducted with a radiolabeled version of the drug allows full characterization, both quantitatively and qualitatively, of the metabolite profile.

When examining the in vitro profile of a new drug it is important to evaluate whether the metabolites were formed through a process that involved reactive intermediates. This may mean they could contribute to various toxicology often associated with reactive species. The vast majority of metabolites are not in this class and are chemically stable after leaving the enzyme active site. For chemically stable metabolites, arguably the most important metabolite property to characterize is on-target pharmacology. This is because the type of metabolic transformations, e.g., hydroxylation or dealkylation of small alkyl groups, do not change the structure dramatically and thus do not change the structure–activity relationship. It is quite common for a stable metabolite to possess some on-target activity but uncommon for the metabolite to possess a unique off-target activity not seen with the parent (Humphreys & Unger, 2006).

In order to characterize plasma samples, especially samples from first-in human trials, there have been published methods that allow activity determination but do not require metabolite synthesis or even isolation (Zhu et al., 2013). Also, there are publications on how to perform relative quantitation of metabolites between species (Gao, Deng, & Obach, 2015; Gao & Obach, 2011) or to get sound quantitative estimates without having metabolite standards (Zhang et al., 2007).

If human data shows that a metabolite reaches the threshold of a major circulating metabolite and/or is produced by a pathway that constitutes >25% of the clearance of parent, then it will require significant characterization. This characterization will almost certainly require some type of synthetic effort to produce a quantity sufficient to fund multiple assays. Also, in some rare cases where there is very low coverage of the human metabolite in plasma of all major toxicology species, the metabolite may need to be synthesized in quantities sufficient to conduct limited duration toxicology studies after administration of the metabolite.

2.3 Late development

Enzymatic transformations have traditionally played a niche but important role in large scale syntheses, whether in late-stage development or commercial processes. Examples of drugs that employ biosynthetic approaches for their production include dihydrocortisone/cortisone and pravastatin. Many fine chemical starting materials are made via biosynthesis. With improvements in technology the role of biosynthesis will continue to play an important role in large scale drug synthesis (Lundemo & Woodley, 2015; Martinez & Rupashinghe, 2013; Urlacher & Eiben, 2006).

3. Directed metabolite biosynthesis

When the need for a metabolite standard arises there are many different pathways that can be followed to reach the goal. Ideally, all potential routes, including synthesis and biosynthesis, can be investigated. In many cases, synthesis will be fairly straightforward and yield the metabolite without large resource commitment. However, some metabolites will require total syntheses that may be as or even more complex than the route to parent. These are the cases where use of biosynthesis methods, with parent as starting material, can yield necessary quantities of metabolite more rapidly and with consumption of far fewer resources.

Another important consideration when choosing a biosynthesis method is the need for robust analysis to make sure the biosynthesized metabolite matches the authentic metabolite derived from the biological source, in most cases formed via a human CYP enzyme. This pertains to any biosynthetic route that involves enzymes that are distinct from the enzyme forming the metabolite of interest, however, is especially true when using microbial systems. Great care should be placed on the analysis of the biosynthesized metabolite to make sure it matches the regio- and stereochemistry of the authentic isolated metabolite sample.

3.1 Metabolite isolation from incubation with expressed enzymes, microsomes, hepatocytes or in vivo

The most straightforward method for biosynthesis is through the use of the enzyme systems already employed to generate early metabolite profiles, i.e., expressed human CYPs, hepatic subcellular fractions, etc. Metabolite yield from incubations of parent with the enzyme system of choice can be quickly optimized with respect to incubation time, parent concentration, enzyme concentration, etc. The process of scale-up to generate sufficient quantities is sometimes challenging as there are often issues with solubility, competing metabolic pathways and overall slow turnover. Cost is often a factor as well if the method of choice employee human microsomes or expressed enzymes. Animal microsomes are a much more cost-efficient path if they produce the desired metabolite in good yield. However, if the quantity of metabolite required for characterization is small, then use of this approach is the simplest and quickest way to biosynthesize and purify metabolites. In general, metabolite quantities in the range of 10–250 μg are reasonable targets using microsome or expressed enzyme incubations (as an example: an incubation with the following conditions would yield 100 μg of product prior to purification: 20 mL incubation volume, compound MW = 500 g/mol, 50 μM compound concentration, 25% yield). Quantities larger than this becomes challenging with these techniques.

This has led to many efforts to introduce incubation systems that allow a variety of different approaches to produce greater quantities of enzyme through hepatocyte expansion; examples include microsomes/hepatocytes from humanized mice (Grompe & Strom, 2013), bioreactors from induced pluripotent stem cells (iPSCs) (Freyer et al., 2016; Yamashita, Takayama, Sakurai, & Mizuguchi, 2018), etc.

3.2 Biosynthesis of metabolites using bioreactors

There are many options for bioreactors that have oxidative metabolism capability. These systems are for the most part centered around various CYP enzymes and are thus typically defined as "CYP biocatalysts intended to support the use of an active form of the CYP and supporting enzymes required to achieve catalysis, under aerobic conditions and in the presence of the required catalytic amounts of reduced NADP(H) cofactor and cofactor recycling system." These systems range from engineered hepatocyte systems to microbial systems in their native form or engineered to express a CYP enzyme.

When considering a system for metabolite synthesis it is important to consider the important drivers that dictate the needs of a metabolite biosynthesis effort. While cost is often an important consideration the main driver typically is completion of synthetic efforts within a timeframe that allows both the clinical and non-clinical programs to continue unhindered. The determination of a metabolite structure when a candidate drug is in late-stage discovery or development, especially if the metabolite is found circulating in human, often leads to a good deal of uncertainty around on- and off-target pharmacology, coverage in toxicology species, etc. This uncertainty remains until the required characterization studies can be completed, which in turn puts pressure on the timelines for metabolite synthesis and dictates the type of system that will be useful for the task.

3.3 Bioreactors with expressed mammalian CYPs

Microbial or insect cell-based systems that express human CYP enzymes are the most straightforward way to transition from liver subcellular fractions to a bioreactor-based biosynthesis. The microbial systems typically use *E. coli*, *S. cerevisiae*, and *P. pastoris* as host. While these systems provide a straightforward method, they are not easily available commercially and to fully implement require licensing fees/agreements or a very large internal effort to derive proprietary systems. Insect cells suffer from high cost of maintenance and lack of sufficient reductase levels. Microbial systems generally suffer from low expression levels. For these reasons, expressed mammalian CYP bioreactors are not a viable option for the majority of drug metabolism scientists.

3.4 Microbial bioreactors

Microbes support an incredible variety of oxidative metabolic transformations, the majority mediated by CYP enzymes. Several microbial enzymes, such as CYP102A1 (commonly referred to as P450BM3) from *Bacillus megaterium* have been studies extensively. The potential of CYP102A1 as a drug biotransformation enzyme is widely acknowledged and has led to the derivation of large mutant libraries. The full CYP enzyme profile of several species/strains, such as *Aspergillus nidulans* and *Cunninghamella elegans*, have been fairly well documented (Kelly, Krasevec, Mullins, & Nelson, 2009; Palmer-Brown, Miranda-CasoLuengo, Wolfe, Byrne, & Murphy, 2019). There have been a number of studies looking at biotransformation reactions catalyzed by *Cunninghamella elegans* (Asha & Vidyavathi, 2009; Gonçalves et al., 2021). Microbial cultures provide high enzyme activities, long-term stability and easier scale-up for the synthesis and purification of metabolites. Microbes have proven to be efficient in select cases in terms of scalability of metabolite production, enzyme activity and costs. A potential downside is that the metabolite profiles from microbial incubations may be complex and analytical resources are required to make sure the microbial metabolite(s) are exact structural matches to the metabolite of interest.

The very significant barrier in the use of microbial bioreactors systems is the issue of rapidly screening strains for the production of a target metabolite. Fungal and bacterial strains may involve very different culture conditions that make simultaneous screening cumbersome. Also, characterized procedures often involve large shake flasks and incubators that are not available in drug metabolism labs. Additionally, it is difficult to maintain sufficient expertise within a drug metabolism function to efficiently use microbial incubations. In some cases, there may be microbiological expertise in other parts of the company that can be applied to metabolite synthesis, but this seems to be very rare in the modern pharmaceutical industry.

The issue with maintenance of complex microbiological facilities could be potentially solved through the establishment of streamlined systems to screen multiple strains at once for production of a target metabolite. While there have been many studies examining the metabolism of drugs by microbes there has been only a few studies that have attempted to define methods for microbe screening and subsequent scale-up. The following methods have examined this problem and present methods that successfully screen for target metabolic activity and then seamlessly transition to scale-up. All of these methods employ plate-based screens of a number of microbial strains shown to have drug metabolizing activity. Quinn et al. (2015) published a method using immobilized *Cunninghamella elegans* with screening accomplished in either 12-well or 96-well plate formats. Li et al. (2008) published a methodology using multiple actinomycetes bacterial strains in a 24-well plate system that was found to yield useful metabolites for a number of drug molecules. Finally, Salter et al. (2019) published a method using both fungi (mostly zygomycete strains) and bacteria (mostly actinomycete strains) purchased from the Hypha Discovery Culture Collection (Hypha Discovery Ltd., Slough, UK).

Importantly, all these methods demonstrated that larger cultures of the strains identified in the screen could be applied directly to allow scale-up to produce >1 mg quantities of metabolite (and in some cases far greater amounts). The following sections details some of the biotransformation reactions studied with these three screening assays.

3.4.1 Examples of microbial-based bioreactors

There have been a wide variety of published reports on the biotransformation of drug by microbes, most with the goal of mimicking a metabolic route found in mammals. While these reports demonstrate the promise of microbial metabolite synthesis, they do not provide a straightforward path for metabolism scientist to accomplish the goal of metabolite synthesis for new drug candidates. The examples illustrated below are from several published methods that provide plate-based microbe screening assay methodology along with direct reaction scale-up procedures.

The method published by Quinn et al. (2015) examined six drugs in a *Cunninghamella elegans* screening system. Known human metabolites of all

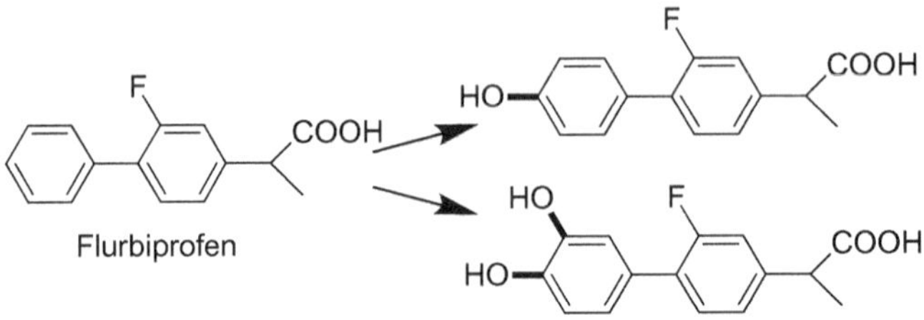

Fig. 2 Metabolism of flurbiprofen to yield major human metabolite by *Cunninghamella elegans* (Amadio et al., 2010; Quinn et al., 2015).

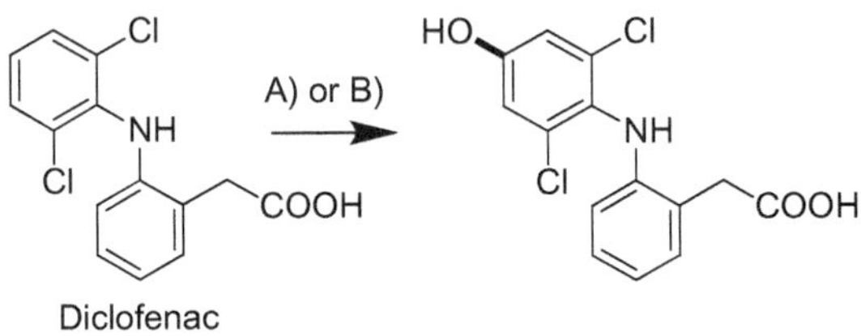

Fig. 3 Metabolism of diclofenac to yield major human metabolite; (A) *Cunninghamella elegans* or (B) *Actinomycetes* sp. (Amadio et al., 2010; Li et al., 2008; Quinn et al., 2015).

six of the drugs were detected and while the fungal system did not produce all of the known metabolites, a majority of the species were detected. Two of the drugs studied, flurbiprofen and diclofenac, and their respective biotransformation products are shown in Figs. 2 and 3 (Amadio, Gordon, & Murphy, 2010; Quinn et al., 2015).

The method published by Li et al. (2008) examined several drugs to demonstrate the capability of a plate-based screening assay with actinomycetes strains. The drugs examined in this study were diclofenac, dasatinib, and BMS-587101. Several strains were identified that produced key human metabolites of all three substrates (diclofenac, Fig. 3 and dasatinib, Fig. 4). In the dasatinib and BMS-587101 examples, both drug candidates were in active development at the time of microbial synthesis and the metabolites produced were used as part of metabolite characterization efforts. This screening method has also been used to produce human metabolite of muraglitazar (Zhang et al., 2006) and BMS-986142 (Fig. 5) (Watterson et al., 2016; Zhao et al., 2017). The regioselectivity demonstrated in the synthesis of the metabolite of BMS-986142 is remarkable. It should be noted that the stereochemistry around the hydroxyl group was never absolutely established but the metabolite matched the authentic standard by chromatographic retention time and LC-MS/MS fragmentation pattern.

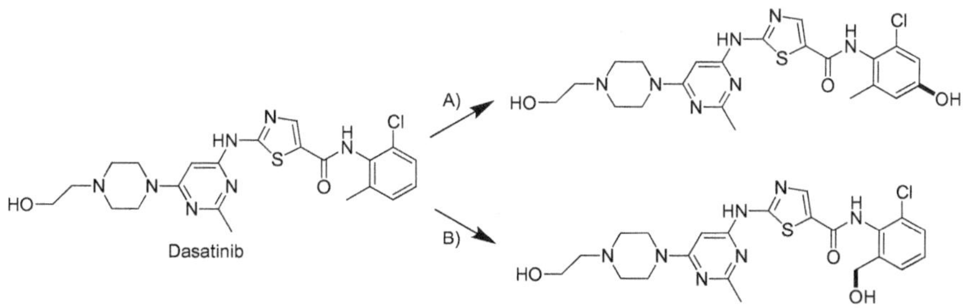

Fig. 4 Metabolism of dasatinib to yield major human metabolites; (A) *Streptomyces griseus* ATCC 10137 (B) *Streptomyces* sp. SC15761 (Li et al., 2008).

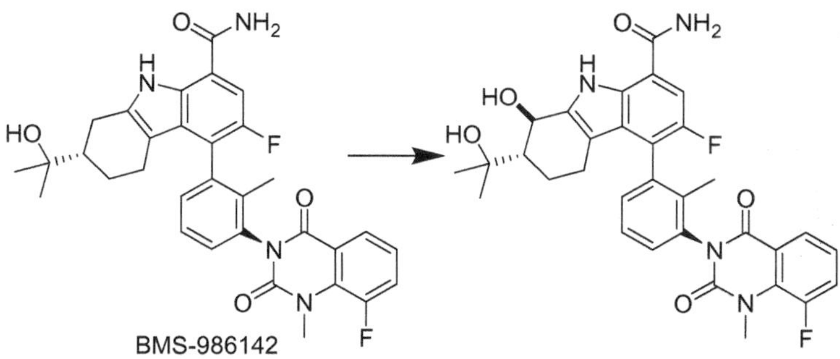

Fig. 5 Metabolism of BMS-986142 to yield major human metabolite by *Streptomyces violascens* (ATCC 31560) (Zhao et al., 2017).

The Salter et al. (2019) method examined a number of drugs that had been in development at either Janssen or Merck & Co. Inc. and had required significant quantities of a particular metabolite synthesized during their development programs. Eight parent molecules were chosen for examination; these parent molecules formed 12 metabolites that had been the target of chemical synthesis efforts (examples of two of these shown in Figs. 6 and 7). The microbial screen was found to produce 8 of the 12 metabolites of interest, and this included both oxidation and conjugation reactions. Several of the metabolites were scaled-up to provide >1 mg quantities. The authors point out that even though one of the target metabolites for scale-up was produced in low yield it was still economically feasible to conduct with microbes as the reagent cost was minimal. These authors also give data on the times for the original chemical synthesis effort for each of the metabolites. The times ranged from 6 to >104 weeks and illustrate the challenges often encountered with chemical synthesis routes.

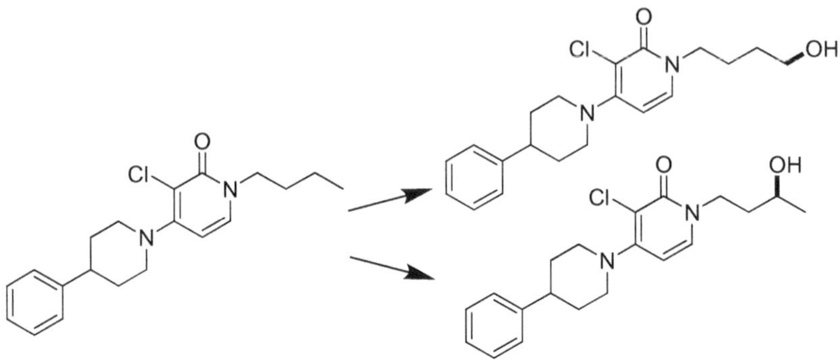

Fig. 6 Metabolism of Janssen positive allosteric metabotropic glutamate 2 receptor modulator to yield major human metabolite by SP7001 (*Amycolatopsis* sp.), SP7043 (*Amycolatopsis lurida*), or SP7045 (*Streptomyces* sp.) (Salter et al., 2019).

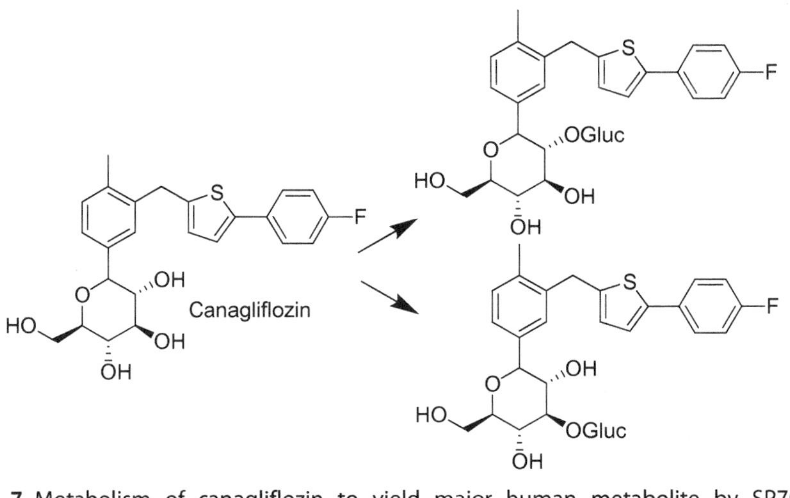

Fig. 7 Metabolism of canagliflozin to yield major human metabolite by SP7045 (*Streptomyces* sp.) (Salter et al., 2019).

4. Conclusion

Information on drug metabolites is important for all aspects of drug discovery and development. Both lead diversification and optimization efforts can be impacted favorably through use of metabolite generating systems as well as detailed understanding of metabolite structure. Once a candidate is selected, then metabolite characterization efforts begin with basic metabolism screening tools. As information from in vitro and in vivo studies is generated there may be a need for additional characterization studies that require synthesis of the metabolite. At that point it is important to consider the goals of the characterization studies and then determine the best methodology to use for synthesis. Chemical and biosynthetic methods should both be considered. One route that can prove to be very effective in the synthesis of metabolite that are challenging to produce through a medicinal chemistry approach is the use of microbial biosynthesis methods. This is especially true if there is a facile screening/scale-up method in place that allows multiple microbial strains to be examined simultaneously with direct scale-up from any incubations found to produce the metabolite of interest.

Conflict of interest statement

The author has no conflict of interest to declare.

References

Amadio, J., Gordon, K., & Murphy, C. D. (2010). Biotransformation of flurbiprofen by Cunninghamella species. *Applied and Environmental Microbiology*, *76*, 6299–6303.

Asha, S., & Vidyavathi, M. (2009). *Cunninghamella*—A microbial model for drug metabolism studies—A review. *Biotechnology Advances*, *27*(1), 16–29.

Augeri, D. J., Robl, J. A., Betebenner, D. A., Magnin, D. R., Khanna, A., Robertson, J. G., et al. (2005). Discovery and preclinical profile of Saxagliptin (BMS-477118): A highly potent, long-acting, orally active dipeptidyl peptidase IV inhibitor for the treatment of type 2 diabetes. *Journal of Medicinal Chemistry*, *48*(15), 5025–5037.

Brodney, M. A., Sharma, R., Lazzaro, J. T., Walker, G. S., & Obach, R. S. (2018). Harnessing biosynthesis and quantitative NMR for late stage functionalization of lead molecules: Application to the M1 positive allosteric modulator (PAM) program. *Bioorganic & Medicinal Chemistry Letters*, *28*(11), 2068–2073.

Cusack, K. P., Koolman, H. F., Lange, U. E., Peltier, H. M., Piel, I., & Vasudevan, A. (2013). Emerging technologies for metabolite generation and structural diversification. *Bioorganic & Medicinal Chemistry Letters*, *23*(20), 5471–5483.

Dalvie, D., Obach, R. S., Kang, P., Prakash, C., Loi, C. M., Hurst, S., et al. (2009). Assessment of three human in vitro systems in the generation of major human excretory and circulating metabolites. *Chemical Research in Toxicology*, *22*, 357–368.

FDA Guidance. (2016). *Guidance for industry: Safety testing of drug metabolites*. Silver Spring, MD: US Department of Health and Human Services FaDA, Center for Drug Evaluation and Research.

Fessner, N. D. (2019). P450 monooxygenases enable rapid late-stage diversification of natural products via C-H bond activation. *ChemCatChem*, *11*(9), 2226–2242.

Freyer, N., Knöspel, F., Strahl, N., Amini, L., Schrade, P., Bachmann, S., et al. (2016). Hepatic differentiation of human induced pluripotent stem cells in a perfused three-dimensional multicompartment bioreactor. *BioResearch Open Access*, *5*(1), 235–248.

Fura, A., Shu, Y. Z., Zhu, M., Hanson, R. L., Roongta, V., & Humphreys, W. G. (2004). Discovering drugs through biological transformation: Role of pharmacologically active metabolites in drug discovery. *Journal of Medicinal Chemistry*, *47*(18), 4339–4351.

Gao, H., Deng, S., & Obach, R. S. (2015). Unbiased scanning method and data banking approach using ultra-high performance liquid chromatography coupled with high-resolution mass spectrometry for quantitative comparison of metabolite exposure in plasma across species analyzed at different dates. *Analytical Chemistry*, *87*(23), 11771–11776.

Gao, H., & Obach, R. S. (2011). Addressing MIST (metabolites in safety testing): Bioanalytical approaches to address metabolite exposures in humans and animals. *Current Drug Metabolism*, *12*(6), 578–586.

Garrigós-Martínez, J., Weninger, A., Montesinos-Seguí, J. L., Schmid, C., Valero, F., Rinnofner, C., et al. (2021). Scalable production and application of Pichia pastoris whole cell catalysts expressing human cytochrome P450 2C9. *Microbial Cell Factories*, *20*(1), 90.

Gonçalves, M. D., Tomiotto-Pellissier, F., de Matos, R. L. N., Assolini, J. P., da Silva Bortoleti, B. T., & Concato, V. M. (2021). Recent advances in biotransformation by *Cunninghamella* species. *Current Drug Metabolism*, *22*(13), 1035–1064.

Griffiths, D. A., Best, D. J., & Jezequel, S. G. (1991). The screening of selected microorganisms for use as models of mammalian drug metabolism. *Applied Microbiology and Biotechnology*, *35*, 373–381.

Grompe, M., & Strom, S. (2013). Mice with human livers. *Gastroenterology*, *145*(6), 1209–1214.

Gumulya, Y., & Gillam, E. M. (2017). Exploring the past and the future of protein evolution with ancestral sequence reconstruction: The 'retro' approach to protein engineering. *The Biochemical Journal*, *474*(1), 1–19.

Hausjell, J., Halbwirth, H., & Spadiut, O. (2018). Recombinant production of eukaryotic cytochrome P450s in microbial cell factories. *Bioscience Reports*, *38*(2), BSR20171290.

Humphreys, W. G., & Unger, S. E. (2006). Safety assessment of drug metabolites: Characterization of chemically stable metabolites. *Chemical Research in Toxicology*, *19*(12), 1564–1569.

Kelly, D. E., Krasevec, N., Mullins, J., & Nelson, D. R. (2009). The CYPome (cytochrome P450 complement) of *aspergillus nidulans*. *Fungal Genetics and Biology*, *46*(Suppl 1), S53–S61.

Li, W., Josephs, J. L., Skiles, G. L., & Humphreys, W. G. (2008). Metabolite generation via microbial biotransformations with actinomycetes: Rapid screening for active strains and biosynthesis of important human metabolites of two development-stage compounds, 5-[(5S,9R)-9-(4-cyanophenyl)-3-(3,5-dichlorophenyl)-1-methyl-2,4-dioxo-1,3,7-triazaspiro[4.4]non7-yl-methyl]-3-thiophenecarboxylic acid (BMS-587101) and dasatinib. *Drug Metabolism and Disposition*, *36*(4), 721–730.

Li, Z., Zhang, W., & Li, S. (2016). Cytochrome P450 enzymes and microbial drug development - a review. *Wei Sheng Wu Xue Bao*, *56*(3), 496–515.

Lundemo, M. T., & Woodley, J. M. (2015). Guidelines for development and implementation of biocatalytic P450 processes. *Applied Microbiology and Biotechnology*, *99*(6), 2465–2483.

Martinez, C. A., & Rupashinghe, S. G. (2013). Cytochrome P450 bioreactors in the pharmaceutical industry: Challenges and opportunities. *Current Topics in Medicinal Chemistry*, *13*(12), 1470–1490.

Masood, M. A., Bazin, M., Bunnage, M. E., Calabrese, A., Cox, M., Fancy, S. A., et al. (2012). Lead diversification 2: Application to P38, gMTP and lead compounds. *Bioorganic & Medicinal Chemistry Letters*, *22*(2), 1255–1262.

Murphy, C. D. (2015). Drug metabolism in microorganisms. *Biotechnology Letters*, *37*(1), 19–28.

Obach, R. S., Walker, G. S., & Brodney, M. A. (2016). Biosynthesis of Fluorinated Analogs of Drugs Using Human Cytochrome P450 Enzymes Followed by Deoxyfluorination and quantitative nuclear magnetic resonance spectroscopy to improve metabolic stability. *Drug Metabolism and Disposition*, *44*(5), 634–646.

Obach, R. S., Walker, G. S., Sharma, R., Jenkinson, S., Tran, T. P., & Stepan, A. F. (2018). Lead diversification at the nanomole scale using liver microsomes and quantitative nuclear magnetic resonance spectroscopy: Application to phosphodiesterase 2 inhibitors. *Journal of Medicinal Chemistry*, *61*(8), 3626–3640.

Palmer-Brown, W., Miranda-CasoLuengo, R., Wolfe, K. H., Byrne, K. P., & Murphy, C. D. (2019). The CYPome of the model xenobiotic-biotransforming fungus *Cunninghamella elegans*. *Scientific Reports*, *9*(1), 9240.

Piska, K., Żelaszczyk, D., Jamrozik, M., Kubowicz-Kwaśny, P., & Pękala, E. (2016). Cunninghamella biotransformation- -similarities to human drug metabolism and its relevance for the drug discovery process. *Current Drug Metabolism*, *17*(2), 107–117.

Quinn, L., Dempsey, R., Casey, E., Kane, A., & Murphy, C. D. (2015). Production of drug metabolites by immobilised *Cunninghamella elegans*: From screening to scale up. *Journal of Industrial Microbiology & Biotechnology*, *42*(5), 799–806.

Rentmeister, A., Arnold, F. H., & Fasan, R. (2009). Chemo-enzymatic fluorination of unactivated organic compounds. *Nature Chemical Biology*, *5*(1), 26–28.

Rosazza, J. P., & Smith, R. V. (1979). Microbial models for drug metabolism. *Advances in Applied Microbiology*, *25*, 169–208.

Rosazza, J. P., Stocklinski, A. W., Gustafson, M. A., Adrian, J., & Smith, R. V. (1975). Microbial models of mammalian metabolism. O-dealkylation of 10,11-dimethoxyaporphine. *Journal of Medicinal Chemistry*, *18*(8), 791–794.

Salter, R., Beshore, D. C., Colletti, S. L., Evans, L., Gong, Y., Helmy, R., et al. (2019). Microbial biotransformation - an important tool for the study of drug metabolism. *Xenobiotica*, *49*(8), 877–886.

Sawayama, A. M., Chen, M. M., Kulanthaivel, P., Kuo, M. S., Hemmerle, H., & Arnold, F. H. (2009). A panel of cytochrome P450 BM3 variants to produce drug metabolites and diversify lead compounds. *Chemistry*, *15*(43), 11723–11729.

Schroer, K., Kittelmann, M., & Lütz, S. (2010). Recombinant human cytochrome P450 monooxygenases for drug metabolite synthesis. *Biotechnology and Bioengineering*, *106*(5), 699–706.

Smith, R. V., Humphrey, D. W., Engel, K. O., & Rosazza, J. P. (1976). Microbial models of mammalian metabolism: Aromatic hydroxylation of isomeric xylenes. *Applied and Environmental Microbiology*, *31*(3), 448–449.

Smith, R. V., & Rosazza, J. P. (1974). Microbial models of mammalian metabolism. Aromatic hydroxylation. *Archives of Biochemistry and Biophysics*, *161*, 551–558.

Urlacher, B. V., & Eiben, S. (2006). Cytochrome P450 monooxygenases: Perspectives for synthetic application. *Trends in Biotechnology*, *24*(7), 324–330.

Vail, R. B., Homann, M. J., Hanna, I., & Zaks, A. (2005). Preparative synthesis of drug metabolites using human cytochrome P450s 3A4, 2C9 and 1A2 with NADPH-P450 reductase expressed in Escherichia coli. *Journal of Industrial Microbiology & Biotechnology*, *32*(2), 67–74.

Venisetty, R. K., & Ciddi, V. (2003). Application of microbial biotransformation for the new drug discovery using natural drugs as substrates. *Current Pharmaceutical Biotechnology*, *4*(3), 153–167.

Walker, G. S., Bauman, J. N., Ryder, T. F., Smith, E. B., Spracklin, D. K., & Obach, R. S. (2014). Biosynthesis of drug metabolites and quantitation using NMR spectroscopy for use in pharmacologic and drug metabolism studies. *Drug Metabolism and Disposition*, *42*(10), 1627–1639.

Watterson, S. H., De Lucca, G. V., Shi, Q., Langevine, C. M., Liu, Q., Batt, D. G., et al. (2016). Discovery of 6-Fluoro-5-(R)-(3-(S)-(8-fluoro-1-methyl-2,4-dioxo-1,2-dihydroquinazolin-3(4H)-yl)-2-methylphenyl)-2-(S)-(2-hydroxypropan-2-yl)-2,3,4,9-tetrahydro-1H-carbazole-8-carboxamide (BMS-986142): A reversible inhibitor of Bruton's tyrosine kinase (BTK) conformationally constrained by two locked Atropisomers. *Journal of Medicinal Chemistry*, *59*(19), 9173–9200.

Yamashita, T., Takayama, K., Sakurai, F., & Mizuguchi, H. (2018). Billion-scale production of hepatocyte-like cells from human induced pluripotent stem cells. *Biochemical and Biophysical Research Communications*, *496*(4), 1269–1275.

Yousuf, M., Jamil, W., & Mammadova, K. (2019). Microbial bioconversion: A Regio-specific method for novel drug design and toxicological study of metabolites. *Current Pharmaceutical Biotechnology*, *20*(14), 1156–1162.

Zhang, R. K., Huang, X., & Arnold, F. H. (2019). Selective CH bond functionalization with engineered heme proteins: New tools to generate complexity. *Current Opinion in Chemical Biology*, *49*, 67–75.

Zhang, D., Raghavan, N., Chando, T., Gambardella, J., Fu, Y., Zhang, D., et al. (2007). LC-MS/MS-based approach for obtaining exposure estimates of metabolites in early clinical trials using radioactive metabolites as reference standards. *Drug Metabolism Letters*, *1*(4), 293–298.

Zhang, D., Zhang, H., Aranibar, N., Hanson, R., Huang, Y., Cheng, P. T., et al. (2006). Structural elucidation of human oxidative metabolites of muraglitazar: Use of microbial bioreactors in the biosynthesis of metabolite standards. *Drug Metabolism and Disposition*, *34*, 267–280.

Zhao, W., Li, W., Liu, A., Li, J., Dai, J., Caceres-Cortes, J., et al. (2017). Characterization of the major metabolites found after plasma metabolite profiling of a BTK Inhibitor, BMS-986142, in FIH studies. In *21st North American ISSX Meeting, P74.*

Zhu, X., Slatter, J. G., Emery, M. G., Deane, M. R., Akrami, A., Zhang, X., et al. (2013). Activity-based exposure comparisons among humans and nonclinical safety testing species in an extensively metabolized drug candidate. *Xenobiotica*, *43*(7), 617–627.

CHAPTER SEVEN

Use of engineered cytochromes P450 for accelerating drug discovery and development

Raine E.S. Thomson[a], Stephlina A. D'Cunha[a], Martin A. Hayes[b], and Elizabeth M.J. Gillam[a,*]

[a]School of Chemistry & Molecular Biosciences, The University of Queensland, Brisbane, QLD, Australia
[b]Compound Synthesis and Management, Discovery Sciences, BioPharmaceuticals R&D AstraZeneca, Mölndal, Sweden
*Corresponding author: e-mail address: e.gillam@uq.edu.au

Contents

Abstract

Numerous steps in drug development, including the generation of authentic metabolites and late-stage functionalization of candidates, necessitate the modification of often complex molecules, such as natural products. While it can be challenging to make the required regio- and stereoselective alterations to a molecule using purely chemical catalysis, enzymes can introduce changes to complex molecules with a high degree of stereo- and regioselectivity. Cytochrome P450 enzymes are biocatalysts of unequalled

Advances in Pharmacology, Volume 95
ISSN 1054-3589
https://doi.org/10.1016/bs.apha.2022.06.001

versatility, capable of regio- and stereoselective functionalization of unactivated C—H bonds by monooxygenation. Collectively they catalyze over 60 different biotransformations on structurally and functionally diverse organic molecules, including natural products, drugs, steroids, organic acids and other lipophilic molecules. This catalytic versatility and substrate range makes them likely candidates for application as potential biocatalysts for industrial chemistry. However, several aspects of the P450 catalytic cycle and other characteristics have limited their implementation to date in industry, including: their lability at elevated temperature, in the presence of solvents, and over lengthy incubation times; the typically low efficiency with which they metabolize non-natural substrates; and their lack of specificity for a single metabolic pathway. Protein engineering by rational design or directed evolution provides a way to engineer P450s for industrial use. Here we review the progress made to date toward engineering the properties of P450s, especially eukaryotic forms, for industrial application, and including the recent expansion of their catalytic repertoire to include non-natural reactions.

Abbreviations

ASR ancestral sequence reconstruction
BAIB bis(acetoxy)-iodobenzene
BI Bayesian inference
CuOOH cumene hydroperoxide
CPR cytochrome P450 reductase
EDA ethyl diazoacetate
epPCR error-prone PCR
JTT Jones-Taylor-Thornton
LSF late-stage functionalization
ML maximum likelihood
MP maximum parsimony
O_2S oxygen surrogate
P450 cytochrome P450
SSM site-saturation mutagenesis
TTN total turnover number.

1. Introduction

The stereo-selective hydroxylation of unactivated C—H bonds in complex organic molecules is one of the most important reactions in the chemical industry, since it allows access to an expanded range of novel, potentially bioactive chemicals (Doyle & Goldberg, 2012; Hartwig, 2016; White & Zhao, 2018). Once a hydroxyl group is introduced into a specific, otherwise-inert position on a molecule, it can serve as a precursor for derivatization in a chemoenzymatic protocol or by further enzymatic modification using enzyme cascades (Durak et al., 2016; France et al., 2017; Lewis et al., 2009; Rentmeister et al., 2009). Performing C—H functionalization in a regio- and stereoselective fashion can be challenging with chemocatalysis alone (Hartwig & Larsen, 2016; Roduner et al., 2013; Shugrue & Miller, 2017). However biological catalysts, i.e., enzymes, offer a way to achieve the desired selectivity, by virtue of their complex and chiral active site topology. The stereo-, regio- and chemospecificity of P450s can be harnessed in industrial applications such as production of pharmaceuticals, drug metabolites, hormones, dyes, and biopolymers, as well as for bioremediation and biosensors (Awan et al., 2016; Gillam & Hayes, 2013; Kumar, 2010; Mousavi et al., 2021; Schachinger et al., 2021). In particular cytochrome P450 enzymes are well known for their ability to selectively hydroxylate an unactivated carbon center in a substrate, on a wide range of potential substrates, which makes them attractive candidates as industrial biocatalysts (Bernhardt & Urlacher, 2014; Bhandari et al., 2021; Fessner, 2019; Li et al., 2020; Rylott et al., 2011; Schneider & Clark, 2013), particularly in the pharmaceutical industry.

In nature, P450s are involved in many complex biosynthetic pathways in microorganisms and plants, including those leading to diverse natural products of interest in drug discovery (Bhattacharya & Yadav, 2018; Cochrane & Vederas, 2014; Ghosh, 2017; Rasool & Mohamed, 2016; Rudolf et al., 2017; Xiao et al., 2019; Zhang et al., 2021). This catalytic versatility allows them to generate a wide range of specific but differentially functionalized products. Thus, plant and microbial P450s collectively represent a rich resource for biocatalysts of specific reactions on natural products and their precursors (Schulz et al., 2012). However P450s are also involved in the degradation of natural products that end up as part of the dietary intake of animals. P450s in animals are involved in the metabolism of plant and microbial secondary metabolites as part of the "chemical defense" system of herbivorous and omnivorous animals (Gillam & Hunter, 2007). Such P450 enzymes responsible for xenobiotic metabolism typically show extraordinary promiscuity, meaning that they can potentially act on a very broad and diverse set of possible substrates (Rendic & Guengerich, 2021), in contrast to the specialized plant and microbial P450s involved in secondary metabolism that have clear biosynthetic functions (Cochrane & Vederas, 2014).

While natural products serve as often potent leads for new drugs (Crag & Newman, 2013), they have been underexplored due to the synthetic challenges involved in both making and modifying them. Difficulties in the stereo- and regioselective modification of often complex, chiral molecules cause bottlenecks in the drug discovery and development pipeline: in the synthesis and optimization of novel drug candidates; the investigation of pharmacological and toxicological profiles of their metabolites; and when characterizing structure-activity relationships of bioactive compounds (Shugrue & Miller, 2017).

2. Lead candidate synthesis and late-stage functionalization of pharmaceutical compounds

Natural biosynthetic P450s have often been used as biocatalysts to accomplish similar chemical reactions as those which occur naturally in the biosynthesis of a natural product (Li et al., 2019; Schulz et al., 2012). In an early engineering effort, wild-type (WT) CYP105AS1 from *Amycolatopsis orientalis* was engineered and introduced into *Penicillium chrysogenum* to produce pravastatin, a cholesterol lowering drug, following stereoselective hydroxylation of the natural product, compactin (McLean et al., 2015). The chemoenzymatic synthesis of a vancomycin aglycone variant was achieved by reconstituting three P450s (OxyA, OxyB, OxyC) *in vitro,* which enabled the formation of all three aromatic crosslinks in the glycopeptide antibiotic (Forneris & Seyedsayamdost, 2018). Another example was the use of P450 CYP71AV1 from the plant *Artemesia annua* in the production of the anti-malarial drug, artemisinin (Paddon et al., 2013; Ro et al., 2006).

However, P450s can also be used for compound diversification using natural lead candidates which can be productively geared toward the development of new therapeutics (Di Nardo & Gilardi, 2020; Li et al., 2019; Zhang & Li, 2017). Recently, attention has focused on using P450s from various sources for late-stage functionalization (LSF) (Fessner, 2019). LSF refers to the introduction of functional chemical groups in the final steps of a chemical synthesis and is usually undertaken in the pharmaceutical industry to optimize the physicochemical properties of an active drug compound (Cernak et al., 2016; Lasso et al., 2021). The decoration and diversification of drug scaffolds is primarily achieved through the functionalization of C—H bonds to generate diversity (Durak et al., 2016). While the concept is not new, most efforts traditionally have been focused on using small molecule chemical catalysts to achieve various difficult chemistries such as methylation, oxygenation, chlorination, fluorination, bromination, amination, ring formation and carbene/nitrene insertion (Lasso et al., 2021; Moir et al., 2019; Shugrue & Miller, 2017; White & Zhao, 2018). However LSF by chemocatalysis often suffers from the limited chemo-, regio- and stereo-selectivity offered by many chemical catalysts. By contrast P450s as promiscuous natural catalysts can carry out C—H bond functionalization in a highly regio- and stereo-specific manner on complex scaffolds under mild conditions (Fessner, 2019). For example, a single mutant (F62L) of $P450_{BM3}$ was utilized to selectively functionalize two sp3 C—H bonds (C9 and C14) in the natural parthenolide carbocyclic backbone, resulting in novel scaffolds with improved anti-leukemic potency against primary acute myeloid leukemia cells and lower toxicity against normal mature and progenitor hematopoietic cells (Kolev et al., 2014). In another example, a panel of human P450s namely CYP3A5, CYP2C9, CYP1A2 and CYP2D6 were used to selectively hydroxylate midazolam, celecoxib, ramelteon, and risperidone followed by deoxyfluorination to produce metabolites that were metabolically more stable than the individual parent compounds (Obach et al., 2016). Similarly, liver microsomes from humans and other species have been utilized to impart structural diversity to drug molecules (Cusack et al., 2013; Obach et al., 2018).

3. Production of drug metabolites

The identification and characterization of drug metabolites form an integral part of the drug development pipeline (Baillie, 2008). Up to 30% of small molecule drug candidates fail in clinical trials due to the inherent toxicity of their metabolites to the study subjects (Guengerich, 2008). Therefore, preparative scale synthesis of drug metabolites is essential and allows the structural identification of metabolites and further pharmacological and toxicological evaluation. With authentic metabolites in hand, an evaluation of potential toxicity and drug-drug interactions is possible, fulfilling the requirements of regulatory guidances (Schadt et al., 2018; Smith & Obach, 2009). Unfortunately, most metabolites are not available commercially and their synthesis is often chemically challenging, so biocatalysis using tissue fractions, microorganisms or recombinant enzymes has come to play a critical role in enabling timely access to metabolites (Shanu-Wilson et al., 2020; Thistlethwaite et al., 2021).

Human P450s such as CYP3A4, CYP2D6, CYP2C9, CYP2C19 and CYP1A2 play prominent roles in drug metabolism. Logically, they can also be used to make authentic drug metabolite standards and microsomal enzyme preparations, pure recombinant P450s (Schiffer et al., 2015; Schroer et al., 2010) as well as intact whole cell systems (Park et al., 2020; Rinnofner et al., 2019; Rushmore et al., 2000) expressing human P450s have been used in small-scale, preparative, metabolite synthesis, e.g., to generate metabolites of testosterone, diclofenac and phenacetin on a 100-mg scale from a few hundred milliliters of culture (Vail et al., 2005).

4. Limitations of P450s as biocatalysts for the pharmaceutical industry

Despite their catalytic potential, the industrial application of P450s is currently limited by several weaknesses including the need for electron transfer partners and expensive cofactors (NADPH), their generally poor catalytic rates on non-native substrates, and the sensitivity of P450s to elevated temperatures and solvent concentrations (Bernhardt & Urlacher, 2014). Moreover they are often expensive to express in recombinant systems, and have little or no reusability, which leads to high production costs (Martinez & Rupashinghe, 2013). Thermostability is especially important in industrial biocatalysts. In industrial chemistry, higher process temperatures are used to increase substrate solubility, minimize microbial contamination, and to promote a more favorable equilibrium (Bommarius & Paye, 2013). Moreover, thermostable enzymes are more durable at ambient temperatures and more amenable to reuse; as the enzyme is usually the most expensive component of a biocatalytic system, this robustness reduces the costs associated with supplying the enzyme and improves yields per unit enzyme. More stable enzymes are also typically more easily expressed in recombinant systems. Tolerance to organic solvents is another important industrial trait. Many organic substrates show limited solubility in water so an increase in organic solvent content allows higher solubility and facilitates substrate loading. Organic solvents also allow for improved product recovery and reduce microbial contamination (Sharma & Kanwar, 2014).

Whole cell systems have been proposed and applied in many cases to circumvent some of these issues (Wachtmeister & Rother, 2016). However, this approach is limited by the solubility and uptake of substrates inside the cell, export of products from the cells, depletion of reducing equivalents, and toxicity of either the substrate or the product to the cells (Duetz et al., 2001).

P450s that can both withstand harsh industrial conditions and carry out industrially relevant reactions efficiently are rare in Nature. Even with advances in genome sequencing and metagenome mining (Furuya & Kino, 2010) it is unlikely that the demands of industrial reactions can be met using natural P450s alone. However, recent advances in protein engineering techniques have made it feasible to optimize enzyme activity and properties (e.g. substrate selectivity, enantioselectivity, thermostability, solvent stability, etc.) to create biocatalysts tailored to specific industrial applications.

5. Progress in changing properties of P450 systems

Natural P450s have evolved as sophisticated catalysts with many properties of interest. In order to develop industrially useful biocatalysts it makes sense to use these "wild" P450s as starting scaffolds to which engineering techniques can be applied (Jung et al., 2011; Schulz et al., 2012). The sheer diversity of P450s in Nature demonstrates the capacity for these enzymes to evolve, indicating the potential to engineer novel activities toward compounds that are not currently substrates as well as to manipulate existing activities. Protein engineering has been used to improve substrate turnover, alter chemo-, regio and stereo-selectivity and catalyze novel reactions not seen in Nature as summarized in Table 1. Indeed P450 enzymes have frequently provided a convenient model system for the development of new engineering methods.

Rational redesign of P450s has been used where information is available on the structure-function relationships of specific enzymes. Where such information is not available, directed evolution approaches have been employed to great effect, including random point mutagenesis (e.g., by error-prone PCR; epPCR), recombinatorial evolution (e.g., by DNA shuffling) or semi-random methods such as saturation mutagenesis at sites considered likely to be determinants of a specific property. (For a detailed compilation of methods, the reader is referred to Gillam et al., 2014). While directed evolution is very powerful in enabling improvements of orders of magnitude in properties of interest and revealing solutions that would not have been considered in rational redesign experiments, it usually requires screening large libraries of mutants. The introduction of structure-guided recombination, e.g., using the SCHEMA algorithm (Voigt et al., 2001) and other computational approaches, has allowed more targeted libraries to be created. Recently, the application of phylogenetic methods, such as ancestral sequence reconstruction (ASR), has allowed the optimization of biophysical properties and, in turn, the activity of enzymes, to tailor them for specific industrial applications (Furukawa et al., 2020; Gumulya & Gillam, 2017; Spence et al., 2021).

Table 1 P450 engineering studies.[a]

Protein	Method[b]	Mutations[c]	Improved property	Reference
$P450_{BM3}$	RD	**R47A**, **Y51F**, **L75T**/K, **L181K**/R, I263K, L437R/K	Increased binding affinity and oxidation of short chain fatty acids (C_4-C_{10})	Ost et al. (2000)
$P450_{BM3}$	SSM, DE	F87X, L188X, A74X **F87V**, **L188Q**, **A74G**	New activity toward novel substrate, indole. Improved activity toward various alkanes and alkanoic acids as well as alicyclic, aromatic and heterocyclic compounds	Li, Schwaneberg, Fischer, and Schmid (2000) Appel, Lutz-Wahl, Fischer, Schwaneberg, and Schmid (2001)
$P450_{BM3}$ (Mutant: F87A)	SSM, DE	P25X, V26X, R47X, Y51X, S72X, A74X, L188X, M354X, **L188K, A74G, RF7F, V26T**	Improved catalytic efficiency toward ω-*p*-nitrophenoxycarboxylic acids of different chain lengths	Li, Ogawa, Schmid, and Shimizu (2001)
$P450_{BM3}$	RD	**R47L**, **Y51F**, **F87A**, **A264G**, M354A, L437A	Increased oxidation of polycyclic aromatic hydrocarbons, increased coupling and altered product distribution	Carmichael and Wong (2001)
$P450_{BM3}$	RM, DE	N/A	Increased activity toward octane	Farinas, Schwaneberg, Glieder, and Arnold (2001)
$P450_{BM3}$	RD	**F87A**	Altered regioselective hydroxylation of myristic acid, lauric acid and capric acid	Cirino and Arnold (2002)
$P450_{BM3}$	RM, DE	**Mutant 139-3: V78A, H138Y, T175I, V178I, A184V, H236Q, E252G, R255S, A290V, A295T, L353V**	Increased turnover rates for oxidation of hydrocarbons of various lengths (C3-C8) as well as epoxidation of various substrates	Glieder et al. (2002) Farinas, Alcalde, and Arnold (2004)
$P450_{BM3}$ (Mutant F87A)	RM, DE	**Mutant 21B3: I58V, H100R, F107L, A135S, M145V, N239H, S274T, K434E, V446I**	Improved hydrogen peroxide (H_2O_2)-driven hydroxylation of 12-*p*-nitrophenoxycarboxylic acid, lauric acid and myristic acid	Cirino and Arnold (2003)

$P450_{BM3}$ (Mutant 21B3)	RM, DS, DE	**Mutant 5H6: L52I, S106R, V145M, A184V, L324I, V340M, I366V, E442K**	Enhanced thermostability	Salazar et al. (2003)
$P450_{BM3}$ (Mutant 139-3)	RM, DS, DE, RD	**Mutant 9-10A: A82L, K94I, Y138H, P142S, I178V, F205C, S226R, A290V, T295A, A328V**	Altered regio- and entioselective hydroxylation of alkanes	Peters, Meinhold, Glieder, and Arnold (2003)
$P450_{BM3}$ (Mutant F87A) and CYP102A2 (Mutant F88A)	SCHEMA		Increased peroxidase activity, and increased hydroxylation rate of allyoxy-benzene. Improved thermostability over CYP102A2	Otey et al. (2004)
$P450_{BM3}$ (Mutant 9-10A)	SSM	A74X, L75X, A78X, F81X, A82X, F87X, T88X, T260X, L263X, I264X, A328X **Mutant 35E11: V78F, A82S, A328F**	New activity toward novel substrate, ethane as well as improved hydroxylation rate and TTN of propane and octane	Meinhold, Peters, Chen, Takahashi, and Arnold (2005)
$P450_{BM3}$	RD	**R47L, F87V, L188Q**	New O-dealkylation activity toward novel substrates; amodiaquine, dextromethorphan, testosterone, acetaminophen, 3,4-methylenedioxymethylamphetamine and alkoxyresorufins	Lussenburg, Babel, Vermeulen, and Commandeur (2005) van Vugt-Lussenburg, Damsten, Maasdijk, Vermeulen, and Commandeur (2006)
$P450_{BM3}$ (Mutant 9-10A)	SSM, DE	A74X, L75X, V78X, F81X, A82X, F87X, T88X, T260X, I263X, A264X, A328X **L75I/W, A78T/F/S, A82T/S/F/I/C/G, F87I/V/L, T88C, T260L/N, A328L/F/M**	Altered hydroxylation regioselectivity and increased hydroxylation rate and TTN of octane, dimethyl ether, hexyl methyl ether	Meinhold, Peters, Hartwick, Hernandez, and Arnold (2006)
$P450_{BM3}$ (Mutant 21B3)	RM	**A82T, S106R, N134D, F205L/S, H239R, E267R, A295S, K306N, E434A**	Improved activity toward propranolol and new activity toward novel substrate phenoxyacetic acid	Bloom et al. (2006)

Continued

Table 1 P450 engineering studies.[a]—cont'd

Protein	Method[b]	Mutations[c]	Improved property	Reference
$P450_{BM3}$ (Mutant 5H6)	RM	**V26A, E35D, A61T, L75R, A74E, W90R, H92R, K98R, S108G, K113E, M118V, D151G, P172A, F173L/V/I, L188Q, D199G, D214Y, D217G, D231E, M237L, L273V, T274S, F275S, D338N, I357T, V366A, E430G, I433F, L437P, F444L, K451E, P461S, H468R**	Improved activity toward propranolol and new activity toward novel substrates 3-phenoxytoluene, naproxen, phenoxyacetic acid and 2-methylbenzofuran	Bloom et al. (2006)
$P450_{BM3}$, CYP102A2, CYP102A3	C		Enhanced thermostability	Otey et al. (2006) Landwehr, Carbone, Otey, Li and Arnold (2007)
$P450_{BM3}$ (Mutant 21B3)	RM, DE	**Mutant 9C1: I102T, L324I, I366V, E442K**	Increased turnover of 12-*p*-nitrophenoxycarboxylic acid using H_2O_2	Otey et al. (2006)
$P450_{BM3}$ (Mutant 9C1)	SSM, RM, DE	A74X, L75X, A78X, F81X, A82X, F87X, T88X, **K24R, R47H, A74H, V78E, A82L/P, A87G**	Produce authentic human metabolites of propanolol	Otey et al. (2006)
$P450_{BM3}$ (Mutant 9-10A)	SSM, DE	A74X, L75X, A78X, F81X, A82X, F87X, T88X, T260X, L263X, I264X, A328X **L75S, A82F/L, F87I/L/V, I263A, A328V**	Increased TTN and epoxidation enantioselectivity of various alkenes	Kubo, Peters, Meinhold, and Arnold (2006)
$P450_{BM3}$, CYP102A2, CYP102A3	C		Enhanced thermostability	Li et al. (2007)
$P450_{BM3}$ (Mutant R47L/F87V/L188Q)	RM, DE	**E64G, F81I, L86I, E143G, E267V**	Improved activity toward dextromethorphan, 3,4-methylenedioxymethylamphetamine and benzyloxyresorufin	van Vugt-Lussenburg et al. (2007)
$P450_{BM3}$ (Mutant 35E11)	RD	**Mutant ETS8: L52I, S106R, M145A, L324I, V340M, I366V, E442K**	Enhanced thermostability	Fasan et al. (2007)

$P450_{BM3}$ (Mutant ETS8)	RM, SSM, DE	A74X, L75X, V78X, A82X, F87X, T88X, L181X, A184X, L188X, T260X, A264X, G265X, T268X, A328X, I401X, L437X, T438X **L52I, A74S, S82G, L188P, V184A, I366V**	Increased coupling and TTN of propane	Fasan et al. (2007)
$P450_{BM3}$ (Mutant F87V)	RD, DE	K69A, **L75A**, **M177A**, **L181A**, **T260A**, I263A, T268A, **L437A**	Improved activity toward various large/bulky substrates	Lewis et al. (2010)
$P450_{BM3}$	RM, DE	**L75P**, **F81L**, **Q189R**, **I263T/A**, **T268A**, **V286E**, **Y305H**	Increased binding affinity for dopamine	Shapiro et al. (2010)
$P450_{BM3}$ (Mutant F87A)	SSM, DE	R47X, T49X, Y51X, V78X, A82X, M185X, L188X, S72X, A74X, L75X, L181X, A184X, T260X, I263X, A328X, A330X, L437X, T438X, V26X, L29X **R47I/Y, T49I/F, Y51I/V, V78L/T/I/V/C, A82F/D/N/G/M, M185N/S/G, L188N/C/G, A330W**	Increased regio- and stereoselectivity in the hydroxylation of testosterone	Kille, Zilly, Acevedo, and Reetz (2011)
$P450_{BM3}$ (Mutant 139-3)	RM	**A221V, H940Q**	Novel activity; steroidal epoxidation based on conversion of progesterone to 16,17-epoxysterol	Jiang, Tu, Bai, and Wang (2013)
$P450_{BM3}$ (Mutant 9-10A-TS-F87V)	RD	L181X, I263X, A328X, L437X, T438X **T268A**, **I263A**, **A328G**, **T438A/S/P** **Mutant $P450_{BM3}$-CIS: 9-10A-TS F87V T268A**	Increased cyclopropanation of styrene via carbene transfer from diazoacetate	Coelho et al. (2013)
$P450_{BM3}$ (Mutant $P450_{BM3}$-CIS)	RD	**P411 mutant: C400S**	Increased cyclopropanation activity toward olefins via carbine transfer	Coelho et al. (2013)
$P450_{BM3}$	Screening of prior mutant libraries	**T268A, T438S, C400S, $P450_{BM3}$-CIS, $P411_{BM3}$-CIS**	Increased TTN and enantioselectivity for the C—H amination of 2,4,6-triethylbenzene-1-sulfonylazide	McIntosh et al. (2013)

Continued

Table 1 P450 engineering studies.[a]—cont'd

Protein	Method[b]	Mutations[c]	Improved property	Reference
P450$_{BM3}$	Screening of prior mutant libraries	**P411$_{BM3}$-CIS, T438S, 1263A**	Increased TTN and enatioselectivity for the sulfimidation of thioanisole via nitrene transfer	Farwell, McIntosh, Hyster, Wang, and Arnold (2014)
P450$_{BM3}$	RM, DS, SSM, DE	Y51X, F87X, A328X, Y334X, D363X **N21S, M30V, Y51H/F, Q55P, N70S, F87I, M119I, M145V, L148S/F, M185H/T, A197V, K202R, D214G, V216A, M237L, N239T, R255S, I263F, Y278C, P301L, G315S, T327N, A328T/V, Y334C, A335V, Y345H, I357V, D363E, V371A, F390L, H408L, D422V,**	Altered regioselectivity in the hydroxylation of palmitic acid	Bruhlmann et al. (2014)
P450$_{BM3}$	RM, C	**R47L, T49S, K59N, C62S, S72C, Q73R/H, F81I, F87V, S89G, N95T, Q110L, Y115C, I122F, I139T, E143G, I153T, L188Q, N186K, N192I, K202Q, I219N, N213D, I259T, E267V/A, T268A, G271D, L272H, V281A, V297A, Y305F, K309R, Y313F, Y334C, A335V, K336E, D351G, D369G, S383R, I401T, Q403K, V413A**	Increased turnover of phenacetin, 7-ethoxycoumarin, 7-etyhoxy-4-trifluoromethylcoumarin, chlorzoxazone and *p*-nitrophenol, simvastatin, lovastatin, fluvastatin, atorvastatin, diclofenac, tamoxifen, propafenone and astemizole	Kang et al. (2014)
P450$_{BM3}$	SSM	L75X, V78X, A82X, L181X, I263X, A328X, A264X, T438X **V78I/F, A82F/I, L181F, I263N, A328F/N, T438I/N**	Increased conversion of cyclohexane to (R)- or (S)-2-hydroxycyclohexanone in a four-step reaction cascade	Li et al. (2016)
P450$_{BM3}$ (Mutant P411$_{BM3}$-CIS T438S)	RD, SSM, DE, screening of prior mutant libraries	A78X, A82X, V87X, L181X, T260X, A268X, A328X, P329X, S400X, S438X **I263F, A328V, V87A, A268G, A82L/I** **Mutant P-4: I263F, V87A, A328V, A268G**	Initiate a sulfimidation/[2,3]-sigmatropic rearrangement sequence by performing imidation of prochiral allylic sulfide to generate allylic sulfimide	Prier, Hyster, Farwell, Huang, and Arnold (2016)

$P450_{BM3}$	Screening of prior mutant libraries	**R47L, Y51F, F87A/V, H171L, A184I, E267V, Q307H, N319Y, A328I, I401P, L437L/V**	Increased hydroxylation activity toward analine derivatives	O'Hanlon, Ren, Morris, Wong, and Robertson (2017)
$P450_{BM3}$ (Mutant P-4, A82L)	SSM, DE	R47X, Y51X, A74X, A78X, S142X, L181X, V184X, G252X, F263X, A264X, E267X, T327X, F393X, G402X **Mutant $P411_{cha}$:A82L, A78V, F263L, E267D**	Enantioselective intermolecular amination of benzylic C—H bonds	Prier, Zhang, Buller, Brinkmann-Chen, and Arnold (2017)
$P450_{BM3}$ (Mutant P-4)	SSM, DE, RD	L52X, D63X, L71X, S72X, A74X, L75X, A78X, A82X, L86X, F87X, T88X, H92X, H100X, M118X, F162X, H171X, M177X, V178X, L181X, L188X, R255X, F261X, I263X, A264X, G265X, E267X, T268X, T269X, T327X, A328X, P329X, A330X, F331X, H361X, F393X, C400X, I401X, T436X, L437X, T438X, L439X **F263Y, A78L, T327I, A74G, L437Q, S438T, T436L, M177L, H266V, N70E, A330Y, I327T, G74P, Q437L** Truncated to remove the FAD domain	Perform novel catalytic activity, alkylation at *a*-amino $C(sp^3)$-H	Zhang et al. (2018)
$P450_{BM3}$	SSM	R47X, Y51X, F87X, L188X **R47D/E, Y51T/M/F/L, F87V, L188D/E/Q/A**	Increased coupling, catalytic efficiency, TTN and altered regioselectivity in the hydroxylation of cetyl-trimethylammonium bromide	Ji et al. (2018)
$P450_{BM3}$ Serine-ligated mutant (P411-CH-C8)	SSM, DE	T327X, E70X, L177X, R226X, Y330X, L401X **T327V, E70T, L177M, R226T, Y330V, L401P**	Increased TTN and entantiospecificity of *a*-amino $C(sp^3)$—H fluoroalkylation	Zhang, Huang, Zhang, and Arnold (2019)
P450cam	RD	**V295I, V247A, Y96F**	Altered regioselectivity of camphor, 1-CH3-norcamphor and norcamphor	Atkins and Sligar (1989)

Continued

Table 1 P450 engineering studies.[a]—cont'd

Protein	Method[b]	Mutations[c]	Improved property	Reference
P450cam	RD	**T185F**	Increased coupling of norcamphor hydroxylation and altered regioselectivity	Paulsen, Filipovic, Sligar, and Ornstein (1993)
P450cam	RD	**Y96A**	New activity toward novel substrate, diphenylmethane	Fowler et al. (1994)
P450cam	RD	**Y96F**, **V247A/L**	Altered regioselectivity toward phenylcyclohexane	Jones, England, Rouch, and Wong (1996)
P450cam	RD	**Y96F/A**	Increased coupling and oxidation rate of alkanes	Stevenson, Westlake, Whittock, and Wong (1996)
P450cam	RD	**Y96F/A**	Tighter binding of styrene and increased coupling of oxidation rate of styrene	Nickerson, Harford-Cross, Fulcher, and Wong (1997)
P450cam	RD	**Y96F/A/V/F/L**	Activity toward novel substrates and altered regioselectivity	Bell, Rouch, and Wong (1997)
P450cam	RD	**Y96G/A/V/F**	Increased coupling and rate of naphthalene and pyrene oxidation	England, Harford-Cross, Stevenson, Rouch, and Wong (1998)
P450cam	RM, DS, DE	**C242F**, **R280L**, **E331K**	Improved activity toward naphthalene and 3-phenylpropionate using H_2O_2	Joo et al. (1999)

P450cam	RD	**F87A/L, Y96A/F**	Increased coupling and rate of oxidation of polycyclic aromatic hydrocarbons plus altered product distribution	Harford-Cross et al. (2000)
P450cam	RD	**F87W, Y96F, F98W, V247L**	Increased coupling and oxidation rates of polychlorinated aromatic compounds	Jones, O'Hare, and Wong (2001)
P450cam	RD	**Y96F, V247L, I395G**	Increased coupling and oxidation rates of diphenylmethane, styrene and ethylbenzene	Bell, Harford-Cross, and Wong (2001)
P450cam	RD	**F87W, Y96F, T101L, V247L**	Increased coupling and oxidation rate of butane and propane	Bell et al. (2002)
P450cam	RD	**F87A/L/W, Y96F, V247L, L224A**	Increased coupling and oxidation rate of (+)-α-pinene and altered product distribution	Bell et al. (2003)
P450cam	RD	**F87W, Y96F, F98W, T101L, V247A/L, L244M, V295I, D297M**, V396L	Increased coupling and oxidation rate of pentane, *n*-butane and propane	Bell et al. (2003)
P450cam	SSM	Y96X, Y98X **Y96A/C/D/H/K, Y98F/H/V/G**	Alternative mutations to those identified by Fowler 1994 that introduce activity toward diphenylmethane	Speight et al. (2004)
P450cam (mutant; F87W/Y96F/T101L/V247L/L1244M)	RD	**T185M, G248A, L294M, L1358P**	Increased coupling and oxidation rate of propane plus new activity toward novel substrate, ethane	Xu et al. (2005)
P450cam	RD	**Y96F/V, T101V, L244A**	New activity toward novel substrate, indole and enhanced activity toward aromatic hydrocarbons coumarin, indoline, quinolone and indene	Manna and Mazumdar (2010)

Continued

Table 1 P450 engineering studies.[a]—cont'd

Protein	Method[b]	Mutations[c]	Improved property	Reference
P450cam	RD, SSM, DE	Y96X, N244X **F87A/F/I/T/V**, **Y96H/M/Q/W**, **T101I/L**, **L244N/Q**, **V247F/I/L**, **V295A/L**, **D297E/I/M/T/V**, **I395H/M/N/V**, **V396A/I**	Increased coupling and altered regioselectivity toward diphenylmethane	Hoffmann, Bonsch, Greiner-Stoffele, and Ballschmiter (2011)
CYP101D2	RD	**Y96A**	Increased binding affinity and oxidation of various hydrophobic substrates	Bell, Yang, Dale, Zhou, and Wong (2013)
P450moxA	RM, DE	**Q87W**, **T115A**, **H132L**, **R191W**, **G294D**	Increased activity toward 7-ethoxycoumarin, diclofenac and naringenin	Kabumoto, Miyazaki, and Arisawa (2009)
P450nov	RM, DE	**L188P**, **F218L**, **L237M**	Increased hydroxylation 3-benzyloxy-2-methyl-4-pyrone	Kozono, Mihara, Minagawa, Hibi, and Ogawa (2017)
CYP105A3 (P450sca-2)	RM	**G52S**, **F89I**, **P159A**, **D269E**, **T323A**, **E370V**	Increased protein expression resulting in greater whole-cell biotransformation of mevastatin to pravastatin	Ba, Li, Zhang, Duan, and Lin (2013)
CYP105A3 (P450sca-2) (Mutant; G52S, F89I, P159A, D269E, T323A, E370V)	SSM, DE	T85X, R77X, V194X, N363X, T119X **T85M/L/V/I/F**, **T119S/N**, **V194C**, **N363H/Y**	Increased rate of conversion of mevastatin to pravastatin	Ba et al. (2013)
P450pyr	SSM, DE	A77X, I82X, I83X, L98X, P99X, N100X, I102X, A103X, S182X, D183X, T185X, T186X, L251X, V254X, G255X, D258X, T259X, L302X, M305X, F403X **Mutant P450pyrTM: A77S**, **I83H**, **M305A/Q**	Increased enantioselective conversion of *N*-benzyl pyrrolidine hydroxylation to (*S*)-*N*-benzyl 3-hydroxypyrrolidine Increased enantioselective conversion of *para*-substituted styrenes to (*R*)-*para*-substituted styrenes	Pham, Pompidor, Liu, Li, and Li (2012) Li, Liu, Pham, and Li (2013)

CYP119	RD	T213A/V/S/F/W, **T214A/V**	Increased catalytic rate of styrene epoxidation using H_2O_2 and enhanced activity supported by putidaredoxin and putidaredoxin reductase	Koo et al. (2000)
CYP119	RD	**T213G**, **T214V**	Increased enantioselectivity and catalytic rate of styrene epoxidation using H_2O_2	Zhang et al. (2014)
CYP119	RD	**T213M**/Y	Increased enantioselective epoxidation of *cis*-β-methylstyrenes	Zhang et al. (2016)
CYP153A13	C	Linked P450 to reductase domains of CYP102A1, CYP102A5 and CYP102D1	Increased hydroxylation of dodecanoic acid	Ahsan, Patil, Jeon, Sung, and Chung (2018)
CYP153A35	SSM	I123X, P128X, L130X, D131X, V132X, M134X, I136X, A219X, Y236X, A239X, L240X, T243X, T292X, L293X, V296X, T301X, L344X, M347X, F445X **D131S/F**	Increased TTN and catalytic efficiency of activity toward palmitic acid	Jung et al. (2018)
CYP260A1	SSM	S225X, S275X, S276X **S276N/I/C/L/V**	Increased regio- and stereo-selective hydroxylation of progesterone to 1α-OH-progesterone and 17α-OH-progesterone	Khatri et al. (2018)
CYP1A2	RM, DE	**E225N**, **Q258H**, **G437D**	Enhanced heterocyclic amine *N*-hydroxylation	Kim and Guengerich (2004b)
CYP1A2	RM, DE	**E163K**, **V193M**, **K170Q**	Tighter binding of 7-methoxyresorufin and increased rate of *O*-demethylation activity	Kim and Guengerich (2004a)
CYP1A1, CYP1A2	DS		Enhanced catalytic rates toward various parent substrates	Johnston et al. (2007)
CYP2A6	RM, RD	L40C, F209T, **L240C**, **N297Q**/H	Increased indole oxidation and novel oxidation of indole-derivatives	Nakamura et al. (2001)

Continued

Table 1 P450 engineering studies.[a]—cont'd

Protein	Method[b]	Mutations[c]	Improved property	Reference
CYP2A6	RM, DE	**F209S**, **S369G**, **E277K**, **A10V**	Increased TTN of nicotine and coumarin	Lee et al. (2014)
CYP2B1	RD	V103I, **I114A**, **F206V**, S294D, **F297G**, **V363L**, I477F, G478V	Altered regioselectivity in progesterone hydroxylation	Kumar et al. (2003)
CYP2B1 Mutant L209A	RM, DE	**V183L**, **F202L**, **L209A**, **S334P**	Enhanced catalytic efficiency toward 7-ethoxy-4-trifluoromethylcoumarin, 7-benzyloxyresorufin, benzphetamine, testosterone, cyclophosphamide and ifosfamide. Increased stereoselectivity of 16α- over 16β-hydroxylation of testosterone	Kumar et al. (2005)
CYP2B1 Mutant: V183L/F202L/L209A/S334P	RM, DE, RD	**K236I**, **D257N**, **L295H**	Enhanced catalytic tolerance to temperature and DMSO	Kumar et al. (2006)
CYP2B6	RD	F58L, M103V, V129L, I154V, M198L, **L264F**, S284H, E350D, Y354H, L390P, T394S	Increased protein expression as well as stability against thermal and chemical denaturation	Kumar et al. (2007)
CYP2B6	RD	V81T, **V234I**, E254A, Y325Q, **P334S**, **I427M**, Q473K	Increased protein expression and thermostability	Talakad et al. (2010)
CYP2B11	RD	I81T, V234I, E254A, Y325Q, **P334S**, I427M, Q473K	Increased protein expression and thermostability	Talakad et al. (2010)
CYP2C9, CYP2C11 and CYP2C19	DS		Increased indole oxidation	Rosic, Huang, Johnston, DeVoss, and Gillam (2007)
CYP2D6	RD	T309V, T312V	Altered regioselectivity and increased CuOOH-supported activity toward multiple substrates	Keizers et al. (2005)

CYP2E1	RD	**T303A**	Increased reaction rate toward multiple substrates	Vaz et al. (1998)
CYP3A4	RM, RD	**L206W**, **F241V**, **F228I**, **T309A/V**/I/F, **T433S**	Enhanced peroxide-supported activity toward 7-benzyloxyquinoline, 7-benzyloxy-4-(trifluoromethyl)coumarin and testosterone	Kumar et al. (2006)
CYP3A4,	RD	**L293P**, **T409R**	Increased whole-cell biotransformation activity toward nifedipine and testosterone	Neunzig et al. (2012)
CYP3A5	RD	**L293P**, **T409R**	Increased whole-cell biotransformation activity toward testosterone and dehydroepiandrosterone	Neunzig et al. (2012)
CYP3A7	RD	**L293P**, **T409R**	Increased whole-cell biotransformation activity toward midazolam, testosterone, dehydroepiandrosterone and luciferin-PFBE	Neunzig et al. (2012)
CYP3A4, CYP3A5, CYP3A7, CYP3A9	DS		Increased production of minor testosterone metabolites	Hunter et al. (2011)
CYP17A1	RD	L105A, F114A, V201A, N202A, I205A, **L206A**, R239A, G297A, G298A, G301A, E305A, T306A, **V366A**, I371A, L482A, **V483A**	Altered regioselectivity in its hydroxylation of progesterone	Morlock et al. (2018)
CYP154E1	RD	L94A/I/F/V, T178F/L/A/G/V, L179A/G/I/V, **L234Q**, L235A, **I238A/V**/L, **G239A**/F/V/S/I, V286A/G/L/T/S, M388Q	Increased activity toward (*E*)-stilbene, (*E*)-2-hydroxystilbene, (*E*)-3-hydroxystilbene, (*E*)-4-hydroxystilbene and pinosylvin	Rühlmann, Antovic, Müller, and Urlacher (2017)

[a]The studies listed are those that focused specifically on engineering rather than deciphering structure-function relationships.
[b]For each study the mutagenesis method is indicated, i.e., rational design (RD), random mutagenesis (RM), site-saturation mutagenesis (SSM), DNA-shuffling (DS) and chimeragenesis (C). Studies that carried out iterative rounds of mutagenesis and screening to achieve successive improvements in the engineered property are described as having involved directed evolution (DE).
[c]All mutations explored in RD and SSM studies are listed, with beneficial mutations shown in bold. Residues mutated by SSM are listed with an X in place of a specific mutation change. In the case of RM studies, only mutations identified as beneficial are listed.

Bacterial P450s, particularly $P450_{BM3}$ and $P450_{cam}$, are arguably the most popular P450s for both rational redesign and directed evolution studies. $P450_{BM3}$ has been particularly popular for several reasons: it is a soluble protein making it easier to purify and reconstitute; it displays superior substrate conversion efficiencies on its native substrates with k_{cat} values of 1000–3000 min^{-1} (Fulco, 1991; Peterson et al., 1997) whereas most eukaryotic P450s have k_{cat} values in the range of ~1–300 min^{-1} (Bernhardt & Urlacher, 2014); and it is self-sufficient by virtue of being a natural, evolutionarily optimized fusion between a haem domain and a reductase domain. In addition, the haem domain of $P450_{BM3}$ has been engineered to utilize H_2O_2 as an oxidant eliminating the need for NAD(P)H or redox partners (Cirino & Arnold, 2003).

Compared with $P450_{BM3}$ and $P450_{cam}$, eukaryotic P450s have been relatively underexplored in engineering studies, despite displaying significantly broader, and arguably more relevant, substrate ranges in the case of drug-metabolizing P450s. To date, there are only a handful of eukaryotic P450s that have been subjected to protein engineering and the majority of these studies have been carried out with the objective of elucidating structure-function relationships (Chen et al., 2004; Parikh et al., 1999; Yun et al., 2000) or as proof-of-concept studies for new methods (Abécassis et al., 2000; Huang et al., 2007). However, with advances in protein engineering, eukaryotic P450s are becoming increasingly promising biocatalytic prospects. Overall, studies have been directed toward enhancing five main properties: (1) catalytic activity toward substrates of interest (substrate specificity); (2) electron transfer from the reductase; (3) ability to be supported by oxygen surrogates; (4) structural stability; and (5) solvent tolerance.

6. Engineering of substrate specificity

$P450_{BM3}$ has been a poster child for many directed evolution efforts geared toward improving substrate specificity and enantioselectivity (Acevedo-Rocha et al., 2018; Agudo et al., 2012; Rea et al., 2012), including the generation of drug metabolites (Kim et al., 2011; Otey, Bandara, et al., 2006; Reinen et al., 2011; Rentmeister et al., 2011; Sawayama et al., 2009; Venkataraman et al., 2014) as listed in Table 1. These have been reviewed extensively previously (Gillam & Hayes, 2013; Girvan & Munro, 2016; Thistlethwaite et al., 2021; Yun et al., 2007) and will not be explored in detail here. However, several themes emerge from these studies. Firstly, certain mutations have been found useful to open up the $P450_{BM3}$ active site and substrate access channel to expand the substrate specificity; secondly certain mutations can shift the equilibrium between the open and closed form of the P450 (Butler et al., 2013); and thirdly, mutations that affect substrate specificity are often remote from the active site, presumably acting by shifting elements of secondary structure rather than directly interacting with the substrates (Axarli et al., 2005). Usefully, the body of work done with $P450_{BM3}$, especially by the Arnold laboratory using the SCHEMA approach to recombinatorial evolution, has generated libraries of P450s that can be screened for activity toward particular substrates (Li et al., 2007; Rentmeister et al., 2011; Sawayama et al., 2009).

While engineering efforts have allowed the substrate scope of $P450_{BM3}$ to be broadened, native bacterial enzymes tend to show more limited substrate scope than promiscuous drug-metabolizing eukaryotic P450s. Whereas bacterial P450s such as $P450_{BM3}$ have been subjected to multiple rounds of mutagenesis to iteratively optimize activity toward particular substrates and reactions, engineering studies using eukaryotic P450s have largely been restricted to "proof of concept" studies used to show how the activity of these enzymes can be tailored (Abécassis et al., 2000; Huang et al., 2007; Hunter et al., 2011; Johnston et al., 2007; Kim & Guengerich, 2004a; Kim et al., 2005; Kumar, Chen, Waxman, & Halpert, 2005; Kumar et al., 2007; Kumar, Sun, et al., 2006; Parikh et al., 1999; Wu et al., 2005). An example is shown in Fig. 1 for CYP3A4 and related forms, which have been used to exemplify several different approaches. However to date, no intensive campaigns directed toward optimization of activities directly applicable to industrial processes have been published to our knowledge.

Several members of the mammalian CYP2 family have been subjected to directed evolution and rational engineering studies to alter activity toward various substrates. Early rational mutagenesis studies relied on information from bacterial P450s (typically $P450_{cam}$ or $P450_{BM3}$), due to the lack of a eukaryotic structure. However, the crystallization of the first mammalian P450, rabbit CYP2C5 (Williams et al., 2000), made better structure prediction possible, and facilitated the engineering of many eukaryotic P450s by rational design using homology models based on the CYP2C5 or other structures. Steroid hydroxylation has been a common target activity for engineering of P450s. Rational design of CYP2B1 was used to alter the regioselectivity of progesterone hydroxylation from 16α- to 21-hydroxylation (Kumar et al., 2003). Seven mutations were selected based on the crystal structure of CYP2C5, a 21-hydroxylase. Likewise, the regioselectivity of bovine CYP17A1 toward progesterone was altered to produce a greater proportion

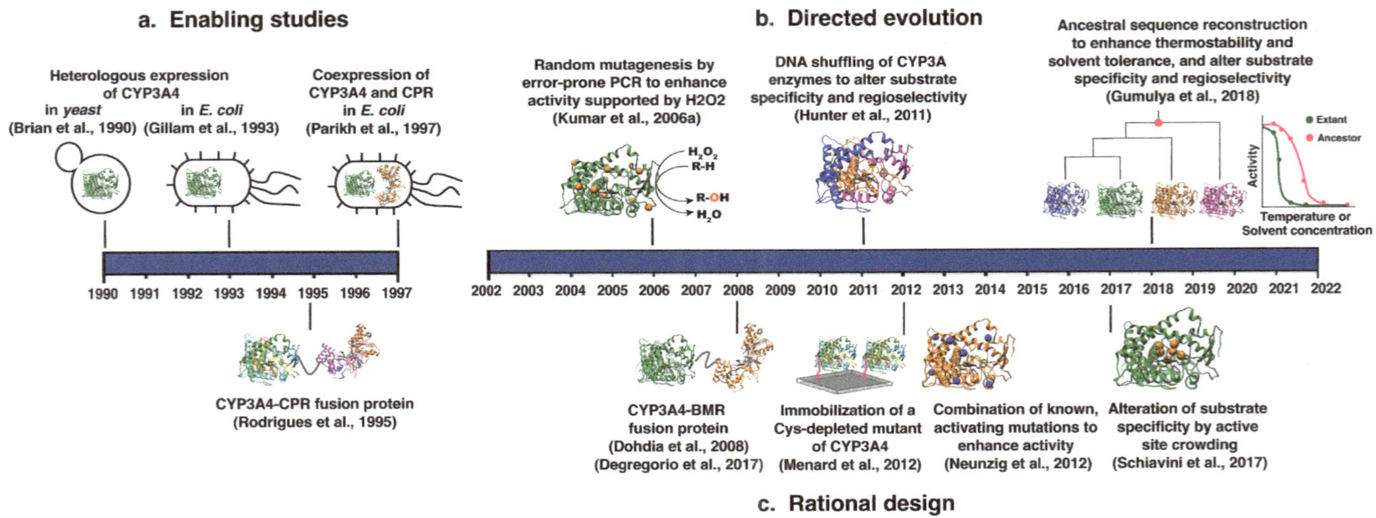

Fig. 1 Approaches used for engineering of CYP3A4 and related CYP3A enzymes. CYP3A4, a major drug-metabolizing human P450, has been the model used in numerous proof-of-principle studies over the last two decades that have exemplified the usefulness of engineering eukaryotic P450s. Milestones in the engineering of CYP3A4 and related enzymes are shown on a timeline from the initial enabling studies (A) where CYP3A4 was expressed in heterologous systems (Brian et al., 1990; Gillam, Baba, Kim, Ohmori, & Guengerich, 1993; Parikh & Guengerich, 1997; Rodrigues et al., 1995), to directed evolution (Gumulya et al., 2018; Hunter et al., 2011; Kumar, Liu, & Halpert, 2006) (B) and rational design experiments (Dodhia et al., 2008; Menard, Huang, Karam, Cosa, & Auclair, 2012)(Degregorio et al., 2017; Neunzig et al., 2012; Schiavini, Cheong, Moitessier, & Auclair, 2017) (C). Only studies where changes were introduced into the protein sequence are shown.

of 16α-hydroxyprogesterone by identifying active site residues from the crystal structures of human CYP17A1 as well as zebrafish CYP17A1 and CYP17A2 (Morlock et al., 2018). Homology-based site directed mutagenesis of CYP2D6 was used to generate a mutant capable of hydroxylating testosterone at the 15α position by replacing the Phe at position 483 with Ile (Smith et al., 1998). Another mutant in which Glu216 (a residue implicated in substrate binding) was changed to Phe, showed 11 times improved specific 6β-testosterone hydroxylation activity.

An interesting approach applied to CYP3A4 has been "active site crowding." CYP3A4 is notorious for showing broad substrate specificity as well as homotropic and heterotropic cooperativity. Multiple residues involved in substrate binding, cooperativity, and regioselectivity were identified by site directed mutagenesis studies then preferentially mutated to bulkier residues such as Tyr, Phe, or Trp to favor oxidation at less sterically hindered positions in substrates (Schiavini et al., 2017).

Early directed evolution studies on eukaryotic P450s focused on CYP1A, CYP2A and CYP2B enzymes. CYP1A2 was subjected to three rounds of mutagenesis and $\sim 10^4$ mutants were screened for improved 7-methoxyresorufin *O*-demethylation activity, revealing a triple mutant that had a k_{cat} that was five times faster than the wildtype (Kim & Guengerich, 2004a). CYP1A2 has also been engineered for enhanced heterocyclic amine *N*-hydroxylation using three rounds of random mutagenesis, which yielded a mutant with a 12-fold enhanced k_{cat}/K_m (Kim & Guengerich, 2004a). CYP2A6 was subjected to random mutagenesis to generate a library that was screened for the oxidation of indole and its derivatives (Nakamura et al., 2001), for the production of indigoids which have applications in dye production and as kinase inhibitors (Guengerich et al., 2004). CYP2A6 was also subjected to four rounds of random mutagenesis and screening toward coumarin and nicotine turnover, which produced a mutant displaying ~7-fold and ~2-fold increases in the total turnover number (TTN), respectively. However, both these substrates also showed a lower binding affinity to the mutant compared to the wild type such that the catalytic efficiency was essentially unchanged (Lee, Kim, et al., 2014).

The substrate promiscuity of mammalian drug-metabolizing P450s is advantageous since it is generally easier to improve an existing activity than to engineer a completely novel one. Therefore the hypothesis was tested that directed evolution could be used to enhance the activity of a P450 while maintaining its substrate versatility. This was done by assessing CYP2B1 activity toward 7-ethoxy-4-trifluoromethylcoumarin, 7-benzyloxyresorufin, benzphetamine and testosterone with the goal of identifying non-active site substitutions that might enhance activity across a panel of structurally diverse substrates (Kumar et al., 2005). While one mutation improved activity toward multiple substrates, overall, differences were seen according to the substrate assessed, support system used (NADPH *vs.* oxygen surrogate) and form of the enzyme used (i.e., N-terminally truncated or full length).

CYP2B enzymes were the target of several studies designed to improve the bioactivation of cyclophosphamide by 4-hydroxylation, and in which both rational and directed evolution approaches were combined (Chen et al., 2004; Kumar et al., 2005; Sun et al., 2007). Initially, residues found to be important in determining substrate specificity in CYP2B enzymes were altered in CYP2B1 (Chen et al., 2004). Two residues were identified that enhanced cyclophosphamide but not ifosfamide activation in CYP2B1, residues which were already present in CYP2B11, a homologue found to be more effective in cyclophosphamide activation. Random mutagenesis was used to identify several mutations that increased cyclophosphamide activation in a CYP2B1 mutant engineered to use hydrogen peroxide as an oxygen surrogate (Kumar et al., 2005). These mutations were then introduced into CYP2B11 (Sun et al., 2007). Again the mutations exerted different effects on the activity toward alternative substrates and routes of metabolism, underscoring the need to optimize for each substrate and reaction individually. Moreover, effects of mutations differed between truncated and full length forms of the enzyme, indicating epistatic interactions dependent on the sequence or structural context.

Recombinatorial evolution of eukaryotic P450s has also been assessed in other proof of concept studies. DNA shuffling was used to create libraries of CYP1A (Johnston et al., 2007), CYP2C (Huang et al., 2007) and CYP3 enzymes (Hunter et al., 2011) from recombination of extant mammalian forms, creating libraries of mutants with different profiles of activity toward marker substrates, which could then be screened for mutants with desired properties, such as enhanced yield of minor products.

7. Engineering catalytic efficiency via the redox system

The requirement by eukaryotic P450s for a redox partner and expensive NADPH cofactor for catalysis is a major limitation for their industrial application. The P450 and CPR can be co-expressed and used in whole cells to take advantage of cofactor regeneration via intermediary metabolism. Rational engineering approaches to alter the cofactor specificity of CPR have mainly focused on mutating residues in the $NADP^+$-binding region of the reductase. Replacement of the door-keeping residue Trp677 to a smaller Ala677 residue has been implicated in providing unobstructed access to NADH to allow the transfer of the first electron (Döhr et al., 2001; Elmore & Porter, 2002; Gutierrez et al., 2000; Sem & Kasper, 1993). While it has proven straightforward to lose the preference for NADPH, creating an NADH-specific CPR that supports P450s has been more challenging (Strohmaier et al., 2019).

Another avenue for reducing the cost of the cofactor is to use non-natural cofactor analogues. To date only a single study has reported engineering P450s to use cheap alternatives to NADPH or NADH (Lo et al., 2017) but this is an interesting prospect for future work, especially in combination with immobilization of such cofactors on solid supports for catalysis in flow (Hartley et al., 2019).

The interaction between the P450 and CPR influences the coupling of cofactor oxidation and substrate monooxygenation; however the drug-metabolizing P450s are typically poorly coupled, as are other P450s acting on non-natural substrates. The highly efficient $P450_{BM3}$, in which the reductase domain is naturally fused to the haem domain, has inspired the creation of fusions between mammalian P450 enzymes and native (human) or non-native (yeast) reductases in an attempt to enhance electron transport (Alterman et al., 1995; Chun et al., 1996; Deeni et al., 2001; Fisher et al., 1992; Murakami et al., 1987; Yabusaki et al., 1988). In most cases, the fusions have been created by joining the P450 C-terminus to a truncated CPR domain via a short linker. The length and sequence of the linker was found to impact the overall efficiency of electron transfer and coupling (Catucci et al., 2022; Hlavica, 2009). Chimeras generated by the fusion of mammalian P450 enzymes and the reductase domain of $P450_{BM3}$ (Fairhead et al., 2005) have exhibited more efficient substrate conversion than reactions supported solely by the $P450_{BM3}$ reductase domain (Rua et al., 2012; Sadeghi & Gilardi, 2013). Engineering of the loop connecting CYP3A4 and the $P450_{BM3}$ reductase domain in a fusion construct led to a two-fold improvement in V_{max} along with a higher coupling efficiency and NADPH oxidation rates, when compared to the original fusion construct (Degregorio et al., 2017).

Engineering of the interaction of the CPR with P450s has been confounded by the lack of a crystal structure of a mammalian P450 in complex with CPR. Without such a structure, the dynamics of the association between the two proteins has been mostly investigated through biophysical and molecular simulation studies (Hedison & Scrutton, 2019; Mukherjee et al., 2021; Sugishima et al., 2014). However, smaller redox proteins such as flavodoxins have been optimized using protein engineering. For example, adrenodoxin was engineered to support bacterial CYP106A2 which resulted in improving the overall activity by 2.5-fold (Sagadin et al., 2019).

Apart from engineering CPR to improve efficiency, P450s can be paired with non-native redox proteins to enhance their activity. When co-expressed with yeast ferredoxin reductase and its ferredoxin homologue (arh1 and etp1^{fd}) respectively, the biotransformation of premedrol by CYP21A1 in whole cells was enhanced (Brixius-Anderko et al., 2015). In a similar example, co-expression in *Schizosaccharomyces pombe* of CYP2D6 with a CPR homolog from fission yeast, and CYP2C9 with a CPR homolog from Bishop's Weed, improved the activity of the respective enzymes when tested with dextromethorphan and diclofenac respectively (Neunzig et al., 2013). Replacing the natural support system of CYP21A2 with a novel sulfite reductase from *Bacillus megaterium* produced a two-fold higher turnover of progesterone (Milhim et al., 2016).

8. Engineering the ability to use oxygen surrogates

Problems in achieving efficient electron transfer can be circumvented by replacing the NADPH-reductase system with oxygen surrogates (O_2Ss) such as H_2O_2, cumene hydroperoxide (CuOOH) or various hypervalent iodine compounds (e.g., bis(acetoxy)-iodobenzene, BAIB), taking advantage of the peroxide shunt pathway to obviate the dependency on redox partners and cofactors (Guengerich, 2018). O_2Ss are considerably cheaper and can generally be used at higher temperatures than the NADPH-reductase system. H_2O_2 is also considered a "green" reagent in the context of industrial catalysis as it is a relatively mild oxidant and its only by-products are water and oxygen (Burek et al., 2019).

O_2Ss have mostly been explored with bacterial P450 forms (Ciaramella et al., 2019; Girvan et al., 2018; Joo, Lin, & Arnold, 1999; Li, Ogawa, Schmid, & Shimizu, 2005; Nguyen, Yeom, & Yun, 2021; Niraula, Kanth, Sohng, & Oh, 2011; Subedi, Kim, Hong, Lee, & Oh, 2021), however several eukaryotic P450s such as CYP1A2 (Anari, Josephy, Henry, & O'Brien, 1997; Hiroya, Murakami, Shimizu, Hatano, & Ortiz de Montellano, 1994), CYP2B1 (Bhakta, Hollenberg, & Wimalasena, 2005), CYP2B4 (Reed, Cawley, & Backes, 2013), CYP2D6 (Chefson, Zhao, & Auclair, 2006) and CYP3A4 (Chefson & Auclair, 2007; Kumar, Liu, & Halpert, 2006) have also been found to work with H_2O_2, CuOOH, tert-butyl hydroperoxide, and/or iodosylbenzene. An investigation with the "big five" drug metabolizing P450s (CYP3A4, CYP2C9, CYP2C19, CYP2D6 and CYP1A2), found that the overall effectiveness of the peroxide-supported reaction was highly dependent on the substrate under investigation and of the oxygen surrogates tested, CuOOH and tert-butyl hydroperoxide performed the best overall (Strohmaier, De Voss, Jurva, Andersson, & Gillam, 2020).

The majority of studies directed toward *engineering* better P450 activity with oxygen donors have focused on bacterial forms (Cirino & Arnold, 2002; Di Nardo & Gilardi, 2012; Glieder, Farinas, & Arnold, 2002), but there are a handful of studies exploring this property in mammalian P450s. Multiple studies have targeted a conserved threonine residue located in the I helix because of its proposed role in dioxygen activation. In early studies this residue was converted to an alanine in CYP2B4 and CYP2E1 (Vaz, McGinnity, & Coon, 1998; Vaz, Pernecky, Raner, & Coon, 1996). CYP2E1 showed an increase in the overall oxidation rate of four substrates, however, the metabolite ratios were significantly different to the wild type (Vaz et al., 1998). Conversely, the CYP2B4 mutant showed decreased activity toward six out of seven substrates assayed across two studies (Vaz et al., 1998, 1996). More recently this threonine residue was mutated to a valine in CYP2D6 (Keizers et al., 2005) resulting in a 4- to 75-fold increase in activity over the wild type toward multiple substrates when using CuOOH. CYP3A4 has also been subjected to random and site-directed mutagenesis (including the conserved threonine to alanine or valine mutations) to enhance H_2O_2-supported metabolism (Kumar et al., 2006). This study yielded a mutant with an 11-fold higher k_{cat}/K_m for oxidation of 7-benzyloxyquinoline than wildtype CYP3A4.

While many P450s, including CYP1A2 (Hiroya et al., 1994), CYP2B1 (Bhakta et al., 2005), CYP2B4 (Kenaan et al., 2013), CYP2D6 (Chefson et al., 2006) and 3A4 (Chefson et al., 2006; Strohmaier et al., 2020) have been found to work with O_2Ss, there are caveats to the use of this system. Although NADPH- and peroxide-supported P450 reactions are usually similar, catalytic rates and metabolites can vary (Anari, Khan, Jatoe, & O'Brien, 1997; Strohmaier et al., 2020). In addition, most P450s are sensitive to oxidative damage by O_2Ss, shortening the lifespan of the enzyme (Wapshott-Stehli & Grunden, 2021). Systems for in situ generation of H_2O_2 may be of use in facilitating the delivery of an oxygen surrogate while limiting the resultant oxidative damage. Increasing the reaction efficiency with oxygen donors and improving the resilience of P450s to oxidative damage should be worthwhile objectives for future protein engineering.

9. Progress in engineering thermostability

In industrial processes, higher temperatures are often desirable to minimize microbial contamination, increase reaction rates and increase substrate solubility (Bommarius & Paye, 2013). In addition, enhanced stability can extend the enzyme half-life, reducing the frequency with which the enzyme needs to be replaced. Attempts to increase thermostability of P450s have thus far focused on the mammalian, xenobiotic metabolizing CYP3, CYP2 and CYP1 subfamilies and the bacterial subfamily, CYP102A (chiefly $P450_{BM3}$).

9.1 Thermostabilization of bacterial P450s

Thermostability studies targeting $P450_{BM3}$ have been reviewed in detail recently (Harris, Thomson, Strohmaier, Gumulya, & Gillam, 2018) so will only be summarized here. Improved thermostability has been achieved using random mutagenesis, DNA-shuffling, chimeragenesis, ancestral sequence reconstruction and *in silico* methods (Fig. 2). In the earliest study reporting the enhancement of P450 thermostability, the starting scaffold used for engineering was the H_2O_2-supported $P450_{BM3}$ mutant, 21B3 ($T_{50} \sim 46\,°C$). This variant, engineered using several rounds of random mutagenesis and recombination, encodes only the haem domain and differs from the wildtype haem domain by 10 mutations. To enhance its thermostability, 21B3 was subjected to five cycles of random mutagenesis, followed by a round of DNA-shuffling with another $P450_{BM3}$ haem domain variant containing the mutation F87A (Salazar, Cirino, & Arnold, 2003). Variant 5H6 ($^{10}T_{50} = 61°C$) was identified that differed from 21B3 at 8 residues (S106R, L52I, V145M, A184V, L324I, V340M, I366V and E442K). The 5H6 variant was subsequently subjected to epPCR with the principal aim of enhancing activity; however, three mutants were identified adventitiously with T_{50} values up to 3 °C higher than 5H6 (Bloom, Labthavikul, Otey, & Arnold, 2006). Several of the mutations identified as beneficial in 5H6 have been used to stabilize other $P450_{BM3}$ variants used in engineering studies (Fasan, Chen, Crook, & Arnold, 2007; Lewis et al., 2010; Shapiro et al., 2010).

The next approach used to stabilize the CYP102A1 haem domain was structure guided recombination using the SCHEMA algorithm (Voigt, Martinez, Wang, Mayo, & Arnold, 2002). A library of over 600 chimeras was created by recombining fragments of the CYP102A haem domain variants CYP102A1 (F87A, $^{10}T_{50} = 55\,°C$), CYP102A2 (F88A, $^{10}T_{50} = 44\,°C$)

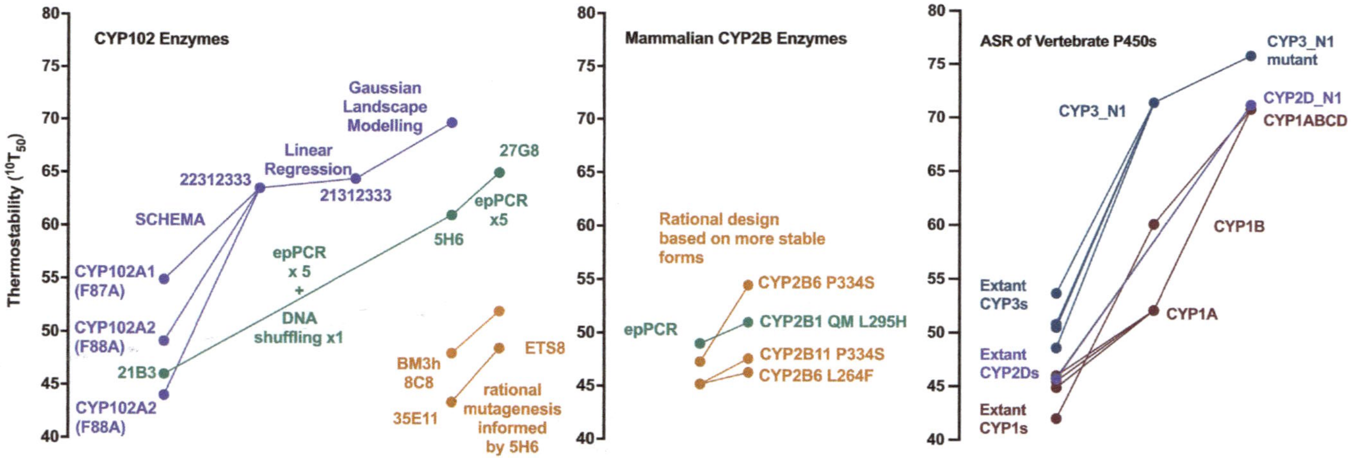

Fig. 2 Engineering of thermostability into P450BM3 and its homologues. Nodes indicate the thermostability ($^{10}T_{50}$) of P450s and their variants used as starting scaffolds (at left) and the most thermostable mutants they gave rise to, using the methods of SCHEMA (Otey et al., 2006), machine learning (Romero et al., 2013), random mutagenesis and DNA-shuffling (Salazar et al., 2003), epPCR (Bloom et al., 2006), rational mutagenesis (Fasan et al., 2007; Shapiro et al., 2010) and ancestral sequence reconstruction (Gumulya et al., 2018, 2019; Harris et al., 2022). Nodes of related variants are connected with a solid line.

and CYP102A3 (F88A, $^{10}T_{50}=49\,°C$) using seven crossover points (Otey et al., 2006). The most stable chimera (22312333) identified from this library had a $^{10}T_{50}$ of 62–63.5 °C (Li et al., 2007; Otey et al., 2006), differing from its closest parent at 84 amino acid positions. The thermostability data from this chimeric library was used as training data subsequently to establish *in silico* methods for predicting novel chimeric sequences with enhanced stability. A linear regression model was used to predict T_{50} values for >6000 chimeras and identified 30 with predicted $^{10}T_{50}$ values $\geq 60\,°C$ (Li et al., 2007). These 30 mutants were constructed and all displayed measured $^{10}T_{50}$ values between 58.5 and 64.4 °C. In a subsequent study, all available chimeric data was used to infer the fitness landscape using Gaussian process regression (Romero, Krause, & Arnold, 2013). An Upper Confidence Bound algorithm was used to iteratively improve the Gaussian process model in regions of the landscape that were predicted to be highly optimized. This method was used to infer and construct 34 sequences, of which 12 had a $^{10}T_{50} \geq 65\,°C$. The most stable variant displayed a $^{10}T_{50}$ of 69.7 °C, making it the most stable CYP102 variant identified to date.

9.2 Thermostabilization of eukaryotic P450 forms

Studies that have used traditional methods of engineering such as random or site-directed mutagenesis to enhance the thermostability of eukaryotic P450s initially focused on the mammalian CYP2B forms to date. In the earliest study, 11 residues conserved in CYP2B1 ($T_m=61\,°C$, thermal denaturation), CYP2B4 ($T_m=59\,°C$) and CYP2B11 ($T_m=51\,°C$) were introduced into CYP2B6 ($T_m=48\,°C$) to increase its stability (Kumar et al., 2007). However, only one of these mutations, L264F, located in the I-helix, resulted in a modest increase in thermostability of 4 °C in a thermal denaturation experiment, and only ~ 1.1 °C when residual activity was measured after a 10 min heat treatment. Similarly, seven residues in CYP2B6 and CYP2B11 were mutated to match the amino acid found in the more stable CYP2B1 and CYP2B4. The mutation P334S improved the T_m of CYP2B6 by ~7 °C and CYP2B11 by ~2 °C (Talakad, Wilderman, Davydov, Kumar, & Halpert, 2010).

In addition to rational design, random mutagenesis has also been used to produce a library of >3000 variants of a CYP2B1 peroxygenase mutant, QM. Two QM variants containing L295H and K236I/D257N mutations showed increases in T_{50} of ~1 °C and ~2 °C, respectively (Kumar et al., 2006).

However, combination of all three mutations reduced the T_{50} by ~6 °C compared to QM. Thus far, studies attempting to increase the thermostability of eukaryotic P450s using random or site-directed mutagenesis have identified relatively few beneficial mutations and have generally only achieved increases in stability of less than 10 °C.

Greater success has been achieved in recent studies using ASR. Improvements in ${}^{10}T_{50}$ of up to 20–25 °C have been achieved routinely in reconstructions of vertebrate P450s from families 1–3 in a single experiment (Gumulya et al., 2018, 2019; Harris et al., 2022), which match or exceed the cumulative improvements (Romero et al., 2013) obtained with CYP102 enzymes via the application of multiple sequential approaches (Fig. 2). The thermostable P450s so created show elevated temperature optima and can be used at temperatures increased substantially over ambient. Importantly, they are also robust templates for further mutagenesis that can lead to alterations in substrate specificity and even greater improvements in stability. Libraries of mutants created from such thermostable forms may prove to be a useful resource for identifying biocatalysts for specific biotransformations.

9.3 Engineering solvent tolerance

Another property that often, but not always, correlates with thermostability, is solvent tolerance. The F87A mutant of $P450_{BM3}$ was evolved using a combination of epPCR and saturation mutagenesis for tolerance to dimethylsulfoxide and tetrahydrofuran, generating a mutant with six- and 3.4 fold improved tolerance to dimethylsulfoxide and tetrahydrofuran respectively, as well as greater resilience to acetone, acetonitrile, ethanol and dimethylformamide (Wong, Arnold, & Schwaneberg, 2004). In similar epPCR experiments on CYP2B1, three mutations were found to confer resistance to DMSO (Kumar et al., 2006). In this study, resistance to solvents was accompanied by improved thermal tolerance, as was also found when ASR was applied to CYP3 enzymes (Gumulya et al., 2018). The ancestral CYP3_N1 enzyme showed markedly better tolerance toward methanol and acetonitrile compared to the extant human form, CYP3A4.

10. Novel chemistry

Over the last decade significant progress has been made toward expanding the reaction scope of P450s to enable new types of chemistry not seen in Nature. Of particular interest is the formation and transfer of reactive carbene and nitrene intermediates for which few if any natural precedents are known. While synthetic methods for carbene and nitrene transfer have been developed that use transition-metals (Davies & Manning, 2008), these small molecule methods lack the chemo-, regio- and stereo-selectivity achievable with an enzyme. The similarity between the high-valent iron-oxene intermediate (Compound I) generated in P450 catalysis and the reactive carbene and nitrene intermediates generated by transition-metal catalysts inspired Arnold and colleagues to investigate whether P450s could be engineered to carry out carbene and nitrene transfers (Brandenberg, Fasan, & Arnold, 2017).

Initially, cyclopropanation of styrene via carbene transfer from a diazo reagent, ethyl diazoacetate (EDA), was used as a model system to screen for this non-natural activity (Coelho, Brustad, Kannan, & Arnold, 2013a). It was observed that under anaerobic conditions in the presence of a reductant and EDA, wildtype $P450_{BM3}$ was able to catalyze trace amounts of styrene cyclopropanation with a total turnover number (TTN) of 5. Screening a library of $P450_{BM3}$ variants revealed that the mutation T268A was key for improving cyclopropanation, increasing the TTN to 323. $P450_{BM3}$-T268A showed strong *trans* selectivity, similar to that seen with hemin alone (TTN=73). In contrast, mutant BM3-CIS, which differs from $P450_{BM3}$ wildtype by 13 mutations (including T26A8) was found to preferentially catalyze *cis*-cyclopropanation (TTN=199). This work led to the identification of many wildtype P450s that showed the promiscuous activity of olefin cyclopropanation using EDA, and equivalent T268A mutations were found to enhance this activity in several of these (Gober et al., 2017, 2016). In addition to the formation of C—C bonds, subsequent screening of $P450_{BM3}$ mutant libraries revealed variants that could also efficiently insert carbenoids into amines and thiols to form C—N and C—S bonds (Chen, Zhang, Brandenberg, Hong, & Arnold, 2018; Wang et al., 2014).

The simplicity of the carbene transfer reactions, with the P450 only requiring activation by a reducing agent, raised the possibility of using these $P450_{BM3}$ variants in whole cell biocatalysis if they could be engineered to be activated by an endogenous reducing agent such as NAD(P)H (Coelho et al., 2013). It was hypothesized that raising the reduction potential of the resting-state enzyme would facilitate NAD(P)H-driven reduction and that substituting the axial cysteine thiolate in $P450_{BM3}$ with the weakly donating serine alcohol would achieve this. A C400S mutation introduced into the $P450_{BM3}$-CIS mutant not only enabled reduction by NAD(P)H but improved the TTN for styrene cyclopropanation four-fold

(Coelho et al., 2013). Mutation of the conserved Cys to Ser also enhanced carbene transfer chemistry in CYP119, CYP15386 and $P450_{cam}$ (Heel, McIntosh, Dodani, Meyerowitz, & Arnold, 2014). Ser-ligated variants are referred to as P411s because of the shift seen in the diagnostic Soret peak of the Fe(II).CO form from 450 nm (Cys-ligated) to 411 nm (Ser-ligated).

After the C400S mutation was shown to enhance carbene transfer activity, the effect of the axial coordinating ligand on cyclopropanation activity was explored further (Wang et al., 2014). His, Met, Tyr and Ala residues were introduced at position 400 in $P450_{BM3}$-T268A, and all enhanced cyclopropanation activity. In particular, the C400H mutant resulted in a ~6-fold greater yield of the cyclopropanated product of styrene, ethyl 2-phenylcyclopropane-1-carboxylate than C400S. The usefulness of these carbene transfer catalysts in pharmaceutical biotransformations was demonstrated using a variant of the His mutant ($P450_{BM3}$-Hstar), generated by two further rounds of site-saturation mutagenesis. $P450_{BM3}$-Hstar could efficiently cyclopropanate acrylamide and was used to produce the chiral precursor to the antidepressant, levomilnacipran, at preparative scale (Wang et al., 2014). A recent publication highlighted the use of P411 mutants for the industrial synthesis of isotopically labeled chiral cyclopropanes starting from ^{13}C-glycine (Sardana et al., 2022).

Mutants derived from the Ser-ligated P411s, particularly P411-CIS, have underpinned the rapid growth in carbene and nitrene transfer biocatalysts over the last few years. Using directed evolution approaches, in particular site-saturation mutagenesis, the repertoire of regio- and stereo-selective transformations that can be accessed using biocatalytic methods has expanded to include many novel chemistries as summarized in Table 2.

Aside from mutagenesis of the amino acid sequence, novel chemistry can also be achieved using P450s in which the native haem is replaced with other metalloporphyrins. Porphyrins containing various transition metal centers (e.g., iron, cobalt, rhodium, ruthenium, iridium etc.) have been found to perform useful reactions abiologically (Che, Lo, Zhou, & Huang, 2011; Lu & Zhang, 2011) and incorporating them into the P450 scaffold could theoretically combine the regio- and stereo-specificity of an enzyme with the catalytic capability of a transition metal. Hartwig and colleagues found iridium-methyl porphyrin (Ir(Me)-PIX) could be incorporated into a CYP119 variant bearing the cofactor-accommodating mutation, C317G. This artificial metalloenzyme could perform an abiological carbene transfer, converting a diazoester to a dihydrobenzofuran, at trace levels (Dydio et al., 2016). Following three rounds of directed evolution using site-directed

Table 2 $P450_{BM3}$ variants engineered for novel carbene and nitrene transfer chemistry.[a]

Starting template[b]	Novel mutations	Model reaction	TTN[c]	Reference
$P450_{BM3}$	T268A	*Trans*-selective cyclopropanation of styrene using EDA as a carbene precursor	323	Coelho et al. (2013)
$P450_{BM3}$	**$P450_{BM3}$-CIS**: V78A, P142S, T175I, A184V, S226R, H236Q, E252G, A290V, L353V, I366V, E442K, F87V, T268A	*Cis*-selective cyclopropanation of styrene using EDA as a carbene precursor	199	Coelho et al. (2013)
$P450_{BM3}$-CIS	**$P411_{BM3}$-CIS**: C400S	*Cis*-selective cyclopropanation of styrene using EDA as a carbene precursor	67,800	Coelho et al. (2013)
$P450_{BM3}$-T268A	C400H	Cyclopropanation of styrene using EDA as a carbene precursor	-	Wang et al. (2014)
$P450_{BM3}$-T268A-C400H	**BM3-Hstar**: L437W, V78M, L181V	Cyclopropanation of acrylamide using EDA as a carbene precursor	-	Wang et al. (2014)
$P450_{BM3}$	**H2-5-F10**: V78A, P142S, T175I, A184V, S226R, H236Q, E252G, A290V, L353V, I366V, E442K, F87V, L75A, I263A, T268A, L437A	Insertion of carbenoid into the N—H bond of aniline using EDA as a carbene precursor	473	Wang, Peck, Renata, and Arnold (2014)
$P411_{BM3}$-CIS		Intramolecular C—H amination of 2,4,6-triethylbenzene-1-sulfonyl azide	680	McIntosh et al. (2013)
$P411_{BM3}$-CIS	T438S, I263A	Sulfimidation of 4-methoxythioanysole using tosyl azide as a nitrene precursor	320	Farwell et al. (2014)

P411$_{BM3}$-CIS	**P-I263F**: I263F, T438S	Intramolecular C—H amination of 2,5-di-*n*-propylbenzenesulfonyl azide	361	Farwell et al. (2014)
P-I263F	A328V, L437V	Aziridination of styrenyl olefins using tosyl azide as a nitrene precursor	1000	Farwell, Zhang, McIntosh, Hyster, and Arnold (2015)
P-1263F	**P-5**: V87A, A328V, A268G, A82I	Sulfimidation/[2,3]-rearrangement of allyl sulfides using tosyl azide as a nitrene precursor	2200	Prier et al. (2016)
P-4 (P-I263F + V87A, A328V, A268G)	**P411$_{CHA}$**: I82L, A78V, F263L, E267D	Amination of benzylic C—H bonds using tosyl azide as a nitrene precursor	–	Prier et al. (2017)
P-4 (A82L)	**P411-CHF**: N70E, A74P, A78L, M177L, F263Y, H266V, A330Y, T436L, S438T, truncation of FAD domain	sp^3 C—H bond alkylation using EDA as a carbene precursor	3750	Zhang et al. (2019)
P411$_{Diane1}$ (P-4 (A82L) + A74G, V78L, M177L, I263Y, T327I, T436L, L437Q)	I327P, Y263W, Q437F	1,2-diamine synthesis through intramolecular amination of sulfamoyl azides	72,000	Yang, Cho, Qi, Liu, and Arnold (2019)
P411-CH-C8	**P411-PFA**: T327V, E70T, L177M, R226T, Y330V, L401P	*R*-selective sp^3 C—H bond fluoroalkylation of N- phenylpyrrolidine using 2,2,2-trifluoro-1-diazoethane or 2,2,3,3,3-pentafluoro-1-diazopropane as a carbene precursor	4070	Zhang et al. (2019)

Continued

Table 2 $P450_{BM3}$ variants engineered for novel carbene and nitrene transfer chemistry.[a]—cont'd

Starting template[b]	Novel mutations	Model reaction	TTN[c]	Reference
P411-CH-C8	**P411-PFA-(*S*)**: T327V, V327T, G74P, Q437L	*S*-selective sp^3 C—H bond fluoroalkylation of a aldehyde-substituted N-aryl pyrrolidine substrate using 2,2,2-trifluoro-1-diazoethane or 2,2,3,3,3-pentafluoro-1-diazopropane as a carbene precursor	1820	Zhang et al. (2019)
$P411_{BM3}$-CIS	**P411-VAC$_{cis}$**: L437F, T438Q, L75Y, L181I	*Cis*-selective cyclopropanation of *N*-vinylphthalimide using EDA as a carbene precursor	35,000	Brandenberg et al. (2018)
$P411_{BM3}$-CIS	**P411-VAC$_{trans}$**: I263G, L437F, V87L, L181R	*Trans*-selective cyclopropanation of *N*-vinylphthalimide using EDA as a carbene precursor	1000	Brandenberg et al. (2018)
P411-VAC$_{cis}$	V87C	*Cis*-selective cyclopropanation of aliphatic alkenes using EDA as a carbene precursor	2900	Knight et al. (2018)
P411-VAC$_{cis}$	V87F	*Trans*-selective cyclopropanation of aliphatic alkenes using EDA as a carbene precursor	2200	Knight et al. (2018)
$P450_{BM3}$	**FL#62**: V78A, F81S, A82V, F87A, P142S, T175I, A180T, A184V, A197V, F205C, S226R, H236Q, E252G, R255S, A290V, L353V	Intramolecular C—H amination of 2,4,6-triisopropyl-benzenesulfonyl azide	388	Singh, Bordeaux, and Fasan (2014)
FL#62	H266F, T268V, P392G	Intramolecular C—H amination of 2,4,6-triisopropyl-benzenesulfonyl azide	14,800	Steck, Kolev, Ren, and Fasan (2020)

FL#62	**I-G1**: S81F, A82T, A87F, V184H	Intramolecular amination of menthol	–	Singh, Kolev, Sutera, and Fasan (2015)
FL#62	**V-D11**: A78Y, F81P, A82A, T180A, A328V **I-B3**: A78F, F81R, V82A, A87V	Intramolecular amination of borneol	–	Singh et al. (2015)
$P411_{BM3}$-CIS	**P411-HF**: V87T, H92F, L181G, N210S, L215Q, I263M, V281L, T438C, K472T, N573D, F646S Q674*	1-methylindole alkylation using EDA as a carbene precursor	18,700	Brandenberg, Chen, and Arnold (2019)
P411-HF	T87A, M263E, A268G, T327P, A328Y, L437M	1-methylindole alkylation using an α-disubstituted carbene precursor, i.e., ethyl 2-diazopropanoate (Me-EDA)	775	Brandenberg, Chen, and Arnold (2019)
P411-HF	M263Y	Cyclopropanation of indene using EDA as a carbene precursor	3990	Brandenberg, Chen, and Arnold (2019)
$P411_{BM3}$-CIS	**P411-IA**: I263Y, T438S, A328V, A82W, A268G, W1046P	1-methylindole amidation using tosyl azide as a nitrene precursor	8400	Brandenberg, Miller, Markel, Ouald Chaib, and Arnold (2019)
P411 $_{BM3}$-CIS	**P411-G8S**: L437F, T438Q, L75Y, L181I	Lactone-carbene insertion into an olefin double bond using α-diazo-γ-lactone as a carbene precursor	11,150	Chen et al. (2018)
P411-G8S	S400C	Lactone-carbene insertion into S—H bonds using α-diazo-γ-lactone as a carbene precursor	2190	Chen et al. (2018)
P411-E10 (P-4 (A82L) + A78V, F263L	V78F, S438A	Cyclobutanation of aromatic alkynes using EDA as a carbene precursor	1880	Chen, Huang, Kan, Zhang, and Arnold (2018)

Continued

Table 2 $P450_{BM3}$ variants engineered for novel carbene and nitrene transfer chemistry.[a]—cont'd

Starting template[b]	Novel mutations	Model reaction	TTN[c]	Reference
P-4	**P411-K10**: A87F, F261G, T237P, S72W, T269L, L437F, A78S, A330V, L188C, T436M	*S*-selective cyclopropenation of aliphatic alkynes using EDA as a carbene precursor	2000	Chen, Huang, Kan, Zhang, and Arnold (2018)
P-4	**P411-C6**: A87W, L437G, T327V, V328Y, F261M, T436H	*R*-selective cyclopropenation of aliphatic alkynes using EDA as a carbene precursor	2960	Chen, Huang, Kan, Zhang, and Arnold (2018)
P411-B2 (P-4 (A82L) +F263M)	**$P411_{APA}$**: G268P, V78M, L437F, T327A, E267D, N395R, S438A	Primary amination of sp^3 C—H bonds in benzylic and allylic substrates using hydroxylamine derivatives as nitrene precursors	3930	Jia, Gao, and Arnold (2020)
P411-C10 (P-4 (A82L) + A78Y, F263L, S438A)	**WIRF**: F263W, Q437I, S72F, L436R	Cyclopropenation of 1-phenylbutyne using EDA as a carbene precursor	2680	Chen and Arnold (2020)
WIRF	**WIRF_GAK**: S332G, G74A, E70K	Cyclopropenation of *para*-substituted aromatic alkynes using EDA as a carbene precursor	5760	Chen and Arnold (2020)
P411-C10 (P-4 (A82L) + A78Y, F263L, S438A)	**L6**: T327V, Q437L, S332A, A87P, A264S **L7**: (L6 + V327P) **L8**: (L7 + E267D) **L9**: (L8 + V328L) **L10**: (L8 + V328R)	Lactone-carbene insertion into analine derivatives using α-diazo-γ-lactone as a carbene precursor	2550 2920 2730 4000 1800	Zhou, Chen, and Arnold (2020)

[a]Details regarding notable mutants generated in various engineering studies are given, including the starting template into which mutations were introduced as well as the novel mutations in the best performing variant.
[b]Many starting templates are the best performing mutants from preceding studies.
[c]The highest TTN achieved for the model reaction in each study is listed.

mutagenesis, the mutant Ir(Me)-CYP119-Max was identified that had a catalytic efficiency 4000 times greater than the iridium containing CYP119-C317G. Furthermore, the rates of reactions catalyzed by Ir(Me)-CYP119-Max at concentrations below K_m were 20-fold greater than those catalyzed by free Ir(Me)-PIX. Subsequent site-saturation mutagenesis generated Ir (Me)-CYP119-Max variants that could perform C—H bond amination of sulfonyl azides (Dydio, Key, Hayashi, Clark, & Hartwig, 2017), cyclopropanation of a broad range of alkenes (Key et al., 2017) and alkylation of C(sp^3)—H bonds with high regio- and enantio-selectivity (Gu, Natoli, Liu, Clark, & Hartwig, 2019).

$P450_{BM3}$ has also been the focus of cofactor substitution studies in which variants were engineered that could selectively incorporate Fe-deuteroporphyrin IX (Fe-DPIX) and Ir(Me)-deuteroporphyrin IX (Ir(Me)-DPIX) in place of haem (Reynolds et al., 2016; Reynolds, Schwochert, McHenry, Watters, & Brustad, 2017). The variant that could efficiently incorporate Fe-DPIX contained mutations in the active site but retained the native Cys at residue 400, whereas to achieve >99% incorporation of Ir(Me)-DPIX, C400G or C400A mutations were introduced. These porphyrin-substituted variants, which both carry the T268A mutation, showed styrene cyclopropanation activity that was comparable to $P450_{BM3}$-T268A.

11. Conclusion

Significant advances have been made in the last few years in respect of engineering P450s for applications in biocatalysis. A clear highlight has been the use of P450s to catalyze reactions for which there is no natural precedent, which has revealed unexpected catalytic versatility that if harnessed effectively, could transform medicinal chemistry. However other successes are also chipping away at the barriers to wide-scale implementation of P450s in drug discovery and development pipelines.

The previously limiting problem of stabilizing the P450 fold has proven the most tractable in recent years. Using ASR to stabilize animal xenobiotic-metabolizing P450s has revealed that the ancestral P450 fold is remarkably resistant to denaturation. More robust enzymes also tend to be more easily expressed, reducing the cost of P450 expression, so off-the-shelf catalysts are coming to be a reality, with libraries of P450s now commercially available for screening for activity toward reactions of interest, engineered from both bacterial and xenobiotic-metabolizing forms. If the correlation with solvent stability holds for more P450s, it should be possible to routinely undertake industrial chemistry at elevated temperatures and high substrate loadings, supported either by a similarly thermostable CPR or by an oxygen surrogate. At present however, highly thermostable redox partners that efficiently support multiple P450s have proven impossible to identify, and this remains a significant limitation to using P450s in both isolated enzyme and whole cell bioreactors.

It remains challenging to identify P450s with high efficiency toward particular reactions and substrates. Libraries can be screened easily for enzymes and once candidate biocatalysts are identified, substrate selectivity can be tuned by directed evolution. However iterative mutagenesis and screening can be resource- and personnel-intensive, depending on the ease of screening for the activity or property of interest and the size of the library required. Therefore, the benefit of extensive directed evolution campaigns needs to be evaluated on a case-by-case basis. Structure-guided strategies are increasingly available to target mutagenesis to more productive and viable areas of sequence space. However ideally protein engineers would like to be able to predict, *a priori*, which mutants would be useful to make novel metabolites. Computational design approaches are yet to be exploited with P450s to any great extent, partly because modelling the heme prosthetic group properly is a recurrent limitation. However advanced protein structure prediction algorithms employing machine learning, such as AlphaFold (Jumper et al., 2021), along with sophisticated docking methods and molecular dynamics, should address this objective in coming years.

A related issue is the problem of improving regioselectivity. To improve yields and reduce work-up costs, it is important to produce the single, desired metabolite free of confounding byproducts. However again this typically requires extensive optimization by directed evolution. Active site crowding strategies or decoy molecules (Polic & Auclair, 2014; Shoji & Watanabe, 2011) could be useful here in limiting the number of possible orientations of the substrate in the active site.

Other lingering problems include optimizing the catalytic efficiency via the coupling to reductase and improving the resilience to reactive oxygen species either released during uncoupling or used to support catalysis in the absence of NADPH. Again improvements in predicting structures should augment our ability to rationally redesign both redox partners to optimize the P450-CPR interaction and also the P450 active site to remove labile residues that could be targets of oxidative injury. Novel cofactors or other means of supplying reducing equivalents, such as electrochemically or light-driven systems (Mellor et al., 2016) may reduce costs and improve the sustainability of industrial P450 biocatalysis.

A final area that is ripe for exploration is the use of immobilized P450 systems (Lee et al., 2014; Weber et al., 2010). Promising results have been obtained to date with synthetic biology approaches but employing P450s in flow would enable increased substrate loading (and thereby yield) by continuous flow and recycling past the biocatalyst. Such systems would also simplify work-up of product, reducing costs and allowing recovery and re-use of the biocatalyst, which is usually the most expensive part of the reaction. However again the increasing availability of stable P450s that are cheap to produce promises a step change in achieving cost-effective, selective biotransformations of complex molecules for many different applications in drug discovery and development.

In conclusion, the application of the full complement of engineering strategies from rational design by site-directed mutagenesis, random and saturation mutagenesis, recombinatorial directed evolution, through to phylogenetic approaches means that libraries of P450s are now commercially available that can be used as "off-the-shelf" reagents for pharmaceutical research. As more is revealed about structure-function relationships in P450s and computational methods for structure prediction become more accurate, drug companies and academic researchers alike can look forward to "designer P450s" for particular reactions becoming a reality.

Acknowledgments

Research in the corresponding author's laboratory at The University of Queensland is supported by Australian Research Council Linkage Project Grant LP170100717 and by AstraZeneca Innovative Medicines and Early Development, Cardiovascular, Renal and Metabolism, Gothenburg. SADC was supported by an International Postgraduate Research Award from the University of Queensland and an Industry Scholarship from AstraZeneca. The authors are grateful to Drs. Ulrik Jurva, Magnus Johansson and Shalini Andersson from AstraZeneca, Gothenburg, for helpful discussions about the pharmaceutical industry perspective.

Author contributions

Raine E.S. Thomson: Investigation, Writing—Original draft preparation, Visualization, Writing—Reviewing and Editing. **Stephlina A. D'Cunha**: Investigation, Writing—Original draft preparation. **Martin A. Hayes:** Investigation, Writing—Reviewing and Editing. **Elizabeth M.J. Gillam:** Investigation, Writing—Original draft preparation, Visualization, Writing—Reviewing and Editing.

Conflict of interest statement

The authors research involves the engineering of thermostable xenobiotic-metabolizing P450s as biocatalysts for application in pharmaceutical and fine chemical synthesis, some of which have been licensed production under the tradename "CYPerior."

References

Abécassis, V., Pompon, D., & Truan, G. (2000). High efficiency family shuffling based on multi-step PCR and in vivo DNA recombination in yeast: statistical and functional analysis of a combinatorial library between human cytochrome P450 1A1 and 1A2. *Nucleic Acids Research*, *28*, e88.

Acevedo-Rocha, C. G., Gamble, C. G., Lonsdale, R., Li, A. T., Nett, N., Hoebenreich, S., et al. (2018). P450-catalyzed regio- and diastereoselective steroid hydroxylation: efficient directed evolution enabled by mutability landscaping. *ACS Catalysis*, *8*, 3395–3410.

Agudo, R., Roiban, G. D., & Reetz, M. T. (2012). Achieving regio- and enantioselectivity of P450-catalyzed Oxidative CH activation of small functionalized molecules by structure-guided directed evolution. *Chembiochem*, *13*, 1465–1473.

Ahsan, M., Patil, M., Jeon, H., Sung, S., & Chung, T. (2018). Biosynthesis of nylon 12 monomer, ω-aminododecanoic acid using artificial self-sufficient P450, AlkJ and ω-TA. *Catalysts*, *8*. https://doi.org/10.3390/catal8090400.

Alterman, M. A., Chaurasia, C. S., Lu, P., Hardwick, J. P., & Hanzlik, R. P. (1995). Fatty acid discrimination and omega-hydroxylation by cytochrome P450 4A1 and a cytochrome P4504A1/NADPH-P450 reductase fusion protein. *Archives of Biochemistry and Biophysics*, *320*, 289–296.

Anari, M. R., Josephy, P. D., Henry, T., & O'Brien, P. J. (1997). Hydrogen peroxide supports human and rat cytochrome P450 1A2-catalyzed 2-amino-3-methylimidazo[4,5-f] quinoline bioactivation to mutagenic metabolites: significance of cytochrome P450 peroxygenase. *Chemical Research in Toxicology*, *10*, 582–588.

Anari, M. R., Khan, S., Jatoe, S. D., & O'Brien, P. J. (1997). Cytochrome P450 dependent xenobiotic activation by physiological hydroperoxides in intact hepatocytes. *European Journal of Drug Metabolism and Pharmacokinetics*, *22*, 305–310.

Appel, D., Lutz-Wahl, S., Fischer, P., Schwaneberg, U., & Schmid, R. D. (2001). A P450BM-3 mutant hydroxylates alkanes, cycloalkanes, arenes and heteroarenes. *Journal of Biotechnology*, *88*, 167–171.

Atkins, W. M., & Sligar, S. G. (1989). Molecular recognition in cytochrome P-450: alteration of regioselective alkane hydroxylation via protein engineering. *Journal of the American Chemical Society*, *111*, 2715–2717.

Awan, A. R., Shaw, W. M., & Ellis, T. (2016). Biosynthesis of therapeutic natural products using synthetic biology. *Advanced Drug Delivery Reviews*, *105*, 96–106.

Axarli, I., Prigipaki, A., & Labrou, N. E. (2005). Engineering the substrate specificity of cytochrome P450 CYP102A2 by directed evolution: production of an efficient enzyme for bioconversion of fine chemicals. *Biomolecular Engineering*, *22*, 81–88.

Ba, L. N., Li, P., Zhang, H., Duan, Y., & Lin, Z. L. (2013). Engineering of a hybrid biotransformation system for cytochrome P450sca-2 in Escherichia coli. *Biotechnology Journal*, *8*, 785–793.

Baillie, T. A. (2008). Metabolism and toxicity of drugs. Two decades of progress in industrial drug metabolism. *Chemical Research in Toxicology*, *21*, 129–137.

Bell, S. G., Stevenson, J. A., Boyd, H. D., Campbell, S., Riddle, A. D., Orton, E. L., et al. (2002). Butane and propane oxidation by engineered cytochrome P450cam. *Chemical Communications*, 490–491.

Bell, S. G., Chen, X. H., Sowden, R. J., Xu, F., Williams, J. N., Wong, L. L., et al. (2003). Molecular recognition in (+)-alpha-pinene oxidation by cytochrome P450(cam). *Journal of the American Chemical Society*, *125*, 705–714.

Bell, S. G., Orton, E., Boyd, H., Stevenson, J. A., Riddle, A., Campbell, S., et al. (2003). Engineering cytochrome P450cam into an alkane hydroxylase. *Dalton Transactions*, 2133–2140.

Bell, S. G., Harford-Cross, C. F., & Wong, L. L. (2001). Engineering the CYP101 system for in vivo oxidation of unnatural substrates. *Protein Engineering*, *14*, 797–802.

Bell, S. G., Rouch, D. A., & Wong, L. L. (1997). Selective aliphatic and aromatic carbon-hydrogen bond activation catalysed by mutants of cytochrome P450(cam). *Journal of Molecular Catalysis B: Enzymatic*, *3*, 293–302.

Bell, S. G., Yang, W., Dale, A., Zhou, W. H., & Wong, L. L. (2013). Improving the affinity and activity of CYP101D2 for hydrophobic substrates. *Applied Microbiology and Biotechnology*, *97*, 3979–3990.

Bernhardt, R., & Urlacher, V. B. (2014). Cytochromes P450 as promising catalysts for biotechnological application: chances and limitations. *Applied Microbiology and Biotechnology*, *98*, 6185–6203.

Bhakta, M. N., Hollenberg, P. F., & Wimalasena, K. (2005). P-450/NADPH/O-2- and P-450/PhIO-catalyzed N-dealkylations are mechanistically distinct. *Journal of the American Chemical Society*, *127*, 1376–1377.

Bhandari, S., Poudel, D. K., Marahatha, R., Dawadi, S., Khadayat, K., Phuyal, S., et al. (2021). Microbial enzymes used in bioremediation. *Journal of Chemistry*, *2021*, 17.

Bhattacharya, S. S., & Yadav, J. S. (2018). Microbial P450 enzymes in bioremediation and drug discovery: emerging potentials and challenges. *Current Protein & Peptide Science*, *19*, 75–86.

Bloom, J. D., Labthavikul, S. T., Otey, C. R., & Arnold, F. H. (2006). Protein stability promotes evolvability. *Proceedings of the National Academy of Sciences of the United States of America*, *103*, 5869–5874.

Bommarius, A. S., & Paye, M. F. (2013). Stabilizing biocatalysts. *Chemical Society Reviews*, *42*, 6534–6565.

Brandenberg, O. F., Prier, C. K., Chen, K., Knight, A. M., Wu, Z., & Arnold, F. H. (2018). Stereoselective enzymatic synthesis of heteroatom-substituted cyclopropanes. *ACS Catalysis*, *8*, 2629–2634.

Brandenberg, O. F., Chen, K., & Arnold, F. H. (2019). Directed evolution of a cytochrome P450 carbene transferase for selective functionalization of cyclic compounds. *Journal of the American Chemical Society*, *141*, 8989–8995.

Brandenberg, O. F., Fasan, R., & Arnold, F. H. (2017). Exploiting and engineering hemoproteins for abiological carbene and nitrene transfer reactions. *Current Opinion in Biotechnology*, *47*, 102–111.

Brandenberg, O. F., Miller, D. C., Markel, U., Ouald Chaib, A., & Arnold, F. H. (2019). Engineering chemoselectivity in hemoprotein-catalyzed indole amidation. *ACS Catalysis*, *9*, 8271–8275.

Brian, W. R., Sari, M. A., Iwasaki, M., Shimada, T., Kaminsky, L. S., & Guengerich, F. P. (1990). Catalytic activities of human liver cytochrome P-450 IIIA4 expressed in Saccharomyces cerevisiae. *Biochemistry*, *29*, 11280–11292.

Brixius-Anderko, S., Schiffer, L., Hannemann, F., Janocha, B., & Bernhardt, R. (2015). A CYP21A2 based whole-cell system in Escherichia coli for the biotechnological production of premedrol. *Microbial Cell Factories*, *14*, 135.

Bruhlmann, F., Fourage, L., Ullmann, C., Haefliger, O. P., Jeckelmann, N., Dubois, C., et al. (2014). Engineering cytochrome P450 BM3 of Bacillus megaterium for terminal oxidation of palmitic acid. *Journal of Biotechnology*, *184*, 17–26.

Burek, B. O., Bormann, S., Hollmann, F., Bloh, J. Z., & Holtmann, D. (2019). Hydrogen peroxide driven biocatalysis. *Green Chemistry*, *21*, 3232–3249.

Butler, C. F., Peet, C., Mason, A. E., Voice, M. W., Leys, D., & Munro, A. W. (2013). Key mutations alter the cytochrome P450 BM3 conformational landscape and remove inherent substrate bias. *Journal of Biological Chemistry*, *288*, 25387–25399.

Carmichael, A. B., & Wong, L.-L. (2001). Protein engineering of Bacillus megaterium CYP102: The oxidation of polycyclic aromatic hydrocarbons. *European Journal of Biochemistry*, *268*, 3117–3125.

Catucci, G., Ciaramella, A., Di Nardo, G., Zhang, C., Castrignano, S., & Gilardi, G. (2022). Molecular Lego of human cytochrome P450: the key role of heme domain flexibility for the activity of the chimeric proteins. *International Journal of Molecular Sciences*, *23*, 16.

Cernak, T., Dykstra, K. D., Tyagarajan, S., Vachal, P., & Krska, S. W. (2016). The medicinal chemist's toolbox for late stage functionalization of drug-like molecules. *Chemical Society Reviews*, *45*, 546–576.

Che, C.-M., Lo, V. K.-Y., Zhou, C.-Y., & Huang, J.-S. (2011). Selective functionalisation of saturated C-H bonds with metalloporphyrin catalysts. *Chemical Society Reviews*, *40*, 1950–1975.

Chefson, A., & Auclair, K. (2007). CYP3A4 activity in the presence of organic cosolvents, ionic liquids, or water-immiscible organic solvents. *Chembiochem*, *8*, 1189–1197.

Chefson, A., Zhao, J., & Auclair, K. (2006). Replacement of the natural cofactors by selected hydrogen peroxide donors or organic peroxides results in improved activity for CYP3A4 and CYP2D6. *Chembiochem*, *7*, 916–919.

Chen, K., & Arnold, F. H. (2020). Engineering cytochrome P450s for enantioselective cyclopropenation of internal alkynes. *Journal of the American Chemical Society*, *142*, 6891–6895.

Chen, C.-S., Lin, J. T., Goss, K. A., He, Y.-A., Halpert, J. R., & Waxman, D. J. (2004). Activation of the anticancer prodrugs cyclophosphamide and ifosfamide: Identification of cytochrome P450 2B enzymes and site-specific mutants with improved enzyme kinetics. *Molecular Pharmacology*, *65*, 1278–1285.

Chen, K., Huang, X. Y., Kan, S. B. J., Zhang, R. K., & Arnold, F. H. (2018). Enzymatic construction of highly strained carbocycles. *Science*, *360*, 71-+.

Chen, K., Zhang, S. Q., Brandenberg, O. F., Hong, X., & Arnold, F. H. (2018). Alternate heme ligation steers activity and selectivity in engineered cytochrome P450-catalyzed carbene-transfer reactions. *Journal of the American Chemical Society*, *140*, 16402–16407.

Chun, Y.-J., Shimada, T., & Guengerich, F. P. (1996). Construction of a human cytochrome P450 1A1:rat NADPH-P450 reductase fusion protein - cDNA expression in Escherichia coli, purification, and catalytic properties of the enzyme in bacterial cells and after purification. *Archives of Biochemistry and Biophysics*, *330*, 48–58.

Ciaramella, A., Catucci, G., Gilardi, G., & Di Nardo, G. (2019). Crystal structure of bacterial CYP116B5 heme domain: New insights on class VII P450s structural flexibility and peroxygenase activity. *International Journal of Biological Macromolecules*, *140*, 577–587.

Cirino, P. C., & Arnold, F. H. (2002). Regioselectivity and activity of cytochrome P450 BM-3 and mutant F87A in reactions driven by hydrogen peroxide. *Advanced Synthesis and Catalysis*, *344*, 932–937.

Cirino, P. C., & Arnold, F. H. (2003). A self-sufficient peroxide-driven hydroxylation biocatalyst. *Angewante Chemie International Edition*, *42*, 3299–3301.

Cochrane, R. V. K., & Vederas, J. C. (2014). Highly Selective but Multifunctional Oxygenases in Secondary Metabolism. *Accounts of Chemical Research*, *47*, 3148–3161.

Coelho, P. S., Wang, Z. J., Ener, M. E., Baril, S. A., Kannan, A., Arnold, F. H., et al. (2013). A serine-substituted P450 catalyzes highly efficient carbene transfer to olefins in vivo. *Nature Chemical Biology*, *9*, 485–U433.

Coelho, P. S., Brustad, E. M., Kannan, A., & Arnold, F. H. (2013). Olefin cyclopropanation via carbene transfer catalyzed by engineered cytochrome P450 enzymes. *Science*, *339*, 307–310.

Cragg, G. M., & Newman, D. J. (2013). Natural products: A continuing source of novel drug leads. *Biochimica et Biophysica Acta-General Subjects*, *1830*, 3670–3695.

Cusack, K. P., Koolman, H. F., Lange, U. E. W., Peltier, H. M., Piel, I., & Vasudevan, A. (2013). Emerging technologies for metabolite generation and structural diversification. *Bioorganic & Medicinal Chemistry Letters*, *23*, 5471–5483.

Davies, H. M. L., & Manning, J. R. (2008). Catalytic C-H functionalization by metal carbenoid and nitrenoid insertion. *Nature*, *451*, 417–424.

Deeni, Y. Y., Paine, M. J. I., Ayrton, A. D., Clarke, S. E., Chenery, R., & Wolf, C. R. (2001). Expression, purification, and biochemical characterization of a human cytochrome P450CYP2D6-NADPH cytochrome P450 reductase fusion protein. *Archives of Biochemistry and Biophysics*, *396*, 16–24.

Degregorio, D., D'Avino, S., Castrignano, S., Di Nardo, G., Sadeghi, S. J., Catucci, G., et al. (2017). Human cytochrome P450 3A4 as a biocatalyst: effects of the engineered linker in modulation of coupling efficiency in 3A4-BMR chimeras. *Frontiers in Pharmacology*, *8*, 13.

Di Nardo, G., & Gilardi, G. (2012). Optimization of the Bacterial Cytochrome P450 BM3 System for the Production of Human Drug Metabolites. *International Journal of Molecular Sciences*, *13*, 15901–15924.

Di Nardo, G., & Gilardi, G. (2020). Natural compounds as pharmaceuticals: the key role of cytochromes P450 reactivity. *Trends in Biochemical Sciences*, *45*, 511–525.

Dodhia, V. R., Sassone, C., Fantuzzi, A., Di Nardo, G., Sadeghi, S. J., & Gilardi, G. (2008). Modulating the coupling efficiency of human cytochrome P450 CYP3A4 at electrode surfaces through protein engineering. *Electrochemistry Communications*, *10*, 1744–1747.

Döhr, O., Paine, M. J. I., Friedberg, T., Roberts, G. C. K., & Wolf, C. R. (2001). Engineering of a functional human NADH-dependent cytochrome P450 system. *Proceedings of the National Academy of Sciences of the United States of America*, *98*, 81–86.

Doyle, M. P., & Goldberg, K. I. (2012). C-H Functionalization. *Accounts of Chemical Research*, *45*, 777.

Duetz, W. A., van Beilen, J. B., & Witholt, B. (2001). Using proteins in their natural environment: potential and limitations of microbial whole-cell hydroxylations in applied biocatalysis. *Current Opinion in Biotechnology*, *12*, 419–425.

Durak, L. J., Payne, J. T., & Lewis, J. C. (2016). Late-stage diversification of biologically active molecules via chemoenzymatic C-H functionalization. *ACS Catalysis*, *6*, 1451–1454.

Dydio, P., Key, H. M., Nazarenko, A., Rha, J. Y. E., Seyedkazemi, V., Clark, D. S., et al. (2016). An artificial metalloenzyme with the kinetics of native enzymes. *Science*, *354*, 102–106.

Dydio, P., Key, H. M., Hayashi, H., Clark, D. S., & Hartwig, J. F. (2017). Chemoselective, Enzymatic C-H Bond Amination Catalyzed by a Cytochrome P450 Containing an Ir(Me)-PIX Cofactor. *Journal of the American Chemical Society*, *139*, 1750–1753.

Elmore, C. L., & Porter, T. D. (2002). Modification of the nucleotide cofactor-binding site of cytochrome P-450 reductase to enhance turnover with NADH in vivo. *Journal of Biological Chemistry*, *277*, 48960–48964.

England, P. A., Harford-Cross, C. F., Stevenson, J. A., Rouch, D. A., & Wong, L. L. (1998). The oxidation of naphthalene and pyrene by cytochrome P450cam. *FEBS Letters*, *424*, 271–274.

Fairhead, M., Giannini, S., Gillam, E. M. J., & Gilardi, G. (2005). Functional characterisation of an engineered multidomain human P450 2E1 by molecular Lego. *Journal of Biological Inorganic Chemistry*, *10*, 842–853.

Farinas, E. T., Alcalde, M., & Arnold, F. (2004). Alkene epoxidation catalyzed by cytochrome P450BM-3 139-3. *Tetrahedron*, *60*, 525–528.

Farinas, E. T., Schwaneberg, U., Glieder, A., & Arnold, F. H. (2001). Directed evolution of a cytochrome P450 monooxygenase for alkane oxidation. *Advanced Synthesis & Catalysis*, *343*, 601–606.

Farwell, C. C., McIntosh, J. A., Hyster, T. K., Wang, Z. J., & Arnold, F. H. (2014). Enantioselective imidation of sulfides via enzyme-catalyzed intermolecular nitrogen-atom transfer. *Journal of the American Chemical Society*, *136*, 8766–8771.
Farwell, C. C., Zhang, R. K., McIntosh, J. A., Hyster, T. K., & Arnold, F. H. (2015). Enantioselective enzyme-catalyzed aziridination enabled by active-site evolution of a cytochrome P450. *ACS Central Science*, *1*, 89–93.
Fasan, R., Chen, M. M., Crook, N. C., & Arnold, F. H. (2007). Engineered alkane-hydroxylating cytochrome P450(BM3) exhibiting nativelike catalytic properties. *Angewandte Chemie. International Edition*, *46*, 8414–8418.
Fessner, N. D. (2019). P450 Monooxygenases enable rapid late-stage diversification of natural products via C-H bond activation. *ChemCatChem*, *11*, 2226–2242.
Fisher, C. W., Shet, M. S., Martin-Wixtrom, C., & Estabrook, R. W. (1992). High-level expression in Escherichia coli of enzymatically active fusion proteins containing the domains of cytochromes P450 and NADPH-P450 reductase flavoprotein. *Proceedings of the National Academy of Sciences of the United States of America*, *89*, 10817–10821.
Forneris, C. C., & Seyedsayamdost, M. R. (2018). In Vitro Reconstitution of OxyC Activity Enables Total Chemoenzymatic Syntheses of Vancomycin Aglycone Variants. *Angewandte Chemie. International Edition*, *57*, 8048–8052.
Fowler, S. M., England, P. A., Westlake, A. C. G., Rouch, D. R., Nickerson, D. P., Blunt, C., et al. (1994). Cytochrome P-450cam monooxygenase can be redesigned to catalyse the regioselective aromatic hydroxylation of diphenylmethane. *ChemComm*, 2761–2762.
France, S. P., Hepworth, L. J., Turner, N. J., & Flitsch, S. L. (2017). Constructing biocatalytic cascades: in vitro and in vivo approaches to de novo multi-enzyme pathways. *ACS Catalysis*, 7, 710–724.
Fulco, A. J. (1991). P450BM-3 and other inducible bacterial P450 cytochromes: biochemistry and regulation. *Annual Review of Pharmacology and Toxicology*, *31*, 177–203.
Furukawa, R., Toma, W., Yamazaki, K., & Akanuma, S. (2020). Ancestral sequence reconstruction produces thermally stable enzymes with mesophilic enzyme-like catalytic properties. *Scientific Reports*, *10*, e15493.
Furuya, T., & Kino, K. (2010). Genome mining approach for the discovery of novel cytochrome P450 biocatalysts. *Applied Microbiology and Biotechnology*, *86*, 991–1002.
Ghosh, S. (2017). Triterpene structural diversification by plant cytochrome P450 enzymes. *Frontiers in Plant Science*, *8*, 15.
Gillam, E. M. J., & Hayes, M. A. (2013). The evolution of cytochrome P450 enzymes as biocatalysts in drug discovery and development. *Current Topics in Medicinal Chemistry*, *13*, 2254–2280.
Gillam, E. M. J., & Hunter, D. J. B. (2007). Chemical defence and exploitation: Biotransformation of xenobiotics by cytochrome P450 enzymes. In A. Sigel, H. Sigel, & R. K. O. Sigel (Eds.), *3. Metal Ions in Life Sciences: The Ubiquitous Roles of Cytochrome P450 Proteins* (pp. 477–560). John Wiley & Sons.
Gillam, E. M. J., Baba, T., Kim, B.-R., Ohmori, S., & Guengerich, F. P. (1993). Expression of modified human cytochrome P450 3A4 in *Escherichia coli* and purification and reconstitution of the enzyme. *Archives of Biochemistry and Biophysics*, *305*, 123–131.
Gillam, E. M. J., Copp, J. N., & Ackerley, D. F. (2014). *Directed evolution library creation methods and protocols. Vol. 1179* (2nd ed.). Humana Press Inc.
Girvan, H. M., & Munro, A. W. (2016). Applications of microbial cytochrome P450 enzymes in biotechnology and synthetic biology. *Current Opinion in Chemical Biology*, *31*, 136–145.
Girvan, H. M., Poddar, H., McLean, K. J., Nelson, D. R., Hollywood, K. A., Levy, C. W., et al. (2018). Structural and catalytic properties of the peroxygenase P450 enzyme CYP152K6 from Bacillus methanolicus. *Journal of Inorganic Biochemistry*, *188*, 18–28.

Glieder, A., Farinas, E. T., & Arnold, F. H. (2002). Laboratory evolution of a soluble, self-sufficient, highly active alkane hydroxylase. *Nature Biotechnology, 20*, 1135–1139.

Gober, J. G., Rydeen, A. E., Gibson-O'Grady, E. J., Leuthaeuser, J. B., Fetrow, J. S., & Brustad, E. M. (2016). Mutating a highly conserved residue in diverse cytochrome P450s facilitates diastereoselective olefin cyclopropanation. *Chembiochem, 17*, 394–397.

Gober, J. G., Ghodge, S. V., Bogart, J. W., Wever, W. J., Watkins, R. R., Brustad, E. M., et al. (2017). P450-mediated non-natural cyclopropanation of dehydroalanine-containing thiopeptides. *ACS Chemical Biology, 12*, 1726–1731.

Gu, Y., Natoli, S. N., Liu, Z., Clark, D. S., & Hartwig, J. F. (2019). Site-selective functionalization of (sp3)C – H bonds catalyzed by artificial metalloenzymes containing an iridium-porphyrin cofactor. *Angewandte Chemie International Edition, 58*, 13954–13960.

Guengerich, F. P. (2008). Cytochrome P450 and chemical toxicology. *Chemical Research in Toxicology, 21*, 70–83.

Guengerich, F. P. (2018). Mechanisms of cytochrome P450-catalyzed oxidations. *ACS Catalysis, 8*, 10964–10976.

Guengerich, F. P., Sorrells, J. L., Schmitt, S., Krauser, J. A., Aryal, P., & Meijer, L. (2004). Generation of new protein kinase inhibitors utilizing cytochrome P450 mutant enzymes for indigoid synthesis. *Journal of Medicinal Chemistry, 47*, 3236–3241.

Gumulya, Y., & Gillam, E. M. J. (2017). Exploring the past and the future of protein evolution with ancestral sequence reconstruction: the 'retro' approach to protein engineering. *Biochemical Journal, 474*, 1–19.

Gumulya, Y., Baek, J.-M., Wun, S.-J., Thomson, R. E. S., Harris, K. L., Hunter, D. J. B., et al. (2018). Engineering highly functional thermostable proteins using ancestral sequence reconstruction. *Nature Catalysis, 1*, 878–888.

Gumulya, Y., Huang, W., D'Cunha, S. A., Richards, K. E., Thomson, R. E. S., Hunter, D. J. B., et al. (2019). Engineering thermostable CYP2D enzymes for biocatalysis using combinatorial libraries of ancestors for directed evolution (CLADE). *ChemCatChem, 11*, 841–850.

Gutierrez, A., Doehr, O., Paine, M., Wolf, C. R., Scrutton, N. S., & Roberts, G. C. K. (2000). Trp-676 facilitates nicotinamide coenzyme exchange in the reductive half-reaction of human cytochrome P450 reductase: Properties of the soluble W676R and W676A mutant reductases. *Biochemistry, 39*, 15990–15999.

Harford-Cross, C. F., Carmichael, A. B., Allan, F. K., England, P. A., Rouch, D. A., & Wong, L.-L. (2000). Protein engineering of cytochrome P450cam (CYP101) for the oxidation of polycyclic aromatic hydrocarbons. *Protein Engineering, 13*, 121–128.

Harris, K. L., Thomson, R. E. S., Gumulya, Y., Foley, G., Carrera-Pacheco, S. E., Syed, P., et al. (2022). Ancestral sequence reconstruction of a cytochrome P450 family involved in chemical defence reveals the functional evolution of a promiscuous, xenobiotic-metabolizing enzyme in vertebrates. *Molecular Biology and Evolution*. in press.

Harris, K. L., Thomson, R. E. S., Strohmaier, S. J., Gumulya, Y., & Gillam, E. M. J. (2018). Determinants of thermostability in the cytochrome P450 fold. *Biochimica et Biophysica Acta - Proteins & Proteomics, 1866*, 97–115.

Hartley, C. J., Williams, C. C., Scoble, J. A., Churches, Q. I., North, A., French, N. G., et al. (2019). Engineered enzymes that retain and regenerate their cofactors enable continuous-flow biocatalysis. *Nature Catalysis, 2*, 1006–1015.

Hartwig, J. F. (2016). Evolution of C-H Bond Functionalization from Methane to Methodology. *Journal of the American Chemical Society, 138*, 2–24.

Hartwig, J. F., & Larsen, M. A. (2016). Undirected, homogeneous C-H bond functionalization: challenges and opportunities. *ACS Central Science, 2*, 281–292.

Hedison, T. M., & Scrutton, N. S. (2019). Tripping the light fantastic in membrane redox biology: linking dynamic structures to function in ER electron transfer chains. *FEBS Journal, 286*, 2004–2017.

Heel, T., McIntosh, J. A., Dodani, S. C., Meyerowitz, J. T., & Arnold, F. H. (2014). Non-natural olefin cyclopropanation catalyzed by diverse cytochrome P450s and other hemoproteins. *Chembiochem*, *15*, 2556–2562.

Hiroya, K., Murakami, Y., Shimizu, T., Hatano, M., & Ortiz de Montellano, P. R. (1994). Differential roles of Glu318 and Thr319 in cytochrome P450 1A2 catalysis supported by NADPH-cytochrome P450 reductase and tert-butyl hydroperoxide. *Archives of Biochemistry and Biophysics*, *310*, 397–401.

Hlavica, P. (2009). Assembly of non-natural electron transfer conduits in the cytochrome P450 system: A critical assessment and update of artificial redox constructs amenable to exploitation in biotechnological areas. *Biotechnology Advances*, *27*, 103–121.

Hoffmann, G., Bonsch, K., Greiner-Stoffele, T., & Ballschmiter, M. (2011). Changing the substrate specificity of P450cam towards diphenylmethane by semi-rational enzyme engineering. *Protein Engineering, Design & Selection*, *24*, 439–446.

Huang, W., Johnston, W. A., Hayes, M. A., De Voss, J. J., & Gillam, E. M. J. (2007). A shuffled CYP2C library with a high degree of structural integrity and functional versatility. *Archives of Biochemistry and Biophysics*, *467*, 193–205.

Hunter, D. J. B., Behrendorff, J. B. Y. H., Johnston, W. A., Hayes, P. Y., Huang, W., Bonn, B., et al. (2011). Facile production of minor metabolites for drug development using a CYP3A shuffled library. *Metabolic Engineering*, *13*, 682–693.

Ji, Y., Mertens, A. M., Gertler, C., Fekiri, S., Keser, M., Sauer, D. F., et al. (2018). Directed omnichange evolution converts P450 BM3 into an alkyltrimethylammonium hydroxylase. *Chemistry*, *24*, 16865–16872.

Jia, Z.-J., Gao, S., & Arnold, F. H. (2020). Enzymatic primary amination of benzylic and allylic C(sp3)-H bonds. *Journal of the American Chemical Society*, *142*, 10279–10283.

Jiang, D., Tu, R., Bai, P., & Wang, Q. H. (2013). Directed evolution of cytochrome P450 for sterol epoxidation. *Biotechnology Letters*, *35*, 1663–1668.

Johnston, W. A., Huang, W., De Voss, J. J., Hayes, M. A., & Gillam, E. M. J. (2007). A shuffled CYP1A library shows both structural integrity and functional diversity. *Drug Metabolism and Disposition*, *35*, 2177–2185.

Jones, N. E., England, P. A., Rouch, D. A., & Wong, L. L. (1996). Engineering the selectivity of aliphatic C-H bond oxidation catalysed by cytochrome P450cam. *Chemical Communications*, 2413–2414.

Jones, J. P., O'Hare, E. J., & Wong, L. L. (2001). Oxidation of polychlorinated benzenes by genetically engineered CYP101 (cytochrome P450cam). *European Journal of Biochemistry*, *268*, 1460–1467.

Joo, H., Lin, Z., & Arnold, F. H. (1999). Laboratory evolution of peroxide-mediated cytochrome P450 hydroxylation. *Nature*, *399*, 670–673.

Jumper, J., Evans, R., Pritzel, A., Green, T., Figurnov, M., Ronneberger, O., et al. (2021). Highly accurate protein structure prediction with AlphaFold. *Nature*, *596*, 583–589.

Jung, E., Park, B., Yoo, H.-W., Kim, J., Choi, K.-Y., & Kim, B.-G. (2018). Semi-rational engineering of CYP153A35 to enhance ω-hydroxylation activity toward palmitic acid. *Applied Microbiology and Biotechnology*, *102*, 169–277.

Jung, S. T., Lauchli, R., & Arnold, F. H. (2011). Cytochrome P450: taming a wild type enzyme. *Current Opinion in Biotechnology*, *22*, 809–817.

Kabumoto, H., Miyazaki, K., & Arisawa, A. (2009). Directed evolution of the actinomycete cytochrome P450 MoxA (CYP105) for enhanced activity. *Bioscience, Biotechnology, and Biochemistry*, *73*, 1922–1927.

Kang, J. Y., Ryu, S. H., Park, S. H., Cha, G. S., Kim, D. H., Kim, K. H., et al. (2014). Chimeric cytochromes P450 engineered by domain swapping and random mutagenesis for producing human metabolites of drugs. *Biotechnology and Bioengineering*, *111*, 1313–1322.

Keizers, P. H., Schraven, L. H., de Graaf, C., Hidestrand, M., Ingelman-Sundberg, M., van Dijk, B. R., et al. (2005). Role of the conserved threonine 309 in mechanism of oxidation by cytochrome P450 2D6. *Biochemical and Biophysical Research Communications*, *338*, 1065–1074.

Kenaan, C., Shea, E. V., Lin, H. L., Zhang, H. M., Pratt-Hyatt, M. J., & Hollenberg, P. F. (2013). Interactions between CYP2E1 and CYP2B4: Effects on affinity for NADPH-cytochrome P450 reductase and substrate metabolism. *Drug Metabolism and Disposition*, *41*, 101–110.

Key, H. M., Dydio, P., Liu, Z., Rha, J. Y. E., Nazarenko, A., Seyedkazemi, V., et al. (2017). Beyond iron: Iridium-containing P450 enzymes for selective cyclopropanations of structurally diverse alkenes. *ACS Central Science*, *3*, 302–308.

Khatri, Y., Jóźwik, I. K., Ringle, M., Ionescu, I. A., Litzenburger, M., Hutter, M. C., et al. (2018). Structure-based engineering of steroidogenic CYP260A1 for stereo- and regioselective hydroxylation of progesterone. *ACS Chemical Biology*, *13*, 1021–1028.

Kille, S., Zilly, F. E., Acevedo, J. P., & Reetz, M. T. (2011). Regio- and stereoselectivity of P450-catalysed hydroxylation of steroids controlled by laboratory evolution. *Nature Chemistry*, *3*, 738–743.

Kim, D., & Guengerich, F. P. (2004a). Enhancement of 7-methoxyresorufin O-demethylation activity of human cytochrome P450 1A2 by molecular breeding. *Archives of Biochemistry and Biophysics*, *432*, 102–108.

Kim, D., & Guengerich, F. P. (2004b). Selection of human cytochrome P450 1A2 mutants with enhanced catalytic activity for heterocyclic amine N-hydroxylation. *Biochemistry*, *43*, 981–988.

Kim, K. H., Kang, J. Y., Kim, D. H., Park, S. H., Park, S. H., Kim, D., et al. (2011). Generation of human chiral metabolites of simvastatin and lovastatin by bacterial CYP102A1 mutants. *Drug Metabolism and Disposition*, *39*, 140–150.

Kim, D., Wu, Z. L., & Guengerich, F. P. (2005). Analysis of coumarin 7-hydroxylation activity of cytochrome P450 2A6 using random mutagenesis. *Journal of Biological Chemistry*, *280*, 40319–40327.

Knight, A. M., Kan, S. B. J., Lewis, R. D., Brandenberg, O. F., Chen, K., & Arnold, F. H. (2018). Diverse engineered heme proteins enable stereodivergent cyclopropanation of unactivated alkenes. *ACS Central Science*, *4*, 372–377.

Kolev, J. N., O'Dwyer, K. M., Jordan, C. T., & Fasan, R. (2014). Discovery of potent parthenolide-based antileukemic agents enabled by late-stage P450-mediated C-H functionalization. *ACS Chemical Biology*, *9*, 164–173.

Koo, L. S., Tschirret-Guth, R. A., Straub, W. E., Moënne-Loccoz, P., Loehr, T. M., & Ortiz de Montellano, P. R. (2000). The active site of the thermophilic CYP119 from sulfolobus solfataricus. *Journal of Biological Chemistry*, *275*, 14112–14123.

Kozono, I., Mihara, K., Minagawa, K., Hibi, M., & Ogawa, J. (2017). Engineering of the cytochrome P450 monooxygenase system for benzyl maltol hydroxylation. *Applied Microbiology and Biotechnology*, *101*, 6651–6658.

Kubo, T., Peters, M. W., Meinhold, P., & Arnold, F. H. (2006). Enantioselective epoxidation of terminal alkenes to (R)- and (S)-epoxides by engineered cytochromes P450BM-3. *Chemistry—a European Journal*, *12*, 1216–1220.

Kumar, S. (2010). Engineering cytochrome P450 biocatalysts for biotechnology, medicine and bioremediation. *Expert Opinion on Drug Metabolism & Toxicology*, *6*, 115–131.

Kumar, S., Sun, L., Halpert, J. R., Negi, S. S., Zhao, Y., & Muralidhara, S. (2007). Rational engineering of human cytochrome P450 2B6 for enhanced expression and stability: Importance of a Leu 264 → Phe substitution. *Molecular Pharmacology*, *72*, 1191–1199.

Kumar, S., Chen, C. S., Waxman, D. J., & Halpert, J. R. (2005). Directed evolution of mammalian cytochrome P450 2B1. Mutations outside of the active site enhance the metabolism of several substrates, including the anticancer prodrugs cyclophosphamide and ifosfamide. *Journal of Biological Chemistry*, *280*, 19569–19575.

Kumar, S., Liu, H., & Halpert, J. R. (2006). Engineering of cytochrome P450 3A4 for enhanced peroxide-mediated substrate oxidation using directed evolution and site-directed mutagenesis. *Drug Metabolism and Disposition*, *34*, 1958–1965.

Kumar, S., Scott, E. E., Liu, H., & Halpert, J. R. (2003). A rational approach to re-engineer cytochrome P450 2B1 regioselectivity based on the crystal structure of cytochrome P450 2C5. *Journal of Biological Chemistry*, *278*, 17178–17184.

Kumar, S., Sun, L., Liu, H., Muralidhara, B. K., & Halpert, J. R. (2006). Engineering mammalian cytochrome P450 2B1 by directed evolution for enhanced catalytic tolerance to temperature and dimethyl sulfoxide. *Protein Engineering Design and Selection*, *19*, 547–554.

Landwehr, M., Carbone, M., Otey, C. R., Li, Y., & Arnold, F. H. (2007). Diversification of catalytic function in a synthetic family of chimeric cytochrome P450s. *Chemistry and Biology*, *14*, 237–238.

Lasso, J. D., Castillo-Pazos, D. J., & Li, C. J. (2021). Green chemistry meets medicinal chemistry: a perspective on modern metal-free late-stage functionalization reactions. *Chemical Society Reviews*, *50*, 10955–10982.

Lee, H., Kim, J. H., Han, S., Lim, Y. R., Park, H. G., Chun, Y. J., et al. (2014). Directed-evolution analysis of human cytochrome P450 2A6 for enhanced enzymatic catalysis. *Journal of Toxicology and Environmental Health-Part a-Current Issues*, 77, 1409–1418.

Lee, J. H., Nam, D. H., Lee, S. H., Park, J. H., Park, S. J., Lee, S. H., et al. (2014). New platform for cytochrome P450 reaction combining in situ immobilization on biopolymer. *Bioconjugate Chemistry*, *25*, 2101–2104.

Lewis, J. C., Bastian, S., Bennett, C. S., Fu, Y., Mitsuda, Y., Chen, M. M., et al. (2009). Chemoenzymatic elaboration of monosaccharides using engineered cytochrome P450(BM3) demethylases. *Proceedings of the National Academy of Sciences of the United States of America*, *106*, 16550–16555.

Lewis, J. C., Mantovani, S. M., Fu, Y., Snow, C. D., Komor, R. S., Wong, C. H., et al. (2010). Combinatorial alanine substitution enables rapid optimization of cytochrome P450(BM3) for selective hydroxylation of large substrates. *Chembiochem*, *11*, 2502–2505.

Li, Y. G., Drummond, D. A., Sawayama, A. M., Snow, C. D., Bloom, J. D., & Arnold, F. H. (2007). A diverse family of thermostable cytochrome P450s created by recombination of stabilizing fragments. *Nature Biotechnology*, *25*, 1051–1056.

Li, A., Ilie, A., Sun, Z., Lonsdale, R., Xu, J.-H., & Reetz, M. T. (2016). Whole-cell-catalyzed multiple regio- and stereoselective functionalizations in cascade reactions enabled by directed evolution. *Angewandte Chemie International Edition*, *55*, 12026–12029.

Li, Z., Jiang, Y. Y., Guengerich, F. P., Ma, L., Li, S. Y., & Zhang, W. (2020). Engineering cytochrome P450 enzyme systems for biomedical and biotechnological applications. *Journal of Biological Chemistry*, *295*, 833–849.

Li, A., Liu, J., Pham, S. Q., & Li, Z. (2013). Engineered P450pyr monooxygenase for asymmetric epoxidation of alkenes with unique and high enantioselectivity. *ChemComm*, *49*, 11572–11575.

Li, Q. S., Ogawa, J., Schmid, R. D., & Shimizu, S. (2001). Engineering cytochrome P450 BM-3 for oxidation of polycyclic aromatic hydrocarbons. *Applied and Environmental Microbiology*, *67*, 5735–5739.

Li, Q. S., Ogawa, J., Schmid, R. D., & Shimizu, S. (2005). Indole hydroxylation by bacterial cytochrome P450 BM-3 and modulation of activity by cumene hydroperoxide. *Bioscience Biotechnology and Biochemistry*, *69*, 293–300.

Li, Q. S., Schwaneberg, U., Fischer, P., & Schmid, R. D. (2000). Directed evolution of the fatty-acid hydyoxylase P450BM-3 into an indole-hydroxylating catalyst. *Chemistry - A European Journal*, *6*, 1531–1536.

Li, F. Z., Zhang, X., & Renata, H. (2019). Enzymatic C-H functionalizations for natural product synthesis. *Current Opinion in Chemical Biology*, *49*, 25–32.

Lo, H. C., Ryan, J. D., Kerr, J. B., Clark, D. S., & Fish, R. H. (2017). Bioorganometallic chemistry: Co-factor regeneration, enzyme recognition of biomimetic 1,4-NADH analogs, and organic synthesis; tandem catalyzed regioselective formation of N-substituted-1,4-dihydronicotinamide derivatives with Cp*Rh(bpy)H (+), coupled to chiral S-alcohol formation with HLADH, and engineered cytochrome P450s, for selective C-H oxidation reactions. *Journal of Organometallic Chemistry*, *839*, 38–52.

Lu, H., & Zhang, X. P. (2011). Catalytic C-H functionalization by metalloporphyrins: Recent developments and future directions. *Chemical Society Reviews*, *40*, 1899–1909.

Lussenburg, B. M. A., Babel, L. C., Vermeulen, N. P. E., & Commandeur, J. N. M. (2005). Evaluation of alkoxyresorufins as fluorescent substrates for cytochrome P450BM3 and site-directed mutants. *Analytical Biochemistry*, *341*, 148–155.

Manna, S. K., & Mazumdar, S. (2010). Tuning the substrate specificity by engineering the active site of cytochrome P450cam: A rational approach. *Dalton Transactions*, *39*, 3115–3123.

Martinez, C. A., & Rupashinghe, S. G. (2013). Cytochrome P450 bioreactors in the pharmaceutical industry: Challenges and opportunities. *Current Topics in Medicinal Chemistry*, *13*, 1470–1490.

McIntosh, J. A., Coelho, P. S., Farwell, C. C., Wang, Z. J., Lewis, J. C., Brown, T. R., et al. (2013). Enantioselective intramolecular C-H amination catalyzed by engineered cytochrome P450 enzymes in vitro and in vivo. *Angewandte Chemie. International Edition*, *52*, 9309–9312.

McLean, K. J., Hans, M., Meijrink, B., van Scheppingen, W. B., Vollebregt, A., Tee, K. L., et al. (2015). Single-step fermentative production of the cholesterol-lowering drug pravastatin via reprogramming of Penicillium chrysogenum. *Proceedings of the National Academy of Sciences of the United States of America*, *112*, 2847–2852.

Meinhold, P., Peters, M. W., Chen, M. M. Y., Takahashi, K., & Arnold, F. H. (2005). Direct conversion of ethane to ethanol by engineered cytochrome P450BM3. *Chembiochem*, *6*, 1765–1768.

Meinhold, P., Peters, M. W., Hartwick, A., Hernandez, A. R., & Arnold, F. H. (2006). Engineering cytochrome P450BM3 for terminal alkane hydroxylation. *Advanced Synthesis & Catalysis*, *348*, 763–772.

Mellor, S. B., Nielsen, A. Z., Burow, M., Motawia, M. S., Jakubauskas, D., Moller, B. L., et al. (2016). Fusion of ferredoxin and cytochrome P450 enables direct light-driven biosynthesis. *ACS Chemical Biology*, *11*, 1862–1869.

Menard, A., Huang, Y., Karam, P., Cosa, G., & Auclair, K. (2012). Site-specific fluorescent labeling and oriented immobilization of a triple mutant of CYP3A4 via C64. *Bioconjugate Chemistry*, *23*, 826–836.

Milhim, M., Gerber, A., Neunzig, J., Hannemann, F., & Bernhardt, R. (2016). A novel NADPH-dependent flavoprotein reductase from Bacillus megaterium acts as an efficient cytochrome P450 reductase. *Journal of Biotechnology*, *231*, 83–94.

Moir, M., Danon, J. J., Reekie, T. A., & Kassiou, M. (2019). An overview of late-stage functionalization in today's drug discovery. *Expert Opinion on Drug Discovery*, *14*, 1137–1149.

Morlock, L. K., Grobe, S., Balke, K., Mauersberger, S., Bottcher, D., & Bornscheuer, U. T. (2018). Protein engineering of the progesterone hydroxylating P450-monooxygenase CYP17A1 alters its regioselectivity. *Chembiochem*, *19*, 1954–1958.

Mousavi, S. M., Hashemi, S. A., Moezzi, S. M. I., Ravan, N., Gholami, A., Lai, C. W., et al. (2021). Recent advances in enzymes for the bioremediation of pollutants. *Biochemistry Research International*, *2021*, 12.

Mukherjee, G., Nandekar, P. P., & Wade, R. C. (2021). An electron transfer competent structural ensemble of membrane-bound cytochrome P450 1A1 and cytochrome P450 oxidoreductase. *Communications Biology*, *4*, 13.

Murakami, H., Yabusaki, Y., Sakaki, T., Shibata, M., & Ohkawa, H. (1987). A genetically engineered P450 monooxygenase: construction of the functional fused enzyme between rat cytochrome P450c and NADPH-cytochrome P450 reductase. *DNA*, *6*, 189–197.

Nakamura, K., Martin, M. V., & Guengerich, F. P. (2001). Random mutagenesis of human cytochrome P450 2A6 and screening with indole oxidation products. *Archives of Biochemistry and Biophysics*, *395*, 25–31.

Neunzig, I., Widjaja, M., Dragan, C.-A., Peters, F., Maurer, H., & Bureik, M. (2012). Engineering of human CYP3A enzymes by combination of activating polymorphic variants. *Applied Biochemistry and Biotechnology*, *168*, 785–796.

Neunzig, I., Widjaja, M., Peters, F. T., Maurer, H. H., Hehn, A., Bourgaud, F., et al. (2013). Coexpression of CPR from various origins enhances biotransformation activity of human CYPs in S. pombe. *Applied Biochemistry and Biotechnology*, *170*, 1751–1766.

Nguyen, T. H. H., Yeom, S. J., & Yun, C. H. (2021). Production of a human metabolite of atorvastatin by bacterial CYP102A1 peroxygenase. *Applied Sciences - Basel*, *11*, 13.

Nickerson, D. P., Harford-Cross, C. F., Fulcher, S. R., & Wong, L.-L. (1997). The catalytic activity of cytochrome P450cam towards styrene oxidation is increased by site-specific mutagenesis. *FEBS Letters*, *405*, 153–156.

Niraula, N. P., Kanth, B. K., Sohng, J. K., & Oh, T. J. (2011). Hydrogen peroxide-mediated dealkylation of 7-ethoxycoumarin by cytochrome P450 (CYP107AJ1) from Streptomyces peucetius ATCC27952. *Enzyme and Microbial Technology*, *48*, 181–186.

O'Hanlon, J. A., Ren, X., Morris, M., Wong, L. L., & Robertson, J. (2017). Hydroxylation of anilides by engineered cytochrome P450BM3. *Organic and Biomolecular Chemistry*, *15*, 8780–8787.

Obach, R. S., Walker, G. S., Sharma, R., Jenkinson, S., Tran, T. P., & Stepan, A. F. (2018). Lead diversification at the nanomole scale using liver microsomes and quantitative nuclear magnetic resonance spectroscopy: application to phosphodiesterase 2 inhibitors. *Journal of Medicinal Chemistry*, *61*, 3626–3640.

Obach, R. S., Walker, G. S., & Brodney, M. A. (2016). Biosynthesis of fluorinated analogs of drugs using human cytochrome P450 enzymes followed by deoxyfluorination and quantitative nuclear magnetic resonance spectroscopy to improve metabolic stability. *Drug Metabolism and Disposition*, *44*, 634–646.

Ost, T. W. B., Miles, C. S., Murdoch, J., Cheung, Y.-F., Reid, G. A., Chapman, S. K., et al. (2000). Rational re-design of the substrate binding site of flavocytochrome P450 BM3. *FEBS Letters*, *486*, 173–177.

Otey, C. R., Silberg, J. J., Voigt, C. A., Endelman, J. B., Bandara, G., & Arnold, F. H. (2004). Functional evolution and structural conservation in chimeric cytochromes P450: Calibrating a structure-guided approach. *Chemistry and Biology*, *11*, 309–318.

Otey, C. R., Landwehr, M., Endelman, J. B., Hiraga, K., Bloom, J. D., & Arnold, F. H. (2006). Structure-guided recombination creates an artificial family of cytochromes P450. *PLoS Biology*, *4*, e112.

Otey, C. R., Bandara, G., Lalonde, J., Takahashi, K., & Arnold, F. H. (2006). Preparation of human metabolites of propranolol using laboratory-evolved bacterial cytochromes P450. *Biotechnology and Bioengineering*, *93*, 494–499.

Paddon, C. J., Westfall, P. J., Pitera, D. J., Benjamin, K., Fisher, K., McPhee, D., et al. (2013). High-level semi-synthetic production of the potent antimalarial artemisinin. *Nature*, *496*, 528–532.

Parikh, A., & Guengerich, F. P. (1997). Expression, purification, and characterization of a catalytically active human cytochrome P450 1A2-rat NADPH-cytochrome P450 reductase fusion protein. *Protein Expression and Purification*, *9*, 346–354.

Parikh, A., Josephy, P. D., & Guengerich, F. P. (1999). Selection and characterization of human cytochrome P450 1A2 mutants with altered catalytic properties. *Biochemistry, 38*, 5283–5289.

Park, H., Park, G., Jeon, W., Ahn, J. O., Yang, Y. H., & Choi, K. Y. (2020). Whole-cell biocatalysis using cytochrome P450 monooxygenases for biotransformation of sustainable bioresources (fatty acids, fatty alkanes, and aromatic amino acids). *Biotechnology Advances, 40*, 22.

Paulsen, M. D., Filipovic, D., Sligar, S. G., & Ornstein, R. L. (1993). Controlling the regiospecificity and coupling of cytochrome P450cam: T185F mutant increases coupling and abolishes 3-hydroxynorcamphor product. *Protein Science, 2*, 357–365.

Peters, M. W., Meinhold, P., Glieder, A., & Arnold, F. H. (2003). Regio- and enantioselective alkane hydroxylation with engineered cytochromes P450 BM-3. *Journal of the American Chemical Society, 125*, 13442–13450.

Peterson, J. A., Sevrioukova, I., Truan, G., & Graham-Lorence, S. E. (1997). P450BM-3: A tale of two domains—Or is it three? *Steroids, 62*, 117–123.

Pham, S. Q., Pompidor, G., Liu, J., Li, X.-D., & Li, Z. (2012). Evolving P450pyr hydroxylase for highly enantioselective hydroxylation at non-activated carbon atom. *ChemComm, 48*, 4618–4620.

Polic, V., & Auclair, K. (2014). Controlling substrate specificity and product regio- and stereo-selectivities of P450 enzymes without mutagenesis. *Bioorganic & Medicinal Chemistry, 22*, 5547–5554.

Prier, C. K., Hyster, T. K., Farwell, C. C., Huang, A., & Arnold, F. H. (2016). Asymmetric enzymatic synthesis of allylic amines: A sigmatropic rearrangement strategy. *Angewandte Chemie. International Edition, 55*, 4711–4715.

Prier, C. K., Zhang, R. J. K., Buller, A. R., Brinkmann-Chen, S., & Arnold, F. H. (2017). Enantioselective, intermolecular benzylic C-H amination catalysed by an engineered iron-haem enzyme. *Nature Chemistry, 9*, 629–634.

Rasool, S., & Mohamed, R. (2016). Plant cytochrome P450s: nomenclature and involvement in natural product biosynthesis. *Protoplasma, 253*, 1197–1209.

Rea, V., Kolkman, A. J., Vottero, E., Stronks, E. J., Ampt, K. A. M., Honing, M., et al. (2012). Active site substitution A82W improves the regioselectivity of steroid hydroxylation by cytochrome P450 BM3 mutants as rationalized by spin relaxation nuclear magnetic resonance studies. *Biochemistry, 51*, 750–760.

Reed, J. R., Cawley, G. F., & Backes, W. L. (2013). Interactions between cytochromes P450 2B4 (CYP2B4) and 1A2 (CYP1A2) lead to alterations in toluene disposition and P450 uncoupling. *Biochemistry, 52*, 4003–4013.

Reinen, J., van Leeuwen, J. S., Li, Y. M., Sun, L. F., Grootenhuis, P. D. J., Decker, C. J., et al. (2011). Efficient screening of cytochrome P450 BM3 mutants for their metabolic activity and diversity toward a wide set of drug-like molecules in chemical space. *Drug Metabolism and Disposition, 39*, 1568–1576.

Rendic, S. P., & Guengerich, F. P. (2021). Human Family 1-4 cytochrome P450 enzymes involved in the metabolic activation of xenobiotic and physiological chemicals: an update. *Archives of Toxicology, 95*, 395–472.

Rentmeister, A., Arnold, F. H., & Fasan, R. (2009). Chemo-enzymatic fluorination of unactivated organic compounds. *Nature Chemical Biology, 5*, 26–28.

Rentmeister, A., Brown, T. R., Snow, C. D., Carbone, M. N., & Arnold, F. H. (2011). Engineered bacterial mimics of human drug metabolizing enzyme CYP2C9. *ChemCatChem, 3*, 1065–1071.

Reynolds, E. W., McHenry, M. W., Cannac, F., Gober, J. G., Snow, C. D., & Brustad, E. M. (2016). An evolved orthogonal enzyme/cofactor pair. *Journal of the American Chemical Society, 138*, 12451–12458.

Reynolds, E. W., Schwochert, T. D., McHenry, M. W., Watters, J. W., & Brustad, E. M. (2017). Orthogonal expression of an artificial metalloenzyme for abiotic catalysis. *Chembiochem, 18*, 2380–2384.

Rinnofner, C., Kerschbaumer, B., Weber, H., Glieder, A., & Winkler, M. (2019). Cytochrome P450 mediated hydroxylation of ibuprofen using Pichia pastoris as biocatalyst. *Biocatalysis and Agricultural Biotechnology*, *17*, 525–528.

Ro, D. K., Paradise, E. M., Ouellet, M., Fisher, K. J., Newman, K. L., Ndungu, J. M., et al. (2006). Production of the antimalarial drug precursor artemisinic acid in engineered yeast. *Nature*, *440*, 940–943.

Rodrigues, A. D., Mulford, O. J., Lee, R. D., Surber, B. W., Kukulka, M. J., Ferrero, J. L., et al. (1995). In vitro metabolism of terfenadine by a purified recombinant fusion protein containing cytochrome P450 3A4 and NADPH-P450 reductase – comparison to human liver microsomes and precision-cut liver-tissue slices. *Drug Metabolism and Disposition*, *23*, 765–775.

Roduner, E., Kaim, W., Sarkar, B., Urlacher, V. B., Pleiss, J., Glaser, R., et al. (2013). Selective catalytic oxidation of C-H bonds with molecular oxygen. *ChemCatChem*, *5*, 82–112.

Romero, P. A., Krause, A., & Arnold, F. H. (2013). Navigating the protein fitness landscape with Gaussian processes. *Proceedings of the National Academy of Sciences of the United States of America*, *110*, E193–E201.

Rosic, N. N., Huang, W., Johnston, W. A., DeVoss, J. J., & Gillam, E. M. J. (2007). Extending the diversity of cytochrome P450 enzymes by DNA family shuffling. *Gene*, *395*, 40–48.

Rua, F., Sadeghi, S. J., Castrignano, S., Di Nardo, G., & Gilardi, G. (2012). Engineering Macaca fascicularis cytochrome P450 2C20 to reduce animal testing for new drugs. *Journal of Inorganic Biochemistry*, *117*, 277–284.

Rudolf, J. D., Chang, C. Y., Ma, M., & Shen, B. (2017). Cytochromes P450 for natural product biosynthesis in Streptomyces: sequence, structure, and function. *Natural Product Reports*, *34*, 1141–1172.

Rühlmann, A., Antovic, D., Müller, T. J. J., & Urlacher, V. B. (2017). Regioselective hydroxylation of stilbenes by engineered cytochrome P450 from *Thermobifida fusca* YX. *Advanced Synthesis and Catalysis*, *359*, 984–994.

Rushmore, T. H., Reider, P. J., Slaughter, D., Assang, C., & Shou, M. (2000). Bioreactor systems in drug metabolism: Synthesis of cytochrome P450-generated metabolites. *Metabolic Engineering*, *2*, 115–125.

Rylott, E. L., Jackson, R. G., Sabbadin, F., Seth-Smith, H. M. B., Edwards, J., Chong, C. S., et al. (2011). The explosive-degrading cytochrome P450 XplA: Biochemistry, structural features and prospects for bioremediation. *Biochimica et Biophysica Acta, Proteins and Proteomics*, *1814*, 230–236.

Sadeghi, S. J., & Gilardi, G. (2013). Chimeric P450 enzymes: activity of artificial redox fusions driven by different reductases for biotechnological applications. *Biotechnology and Applied Biochemistry*, *60*, 102–110.

Sagadin, T., Riehm, J., Putkaradze, N., Hutter, M. C., & Bernhardt, R. (2019). Novel approach to improve progesterone hydroxylation selectivity by CYP106A2 via rational design of adrenodoxin binding. *FEBS Journal*, *286*, 1240–1249.

Salazar, O., Cirino, P. C., & Arnold, F. H. (2003). Thermostabilization of a cytochrome P450 peroxygenase. *Chembiochem*, *4*, 891–893.

Sardana, M., Mühlfenzl, K. S., Wenker, S. T. M., Åkesson, C., Hayes, M. A., Elmore, C. S., & Pithani, S. (2022). Exploring the enzyme-catalyzed synthesis of isotope labeled cyclopropanes. *Journal of Labelled Compounds and Radiopharmaceuticals*, *65*, 86–100.

Sawayama, A. M., Chen, M. M. Y., Kulanthaivel, P., Kuo, M. S., Hemmerle, H., & Arnold, F. H. (2009). A panel of cytochrome P450 BM3 variants to produce drug metabolites and diversify lead compounds. *Chemistry—a European Journal*, *15*, 11723–11729.

Schachinger, F., Chang, H. C., Scheiblbrandner, S., & Ludwig, R. (2021). Amperometric Biosensors Based on Direct Electron Transfer Enzymes. *Molecules*, *26*, 32.

Schadt, S., Bister, B., Chowdhury, S. K., Funk, C., Hop, C., Humphreys, W. G., et al. (2018). A Decade in the MIST: learnings from investigations of drug metabolites in drug development under the "Metabolites in Safety Testing" regulatory guidance. *Drug Metabolism and Disposition*, *46*, 865–878.

Schiavini, P., Cheong, K. J., Moitessier, N., & Auclair, K. (2017). Active site crowding of cytochrome P450 3A4 as a strategy to alter its selectivity. *Chembiochem*, *18*, 248–252.

Schiffer, L., Anderko, S., Hobler, A., Hannemann, F., Kagawa, N., & Bernhardt, R. (2015). A recombinant CYP11B1 dependent Escherichia coli biocatalyst for selective cortisol production and optimization towards a preparative scale. *Microbial Cell Factories*, *14*, 25.

Schneider, E., & Clark, D. S. (2013). Cytochrome P450 (CYP) enzymes and the development of CYP biosensors. *Biosensors and Bioelectronics*, *39*, 1–13.

Schroer, K., Kittelmann, M., & Lutz, S. (2010). Recombinant human cytochrome P450 monooxygenases for drug metabolite synthesis. *Biotechnology and Bioengineering*, *106*, 699–706.

Schulz, S., Girhard, M., & Urlacher, V. B. (2012). Biocatalysis: key to selective oxidations. *ChemCatChem*, *4*, 1889–1895.

Sem, D. S., & Kasper, C. B. (1993). Interaction with arginine 597 of NADPH-cytochrome P-450 oxidoreductase is a primary source of the uniform binding energy used to discriminate between NADPH and NADH. *Biochemistry*, *32*, 11548–11558.

Shanu-Wilson, J., Evans, L., Wrigley, S., Steele, J., Atherton, J., & Boer, J. (2020). Biotransformation: impact and application of metabolism in drug discovery. *ACS Medicinal Chemistry Letters*, *11*, 2087–2107.

Shapiro, M. G., Westmeyer, G. G., Romero, P. A., Szablowski, J. O., Kuster, B., Shah, A., et al. (2010). Directed evolution of a magnetic resonance imaging contrast agent for noninvasive imaging of dopamine. *Nature Biotechnology*, *28*, 264–U120.

Sharma, S., & Kanwar, S. S. (2014). *Organic solvent tolerant lipases and applications* (p. 15). Scientific World Journal.

Shoji, O., & Watanabe, Y. (2011). Design of H2O2-dependent oxidation catalyzed by hemoproteins. *Metallomics*, *3*, 379–388.

Shugrue, C. R., & Miller, S. J. (2017). Applications of nonenzymatic catalysts to the alteration of natural products. *Chemical Reviews*, *117*, 11894–11951.

Singh, R., Bordeaux, M., & Fasan, R. (2014). P450-catalyzed intramolecular sp3 C–H amination with arylsulfonyl azide substrates. *ACS Catalysis*, *4*, 546–552.

Singh, R., Kolev, J. N., Sutera, P. A., & Fasan, R. (2015). Enzymatic C(sp3)-H amination: P450-catalyzed conversion of carbonazidates into oxazolidinones. *ACS Catalysis*, *5*, 1685–1691.

Smith, D. A., & Obach, R. S. (2009). Metabolites in Safety Testing (MIST): considerations of mechanisms of toxicity with dose, abundance, and duration of treatment. *Chemical Research in Toxicology*, *22*, 267–279.

Smith, G., Modi, S., Pillai, I., Lian, L. Y., Sutcliffe, M. J., Pritchard, M. P., et al. (1998). Determinants of the substrate specificity of human cytochrome P-450 CYP2D6: design and construction of a mutant with testosterone hydroxylase activity. *Biochemical Journal*, *331*, 783–792.

Speight, R. E., Hancock, F. E., Winkel, C., Bevinakatti, H. S., Sarkar, M., Flitsch, S. L., et al. (2004). Rapid identification of cytochrome P450(cam) variants by in vivo screening of active site libraries. *Tetrahedron-Asymmetry*, *15*, 2829–2831.

Spence, M. A., Kaczmarski, J. A., Saunders, J. W., & Jackson, C. J. (2021). Ancestral sequence reconstruction for protein engineers. *Current Opinion in Structural Biology*, *69*, 131–141.

Steck, V., Kolev, J. N., Ren, X., & Fasan, R. (2020). Mechanism-guided design and discovery of efficient cytochrome P450-derived C-H amination biocatalysts. *Journal of the American Chemical Society*, *142*, 10343–10357.
Stevenson, J. A., Westlake, A. C. G., Whittock, C., & Wong, L. L. (1996). The catalytic oxidation of linear and branched alkanes by cytochrome P450(cam). *Journal of the American Chemical Society*, *118*, 12846–12847.
Strohmaier, S. J., De Voss, J. J., Jurva, U., Andersson, S., & Gillam, E. M. J. (2020). Oxygen surrogate systems for supporting human drug-metabolizing cytochrome P450 enzymes. *Drug Metabolism and Disposition*, *48*, 432–437.
Strohmaier, S. J., Huang, W., Baek, J.-M., Hunter, D. J. B., & Gillam, E. M. J. (2019). Rational evolution of the cofactor-binding site of cytochrome P450 reductase yields variants with increased activity towards specific cytochrome P450 enzymes. *FEBS Journal*, *286*, 4473–4493.
Subedi, P., Kim, K. H., Hong, Y. S., Lee, J. H., & Oh, T. J. (2021). Enzymatic characterization and comparison of two steroid hydroxylases CYP154C3-1 and CYP154C3-2 from Streptomyces species. *Journal of Microbiology and Biotechnology*, *31*, 464–474.
Sugishima, M., Sato, H., Higashimoto, Y., Harada, J., Wada, K., Fukuyama, K., et al. (2014). Structural basis for the electron transfer from an open form of NADPH-cytochrome P450 oxidoreductase to heme oxygenase. *Proceedings of the National Academy of Sciences of the United States of America*, *111*, 2524–2529.
Sun, L., Chen, C. S., Waxman, D. J., Liu, H., Halpert, J. R., & Kumar, S. (2007). Re-engineering cytochrome P450 2B11dH for enhanced metabolism of several substrates including the anti-cancer prodrugs cyclophosphamide and ifosfamide. *Archives of Biochemistry and Biophysics*, *458*, 167–174.
Talakad, J. C., Wilderman, P. R., Davydov, D. R., Kumar, S., & Halpert, J. R. (2010). Rational engineering of cytochromes P450 2B6 and 2B11 for enhanced stability: Insights into structural importance of residue 334. *Archives of Biochemistry and Biophysics*, *494*, 151–158.
Thistlethwaite, S., Jeffreys, L. N., Girvan, H. M., McLean, K. J., & Munro, A. W. (2021). A promiscuous bacterial P450: the unparalleled diversity of BM3 in pharmaceutical metabolism. *International Journal of Molecular Sciences*, *22*, 11380.
Vail, R. B., Homann, M. J., Hanna, I., & Zaks, A. (2005). Preparative synthesis of drug metabolites using human cytochrome P450s 3A4, 2C9 and 1A2 with NADPH-P450 reductase expressed in Escherichia coli. *Journal of Industrial Microbiology & Biotechnology*, *32*, 67–74.
van Vugt-Lussenburg, B. M. A., Stjernschantz, E., Lastdrager, J., Oostenbrink, C., Vermeulen, N. P. E., & Commandeur, J. N. M. (2007). Identification of critical residues in novel drug metabolizing mutants of cytochrome P450 BM3 using random mutagenesis. *Journal of Medicinal Chemistry*, *50*, 455–461.
van Vugt-Lussenburg, B. M. A., Damsten, M. C., Maasdijk, D. M., Vermeulen, N. P. E., & Commandeur, J. N. M. (2006). Heterotropic and homotropic cooperativity by a drug-metabolising mutant of cytochrome P450BM3. *Biochemical and Biophysical Research Communications*, *346*, 810–818.
Vaz, A. D. N., McGinnity, D. F., & Coon, M. J. (1998). Epoxidation of olefins by cytochrome P450: Evidence from site-specific mutagenesis for hydroperoxo-iron as an electrophilic oxidant. *Proceedings of the National Academy of Sciences of the United States of America*, *95*, 3555–3560.
Vaz, A. D. N., Pernecky, S. J., Raner, G. M., & Coon, M. J. (1996). Peroxo-iron and oxenoid-iron species as alternative oxygenating agents in cytochrome P450-catalyzed reactions: Switching by threonine-302 to alanine mutagenesis of cytochrome P450 2B4. *Proceedings of the National Academy of Sciences of the United States of America*, *93*, 4644–4648.

Venkataraman, H., Verkade-Vreeker, M. C. A., Capoferri, L., Geerke, D. P., Vermeulen, N. P. E., & Commandeur, J. N. M. (2014). Application of engineered cytochrome P450 mutants as biocatalysts for the synthesis of benzylic and aromatic metabolites of fenamic acid NSAIDs. *Bioorganic & Medicinal Chemistry*, *22*, 5613–5620.

Voigt, C. A., Martinez, C., Wang, Z. G., Mayo, S. L., & Arnold, F. H. (2002). Protein building blocks preserved by recombination. *Nature Structural Biology*, *9*, 553–558.

Voigt, C. A., Mayo, S. L., Arnold, F. H., & Wang, Z. G. (2001). Computational method to reduce the search space for directed protein evolution. *Proceedings of the National Academy of Sciences of the United States of America*, *98*, 3778–3783.

Wachtmeister, J., & Rother, D. (2016). Recent advances in whole cell biocatalysis techniques bridging from investigative to industrial scale. *Current Opinion in Biotechnology*, *42*, 169–177.

Wang, Z. J., Renata, H., Peck, N. E., Farwell, C. C., Coelho, P. S., & Arnold, F. H. (2014). Improved cyclopropanation activity of histidine-ligated cytochrome P450 enables the enantioselective formal synthesis of levomilnacipran. *Angewandte Chemie. International Edition*, *53*, 6810–6813.

Wang, Z. J., Peck, N. E., Renata, H., & Arnold, F. H. (2014). Cytochrome P450-catalyzed insertion of carbenoids into N-H bonds. *Chemical Science*, *5*, 598–601.

Wapshott-Stehli, H. L., & Grunden, A. M. (2021). In situ H2O2 generation methods in the context of enzyme biocatalysis. *Enzyme and Microbial Technology*, *145*, 16.

Weber, E., Sirim, D., Schreiber, T., Thomas, B., Pleiss, J., Hunger, M., et al. (2010). Immobilization of P450 BM-3 monooxygenase on mesoporous molecular sieves with different pore diameters. *Journal of Molecular Catalysis B: Enzymatic*, *64*, 29–37.

White, M. C., & Zhao, J. P. (2018). Aliphatic C-H oxidations for late-stage functionalization. *Journal of the American Chemical Society*, *140*, 13988–14009.

Williams, P. A., Cosme, J., Sridhar, V., Johnson, E. F., & McRee, D. E. (2000). Mammalian microsomal cytochrome P450 monooxygenase: structural adaptations for membrane binding and functional diversity. *Molecular Cell*, *5*, 121–131.

Wong, T. S., Arnold, F. H., & Schwaneberg, U. (2004). Laboratory evolution of cytochrome P450 BM-3 monooxygenase for organic cosolvents. *Biotechnology and Bioengineering*, *85*, 351–358.

Wu, Z. L., Podust, L. M., & Guengerich, F. P. (2005). Expansion of substrate specificity of cytochrome P450 2A6 by random and site-directed mutagenesis. *Journal of Biological Chemistry*, *280*, 41090–41100.

Xiao, H., Zhang, Y., & Wang, M. (2019). Discovery and engineering of cytochrome P450s for terpenoid biosynthesis. *Trends in Biotechnology*, *37*, 618–631.

Xu, F., Bell, S. G., Lednik, J., Insley, A., Rao, Z. H., & Wong, L. L. (2005). The heme monooxygenase cytochrome P450(cam) can be engineered to oxidize ethane to ethanol. *Angewandte Chemie. International Edition*, *44*, 4029–4032.

Yabusaki, Y., Murakami, H., Sakaki, T., Shibata, M., & Ohkawa, H. (1988). Genetically engineered modification of P450 monooxygenases - Functional analysis of the amino-terminal hydrophobic region and hinge region of the P450/reductase fused enzyme. *DNA*, *7*, 701–711.

Yang, Y., Cho, I., Qi, X., Liu, P., & Arnold, F. H. (2019). An enzymatic platform for the asymmetric amination of primary, secondary and tertiary C(sp3)–H bonds. *Nature Chemistry*, *11*, 987–993.

Yun, C. H., Kim, K. H., Kim, D. H., Jung, H. C., & Pan, J. G. (2007). The bacterial P450BM3: a prototype for a biocatalyst with human P450 activities. *Trends in Biotechnology*, *25*, 289–298.

Yun, C. H., Miller, G. P., & Guengerich, F. P. (2000). Rate-determining steps in phenacetin oxidations by human cytochrome P450 1A2 and selected mutants. *Biochemistry*, *39*, 11319–11329.

Zhang, X. W., & Li, S. Y. (2017). Expansion of chemical space for natural products by uncommon P450 reactions. *Natural Product Reports*, *34*, 1061–1089.
Zhang, C., Li, J., Yang, B., He, F., Yang, S.-Y., Yu, X.-Q., et al. (2014). Enhanced turnover rate and enantioselectivity in the asymmetric epoxidation of styrene by new T213G mutants of CYP119. *RSC Advances*, *4*, 27526–27531.
Zhang, C., Liu, P. X., Huang, L. Y., Wei, S. P., Wang, L., Yang, S. Y., et al. (2016). Engineering P450 peroxygenase to catalyze highly enantioselective epoxidation of cis-beta-methylstyrenes. *Chemistry - A European Journal*, *22*, 10969–10975.
Zhang, R. K., Chen, K., Huang, X., Wohlschlager, L., Renata, H., & Arnold, F. H. (2018). Enzymatic assembly of carbon–carbon bonds via iron-catalysed sp3 C–H functionalization. *Nature*, *565*, 67–72.
Zhang, X. W., Guo, J. W., Cheng, F. Y., & Li, S. Y. (2021). Cytochrome P450 enzymes in fungal natural product biosynthesis. *Natural Product Reports*, *38*, 1072–1099.
Zhang, J., Huang, X., Zhang, R. K., & Arnold, F. H. (2019). Enantiodivergent a-amino C-H fluoroalkylation catalyzed by engineered cytochrome P450s. *Journal of the American Chemical Society*, *141*, 9798–9802.
Zhou, A. Z., Chen, K., & Arnold, F. H. (2020). Enzymatic lactone-carbene C–H insertion to build contiguous chiral centers. *ACS Catalysis*, *10*, 5393–5398.

CHAPTER EIGHT

Assessing cytochrome P450 function using genetically engineered mouse models

Sarrah L. Hannon and Xinxin Ding*

Department of Pharmacology and Toxicology, Ken R. Coit College of Pharmacy, The University of Arizona, Tucson, AZ, United States

*Corresponding author: e-mail address: xding@pharmacy.arizona.edu

Contents

Abstract

The ability to knock out and/or humanize different genes in experimental animals, globally or in cell- and tissue-specific patterns, has revolutionized scientific research in many areas. Genetically engineered mouse models, including knockout models, transgenic models, and humanized models, have played important roles in revealing the in vivo functions of various cytochrome P450 (CYP) enzymes. These functions are very diverse, ranging from the biotransformation of drugs and other xenobiotics, events that often dictate their pharmacokinetic or toxicokinetic properties and the associated therapeutic or adverse actions, to the metabolism of endogenous compounds, such as steroid hormones and other bioactive substances, that may determine susceptibility to many diseases, such as cancer and metabolic diseases. In this review, we provide a comprehensive list of *Cyp*-knockout, human CYP-transgenic, and CYP-humanized mouse models that target genes in the *CYP1–4* gene families, and highlight their utility in assessing the in vivo metabolism, bioactivation, and toxicity of various xenobiotic compounds, including therapeutic agents and chemical carcinogens. We aim to showcase the advantages of utilizing these mouse models for in vivo drug metabolism and toxicology studies, and to encourage and facilitate greater utility of engineered mouse

Advances in Pharmacology, Volume 95
ISSN 1054-3589
https://doi.org/10.1016/bs.apha.2022.05.008

models to further improve our knowledge of the in vivo functions of various P450 enzymes, which is integral to our ability to develop safer and more effective therapeutics and to identify individuals predisposed to adverse drug reactions or environmental diseases.

Abbreviations

APAP	acetaminophen
AαC	2-amino-9H-pyrido[2,3-b]indole
BaP	benzo[*a*]pyrene
CPR	NADPH-cytochrome P450 reductase
dGC8-AαC	*N*-(deoxyguanosin-8-yl)-2-amino-9H-pyrido[2,3-b]indole
DMBA	7,12-dimethylbenz(*a*)anthracene
GSH	reduced glutathione
HAA	heterocyclic amines
MDZ	midazolam
NA	naphthalene
NAPQI	*N*-acetyl-p-benzoquinone imine
NNK	4-(methylnitrosoamino)-1-(3-pyridyl)-1-butanone
P450 or CYP	cytochrome P450
PA	pyrrolizidine alkaloids
PAH	polycyclic aromatic hydrocarbons
PhIP	2-amino-1-methyl-6-phenylimidazo[4,5-b]pyridine
ROS	reactive oxygen species
WT	wild-type

1. Introduction

Cytochrome P450 (P450 or CYP) enzymes are responsible for the bulk of phase I biotransformation of xenobiotic compounds. P450 substrate specificity and catalytic efficiency can be readily assessed in vitro, for example, through assays that use recombinant human P450 enzymes. However, the role of P450-mediated metabolism in the fate or actions of a substrate in vivo is complicated to predict, given the existence of so many different P450 isoforms and non-CYP biotransformation enzymes, often with overlapping substrate specificity, the many physiological, pathological, dietary, and environmental factors that can modify CYP gene expression, and the complicated relationships between phase I and phase II metabolism or between metabolism and excretion. Though pharmacological approaches have been commonly used to deduce the function of a given P450, the general lack of stringent specificity by P450 inhibitors weakens the conclusions reached in these in vivo studies. The advent of *Cyp* knockout mouse models was a game-changer in this regard. Comparisons between a knockout mouse and its wild-type (WT) controls for in vivo metabolism, pharmacokinetics, and toxicity of a given drug or other xenobiotic substrate can provide straightforward answers to many questions important in preclinical drug discovery or mechanistic toxicology, such as "whether P450s are involved," "which specific P450 isoform is the most important for the selected experimental endpoints," and "are P450-mediated metabolism more important for protection (via disposition and detoxification) or for toxification (via bioactivation)."

The well-known species differences between rodents and humans in P450 expression and activity necessitate studies that directly examine function of human P450 enzymes in an in vivo environment, under conditions that simulate human exposure/treatment or can demonstrate exposure/treatment-induced adverse effects. Thus, human CYP transgenic mice have been valuable, for examples, for modeling human-specific metabolic pathways, depicting potential for drug–drug interactions through inhibition or induction of the human CYPs, and understanding mechanisms of regulation of human CYPs by various external or internal factor.

The coexistence of mouse and human CYPs in a human CYP-transgenic mouse complicates analysis of the functions of the human CYP, as the mouse CYP enzymes are often more abundant or may possess metabolic activities that are too high to permit detection of activities of the human CYPs. Thus, CYP-humanized mice are created, where the orthologous mouse CYPs are removed, replaced with the human CYP. The "humanization" does not stop at the CYPs, as important nuclear receptors are also found to have species differences, such as PXR, and it is feasible to double or multiple "humanize" for selected CYPs and nuclear receptors (Ma et al., 2008). To make the models more like a human, who has not just one CYP, but the whole complement of CYPs, multiple CYPs were introduced into one mouse model, to study potential interactions (e.g., competition or cooperation) among coexisting CYPs. Other models, where the NADPH-cytochrome P450 reductase (CPR or POR) gene is knocked out in a tissue-specific fashion, thus silencing all microsomal CYPs (Gu et al., 2003; Henderson et al., 2003), or where most of the mouse liver is replaced by human hepatocytes (Bissig et al., 2018), have also been produced and found to offer unique advantages.

The topic of P450 transgenic mice has been reviewed often, for examples, (Buters, Doehmer, & Gonzalez, 1999; Cheung & Gonzalez, 2008;

Ghanayem, Wang, & Sumner, 2000; Gonzalez, 2004; Gonzalez & Yu, 2006; Henderson & Wolf, 2003; Jiang, Gonzalez, & Yu, 2011; Scheer & Wolf, 2014; van Waterschoot & Schinkel, 2011), but few review articles have appeared in recent years (Bissig et al., 2018; Reed, Arlt, & Phillips, 2018). In this chapter, we provide a comprehensive list (Section 2) of *Cyp*-knockout, human CYP-transgenic, and CYP-humanized mouse models for the *CYP1*, *CYP2*, *CYP3*, and *CYP4* gene families, which are best known for the metabolism of xenobiotics. Many mouse models have also been reported for genes in the *CYP7-CYP51* families (Lorbek, Lewinska, & Rozman, 2012), which are specialized for the metabolism and homeostasis of endogenous compounds, such as cholesterol and steroid hormones; but we will not be able to discuss those due to space limitation. We will also not include studies using rat models. However, we recognize that, though human CYP-transgenic or CYP-knockout rat models are still not commonly used, there has been increasing interest in their production and utility (Lu et al., 2021).

We will first briefly describe examples of utility of the mouse models for in vivo metabolism, pharmacokinetics and toxicity studies of therapeutics (Section 3). Then, we will provide a more complete account of the application of these models for studies on the in vivo metabolism and toxicity of known or suspected chemical carcinogens (Section 4), a topic of current research focus of the authors' laboratory. Overall, we hope to showcase the advantages of utilizing these mouse models for in vivo drug metabolism and toxicology studies, highlighting unique insights gained.

2. Available mouse models

The first report of a P450 knockout mouse model appeared in 1995, for a *Cyp1a2*-null mouse (Pineau et al., 1995). Several other *Cyp*-knockout and the first human CYP cDNA transgenic models were reported the next year, for *Cyp2e1*-null (Lee, Buters, Pineau, Fernandez-Salguero, & Gonzalez, 1996), *Cyp7a1*-null (Ishibashi, Schwarz, Frykman, Herz, & Russell, 1996), and a new *Cyp1a2*-null (Liang et al., 1996), as well as a CYP3A7 cDNA transgenic (Li et al., 1996) and a CYP19A1 cDNA transgenic mouse (Tekmal et al., 1996). Since then, many mouse models have been reported.

The null mouse models reported to date (to the best of our knowledge) for *Cyp* gene families 1–4 are summarized in Table 1. These include single gene knockouts, such as *Cyp1b1*-null (Buters, Sakai, et al., 1999); multiple *Cyp* gene knockouts, made possible because two *Cyp* genes are located in

Table 1 Knockout mouse models for the *Cyp1–4* gene families.

Mouse model	References
Cyp1-null (*Cyp1a1/1a2/1b1*-null)	Dragin et al. (2008)
Cyp1a-null	Dragin, Uno, Wang, Dalton, and Nebert (2007)
Cyp1a1-null	Dalton et al. (2000)
Cyp1a2-null	Liang et al. (1996), Pineau et al. (1995)
Cyp1b1-null	Buters et al. (1999)
Cyp1a1/1b1-null	Uno et al. (2006)
Cyp1a2/1b1-null	Uno et al. (2006)
Cyp2a5-null	Zhou et al. (2010)
Cyp2a(4/5)bgs-null	Wei et al. (2013)
Cyp2abfgs-null	Li, Megaraj, Wei, and Ding (2014)
Cyp2a12/2c70-null	Honda et al. (2020)
Cyp2a12-null	Honda et al. (2020)
Cyp2b-null (RNAi)	Damiri, Holle, Yu, and Baldwin (2012)
Cyp2b9/10/13-null	Kumar et al. (2017)
Cyp2c-null	Scheer et al. (2012)
Cyp2c/2d/3a-null	Scheer et al. (2014)
Cyp2c/2d/3a-null select	Hough, Nalwalk, Ding, and Scheer (2015)
Cyp2c44-null	Pozzi et al. (2010)
Cyp2c70-null	de Boer et al. (2020)
Cyp2a12/2c70-null	Honda et al. (2020)
Cyp2d-null	Scheer et al. (2012)
Cyp2e1-null	Lee et al. (1996)
Cyp2f2-null	Li et al. (2011)
Cyp2g1-null	Zhuo et al. (2004)
Cyp2g1-null/*Cyp2a5*-low	Zhou et al. (2011)
Cyp2j-null	Zhou et al. (2013)
Cyp2j5-null	Athirakul et al. (2008)
Cyp2r1-null	Zhu, Ochalek, Kaufmann, Jones, and Deluca (2013)

Continued

Table 1 Knockout mouse models for the *Cyp1–4* gene families.—cont'd

Mouse model	References
Cyp2u1-null	Pujol et al. (2021)
Cyp3a-null	van Herwaarden et al. (2007)
Cyp4a10-null	Nakagawa et al. (2006)
Cyp4a14-null	Holla et al. (2001)
Cyp4b1-null	Parkinson, Liggitt, Rettie, and Kelly (2013)
Cyp4f14-null	Bardowell, Duan, Manor, Swanson, and Parker (2012)
Cyp4f18-null	Winslow et al. (2014)
Cyp4f39-null	Miyamoto, Itoh, Sawai, Sassa, and Kihara (2020)
Cyp4v3-null	Lockhart, Nakano, Rettie, and Kelly (2014)
Cyp4x1-null	Kharkwal et al. (2017)

close proximity to allow for simultaneous deletion, as in *Cyp1a1/1a2*-null (Dragin et al., 2007), or were produced through crossbreeding between two, or among multiple, knockout strains, as in *Cyp1a1/1b1*-null (Uno et al., 2006), or through the use of RNAi (Damiri et al., 2012) or the Crispr/Cas9 system (Kumar et al., 2017); and *Cyp* gene cluster nulls, generated through DNA recombinase (e.g., Cre/LoxP)-based genetic engineering, as in *Cyp2abfgs*-null (Li, Megaraj, et al., 2014). Collectively, these models cover most of the mouse *Cyp* genes in families 1–4. Not included in the table are mouse models that target the *Cpr* gene, which have also been valuable for assessing functions of microsomal P450 enzymes (Gu et al., 2003; Henderson et al., 2003; Wei et al., 2010; Wu et al., 2005).

Reported human CYP-transgenic mouse models for the *CYP1–4* gene families are summarized in Table 2. Some of these are single *CYP* transgenic, as in *CYP2D6* transgenic (Corchero et al., 2001). Other models contain more than one human *CYP* gene, as in *CYP2A13/2B6/2F1* transgenic (Wei et al., 2012); the fact that these genes are in close proximity to each other made it convenient, or in some cases necessary for proper transgene expression, to insert them as one unit into the mouse genome. Notably, cDNA-based transgenic strains use surrogate promoters to drive gene expression in one or more tissues; they differ from the gene-based transgenic

Table 2 Human CYP transgenic mouse models for the *CYP1–4* gene families.

Mouse model	References
CYP1A2 (cDNA) transgenic	Ueno et al. (2000)
CYP1A1/1A2 transgenic	Jiang et al. (2005)
CYP1B1 (cDNA) transgenic	Hwang et al. (2001)
CYP2A6 (cDNA) transgenic	Zhang et al. (2005)
CYP2A13/2B6/2F1 transgenic	Wei et al. (2012)
CYP2A13 transgenic	Jia et al. (2014)
CYP2C8 (cDNA) transgenic	Lee et al. (2010)
CYP2C9 (cDNA) transgenic	Scheer, Kapelyukh, Chatham, et al. (2012)
CYP2C18/2C19 transgenic	Lofgren et al. (2008)
CYP2D6 transgenic (3 models)	Cheng et al. (2013), Corchero et al. (2001), Scheer, Kapelyukh, McEwan, et al. (2012)
CYP2D6/3A4 transgenic	Felmlee, Lon, Gonzalez, and Yu (2008)
CYP1A/2D6/2E1/3A4/7 transgenic	Cheung and Gonzalez (2008)
CYP2E1 (cDNA) transgenic	Morgan, French, and Morgan (2002)
CYP2E1 transgenic	Cheung et al. (2005)
CYP2J2 (cDNA) transgenic (3 models)	Lee et al. (2010), Seubert et al. (2004), Xiao et al. (2004)
CYP3A transgenic	Abe et al. (2017), Kazuki et al. (2013)
CYP3A4 transgenic	Granvil et al. (2003)
CYP3A4 (cDNA)-transgenic (2 models)	van Herwaarden et al. (2005, 2007)
CYP3A7 transgenic	Li et al. (1996)
CYP3A4/7 transgenic (3 models)	Cheung et al. (2006), Hasegawa et al. (2011), Ma et al. (2008)
CYP4A11 transgenic	Savas et al. (2009)
CYP4A12 (cDNA) transgenic	Gilani et al. (2020)
CYP4B1 (cDNA) transgenic	Imaoka et al. (2001)
CYP4F2 (cDNA) transgenic (2 models)	Lai, Liu, Wu, Liu, and Zhao (2012), Liu et al. (2009)

strains, which retain the authentic human *CYP* promoter and at least some of the regulatory elements that govern their expression. Table 2 also includes models that express multiple human CYP genes, as in *CYP1A/2D6/2E1/3A4/7* transgenic, which were produced through crossbreeding among multiple CYP-transgenic mouse strains.

CYP-humanized mouse models are defined here as those that produce human CYPs from a mouse genome that no longer contain the orthologous mouse *Cyp(s)*. However, given the disparity between mouse and human CYP in the number of genes within each gene subfamily, it is not always straightforward to designate mouse orthologs for a given human CYP. The *Cyp* gene cluster knockout models have made it easier, though "humanized" models that use targeted, single *Cyp* knockout as strain background can also be informative, e.g., CYP2A13/2B6/2F1-transgenic on *Cyp2a5*-null (Megaraj et al., 2014). The possible combinations of transgenic and null mice that can be used for "humanization" are large and can be readily made through crossbreeding. Thus, only the most straightforward CYP-humanized mouse models for the *CYP1–4* gene families are shown in Table 3.

Table 3 Examples of CYP-humanized mouse models for the *CYP1–4* gene families.

Mouse model	References
CYP1A1/1A2-humanized on *Cyp1a1/1a2*-null	Dragin et al. (2007)
CYP1B1-humanized on *Cyp1b1*-null	Li et al. (2014)
CYP2A13-humanized on *Cyp2abfgs*-null	Li et al. (2017)
CYP2A13/2B6/2F1-humanized on *Cyp2abfgs*-null	Li et al. (2017)
CYP2C9/2D6/3A4/3A7-humanized on *Cyp2c/2d/3a*-null	Scheer et al. (2015)
CYP2C9-humanized on *Cyp2c-null*	Scheer, Kapelyukh, Chatham, et al. (2012)
CYP2D6-humanized on *Cyp2d*-null	Scheer, Kapelyukh, McEwan, et al. (2012)
CYP2E1-humanized on *Cyp2e1*-null	Cheung et al. (2005)
CYP2J2-humanized on *Cyp2j*-null	Zhou et al. (2013)
CYP3A-humanized on *Cyp3a*-null	Abe et al. (2017)
CYP3A4-humanized on *Cyp3a*-null	van Herwaarden et al. (2007)

3. Assessing CYP function in the in vivo metabolism and toxicity of therapeutic drugs

A major application of CYP knockout, transgenic, and humanized mouse models has been to study in vivo metabolism and pharmacokinetics of drugs. A literature review identified more than 100 publications that fall into this category. Due to space limitation, we have opted to show only selected studies published in the last 5 years in Table 4. It is believed that many more (unpublished) studies are carried out during preclinical development of drug candidates. Two of the commonly studied drugs are highlighted below to illustrate the types of insights gained from the utility of one or more engineered mouse models.

Table 4 Pharmaceuticals evaluated with *Cyp*-null, human CYP-transgenic, or CYP-humanized mice for in vivo metabolism and pharmacokinetics (2017–2022).

Drug	Mouse model	References
Imiquimod	*Cyp1a*-null	Mescher et al. (2019)
Docataxel, Reprotrectinob, Selitrectinib, Lorlatinib, Galunisertib, Quizartinib, Triazolam	*Cyp3a*-null	Li, Sparidans, Lebre, Beijnen, & Schinkel (2021), Li et al. (2021, 2019, 2018, 2020), Wang et al. (2019), Minegishi et al. (2019)
Caffeine, Midazolam, Tolbutamide, Rifampin, Debrisoquine, Dextromethorphan, Darafenib, Sulfaphenazole	CAR/PXR/CYP1A/2C9/2D6/3A4/3A7-humanized	Henderson et al. (2019)
Rifampin, Triazolam	PXR/CYP3A4-humanized	Kobayashi et al. (2019)
Tamoxifen	*Cyp2d*-null, CYP2D6-transgenic, CYP2D6-humanized	Konstandi, Andriopoulou, Cheng, and Gonzalez (2020), MacLeod, McLaughlin, Henderson, and Wolf (2017)

Continued

Table 4 Pharmaceuticals evaluated with *Cyp*-null, human CYP-transgenic, or CYP-humanized mice for in vivo metabolism and pharmacokinetics (2017–2022).—cont'd

Drug	Mouse model	References
Osimertinib	*Cyp2c*-null, *Cyp2d*-null, *Cyp3a*-null, *Cyp2c/2d*-null, CYP2D6.2-humanized, PXR/CAR/ CYP3A4/3A7-humanized, CYP1A-humanized	MacLeod et al. (2018)
Harmine	CYP2D6-transgenic	Stocco et al. (2020)
Propranolol	CYP2D6-transgenic, PXR/CAR/ CYP3A4/3A7-humanized	Stocco et al. (2020), Tolledo, Stocco, Miksys, Gonzalez, and Tyndale (2020), Tolledo, Miksys, Gonzalez, and Tyndale (2020), Ly et al. (2021)
Triazolam	CYP3A-humanized	Minegishi et al. (2019)
Docataxel	*Cyp3a/p-gp*-null	Hendrikx et al. (2020)
Gefitinib, Alprazolam, Bosutibiv, Crizotinib, Dasatinib, Ibrutinib Regorafenib, Sorafenib, Vandetinib, Triazolam	CYP3A4/3A7-humanized	Ly, Messick, Qin, Takahashi, and Choo (2017)
Efavirenz, Rifampin	PXR/CAR/ CYP3A4/3A7-humanized	Ly et al. (2021)
Gentamicin	Cpr-low	Ding et al. (2020)
Niclosamide	LCN, IECN	Fan, Li, Ding, and Zhang (2019)

Pentobarbital, a barbiturate hypnotic drug, is a convenient probe for in vivo metabolism because of its easily measured phenotype—sleeping time. The administration of pentobarbital to mouse models with liver-specific deletion of P450 reductase (named HRN or LCN by different groups) (Gu et al., 2003; Henderson et al., 2003) resulted in significantly increased sleeping time compared to WT mice, confirming the essential role of hepatic P450 enzymes in the metabolic disposition of this drug. *Cyp2a(4/5)bgs*-null mice treated with pentobarbital had a significant increase in sleeping time as well, compared to WT mice, indicating a specific role of the *Cyp2a(4/5)bgs* genes in pentobarbital clearance (Wei et al., 2013).

Midazolam (MDZ), a benzodiazepine most commonly used as an anxiolytic before surgical or other procedures, is widely used as a CYP3A probe. *Cyp3a*-null hepatic microsomes in vitro and *Cyp3a*-null mice in vivo still metabolized MDZ, suggesting the involvement of other enzymes (van Waterschoot et al., 2008). MDZ also showed an increase in the area under the concentration-time curve in *Cyp2c*-null mice, with a larger increase after pretreatment with troleandomycin (a CYP3A inhibitor), indicating CYP2C involvement in MDZ metabolism (Grimsley et al., 2013). Later models with humanization of multiple CYP enzymes and nuclear receptors (specifically CAR and PXR in the case of CYP3A) have been shown to be more accurate representations of human metabolism, with potentially greater utility in clinical drug development and testing (Henderson et al., 2019; Scheer et al., 2015).

A number of studies have also utilized engineered mouse models to identify possible roles and mechanisms of drug-induced tissue toxicity, though the number is much lower than that of drug metabolism and pharmacokinetics studies. These studies are more challenging to conduct, as the toxic mechanisms and endpoints are diverse. A few examples are highlighted below.

Acetaminophen (APAP), a commonly used over-the-counter pain reliever, is widely known for its potential hepatotoxicity and has been one of the most studied drugs for mechanisms of toxicity. APAP-related liver damage is associated with the generation of the reactive metabolite *N*-acetyl-*p*-benzoquinone imine (NAPQI) by P450 enzymes and NAPQI's subsequent depletion of reduced glutathione (GSH). GSH depletion can result in mitochondrial oxidative and nitrosative stress, eventually leading to cell death. Studies on the role of various P450 enzymes in the in vivo metabolism and toxicity of APAP represent some of the earliest examples of application of P450 knockout mouse models. *Cyp2e1*-null mice, as well as *Cyp1a2/Cyp2e1* double null mice, were resistant to APAP-induced liver necrosis and protein adduct formation (Abdelmegeed, Moon, Chen, Gonzalez, & Song, 2010; Lee et al., 1996; Zaher et al., 1998). Whereas, APAP was hepatotoxic and even fatal in *Cyp1a2*-null mice compared to WT mice (Tonge et al., 1998), a result suggesting that the involvement of CYP1A2 was minimal compared to the involvement of CYP2E1. CYP2E1-humanized mice exposed to APAP exhibited increased hepatocyte necrosis compared to WT mice, a finding confirming role of human CYP2E1 in APAP hepatotoxicity (Cheung et al., 2005).

APAP causes toxicity in liver as well as extrahepatic tissues. The organ contributions to APAP toxicity was examined using HRN and LCN mouse models. HRN mice had unchanged levels of hepatic GSH after administration of APAP, compared to a 90% decrease in WT mice, data consistent with a role of hepatic APAP metabolites in liver toxicity (Henderson et al., 2003). Loss of hepatic APAP metabolism in the LCN mice had tissue-specific impact on APAP toxicity in the lung, kidney, and the nasal cavity, with decreases in toxicity, compared to WT mice, in the lung, kidney, and lateral nasal glands (LNG), but not in the nasal olfactory and respiratory mucosa, results that show the potential of liver-generated APAP metabolites to cause toxicity in selected extrahepatic organs (Gu et al., 2005).

Studies using *Cyp1a2*-null mice and recombinant CYP2A5 and CYP2G1, which are dominantly (CYP2A5) or specifically (CYP2G1) expressed in the olfactory mucosa, suggested that both enzymes might contribute to APAP bioactivation in this tissue (Genter et al., 1998; Gu et al., 1998). However, further studies of a *Cyp2g1*-null/*Cyp2a5*-low mouse indicated that CYP2A5 and CYP2G1 may not play a central role in APAP-induced toxicity in the olfactory mucosa (Zhuo et al., 2004). Interestingly, studies of APAP toxicity in the LNG of the *Cyp2g1*-null/*Cyp2a5*-low mice (Zhuo et al., 2004) and subsequently generated *Cyp2g1*-null mice (Zhou et al., 2011) and *Cyp2a5*-null mice led to the intriguing finding that CYP2A5 regulates testosterone levels in the LNG of the male mice, which in turn regulates the expression of salivary androgen-binding protein (ABP). Upregulation of ABP expression in the *Cyp2a5*-null mice increases resistance to APAP toxicity in the LNG due to the ability of ABP to quench reactive APAP metabolites (Zhou et al., 2011). Notably, though human CYP2A6 has similar substrate specificity to its mouse ortholog, CYP2A5, this intriguing CYP2A-testosterone-ABP defensive mechanism unlikely exists in humans as the human *ABPs* are all pseudogenes.

Cisplatin, a chemotherapeutic, is widely established as nephrotoxic. Cisplatin accumulates in the kidney where, through a series of reactions, it is metabolized into a reactive thiol compound and transported to the proximal tubule cells and, through a multitude of pathways, induces cell death (Miller, Tadagavadi, Ramesh, & Reeves, 2010). When exposed to cisplatin, *Cyp2e1*-null mice showed protection against renal injuries, with a decrease in reactive oxygen species (ROS), cytotoxicity, and apoptosis, a result indicating role of CYP2E1 in cisplatin bioactivation in vivo.

Thalidomide, originally prescribed for nausea in pregnant women, is one of the most widely known failures of preclinical drug safety testing. Thalidomide proved to be a teratogen, causing birth defects in thousands of children in the late 1950s and early 1960s. Testing in rodents did not reveal the teratogenicity of thalidomide and it wasn't until the generation of a CYP3A-humanized mouse that its etiology began to be understood. Embryos of CYP3A-humanized mouse (on a *Cyp3a*-null background), which expresses CYP3A in the placenta, developed limb abnormalities after treatment with thalidomide (Kazuki et al., 2016). Further identification of targets for protein adduction by metabolites of thalidomide in maternal liver and whole fetal tissue homogenates in this model suggested a possible mechanism for the toxicity of thalidomide (Yamazaki et al., 2016).

4. Assessing the function of CYPs in the in vivo metabolism, bioactivation, and toxicity of known or suspected chemical carcinogens

There is an abundance of in vitro data demonstrating the ability of various P450 enzymes, particularly those in the CYP1–4 gene families, to metabolize countless carcinogens. The consequence of metabolism is often bioactivation, producing reactive metabolites that are intermediate or ultimate carcinogens. Conversely, there are far fewer reports of in vivo studies where the relationship between the activity of a given P450 and the tumorigenicity or other cancer-related toxic endpoints of a chemical carcinogen has been established in animal models.

Chemical carcinogenesis is a complicated process that is still not fully understood. However, for many pro-carcinogens, it is clear that the initial bioactivation by P450 or other biotransformation enzymes is the essential, enabling step. Metabolism of a carcinogen can lead to detoxification or bioactivation. Thus, the outcome of metabolism can be protective or damaging, depending on the in vivo environment where the metabolism occurs; the deciding factors may include the rate of metabolism, the specific metabolites formed, the fate or reactivity of the metabolites, and the cellular defense mechanisms. The nature and abundance of the reactive metabolites can dictate their ability to form adducts with DNA or other important molecules, which in turn may influence the occurrence of mutations, increases in cell proliferation, and tumor initiation. Conversely, metabolic disposition can prevent carcinogens from reaching the target organ or cellular sites, or facilitate their removal from the body, thus reducing the risks of carcinogenesis in exposed individuals. Therefore, the importance of carcinogen metabolism by a given enzyme or groups of enzymes may not be readily predicted from their in vitro activity, and studies using knockout and humanized mouse models are essential, not only for dissecting carcinogen metabolic pathways in vivo, but also for establishing the mechanistic links between carcinogen metabolites and various cancer-related toxic endpoints, ranging from DNA damages to tumor formation.

Many polycyclic aromatic hydrocarbons (PAH), such as 7,12-dimethylbenz(*a*)anthracene (DMBA), have been established to be genotoxic carcinogens. DMBA is a component of cigarette smoke and forms primarily hydroxy and diol metabolites and epoxide intermediates capable of adducting to DNA (Miyata, Furukawa, Takahashi, Gonzalez, & Yamazoe, 2001; Smolarek et al., 1987). Both CYP1A1 and CYP1B1 can bioactivate DMBA in vitro; however, *Cyp1b1*-null mice had much reduced incidence (7.5%) of malignant lymphomas when treated with DMBA, compared to a 70% tumor incidence rate in DMBA-treated WT mice (Buters, Sakai, et al., 1999). This study demonstrated a pivotal role of CYP1B1, rather than CYP1A1, in mediating DMBA's carcinogenicity.

DMBA is also a breast carcinogen. The relationship between CYP-mediated bioactivation and detoxification in the microenvironment of the mammary gland has also been examined for DMBA. When the *Cpr* gene was selectively knocked out from the mammary epithelial cells, but not stromal cells, the resulting mammary epithelium-specific Cpr-null (MEpi-Cpr-null) mice had significantly higher levels of DMBA, greater induction of CYP1B1 expression, and greater abundance of DMBA-DNA adducts in the mammary gland, compared to those in WT mice, following systemic exposure to DMBA (Lin et al., 2012). Notably, hepatic and blood levels of DMBA were not different between the null and control mouse strains, a result consistent with a breast tissue-specific *Cpr* knockout. These results suggested that CYP-mediated DMBA metabolism in mammary epithelial cells played an important role in removing DMBA from the tissue and implied that both stromal and epithelial P450 enzymes, particularly CYP1B1, mediate DMBA bioactivation and genotoxicity in the mammary glands. In that connection, the role of CYP1B1 in DMBA bioactivation and target tissue toxicity was also established for the bone marrow. *Cyp1b1*-null mice were resistant to DMBA toxic effects, including bone marrow cytotoxicity and induction of preleukemia, and, unlike WT mice, their bone marrow did not contain detectable amounts of the DNA adducts with DMBA dihydrodiol epoxide (Heidel et al., 1999, 2000).

Benzo[*a*]pyrene (BaP) is another PAH carcinogen that has been intensively studied. BaP is a pollutant resulting from incomplete combustion. It forms radical cation, diol epoxide, and *o*-quinone reactive metabolites capable of intercalating into DNA. The roles of mouse and human CYP1A1 and CYP1A2 in BaP in vivo metabolism and toxicity have been examined using knockout and humanized mouse models (Dragin et al., 2007). BaP was administered orally to WT mice, as well as four separate transgenic mouse models, *Cyp1a1*-null, *Cyp1a2*-null, *Cyp1a1/1a2*-null, and CYP1A1/1A2-humanized (on *Cyp1a1/1a2*-null background), to elucidate the specific contributions of each of these CYP1A enzymes to BaP disposition and toxicity in vivo. It was an important finding that *Cyp1a1*-null mice and *Cyp1a1/1a2*-null mice exhibited significant elevation in circulating BaP levels, whereas *Cyp1a2*-null mice and CYP1A1/1A2-humanized mice had BaP levels that were similar to those found in WT mice. Furthermore, whereas the *Cyp1a1*-null and *Cyp1a1/1a2*-null mice had larger livers, smaller spleen and thymus, elevated hepatotoxicity, and leukocytopenia, the *Cyp1a2*-null mice did not exhibit these phenotypes and the CYP1A1/1A2-humanized mice showed partial rescue from BaP toxicity (Dragin et al., 2007). These results illustrated the complicated relationship between bioactivation and detoxification in the context of toxicokinetics, that while CYP1A1 can bioactivate BaP, its capacity to eliminate BaP, through bioactivation and subsequent phase II metabolism, can reduce BaP tissue burden and avoid BaP toxicity in target tissues. The fact that CYP1A2 is predominantly expressed in the liver and not expressed in the intestine also suggested unique importance of intestinal CYP1A1 in the protection against orally ingested BaP. This specific contribution of intestinal BaP metabolism was validated in further studies using tissue-specific *Cpr* knockout mouse models. BaP was administered orally or intraperitoneally (i.p.) to WT mice, as well as mice with tissue-specific knockouts of *Cpr* in the liver (LCN) or intestinal epithelium (intestinal epithelium-specific Cpr-null, or IECN). The IECN mice, but not the LCN mice, had significantly lower clearance rates of oral BaP in blood compared to WT; conversely, the three mouse strains had similar clearance rates when BaP was administered i.p. (Fang & Zhang, 2010). These results indicated that intestinal P450 enzymes played a greater role in the first-pass clearance of orally administered BaP than those in the liver. Consistent with the protective role of CYP1A1 against BaP toxicity, mice with a knockout of *Cyp1a1* developed adenocarcinoma on their proximal small intestine within just 8–12 weeks of oral feeding with BaP; whereas, mice with both *Cyp1a1* and *Cyp1b1* knocked out developed preputial gland duct squamous cell carcinoma within 12 weeks (Galvez-Peralta, Shi, Chen, Miller, & Nebert, 2013).

Well-done cooked meat contains compounds known as heterocyclic amines (HAA), with 2-amino-1-methyl-6-phenylimidazo[4,5-b]pyridine (PhIP) being a well-known example. PhIP is a commonly studied genotoxic HAA carcinogen shown to form adducts with DNA in vivo, though it may act through non-genotoxic carcinogenesis mechanisms as well (Gooderham, Creton, Lauber, & Zhu, 2007). CYP1A2 is known to be a highly active enzyme in bioactivating PhIP via the N2-hydroxyaltion pathway, which is thought to underly the ability of PhIP to induce lymphoma and liver and lung tumors in mice. However, in vivo bioassay performed with PhIP in WT and *Cyp1a2*-null mice showed that mouse CYP1A2 was not responsible for the tumorigenesis seen in the WT mice (Kimura et al., 2003). Conversely, a regimen of oral PhIP plus dextran sodium sulfate in drinking water induced tumorigenesis in the colon of a CYP1A-humanized mouse model (expressing human CYP1A1 and CYP1A2, but not mouse CYP1A1 or CYP1A2), but not in WT mice (Cheung, Loy, Li, Liu, & Yang, 2011), a result suggesting greater potential for human CYP1A enzymes to contribute to dietary carcinogen (such as PhIP)-induced colon cancer in people. The abilities of human CYP1A to mediate PhIP-induced prostate cancer (Li et al., 2012) and, with introduction of concurrent obesity, small intestinal cancer (Wang et al., 2016) have also been demonstrated using the CYP1A-humanized mouse model.

The role of hepatic and intestinal P450 enzymes in the in vivo metabolism and bioactivation of 2-amino-9H-pyrido[2,3-b]indole (AαC), another HAA carcinogen, was examined using LCN mice and IECN mice (Turesky et al., 2015). Hepatic, but not intestinal, P450 was found to be important for the detoxification of orally ingested AαC as higher levels of AαC DNA adduct, N-(deoxyguanosin-8-yl)-2-amino-9H-pyrido[2,3-b]indole (dGC8-AαC), were detected in several extrahepatic tissues of LCN mice, compared to WT mice. Hepatic P450 was also found to partially contribute to hepatic dG-C8-AαC formation, though they were not essential for DNA adduct formation in extrahepatic tissues.

Many nitrosamine carcinogens found in tobacco smoke, such as NNK [4-(methylnitrosoamino)-1-(3-pyridyl)-1-butanone], require P450 for bioactivation. NNK is a tobacco-specific nitrosamine and a lung carcinogen. The essential role of lung, but not liver, P450 enzymes in mediating NNK-induced lung tumorigenesis was convincingly demonstrated using a lung-*Cpr*-null mouse model (Weng et al., 2007). Subsequently, the specific roles of mouse CYP2A, 2B, 2F2, and 2S1 enzymes in NNK-induced lung tumorigenesis was established using *Cyp2abfgs*-null mice (Li, Megaraj, et al., 2014). Furthermore, the ability of human CYP2A13 to mediate NNK-induced lung tumorigenesis was recognized by using a CYP2A13/2B6/2F1-humanized mice on a *Cyp2a5*-null background (Megaraj et al., 2014).

A series of studies have been conducted to identify the CYP enzymes important in the toxicity of naphthalene (NA) in the respiratory tract. NA, the simplest of the PAHs, is a commonly occurring environmental pollutant and possible human carcinogen that is known to cause tumors in the nose in rats and in the lungs in mice. A number of CYP enzymes, such as CYP1A, CYP2A, and CYP2F, are known to bioactivate NA in vitro, producing highly reactive NA oxide, which can be further metabolized to form reactive quinone metabolites or more stable hydroxy metabolites. A suspected role of CYP1A1 and CYP1A2 in mediating NA's olfactory toxicity was rejected by studies using *Cyp1a1*-null and *Cyp1a2*-null mice, which were as sensitive as WT mice to NA-induced cytotoxicity in the olfactory mucosa (Genter et al., 2006). Studies comparing *Cyp2f2*-null mice and WT mice produced strong evidence that CYP2F2, expressed in both the liver and the respiratory tract, and having the highest catalytic efficiency in the formation of NA-GSH from NA among all known CYPs studied, is the major enzyme responsible for NA-induced toxicity in lung airways, though it was not essential for NA-induced cytotoxicity in the olfactory mucosa (Li et al., 2011). A further study using *Cyp2a5*-null mice revealed that, whereas CYP2A5, expressed abundantly in the olfactory mucosa, as well as in the lung and liver, had minimal contribution to NA-induced lung toxicity in mice following i.p. NA administration, it was essential for NA-induced cytotoxicity in the olfactory mucosa (Hu et al., 2014). These studies showed tissue-specific contributions of individual CYP enzymes to xenobiotic toxicity and highlighted the need to consider relative enzyme levels as well as catalytic properties of individual CYP isoforms when predicting toxicity risks from NA and other bioactivated xenobiotics. Further studies using *Cyp2abfgs*-null and CYP2A13/2B6/2F1-humanized mice showed that expression of human CYP2A13 and CYP2F1 in the nasal mucosa and respiratory tract increased NA-mediated damage in the olfactory mucosa and terminal bronchioles of the humanized mice, compared to the *Cyp2abfgs*-null mice (Li et al., 2017). Additionally, studies using LCN mice (Kovalchuk et al., 2017), lung-Cpr-null mice (Kovalchuk, Zhang, Van Winkle, & Ding, 2020), and *Cyp2abfgs*-null/LCN mice

(Kovalchuk, Zhang, Kelty, Van Winkle, & Ding, 2019) revealed the ability of hepatic P450-generated NA metabolites to contribute to its lung toxicity, while confirming the important role of hepatic P450 in the disposition of NA even following inhalation NA exposure, as well as the importance of target tissue bioactivation in NA's lung toxicity.

NA is believed to cause cancer by mostly a non-genotoxic mechanism, through repeated cycles of tissue injury and repair, though NA can form DNA adducts and the involvement of a genotoxic mechanism is still possible (Buchholz et al., 2019; Carratt et al., 2019). Many other chemicals can induce cancer through non-genotoxic mechanisms. P450-catalyzed metabolism of these compounds may result in elevated levels of ROS, which can cause oxidation of DNA as well as changes to basic cellular functions such as proliferation, apoptosis, and senescence. As well, bioactivation of a variety of environmental or dietary toxicants may result in depletion of cellular antioxidants, acute cytotoxicity, necrosis, or other forms of cell death, which may lead to tissue disrepair and possibly carcinogenesis. Thus, studies that identify P450 contributions to acute toxicity, including connections between metabolic events or pathways and direct or indirect toxic endpoints that can contribute to carcinogenesis, are valuable for understanding mechanisms of chemical carcinogenesis as well as other diseases of an environmental origin.

In addition to NA, several respiratory toxicants have been studied utilizing P450 knockout mouse models. For example, the complexity of tissue specific CYP-mediated xenobiotic metabolism was illustrated by studies on the bioactivation of 3-methylindole, a lung and nasal toxicant present in tobacco smoke, using *Cyp2a5*-null and *Cyp2f2*-null mice (Zhou et al., 2012). While CYP2A5 and CYP2F2 both can metabolize 3-methylindole through either epoxidation or dehydrogenation pathways, they produce different metabolites (with CYP2F2 favoring reactive iminium ions and CYP2A5 favoring more stable derivatives), and, as in the case with NA, show tissue-specific dominance in the overall metabolism (CYP2A5 in the olfactory mucosa and CYP2F2 in the lung).

The toxicity of several ROS-inducing compounds has been studied using *Cyp2e1*-null and CYP2E1-humanized mice. Acrylonitrile, a compound used in the manufacture of plastics, is metabolized to reactive epoxide metabolites by P450 enzymes. Acrylonitrile exposure results in oxidative DNA damage and increased levels of ROS (Pu, Kamendulis, & Klaunig, 2009). Comparisons of metabolite profiles in WT and *Cyp2e1*-null mice following exposure to radiolabeled acrylonitrile or methacrylonitrile revealed a major role for CYP2E1 in the bioactivation, and potentially carcinogenesis, of these acrylonitrile-related compounds (Ghanayem, Sanders, Chanas, Burka, & Gonzalez, 1999; Sumner et al., 1999).

Urethane, also known as ethyl carbamate, is an industrial compound that can be generated in yeast-fermented beverages and foods. The majority of urethane is metabolized to ethanol, ammonia and carbon dioxide by microsomal esterases; but a small portion is metabolized to vinyl carbamate and hydroxycarbamates by P450. Its metabolism by P450 increases ROS and could result in the formation of DNA, RNA, and protein adducts (Gowd, Su, Karlovsky, & Chen, 2018; Sakano, Oikawa, Hiraku, & Kawanishi, 2002). Urethane-exposed *Cyp2e1*-null mice had significantly fewer liver hemangiomas and hemangiosarcomas, lung bronchoalveolar adenomas and carcinomas, and hyperplasia and adenomas in Harderian gland compared to WT (Ghanayem, 2007). These results suggested that CYP2E1 is responsible for urethane bioactivation and contributes to urethane carcinogenesis in mice.

Benzene exposure and its induction of acute myeloid leukemia has been well documented. Benzene metabolites cause an increase in ROS and likely cause chromosomal aberrations through the inhibition of DNA topoisomerase II. *Cyp2e1*-null mice was resistant to benzene's cytotoxicity and genotoxicity, whereas WT mice experienced severe toxicity after exposure (Valentine et al., 1996). Overall urinary metabolites in the null mice were reduced compared to WT and the overall metabolite profiles were different.

Exposure to carbon tetrachloride, previously used as a refrigerant and cleaning agent, can result in liver toxicity due to its metabolism into a trichloromethyl radical by CYP2E1; the radical binds to lipids causing lipid peroxidation and increasing ROS (Palmer & Phillips, 2007; Slater, Cheeseman, & Ingold, 1985). *Cyp2e1*-null mice exposed to carbon tetrachloride do not show signs of liver toxicity, while there is clear liver damage in WT-exposed mice (Wong, Chan, & Lee, 1998).

The mechanism of chloroform carcinogenicity is not clear, but none of its metabolites appear to be genotoxic; cytotoxicity following metabolism by CYP2E1 and the subsequent increase in cell proliferation was the predominating hypothesis (Butterworth et al., 1995; Templin et al., 1996). The role of CYP2E1 was confirmed by comparing toxicity in chloroform-exposed WT and *Cyp2e1*-null mice (Constan et al., 1999). The protective role of hepatic P450-mediated chloroform disposition against chloroform-induce renal toxicity was revealed by studies on liver-Cpr-null mice, which were more sensitive than WT mice in the formation of kidney lesions and had higher levels of chloroform remaining in their tissues (Fang et al., 2008). The implied ability of renal P450 to bioactivate chloroform in situ and mediate its toxicity was confirmed in subsequent studies using proximal tubule-specific Cpr-null(PTCN) mice, Cpr-low mice, and extra-proximal tubule-Cpr-low (XPT-CL) mice (which had global suppression of Cpr activity in all extra-proximal tubular tissues); there was less severe toxicity in the PTCN and Cpr-low models compared to WT and XPT-CL, but there were no significant differences in chloroform levels in blood or tissues in any of the models (Liu et al., 2013).

Pyrrolizidine alkaloids (PAs) are common phytotoxins found in many plant species and they are contaminants in foods and herbal products. PAs cause liver toxicity as well as lung and kidney toxicity. Contrary to the lack of dependency of chloroform renal toxicity on hepatic P450-mediated chloroform metabolism, hepatic P450-mediated PA bioactivation seems to have an essential role in PA's toxicity in liver as well as lung and kidney, as was demonstrated by studies using the liver-Cpr-null mice (He et al., 2021; Yao et al., 2014).

5. Conclusion

The vast collection of *Cyp*-null, human CYP-transgenic, and CYP-humanized mouse models is an invaluable resource for fundamental as well as translational research in pharmacology and toxicology. With the recent advances in gene editing technology (Khalil, 2020), and the ability to combine different strains through crossbreeding, it is quite possible to generate more complex mouse models that represent even broader aspects of human xenobiotic metabolism. Studies that utilized these mouse models have made huge contributions to our current understanding of the in vivo functions of many mouse and human CYP enzymes in the metabolism, disposition, and bioactivation of hundreds of xenobiotic compounds, providing foundational knowledge for the prediction and control of drug bioavailability, drug–drug interactions, and drug toxicity, as well as the prevention of carcinogenesis by environmental chemicals. Most of these mouse models are available to the research and development community, and increases in their utility will help to further improve our knowledge of the in vivo functions of various P450 enzymes, which is integral to our ability to develop safer and more effective therapeutics and to identify individuals predisposed to adverse drug reactions or environmental diseases.

Acknowledgments

We would like to thank Lisa Tran and Dr. Qing-Yu Zhang for reading the manuscript. Research in the authors' laboratory was supported in part by grants from the National Institutes of Health (P30 CA023074, P30 ES006694, P42 ES004940, R01 CA092596, R01 ES014901, R01 ES020867, and R01 ES031529). SLH is supported by NIH grant T32 ES007091.

Conflict of interest statement

The authors do not have any conflict of interest to declare.

References

Abdelmegeed, M. A., Moon, K. H., Chen, C., Gonzalez, F. J., & Song, B. J. (2010). Role of cytochrome P450 2E1 in protein nitration and ubiquitin-mediated degradation during acetaminophen toxicity. *Biochemical Pharmacology*, *79*(1), 57–66. https://doi.org/10.1016/j.bcp.2009.07.016.

Abe, S., Kobayashi, K., Oji, A., Sakuma, T., Kazuki, K., Takehara, S., et al. (2017). Modification of single-nucleotide polymorphism in a fully humanized CYP3A mouse by genome editing technology. *Scientific Reports*, 7(1), 15189. https://doi.org/10.1038/s41598-017-15033-0.

Athirakul, K., Bradbury, J. A., Graves, J. P., DeGraff, L. M., Ma, J., Zhao, Y., et al. (2008). Increased blood pressure in mice lacking cytochrome P450 2J5. *The FASEB Journal*, *22*(12), 4096–4108. https://doi.org/10.1096/fj.08-114413.

Bardowell, S. A., Duan, F., Manor, D., Swanson, J. E., & Parker, R. S. (2012). Disruption of mouse cytochrome p450 4f14 (Cyp4f14 gene) causes severe perturbations in vitamin E metabolism. *The Journal of Biological Chemistry*, *287*(31), 26077–26086. https://doi.org/10.1074/jbc.M112.373597.

Bissig, K. D., Han, W., Barzi, M., Kovalchuk, N., Ding, L., Fan, X., et al. (2018). P450-humanized and human liver chimeric mouse models for studying xenobiotic metabolism and toxicity. *Drug Metabolism and Disposition*, *46*(11), 1734–1744. https://doi.org/10.1124/dmd.118.083303.

Buchholz, B. A., Carratt, S. A., Kuhn, E. A., Collette, N. M., Ding, X., & Van Winkle, L. S. (2019). Naphthalene DNA adduct formation and tolerance in the lung. *Nuclear Instruments and Methods in Physics Research B*, *438*, 119–123. https://doi.org/10.1016/j.nimb.2018.07.004.

Buters, J. T., Doehmer, J., & Gonzalez, F. J. (1999). Cytochrome P450-null mice. *Drug Metabolism Reviews*, *31*(2), 437–447. https://doi.org/10.1081/dmr-100101929.

Buters, J. T., Sakai, S., Richter, T., Pineau, T., Alexander, D. L., Savas, U., et al. (1999). Cytochrome P450 CYP1B1 determines susceptibility to 7, 12-dimethylbenz[a] anthracene-induced lymphomas. *Proceedings of the National Academy of Sciences of the United States of America*, *96*(5), 1977–1982. https://doi.org/10.1073/pnas.96.5.1977.

Butterworth, B. E., Templin, M. V., Borghoff, S. J., Conolly, R. B., Kedderis, G. L., & Wolf, D. C. (1995). The role of regenerative cell proliferation in chloroform-induced cancer. *Toxicology Letters*, *82-83*, 23–26. https://doi.org/10.1016/0378-4274(95)03543-5.

Carratt, S. A., Hartog, M., Buchholz, B. A., Kuhn, E. A., Collette, N. M., Ding, X., et al. (2019). Naphthalene genotoxicity: DNA adducts in primate and mouse airway explants. *Toxicology Letters*, *305*, 103–109. https://doi.org/10.1016/j.toxlet.2019.01.009.

Cheng, J., Zhen, Y., Miksys, S., Beyoglu, D., Krausz, K. W., Tyndale, R. F., et al. (2013). Potential role of CYP2D6 in the central nervous system. *Xenobiotica*, *43*(11), 973–984. https://doi.org/10.3109/00498254.2013.791410.

Cheung, C., & Gonzalez, F. J. (2008). Humanized mouse lines and their application for prediction of human drug metabolism and toxicological risk assessment. *The Journal of Pharmacology and Experimental Therapeutics*, *327*(2), 288–299. https://doi.org/10.1124/jpet.108.141242.

Cheung, C., Loy, S., Li, G. X., Liu, A. B., & Yang, C. S. (2011). Rapid induction of colon carcinogenesis in CYP1A-humanized mice by 2-amino-1-methyl-6-phenylimidazo [4,5-b]pyridine and dextran sodium sulfate. *Carcinogenesis*, *32*(2), 233–239. https://doi.org/10.1093/carcin/bgq235.

Cheung, C., Yu, A. M., Chen, C. S., Krausz, K. W., Byrd, L. G., Feigenbaum, L., et al. (2006). Growth hormone determines sexual dimorphism of hepatic cytochrome P450 3A4 expression in transgenic mice. *The Journal of Pharmacology and Experimental Therapeutics*, *316*(3), 1328–1334. https://doi.org/10.1124/jpet.105.094367.

Cheung, C., Yu, A. M., Ward, J. M., Krausz, K. W., Akiyama, T. E., Feigenbaum, L., et al. (2005). The cyp2e1-humanized transgenic mouse: Role of cyp2e1 in acetaminophen hepatotoxicity. *Drug Metabolism and Disposition*, *33*(3), 449–457. https://doi.org/10.1124/dmd.104.002402.

Constan, A. A., Sprankle, C. S., Peters, J. M., Kedderis, G. L., Everitt, J. I., Wong, B. A., et al. (1999). Metabolism of chloroform by cytochrome P450 2E1 is required for induction of toxicity in the liver, kidney, and nose of male mice. *Toxicology and Applied Pharmacology*, *160*(2), 120–126. https://doi.org/10.1006/taap.1999.8756.

Corchero, J., Granvil, C. P., Akiyama, T. E., Hayhurst, G. P., Pimprale, S., Feigenbaum, L., et al. (2001). The CYP2D6 humanized mouse: Effect of the human CYP2D6 transgene and HNF4alpha on the disposition of debrisoquine in the mouse. *Molecular Pharmacology*, *60*(6), 1260–1267. https://doi.org/10.1124/mol.60.6.1260.

Dalton, T. P., Dieter, M. Z., Matlib, R. S., Childs, N. L., Shertzer, H. G., Genter, M. B., et al. (2000). Targeted knockout of Cyp1a1 gene does not alter hepatic constitutive expression of other genes in the mouse [ah] battery. *Biochemical and Biophysical Research Communications*, *267*(1), 184–189. https://doi.org/10.1006/bbrc.1999.1913.

Damiri, B., Holle, E., Yu, X., & Baldwin, W. S. (2012). Lentiviral-mediated RNAi knockdown yields a novel mouse model for studying Cyp2b function. *Toxicological Sciences: An Official Journal of the Society of Toxicology*, *125*(2), 368–381. https://doi.org/10.1093/toxsci/kfr309.

de Boer, J. F., Verkade, E., Mulder, N. L., de Vries, H. D., Huijkman, N., Koehorst, M., et al. (2020). A human-like bile acid pool induced by deletion of hepatic Cyp2c70 modulates effects of FXR activation in mice. *Journal of Lipid Research*, *61*(3), 291–305. https://doi.org/10.1194/jlr.RA119000243.

Ding, L., Li, L., Liu, S., Bao, X., Dickman, K. G., Sell, S. S., et al. (2020). Proximal tubular vacuolization and hypersensitivity to drug-induced nephrotoxicity in male mice with decreased expression of the NADPH-cytochrome P450 reductase. *Toxicological Sciences*, *173*(2), 362–372. https://doi.org/10.1093/toxsci/kfz225.

Dragin, N., Shi, Z., Madan, R., Karp, C. L., Sartor, M. A., Chen, C., et al. (2008). Phenotype of the Cyp1a1/1a2/1b1 −/− triple-knockout mouse. *Molecular Pharmacology*, *73*(6), 1844–1856. https://doi.org/10.1124/mol.108.045658.

Dragin, N., Uno, S., Wang, B., Dalton, T. P., & Nebert, D. W. (2007). Generation of 'humanized' hCYP1A1_1A2_Cyp1a1/1a2(−/−) mouse line. *Biochemical and Biophysical Research Communications*, *359*(3), 635–642. https://doi.org/10.1016/j.bbrc.2007.05.202.

Fan, X., Li, H., Ding, X., & Zhang, Q.-Y. (2019). Contributions of hepatic and intestinal metabolism to the disposition of Niclosamide, a repurposed drug with poor bioavailability. *Drug Metabolism and Disposition*, *47*(7), 756–763. https://doi.org/10.1124/dmd.119.086678.

Fang, C., Behr, M., Xie, F., Lu, S., Doret, M., Luo, H., et al. (2008). Mechanism of chloroform-induced renal toxicity: Non-involvement of hepatic cytochrome P450-dependent metabolism. *Toxicology and Applied Pharmacology*, *227*(1), 48–55. https://doi.org/10.1016/j.taap.2007.10.014.

Fang, C., & Zhang, Q. Y. (2010). The role of small-intestinal P450 enzymes in protection against systemic exposure of orally administered benzo[a]pyrene. *The Journal of Pharmacology and Experimental Therapeutics*, *334*(1), 156–163. https://doi.org/10.1124/jpet.110.167742.

Felmlee, M. A., Lon, H. K., Gonzalez, F. J., & Yu, A. M. (2008). Cytochrome P450 expression and regulation in CYP3A4/CYP2D6 double transgenic humanized mice. *Drug Metabolism and Disposition*, *36*(2), 435–441. https://doi.org/10.1124/dmd.107.018838.

Galvez-Peralta, M., Shi, Z., Chen, J., Miller, M. L., & Nebert, D. W. (2013). Oral benzo[a]pyrene in Cyp1a1/1b1(−/−) double-knockout mice: Microarray analysis during squamous cell carcinoma formation in preputial gland duct. *International Journal of Cancer*, *132*(9), 2065–2075. https://doi.org/10.1002/ijc.27897.

Genter, M. B., Liang, H. C., Gu, J., Ding, X., Negishi, M., McKinnon, R. A., et al. (1998). Role of CYP2A5 and 2G1 in acetaminophen metabolism and toxicity in the olfactory mucosa of the Cyp1a2(−/−) mouse. *Biochemical Pharmacology*, *55*(11), 1819–1826. https://doi.org/10.1016/s0006-2952(98)00004-5.

Genter, M. B., Marlowe, J., Kevin Kerzee, J., Dragin, N., Puga, A., Dalton, T. P., et al. (2006). Naphthalene toxicity in mice and aryl hydrocarbon receptor-mediated CYPs. *Biochemical and Biophysical Research Communications*, *348*(1), 120–123. https://doi.org/10.1016/j.bbrc.2006.07.025.

Ghanayem, B. I. (2007). Inhibition of urethane-induced carcinogenicity in cyp2e1 −/− in comparison to cyp2e1 +/+ mice. *Toxicological Sciences: An Official Journal of the Society of Toxicology*, *95*(2), 331–339. https://doi.org/10.1093/toxsci/kfl158.

Ghanayem, B. I., Sanders, J. M., Chanas, B., Burka, L. T., & Gonzalez, F. J. (1999). Role of cytochrome P-450 2E1 in methacrylonitrile metabolism and disposition. *The Journal of Pharmacology and Experimental Therapeutics*, *289*(2), 1054–1059 (Retrieved from https://www.ncbi.nlm.nih.gov/pubmed/10215687).

Ghanayem, B. I., Wang, H., & Sumner, S. (2000). Using cytochrome P-450 gene knock-out mice to study chemical metabolism, toxicity, and carcinogenicity. *Toxicologic Pathology*, *28*(6), 839–850. https://doi.org/10.1177/019262330002800613.

Gilani, A., Agostinucci, K., Pascale, J. V., Hossain, S., Kandhi, S., Pandey, V., et al. (2020). Proximal tubular-targeted overexpression of the Cyp4a12-20-HETE synthase promotes salt-sensitive hypertension in male mice. *American Journal of Physiology. Regulatory, Integrative and Comparative Physiology*. https://doi.org/10.1152/ajpregu.00089.2020.

Gonzalez, F. J. (2004). Cytochrome P450 humanised mice. *Human Genomics*, *1*(4), 300–306. https://doi.org/10.1186/1479-7364-1-4-300.

Gonzalez, F. J., & Yu, A. M. (2006). Cytochrome P450 and xenobiotic receptor humanized mice. *Annual Review of Pharmacology and Toxicology*, *46*(1), 41–64. https://doi.org/10.1146/annurev.pharmtox.45.120403.100007.

Gooderham, N. J., Creton, S., Lauber, S. N., & Zhu, H. (2007). Mechanisms of action of the carcinogenic heterocyclic amine PhIP. *Toxicology Letters*, *168*(3), 269–277. https://doi.org/10.1016/j.toxlet.2006.10.022.

Gowd, V., Su, H., Karlovsky, P., & Chen, W. (2018). Ethyl carbamate: An emerging food and environmental toxicant. *Food Chemistry*, *248*, 312–321. https://doi.org/10.1016/j.foodchem.2017.12.072.

Granvil, C. P., Yu, A. M., Elizondo, G., Akiyama, T. E., Cheung, C., Feigenbaum, L., et al. (2003). Expression of the human CYP3A4 gene in the small intestine of transgenic mice: In vitro metabolism and pharmacokinetics of midazolam. *Drug Metabolism and Disposition*, *31*(5), 548–558. https://doi.org/10.1124/dmd.31.5.548.

Grimsley, A., Gallagher, R., Hutchison, M., Pickup, K., Wilson, I. D., & Samuelsson, K. (2013). Drug-drug interactions and metabolism in cytochrome P450 2C knockout mice: Application to troleandomycin and midazolam. *Biochemical Pharmacology*, *86*(4), 529–538. https://doi.org/10.1016/j.bcp.2013.05.015.

Gu, J., Cui, H., Behr, M., Zhang, L., Zhang, Q. Y., Yang, W., et al. (2005). In vivo mechanisms of tissue-selective drug toxicity: Effects of liver-specific knockout of the NADPH-cytochrome P450 reductase gene on acetaminophen toxicity in kidney, lung, and nasal mucosa. *Molecular Pharmacology*, *67*(3), 623–630. https://doi.org/10.1124/mol.104.007898.

Gu, J., Weng, Y., Zhang, Q. Y., Cui, H., Behr, M., Wu, L., et al. (2003). Liver-specific deletion of the NADPH-cytochrome P450 reductase gene: Impact on plasma cholesterol homeostasis and the function and regulation of microsomal cytochrome P450 and heme oxygenase. *The Journal of Biological Chemistry*, *278*(28), 25895–25901. https://doi.org/10.1074/jbc.M303125200.

Gu, J., Zhang, Q. Y., Genter, M. B., Lipinskas, T. W., Negishi, M., Nebert, D. W., et al. (1998). Purification and characterization of heterologously expressed mouse CYP2A5 and CYP2G1: Role in metabolic activation of acetaminophen and 2,6-dichlorobenzonitrile in mouse olfactory mucosal microsomes. *The Journal of Pharmacology and Experimental Therapeutics*, *285*(3), 1287–1295 (Retrieved from https://www.ncbi.nlm.nih.gov/pubmed/9618435).

Hasegawa, M., Kapelyukh, Y., Tahara, H., Seibler, J., Rode, A., Krueger, S., et al. (2011). Quantitative prediction of human pregnane X receptor and cytochrome P450 3A4 mediated drug-drug interaction in a novel multiple humanized mouse line. *Molecular Pharmacology*, *80*(3), 518–528. https://doi.org/10.1124/mol.111.071845.

He, Y., Lian, W., Ding, L., Fan, X., Ma, J., Zhang, Q. Y., et al. (2021). Lung injury induced by pyrrolizidine alkaloids depends on metabolism by hepatic cytochrome P450s and blood transport of reactive metabolites. *Archives of Toxicology*, *95*(1), 103–116. https://doi.org/10.1007/s00204-020-02921-0.

Heidel, S. M., Holston, K., Buters, J. T. M., Gonzalez, F. J., Jefcoate, C. R., & Czupyrynski, C. J. (1999). Bone marrow stromal cell cytochrome P450B1 is required for pre-B cell apoptosis induced by 7,12-Dimethylbenz[a]anthracene. *Molecular Pharmacology*, *56*, 1317–1323.

Heidel, S. M., MacWilliams, P. S., Baird, W. M., Dashwood, W. M., Buters, J. T. M., Gonzalez, F. J., et al. (2000). Cytochrome P450B1 mediates induction of bone marrow cytotoxicity and preleukemia cells in mice treated with 7,12-Dimethylbenz[*a*]anthracene. *Cancer Research*, *60*, 3454–3460.

Henderson, C. J., Kapelyukh, Y., Scheer, N., Rode, A., McLaren, A. W., MacLeod, A. K., et al. (2019). An extensively humanized mouse model to predict pathways of drug disposition and drug/drug interactions, and to facilitate Design of Clinical Trials. *Drug Metabolism and Disposition*, *47*(6), 601–615. https://doi.org/10.1124/dmd.119.086397.

Henderson, C. J., Otto, D. M., Carrie, D., Magnuson, M. A., McLaren, A. W., Rosewell, I., et al. (2003). Inactivation of the hepatic cytochrome P450 system by conditional deletion of hepatic cytochrome P450 reductase. *The Journal of Biological Chemistry*, *278*(15), 13480–13486. https://doi.org/10.1074/jbc.M212087200.

Henderson, C. J., & Wolf, C. R. (2003). Transgenic analysis of human drug-metabolizing enzymes: Preclinical drug development and toxicology. *Molecular Interventions*, *3*(6), 331–343. https://doi.org/10.1124/mi.3.6.331.

Hendrikx, J., Stuurman, F. E., Song, J. Y., de Weger, V. A., Lagas, J. S., Rosing, H., et al. (2020). No relation between docetaxel administration route and high-grade diarrhea incidence. *Pharmacology Research & Perspectives*, *8*(4), e00633. https://doi.org/10.1002/prp2.633.

Holla, V. R., Adas, F., Imig, J. D., Zhao, X., Price, E., Jr., Olsen, N., et al. (2001). Alterations in the regulation of androgen-sensitive Cyp 4a monooxygenases cause hypertension.

Proceedings of the National Academy of Sciences of the United States of America, 98(9), 5211–5216. https://doi.org/10.1073/pnas.081627898.

Honda, A., Miyazaki, T., Iwamoto, J., Hirayama, T., Morishita, Y., Monma, T., et al. (2020). Regulation of bile acid metabolism in mouse models with hydrophobic bile acid composition. *Journal of Lipid Research, 61*(1), 54–69. https://doi.org/10.1194/jlr.RA119000395.

Hough, L. B., Nalwalk, J. W., Ding, X., & Scheer, N. (2015). Opioid analgesia in P450 gene cluster knockout mice: A search for analgesia-relevant isoforms. *Drug Metabolism and Disposition, 43*(9), 1326–1330. https://doi.org/10.1124/dmd.115.065490.

Hu, J., Sheng, L., Li, L., Zhou, X., Xie, F., D'Agostino, J., et al. (2014). Essential role of the cytochrome P450 enzyme CYP2A5 in olfactory mucosal toxicity of naphthalene. *Drug Metabolism and Disposition, 42*(1), 23–27. https://doi.org/10.1124/dmd.113.054429.

Hwang, D. Y., Chae, K. R., Shin, D. H., Hwang, J. H., Lim, C. H., Kim, Y. J., et al. (2001). Xenobiotic response in humanized double transgenic mice expressing tetracycline-controlled transactivator and human CYP1B1. *Archives of Biochemistry and Biophysics, 395*(1), 32–40. https://doi.org/10.1006/abbi.2001.2542.

Imaoka, S., Hayashi, K., Hiroi, T., Yabusaki, Y., Kamataki, T., & Funae, Y. (2001). A transgenic mouse expressing human CYP4B1 in the liver. *Biochemical and Biophysical Research Communications, 284*(3), 757–762. https://doi.org/10.1006/bbrc.2001.5055.

Ishibashi, S., Schwarz, M., Frykman, P. K., Herz, J., & Russell, D. W. (1996). Disruption of cholesterol 7alpha-hydroxylase gene in mice. I. Postnatal lethality reversed by bile acid and vitamin supplementation. *The Journal of Biological Chemistry, 271*(30), 18017–18023. https://doi.org/10.1074/jbc.271.30.18017.

Jia, K., Li, L., Liu, Z., Hartog, M., Kluetzman, K., Zhang, Q. Y., et al. (2014). Generation and characterization of a novel CYP2A13--transgenic mouse model. *Drug Metabolism and Disposition, 42*(8), 1341–1348. https://doi.org/10.1124/dmd.114.059188.

Jiang, Z., Dalton, T. P., Jin, L., Wang, B., Tsuneoka, Y., Shertzer, H. G., et al. (2005). Toward the evaluation of function in genetic variability: Characterizing human SNP frequencies and establishing BAC-transgenic mice carrying the human CYP1A1_CYP1A2 locus. *Human Mutation, 25*(2), 196–206. https://doi.org/10.1002/humu.20134.

Jiang, X. L., Gonzalez, F. J., & Yu, A. M. (2011). Drug-metabolizing enzyme, transporter, and nuclear receptor genetically modified mouse models. *Drug Metabolism Reviews, 43*(1), 27–40. https://doi.org/10.3109/03602532.2010.512294.

Kazuki, Y., Akita, M., Kobayashi, K., Osaki, M., Satoh, D., Ohta, R., et al. (2016). Thalidomide-induced limb abnormalities in a humanized CYP3A mouse model. *Scientific Reports, 6*(1), 21419. https://doi.org/10.1038/srep21419.

Kazuki, Y., Kobayashi, K., Aueviriyavit, S., Oshima, T., Kuroiwa, Y., Tsukazaki, Y., et al. (2013). Trans-chromosomic mice containing a human CYP3A cluster for prediction of xenobiotic metabolism in humans. *Human Molecular Genetics, 22*(3), 578–592. https://doi.org/10.1093/hmg/dds468.

Khalil, A. M. (2020). The genome editing revolution: Review. *Journal, Genetic Engineering & Biotechnology, 18*(1), 68. https://doi.org/10.1186/s43141-020-00078-y.

Kharkwal, H., Batool, F., Koentgen, F., Bell, D. R., Kendall, D. A., Ebling, F. J. P., et al. (2017). Generation and phenotypic characterisation of a cytochrome P450 4x1 knockout mouse. *PLoS One, 12*(12), e0187959. https://doi.org/10.1371/journal.pone.0187959.

Kimura, S., Kawabe, M., Yu, A., Morishima, H., Fernandez-Salguero, P., Hammons, G. J., et al. (2003). Carcinogenesis of the food mutagen PhIP in mice is independent of CYP1A2. *Carcinogenesis, 24*(3), 583–587. https://doi.org/10.1093/carcin/24.3.583.

Kobayashi, K., Kuze, J., Abe, S., Takehara, S., Minegishi, G., Igarashi, K., et al. (2019). CYP3A4 induction in the liver and intestine of Pregnane X receptor/CYP3A-humanized mice: Approaches by mass spectrometry imaging and portal blood analysis. *Molecular Pharmacology, 96*(5), 600–608. https://doi.org/10.1124/mol.119.117333.

Konstandi, M., Andriopoulou, C. E., Cheng, J., & Gonzalez, F. J. (2020). Sex steroid hormones differentially regulate CYP2D in female wild-type and CYP2D6-humanized mice. *The Journal of Endocrinology*, *245*(2), 301–314. https://doi.org/10.1530/JOE-19-0561.

Kovalchuk, N., Kelty, J., Li, L., Hartog, M., Zhang, Q.-Y., Edwards, P., et al. (2017). Impact of hepatic P450-mediated biotransformation on the disposition and respiratory tract toxicity of inhaled naphthalene. *Toxicology and Applied Pharmacology*, *329*, 1–8. https://doi.org/10.1016/j.taap.2017.05.015.

Kovalchuk, N., Zhang, Q. Y., Kelty, J., Van Winkle, L., & Ding, X. (2019). Toxicokinetic interaction between hepatic disposition and pulmonary bioactivation of inhaled naphthalene studied using Cyp2abfgs-null and CYP2A13/2F1-humanized mice with deficient hepatic cytochrome P450 activity. *Drug Metabolism and Disposition*, *47*(12), 1469–1478. https://doi.org/10.1124/dmd.119.088930.

Kovalchuk, N., Zhang, Q. Y., Van Winkle, L., & Ding, X. (2020). Contribution of pulmonary CYP-mediated bioactivation of naphthalene to airway epithelial injury in the lung. *Toxicological Sciences: An Official Journal of the Society of Toxicology*, *177*(2), 334–346. https://doi.org/10.1093/toxsci/kfaa114.

Kumar, R., Mota, L. C., Litoff, E. J., Rooney, J. P., Boswell, W. T., Courter, E., et al. (2017). Compensatory changes in CYP expression in three different toxicology mouse models: CAR-null, Cyp3a-null, and Cyp2b9/10/13-null mice. *PLoS One*, *12*(3), e0174355. https://doi.org/10.1371/journal.pone.0174355.

Lai, G., Liu, X., Wu, J., Liu, H., & Zhao, Y. (2012). Evaluation of CMV and KAP promoters for driving the expression of human CYP4F2 in transgenic mice. *International Journal of Molecular Medicine*, *29*(1), 107–112. https://doi.org/10.3892/ijmm.2011.787.

Lee, S. S., Buters, J. T., Pineau, T., Fernandez-Salguero, P., & Gonzalez, F. J. (1996). Role of CYP2E1 in the hepatotoxicity of acetaminophen. *The Journal of Biological Chemistry*, *271*(20), 12063–12067. https://doi.org/10.1074/jbc.271.20.12063.

Lee, C. R., Imig, J. D., Edin, M. L., Foley, J., DeGraff, L. M., Bradbury, J. A., et al. (2010). Endothelial expression of human cytochrome P450 epoxygenases lowers blood pressure and attenuates hypertension-induced renal injury in mice. *The FASEB Journal*, *24*(10), 3770–3781. https://doi.org/10.1096/fj.10-160119.

Li, L., Carratt, S., Hartog, M., Kovalchik, N., Jia, K., Wang, Y., et al. (2017). Human CYP2A13 and CYP2F1 mediate naphthalene toxicity in the lung and nasal mucosa of CYP2A13/2F1-humanized mice. *Environmental Health Perspectives*, *125*(6), 067004. https://doi.org/10.1289/EHP844.

Li, F., Jiang, C., Larsen, M. C., Bushkofsky, J., Krausz, K. W., Wang, T., et al. (2014). Lipidomics reveals a link between CYP1B1 and SCD1 in promoting obesity. *Journal of Proteome Research*, *13*(5), 2679–2687. https://doi.org/10.1021/pr500145n.

Li, L., Megaraj, V., Wei, Y., & Ding, X. (2014). Identification of cytochrome P450 enzymes critical for lung tumorigenesis by the tobacco-specific carcinogen 4-(methylnitrosamino)-1-(3-pyridyl)-1-butanone (NNK): Insights from a novel Cyp2abfgs-null mouse. *Carcinogenesis*, *35*(11), 2584–2591. https://doi.org/10.1093/carcin/bgu182.

Li, W., Sparidans, R. W., Lebre, M. C., Beijnen, J. H., & Schinkel, A. H. (2021). ABCB1 and ABCG2 control brain accumulation and intestinal disposition of the novel ROS1/TRK/ALK inhibitor Repotrectinib, while OATP1A/1B, ABCG2, and CYP3A limit its Oral availability. *Pharmaceutics*, *13*(11). https://doi.org/10.3390/pharmaceutics13111761.

Li, W., Sparidans, R. W., Martins, M. L. F., El-Lari, M., Lebre, M. C., van Tellingen, O., et al. (2021). ABCB1 and ABCG2 restrict brain and testis accumulation and, alongside CYP3A, limit Oral availability of the novel TRK inhibitor Selitrectinib. *Molecular Cancer Therapeutics*, *20*(6), 1173–1182. https://doi.org/10.1158/1535-7163.MCT-20-0705.

Li, W., Sparidans, R. W., Wang, Y., Lebre, M. C., Beijnen, J. H., & Schinkel, A. H. (2019). Oral coadministration of elacridar and ritonavir enhances brain accumulation and oral availability of the novel ALK/ROS1 inhibitor lorlatinib. *European Journal of Pharmaceutics and Biopharmaceutics*, *136*, 120–130. https://doi.org/10.1016/j.ejpb.2019.01.016.

Li, W., Sparidans, R. W., Wang, Y., Lebre, M. C., Wagenaar, E., Beijnen, J. H., et al. (2018). P-glycoprotein (MDR1/ABCB1) restricts brain accumulation and cytochrome P450-3A (CYP3A) limits oral availability of the novel ALK/ROS1 inhibitor lorlatinib. *International Journal of Cancer*, *143*(8), 2029–2038. https://doi.org/10.1002/ijc.31582.

Li, W., Tibben, M., Wang, Y., Lebre, M. C., Rosing, H., Beijnen, J. H., et al. (2020). P-glycoprotein (MDR1/ABCB1) controls brain accumulation and intestinal disposition of the novel TGF-beta signaling pathway inhibitor galunisertib. *International Journal of Cancer*, *146*(6), 1631–1642. https://doi.org/10.1002/ijc.32568.

Li, G., Wang, H., Liu, A. B., Cheung, C., Reuhl, K. R., Bosland, M. C., et al. (2012). Dietary carcinogen 2-amino-1-methyl-6-phenylimidazo[4,5-b]pyridine-induced prostate carcinogenesis in CYP1A-humanized mice. *Cancer Prevention Research (Philadelphia, Pa.)*, *5*(7), 963–972. https://doi.org/10.1158/1940-6207.CAPR-12-0023.

Li, L., Wei, Y., Van Winkle, L., Zhang, Q. Y., Zhou, X., Hu, J., et al. (2011). Generation and characterization of a Cyp2f2-null mouse and studies on the role of CYP2F2 in naphthalene-induced toxicity in the lung and nasal olfactory mucosa. *The Journal of Pharmacology and Experimental Therapeutics*, *339*(1), 62–71. https://doi.org/10.1124/jpet.111.184671.

Li, Y., Yokoi, T., Kitamura, R., Sasaki, M., Gunji, M., Katsuki, M., et al. (1996). Establishment of transgenic mice carrying human fetus-specific CYP3A7. *Archives of Biochemistry and Biophysics*, *329*(2), 235–240. https://doi.org/10.1006/abbi.1996.0214.

Liang, H. C., Li, H., McKinnon, R. A., Duffy, J. J., Potter, S. S., Puga, A., et al. (1996). Cyp1a2(−/−) null mutant mice develop normally but show deficient drug metabolism. *Proceedings of the National Academy of Sciences of the United States of America*, *93*(4), 1671–1676. https://doi.org/10.1073/pnas.93.4.1671.

Lin, Y., Yao, Y., Liu, S., Wang, L., Moorthy, B., Xiong, D., et al. (2012). Role of mammary epithelial and stromal P450 enzymes in the clearance and metabolic activation of 7,12-dimethylbenz(a)anthracene in mice. *Toxicology Letters*, *212*(2), 97–105. https://doi.org/10.1016/j.toxlet.2012.05.005.

Liu, S., Yao, Y., Lu, S., Aldous, K., Ding, X., Mei, C., et al. (2013). The role of renal proximal tubule P450 enzymes in chloroform-induced nephrotoxicity: Utility of renal specific P450 reductase knockout mouse models. *Toxicology and Applied Pharmacology*, *272*(1), 230–237. https://doi.org/10.1016/j.taap.2013.05.022.

Liu, X., Zhao, Y., Wang, L., Yang, X., Zheng, Z., Zhang, Y., et al. (2009). Overexpression of cytochrome P450 4F2 in mice increases 20-hydroxyeicosatetraenoic acid production and arterial blood pressure. *Kidney International*, *75*(12), 1288–1296. https://doi.org/10.1038/ki.2009.67.

Lockhart, C. M., Nakano, M., Rettie, A. E., & Kelly, E. J. (2014). Generation and characterization of a murine model of Bietti crystalline dystrophy. *Investigative Ophthalmology & Visual Science*, *55*(9), 5572–5581. https://doi.org/10.1167/iovs.13-13717.

Lofgren, S., Baldwin, R. M., Hiratsuka, M., Lindqvist, A., Carlberg, A., Sim, S. C., et al. (2008). Generation of mice transgenic for human CYP2C18 and CYP2C19: Characterization of the sexually dimorphic gene and enzyme expression. *Drug Metabolism and Disposition*, *36*(5), 955–962. https://doi.org/10.1124/dmd.107.019349.

Lorbek, G., Lewinska, M., & Rozman, D. (2012). Cytochrome P450s in the synthesis of cholesterol and bile acids- -from mouse models to human diseases. *The FEBS Journal*, *279*(9), 1516–1533. https://doi.org/10.1111/j.1742-4658.2011.08432.x.

Lu, J., Liu, J., Guo, Y., Zhang, Y., Xu, Y., & Wang, X. (2021). CRISPR-Cas9: A method for establishing rat models of drug metabolism and pharmacokinetics. *Acta Pharmaceutica Sinica B, 11*(10), 2973–2982. https://doi.org/10.1016/j.apsb.2021.01.007.

Ly, J. Q., Messick, K., Qin, A., Takahashi, R. H., & Choo, E. F. (2017). Utility of CYP3A4 and PXR-CAR-CYP3A4/3A7 transgenic mouse models to assess the magnitude of CYP3A4 mediated drug–drug interactions. *Molecular Pharmaceutics, 14*(5), 1754–1759. https://doi.org/10.1021/acs.molpharmaceut.7b00006.

Ly, J. Q., Wong, S., Liu, L., Li, R., Messick, K., & Chang, J. H. (2021). Investigating the utility of humanized Pregnane X receptor-constitutive androstane receptor-CYP3A4/7 mouse model to assess CYP3A-mediated induction. *Drug Metabolism and Disposition, 49*(7), 540–547. https://doi.org/10.1124/dmd.121.000439.

Ma, X., Cheung, C., Krausz, K. W., Shah, Y. M., Wang, T., Idle, J. R., et al. (2008). A double transgenic mouse model expressing human pregnane X receptor and cytochrome P450 3A4. *Drug Metabolism and Disposition, 36*(12), 2506–2512. https://doi.org/10.1124/dmd.108.022723.

MacLeod, A. K., Lin, D., Huang, J. T., McLaughlin, L. A., Henderson, C. J., & Wolf, C. R. (2018). Identification of novel pathways of Osimertinib disposition and potential implications for the outcome of lung cancer therapy. *Clinical Cancer Research, 24*(9), 2138–2147. https://doi.org/10.1158/1078-0432.CCR-17-3555.

MacLeod, A. K., McLaughlin, L. A., Henderson, C. J., & Wolf, C. R. (2017). Application of mice humanized for CYP2D6 to the study of tamoxifen metabolism and drug-drug interaction with antidepressants. *Drug Metabolism and Disposition, 45*(1), 17–22. https://doi.org/10.1124/dmd.116.073437.

Megaraj, V., Zhou, X., Xie, F., Liu, Z., Yang, W., & Ding, X. (2014). Role of CYP2A13 in the bioactivation and lung tumorigenicity of the tobacco-specific lung procarcinogen 4-(methylnitrosamino)-1-(3-pyridyl)-1-butanone: In vivo studies using a CYP2A13-humanized mouse model. *Carcinogenesis, 35*(1), 131–137. https://doi.org/10.1093/carcin/bgt269.

Mescher, M., Tigges, J., Rolfes, K. M., Shen, A. L., Yee, J. S., Vogeley, C., et al. (2019). The toll-like receptor agonist imiquimod is metabolized by aryl hydrocarbon receptor-regulated cytochrome P450 enzymes in human keratinocytes and mouse liver. *Archives of Toxicology, 93*(7), 1917–1926. https://doi.org/10.1007/s00204-019-02488-5.

Miller, R. P., Tadagavadi, R. K., Ramesh, G., & Reeves, W. B. (2010). Mechanisms of cisplatin nephrotoxicity. *Toxins, 2*(11), 2490–2518. https://doi.org/10.3390/toxins2112490.

Minegishi, G., Kazuki, Y., Yamasaki, Y., Okuya, F., Akita, H., Oshimura, M., et al. (2019). Comparison of the hepatic metabolism of triazolam in wild-type andCyp3a-knockout mice for understanding CYP3A-mediated metabolism inCYP3A-humanised mice in vivo. *Xenobiotica, 49*(11), 1303–1310. https://doi.org/10.1080/00498254.2018.1560516.

Miyamoto, M., Itoh, N., Sawai, M., Sassa, T., & Kihara, A. (2020). Severe skin permeability barrier dysfunction in knockout mice deficient in a fatty acid omega-hydroxylase crucial to Acylceramide production. *The Journal of Investigative Dermatology, 140*(2), 319–326 e314. https://doi.org/10.1016/j.jid.2019.07.689.

Miyata, M., Furukawa, M., Takahashi, K., Gonzalez, F. J., & Yamazoe, Y. (2001). Mechanism of 7,12-dimethylbenz[a]anthracene-induced immunotoxicity: Role of metabolic activation at the target organ. *Japanese Journal of Pharmacology, 86*(3), 302–309. https://doi.org/10.1254/jjp.86.302.

Morgan, K., French, S. W., & Morgan, T. R. (2002). Production of a cytochrome P450 2E1 transgenic mouse and initial evaluation of alcoholic liver damage. *Hepatology, 36*(1), 122–134. https://doi.org/10.1053/jhep.2002.33720.

Nakagawa, K., Holla, V. R., Wei, Y., Wang, W. H., Gatica, A., Wei, S., et al. (2006). Salt-sensitive hypertension is associated with dysfunctional Cyp4a10 gene and kidney epithelial sodium channel. *The Journal of Clinical Investigation, 116*(6), 1696–1702. https://doi.org/10.1172/JCI27546.

Palmer, R. B., & Phillips, S. D. (2007). Chlorinated hydrocarbons. In M. W. Shannon, S. W. Borron, & M. J. Burns (Eds.), *Haddad and Winchester's clinical management of poisoning and drug overdose* (pp. 1347–1361). Philadelphia: W.B. Saunders.

Parkinson, O. T., Liggitt, H. D., Rettie, A. E., & Kelly, E. J. (2013). Generation and characterization of a Cyp4b1 null mouse and the role of CYP4B1 in the activation and toxicity of Ipomeanol. *Toxicological Sciences: An Official Journal of the Society of Toxicology*, *134*(2), 243–250. https://doi.org/10.1093/toxsci/kft123.

Pineau, T., Fernandez-Salguero, P., Lee, S. S., McPhail, T., Ward, J. M., & Gonzalez, F. J. (1995). Neonatal lethality associated with respiratory distress in mice lacking cytochrome P450 1A2. *Proceedings of the National Academy of Sciences of the United States of America*, *92*(11), 5134–5138. https://doi.org/10.1073/pnas.92.11.5134.

Pozzi, A., Popescu, V., Yang, S., Mei, S., Shi, M., Puolitaival, S. M., et al. (2010). The anti-tumorigenic properties of peroxisomal proliferator-activated receptor alpha are arachidonic acid epoxygenase-mediated. *The Journal of Biological Chemistry*, *285*(17), 12840–12850. https://doi.org/10.1074/jbc.M109.081554.

Pu, X., Kamendulis, L. M., & Klaunig, J. E. (2009). Acrylonitrile-induced oxidative stress and oxidative DNA damage in male Sprague-Dawley rats. *Toxicological Sciences: An Official Journal of the Society of Toxicology*, *111*(1), 64–71. https://doi.org/10.1093/toxsci/kfp133.

Pujol, C., Legrand, A., Parodi, L., Thomas, P., Mochel, F., Saracino, D., et al. (2021). Implication of folate deficiency in CYP2U1 loss of function. *The Journal of Experimental Medicine*, *218*(11). https://doi.org/10.1084/jem.20210846.

Reed, L., Arlt, V. M., & Phillips, D. H. (2018). The role of cytochrome P450 enzymes in carcinogen activation and detoxication: An in vivo-in vitro paradox. *Carcinogenesis*, *39*(7), 851–859. https://doi.org/10.1093/carcin/bgy058.

Sakano, K., Oikawa, S., Hiraku, Y., & Kawanishi, S. (2002). Metabolism of carcinogenic urethane to nitric oxide is involved in oxidative DNA damage. *Free Radical Biology & Medicine*, *33*(5), 703–714. https://doi.org/10.1016/s0891-5849(02)00969-3.

Savas, U., Machemer, D. E. W., Hsu, M. H., Gaynor, P., Lasker, J. M., Tukey, R. H., et al. (2009). Opposing roles of peroxisome proliferator-activated receptor alpha and growth hormone in the regulation of CYP4A11 expression in a transgenic mouse model. *The Journal of Biological Chemistry*, *284*(24), 16541–16552. https://doi.org/10.1074/jbc.M902074200.

Scheer, N., Kapelyukh, Y., Chatham, L., Rode, A., Buechel, S., & Wolf, C. R. (2012). Generation and characterization of novel cytochrome P450 Cyp2c gene cluster knockout and CYP2C9 humanized mouse lines. *Molecular Pharmacology*, *82*(6), 1022–1029. https://doi.org/10.1124/mol.112.080036.

Scheer, N., Kapelyukh, Y., McEwan, J., Beuger, V., Stanley, L. A., Rode, A., et al. (2012). Modeling human cytochrome P450 2D6 metabolism and drug-drug interaction by a novel panel of knockout and humanized mouse lines. *Molecular Pharmacology*, *81*(1), 63–72. https://doi.org/10.1124/mol.111.075192.

Scheer, N., Kapelyukh, Y., Rode, A., Oswald, S., Busch, D., McLaughlin, L. A., et al. (2015). Defining human pathways of drug metabolism in vivo through the development of a multiple humanized mouse model. *Drug Metabolism and Disposition*, *43*(11), 1679–1690. https://doi.org/10.1124/dmd.115.065656.

Scheer, N., McLaughlin, L. A., Rode, A., Macleod, A. K., Henderson, C. J., & Wolf, C. R. (2014). Deletion of 30 murine cytochrome p450 genes results in viable mice with compromised drug metabolism. *Drug Metabolism and Disposition*, *42*(6), 1022–1030. https://doi.org/10.1124/dmd.114.057885.

Scheer, N., & Wolf, C. R. (2014). Genetically humanized mouse models of drug metabolizing enzymes and transporters and their applications. *Xenobiotica*, *44*(2), 96–108. https://doi.org/10.3109/00498254.2013.815831.

Seubert, J., Yang, B., Bradbury, J. A., Graves, J., Degraff, L. M., Gabel, S., et al. (2004). Enhanced postischemic functional recovery in CYP2J2 transgenic hearts involves mitochondrial ATP-sensitive K+ channels and p42/p44 MAPK pathway. *Circulation Research*, *95*(5), 506–514. https://doi.org/10.1161/01.RES.0000139436.89654.c8.

Slater, T. F., Cheeseman, K. H., & Ingold, K. U. (1985). Carbon tetrachloride toxicity as a model for studying free-radical mediated liver injury. *Philosophical Transactions of the Royal Society of London. Series B, Biological Sciences*, *311*(1152), 633–645. https://doi.org/10.1098/rstb.1985.0169.

Smolarek, T. A., Morgan, S. L., Moynihan, C. G., Lee, H., Harvey, R. G., & Baird, W. M. (1987). Metabolism and DNA adduct formation of benzo[a]pyrene and 7,12-dimethylbenz[a]anthracene in fish cell lines in culture. *Carcinogenesis*, *8*(10), 1501–1509. https://doi.org/10.1093/carcin/8.10.1501.

Stocco, M. R., Tolledo, C., Wadji, F. B., Gonzalez, F. J., Miksys, S., & Tyndale, R. F. (2020). Human CYP2D6 in the brain is protective against Harmine-induced neurotoxicity: Evidence from humanized CYP2D6 transgenic mice. *Molecular Neurobiology*, *57*(11), 4608–4621. https://doi.org/10.1007/s12035-020-02050-w.

Sumner, S. C., Fennell, T. R., Moore, T. A., Chanas, B., Gonzalez, F., & Ghanayem, B. I. (1999). Role of cytochrome P450 2E1 in the metabolism of acrylamide and acrylonitrile in mice. *Chemical Research in Toxicology*, *12*(11), 1110–1116. https://doi.org/10.1021/tx990040k.

Tekmal, R. R., Ramachandra, N., Gubba, S., Durgam, V. R., Mantione, J., Toda, K., et al. (1996). Overexpression of int-5/aromatase in mammary glands of transgenic mice results in the induction of hyperplasia and nuclear abnormalities. *Cancer Research*, *56*(14), 3180–3185 (Retrieved from https://www.ncbi.nlm.nih.gov/pubmed/8764102).

Templin, M. V., Jamison, K. C., Sprankle, C. S., Wolf, D. C., Wong, B. A., & Butterworth, B. E. (1996). Chloroform-induced cytotoxicity and regenerative cell proliferation in the kidneys and liver of BDF1 mice. *Cancer Letters*, *108*(2), 225–231. https://doi.org/10.1016/s0304-3835(96)04427-8.

Tolledo, E. C., Miksys, S., Gonzalez, F. J., & Tyndale, R. F. (2020). Propranolol is a mechanism-based inhibitor of CYP2D and CYP2D6 in humanized CYP2D6-transgenic mice: Effects on activity and drug responses. *British Journal of Pharmacology*, *177*(3), 701–712. https://doi.org/10.1111/bph.14884.

Tolledo, C., Stocco, M. R., Miksys, S., Gonzalez, F. J., & Tyndale, R. F. (2020). Human CYP2D6 is functional in brain in vivo: Evidence from humanized CYP2D6 transgenic mice. *Molecular Neurobiology*, *57*(6), 2509–2520. https://doi.org/10.1007/s12035-020-01896-4.

Tonge, R. P., Kelly, E. J., Bruschi, S. A., Kalhorn, T., Eaton, D. L., Nebert, D. W., et al. (1998). Role of CYP1A2 in the hepatotoxicity of acetaminophen: Investigations using *Cyp1a2* null mice. *Toxicology and Applied Pharmacology*, *153*, 102–108.

Turesky, R. J., Konorev, D., Fan, X., Tang, Y., Yao, L., Ding, X., et al. (2015). Effect of cytochrome P450 reductase deficiency on 2-amino-9H-pyrido[2,3-b]indole metabolism and DNA adduct formation in liver and extrahepatic tissues of mice. *Chemical Research in Toxicology*, *28*(12), 2400–2410. https://doi.org/10.1021/acs.chemrestox.5b00405.

Ueno, T., Tamura, S., Frels, W. I., Shou, M., Gonzalez, F. J., & Kimura, S. (2000). A transgenic mouse expressing human CYP1A2 in the pancreas. *Biochemical Pharmacology*, *60*(6), 857–863. https://doi.org/10.1016/s0006-2952(00)00389-0.

Uno, S., Dalton, T. P., Dragin, N., Curran, C. P., Derkenne, S., Miller, M. L., et al. (2006). Oral benzo[a]pyrene in Cyp1 knockout mouse lines: CYP1A1 important in detoxication, CYP1B1 metabolism required for immune damage independent of total-body burden and clearance rate. *Molecular Pharmacology*, *69*(4), 1103–1114. https://doi.org/10.1124/mol.105.021501.

Valentine, J. L., Lee, S. S., Seaton, M. J., Asgharian, B., Farris, G., Corton, J. C., et al. (1996). Reduction of benzene metabolism and toxicity in mice that lack CYP2E1 expression. *Toxicology and Applied Pharmacology*, *141*(1), 205–213. https://doi.org/10.1006/taap.1996.0277.

van Herwaarden, A. E., Smit, J. W., Sparidans, R. W., Wagenaar, E., van der Kruijssen, C. M., Schellens, J. H., et al. (2005). Midazolam and cyclosporin a metabolism in transgenic mice with liver-specific expression of human CYP3A4. *Drug Metabolism and Disposition*, *33*(7), 892–895. https://doi.org/10.1124/dmd.105.004721.

van Herwaarden, A. E., Wagenaar, E., van der Kruijssen, C. M., van Waterschoot, R. A., Smit, J. W., Song, J. Y., et al. (2007). Knockout of cytochrome P450 3A yields new mouse models for understanding xenobiotic metabolism. *The Journal of Clinical Investigation*, *117*(11), 3583–3592. https://doi.org/10.1172/JCI33435.

van Waterschoot, R. A., & Schinkel, A. H. (2011). A critical analysis of the interplay between cytochrome P450 3A and P-glycoprotein: Recent insights from knockout and transgenic mice. *Pharmacological Reviews*, *63*(2), 390–410. https://doi.org/10.1124/pr.110.002584.

van Waterschoot, R. A., van Herwaarden, A. E., Lagas, J. S., Sparidans, R. W., Wagenaar, E., van der Kruijssen, C. M., et al. (2008). Midazolam metabolism in cytochrome P450 3A knockout mice can be attributed to up-regulated CYP2C enzymes. *Molecular Pharmacology*, *73*(3), 1029–1036. https://doi.org/10.1124/mol.107.043869.

Wang, J., Gan, C., Retmana, I. A., Sparidans, R. W., Li, W., Lebre, M. C., et al. (2019). P-glycoprotein (MDR1/ABCB1) and breast cancer resistance protein (BCRP/ABCG2) limit brain accumulation of the FLT3 inhibitor quizartinib in mice. *International Journal of Pharmaceutics*, *556*, 172–180. https://doi.org/10.1016/j.ijpharm.2018.12.014.

Wang, H., Liu, A., Kuo, Y., Chi, E., Yang, X., Zhang, L., et al. (2016). Obesity promotes PhIP-induced small intestinal carcinogenesis in hCYP1A-db/db mice: Involvement of mutations and DNA hypermethylation of Apc. *Carcinogenesis*, *37*(7), 723–730. https://doi.org/10.1093/carcin/bgw054.

Wei, Y., Li, L., Zhou, X., Zhang, Q. Y., Dunbar, A., Liu, F., et al. (2013). Generation and characterization of a novel Cyp2a(4/5)bgs-null mouse model. *Drug Metabolism and Disposition*, *41*(1), 132–140. https://doi.org/10.1124/dmd.112.048736.

Wei, Y., Wu, H., Li, L., Liu, Z., Zhou, X., Zhang, Q. Y., et al. (2012). Generation and characterization of a CYP2A13/2B6/2F1-transgenic mouse model. *Drug Metabolism and Disposition*, *40*(6), 1144–1150. https://doi.org/10.1124/dmd.112.044826.

Wei, Y., Zhou, X., Fang, C., Li, L., Kluetzman, K., Yang, W., et al. (2010). Generation of a mouse model with a reversible hypomorphic cytochrome P450 reductase gene: Utility for tissue-specific rescue of the reductase expression, and insights from a resultant mouse model with global suppression of P450 reductase expression in extrahepatic tissues. *The Journal of Pharmacology and Experimental Therapeutics*, *334*(1), 69–77. https://doi.org/10.1124/jpet.110.167411.

Weng, Y., Fang, C., Turesky, R. J., Behr, M., Kaminsky, L. S., & Ding, X. (2007). Determination of the role of target tissue metabolism in lung carcinogenesis using conditional cytochrome P450 reductase-null mice. *Cancer Research*, *67*(16), 7825–7832. https://doi.org/10.1158/0008-5472.CAN-07-1006.

Winslow, V., Vaivoda, R., Vasilyev, A., Dombkowski, D., Douaidy, K., Stark, C., et al. (2014). Altered leukotriene B4 metabolism in CYP4F18-deficient mice does not impact inflammation following renal ischemia. *Biochimica et Biophysica Acta*, *1841*(6), 868–879. https://doi.org/10.1016/j.bbalip.2014.03.002.

Wong, F. W., Chan, W. Y., & Lee, S. S. (1998). Resistance to carbon tetrachloride-induced hepatotoxicity in mice which lack CYP2E1 expression. *Toxicology and Applied Pharmacology*, *153*(1), 109–118. https://doi.org/10.1006/taap.1998.8547.

Wu, L., Gu, J., Cui, H., Zhang, Q. Y., Behr, M., Fang, C., et al. (2005). Transgenic mice with a hypomorphic NADPH-cytochrome P450 reductase gene: Effects on development, reproduction, and microsomal cytochrome P450. *The Journal of Pharmacology and Experimental Therapeutics*, *312*(1), 35–43. https://doi.org/10.1124/jpet.104.073353.

Xiao, Y. F., Ke, Q., Seubert, J. M., Bradbury, J. A., Graves, J., Degraff, L. M., et al. (2004). Enhancement of cardiac L-type Ca2+ currents in transgenic mice with cardiac-specific overexpression of CYP2J2. *Molecular Pharmacology*, *66*(6), 1607–1616. https://doi.org/10.1124/mol.104.004150.

Yamazaki, H., Suemizu, H., Kazuki, Y., Oofusa, K., Kuribayashi, S., Shimizu, M., et al. (2016). Assessment of protein binding of 5-Hydroxythalidomide bioactivated in humanized mice with human P450 3A-chromosome or hepatocytes by two-dimensional electrophoresis/accelerator mass spectrometry. *Chemical Research in Toxicology*, *29*(8), 1279–1281. https://doi.org/10.1021/acs.chemrestox.6b00210.

Yao, J., Li, C. G., Gong, L. K., Feng, C. C., Li, C. Z., Gao, M., et al. (2014). Hepatic cytochrome P450s play a major role in monocrotaline-induced renal toxicity in mice. *Acta Pharmacologica Sinica*, *35*(2), 292–300. https://doi.org/10.1038/aps.2013.145.

Zaher, H., Buters, J. T., Ward, J. M., Bruno, M. K., Lucas, A. M., Stern, S. T., et al. (1998). Protection against acetaminophen toxicity in CYP1A2 and CYP2E1 double-null mice. *Toxicology and Applied Pharmacology*, *152*(1), 193–199. https://doi.org/10.1006/taap.1998.8501.

Zhang, Q. Y., Gu, J., Su, T., Cui, H., Zhang, X., D'Agostino, J., et al. (2005). Generation and characterization of a transgenic mouse model with hepatic expression of human CYP2A6. *Biochemical and Biophysical Research Communications*, *338*(1), 318–324. https://doi.org/10.1016/j.bbrc.2005.08.086.

Zhou, G. L., Beloiartsev, A., Yu, B., Baron, D. M., Zhou, W., Niedra, R., et al. (2013). Deletion of the murine cytochrome P450 Cyp2j locus by fused BAC-mediated recombination identifies a role for Cyp2j in the pulmonary vascular response to hypoxia. *PLoS Genetics*, *9*(11), e1003950. https://doi.org/10.1371/journal.pgen.1003950.

Zhou, X., D'Agostino, J., Li, L., Moore, C. D., Yost, G. S., & Ding, X. (2012). Respective roles of CYP2A5 and CYP2F2 in the bioactivation of 3-methylindole in mouse olfactory mucosa and lung: Studies using Cyp2a5-null and Cyp2f2-null mouse models. *Drug Metabolism and Disposition*, *40*(4), 642–647. https://doi.org/10.1124/dmd.111.044081.

Zhou, X., Wei, Y., Xie, F., Laukaitis, C. M., Karn, R. C., Kluetzman, K., et al. (2011). A novel defensive mechanism against acetaminophen toxicity in the mouse lateral nasal gland: Role of CYP2A5-mediated regulation of testosterone homeostasis and salivary androgen-binding protein expression. *Molecular Pharmacology*, *79*(4), 710–723. https://doi.org/10.1124/mol.110.070045.

Zhou, X., Zhuo, X., Xie, F., Kluetzman, K., Shu, Y. Z., Humphreys, W. G., et al. (2010). Role of CYP2A5 in the clearance of nicotine and cotinine: Insights from studies on a Cyp2a5-null mouse model. *The Journal of Pharmacology and Experimental Therapeutics*, *332*(2), 578–587. https://doi.org/10.1124/jpet.109.162610.

Zhu, J. G., Ochalek, J. T., Kaufmann, M., Jones, G., & Deluca, H. F. (2013). CYP2R1 is a major, but not exclusive, contributor to 25-hydroxyvitamin D production in vivo. *Proceedings of the National Academy of Sciences of the United States of America*, *110*(39), 15650–15655. https://doi.org/10.1073/pnas.1315006110.

Zhuo, X., Gu, J., Behr, M. J., Swiatek, P. J., Cui, H., Zhang, Q. Y., et al. (2004). Targeted disruption of the olfactory mucosa-specific Cyp2g1 gene: Impact on acetaminophen toxicity in the lateral nasal gland, and tissue-selective effects on Cyp2a5 expression. *The Journal of Pharmacology and Experimental Therapeutics*, *308*(2), 719–728. https://doi.org/10.1124/jpet.103.060301.

CHAPTER NINE

Expression and functional activity of cytochrome P450 enzymes in human hepatocytes with sustainable reproducibility for *in vitro* phenotyping studies

Pamela Bachour-El Azzi[a], Christophe Chesné[a,*], and Shotaro Uehara[b]
[a]Biopredic International SARL, Saint Grégoire, France
[b]Central Institute for Experimental Animals, Kawasaki, Kanagawa, Japan
*Corresponding author: e-mail address: c.chesne@wepredic.com

Contents

Abstract

Primary human hepatocytes are an essential *in vitro* tool for evaluating drug metabolism, drug–drug interactions, and hepatotoxicity. This model is considered as the gold standard in matter of DMPK studies in both industrial and academic research. The primary human hepatocytes are used either in suspension or in monolayer, as fresh or frozen cells. However, the use of this model is limited due to the lack of availability, rapid loss of functionality, high cost as well as the variable hepatocyte plating efficiencies in culture and the limited stock of hepatocytes derived from the same origin. Chimeric TK-NOG mice with humanized livers (humanized liver mice) are an attractive platform for drug metabolism and toxicity, which were produced by transplanting human hepatocytes into immunodeficient mice with injured livers. Here, we show that, using humanized mouse liver, *in vivo* human hepatocyte repopulation was over ~100-fold enabling the continuous and abundant use of human hepatocytes of the same origin and improving their plateability. In our latest cell preparations, hepatocytes isolated from humanized liver mice (Hu-Liver cells) exhibited high purity (ratio of HLA-positive cells: 92 ± 3%), good viability

Advances in Pharmacology, Volume 95
ISSN 1054-3589
https://doi.org/10.1016/bs.apha.2022.05.009

(75 ± 12%), and yield (1.0 × 10^8 cells/mouse). Human hepatic drug metabolizing enzymes, transporters, and nuclear receptors genes were expressed in humanized mouse liver. Drug-metabolizing activities in Hu-Liver cells were comparable to or higher than those in primary human hepatocytes. An extensive P450-dependent human drug metabolism was observed in Hu-Liver cells. CYP1A2, CYP2B6, and CYP3A4/5 activities/mRNA in Hu-Liver cells were induced by the hepatocyte exposure to typical human P450 inducers, omeprazole, phenobarbital, and rifampicin, respectively. Finally, Human albumin secretion and CYP3A-mediated drug oxidation activity were maintained over 4-weeks. Altogether, the expression level of pharmacokinetics-related genes, enzyme activity, human-typed drug metabolism, and inducibility of P450 in Hu-Liver cells make from humanized mouse liver a relevant and robust model for *in vitro* preclinical studies, including drug metabolism, pharmacokinetics, and toxicology studies.

Abbreviations

CYP	general term for cytochrome P450 (EC 1.14.14.1)
GAPDH	glyceraldehyde-3-phosphate dehydrogenase
HLA	human leukocyte antigen
HSVtk	herpes simplex virus type 1 thymidine kinase
iPSC	induced pluripotent stem cells
LC-MS/MS	liquid chromatography–tandem mass spectrometry
NOG	NOD/Shi-scid IL2 receptor gamma-null mice
qPCR	quantitative polymerase chain reaction
SD	standard deviation
TK, HSVtk	TKm30, HSVtk mutant 30 clone
UGT	uridine 5′-diphospho-glucuronosyltransferases

1. Introduction

Human hepatocytes have become the "gold standard" for preclinical assessment of human-specific drug properties, including P450 induction, hepatic metabolism, and toxicity of drugs *in vitro* (Godoy et al., 2013; Li, 2007). Considering the key role of P450s in drug–drug interactions, the induction potency of P450 should be assessed using *in vitro* models as part of the standard drug interaction study protocol in the U.S. Food and Drug Administration guidance, the European Medicines Agency guideline, and the Ministry of Health, Labor and Welfare of Japan guideline. Freshly isolated human hepatocytes are not available on a regular basis, whereas cryopreserved hepatocytes have many drawbacks, including low availability, rapid loss of hepatic functions either in suspension (few hours after isolation) or in monolayer (few days after seeding), high cost, limited lot supply, inter-individual variability, and different levels of attachment efficiency and confluence (Alexandre et al., 2012). Although alternative cell models, such as the hepatoma-derived HepG2 (Bouma, Rogier, Verthier, Labarre, &

Feldmann, 1989) and the immortalized Fa2N-4 (Mills, Rose, Sadagopan, Sahi, & de Morais, 2004) have been developed, the use of these cells for drug safety assessment and drug–drug interactions remains questionable due to the low or absent expression of drug-metabolizing enzyme genes, low metabolic functionality, and/or poor inducibility of P450 enzymes (Gerets et al., 2012; Hariparsad, Carr, Evers, & Chu, 2008; Wilkening, Stahl, & Bader, 2003). Another model of hepatocytes derived from human induced pluripotent stem cells (iPSCs) can be generated from virtually any donor and differentiated, using diverse reprogramming techniques (Raab, Klingenstein, Liebau, & Linta, 2014; Suter-Dick et al., 2015). iPSC-derived hepatocytes were shown to have sustainable function on long-term culture, and they correlate genetically more closely to primary human hepatocytes than most cell lines (Gao & Liu, 2017). However, the major drawback of these cells is that their phenotype remains partially fetal (Luce, Messina, Duclos-Vallée, & Dubart-Kupperschmitt, 2021). Interestingly, HepaRG cell line is an exception that overcomes the drawbacks of the aforementioned models. Derived from human liver carcinoma 20 years ago, HepaRG cells have been used to set up an appropriate cell bank ensuring the use of a sustainable model for several decades. HepaRG cells were shown to express phase I and II enzymes, functional hepatobiliary transporters, nuclear receptors, and many other hepatic functions, similarly to those in human primary hepatocytes (Aninat et al., 2006; Josse et al., 2008; Turpeinen et al., 2009). These expressions can remain relatively stable for up to 4 weeks, making the HepaRG cell model suitable for chronic exposure assessment (Antherieu et al., 2010). Moreover, the expression and activity of main P450 enzymes have been shown to be significantly induced following exposure of HepaRG cells to prototypical inducers (Antherieu et al., 2010).

As no model is perfect, HepaRG still has its own limitations. Indeed, HepaRG cells require a relatively long period of time to differentiate, express low level of CYP2D6, and represent a single donor, limiting thereby the interdonor variability evaluation. Despite all this, the HepaRG functionality associated with the consistent and reproducible results, the large availability as well as the ability to culture these cells under different modes, make them the best surrogate of primary human hepatocytes. However, there is still a need for an *in vitro* model that overcomes the limitations of the currently available hepatocyte models, closely mimics the *in vivo* situation and is sustainable. Hu-liver cells would constitute an alternative of the existing hepatocyte lines and a complementary model to HepaRG cell line.

Uehara et al. have established an *in vivo* cell expansion technology using humanized mice liver (Fig. 1) (Uehara, Higuchi, Yoneda, Yamazaki, & Suemizu, 2019). Hepatocytes from humanized mice liver (Hu-Liver cells)

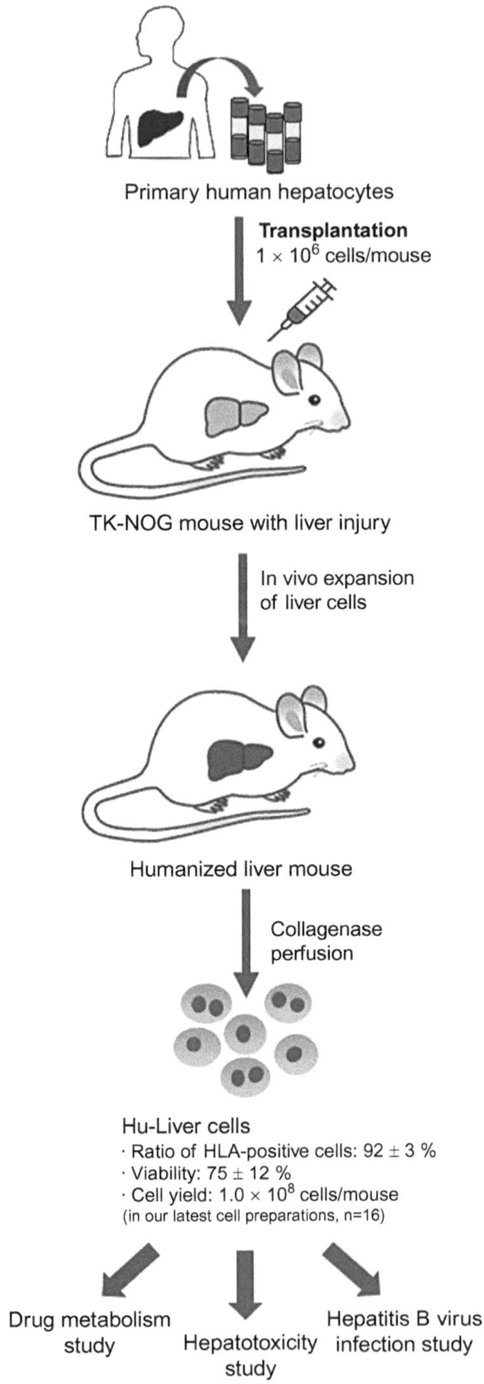

Fig. 1 Preparation of Hu-Liver cells from humanized mouse liver.

have enabled the extensive supply of plateable primary human hepatocytes from a same donor (Uehara et al., 2019). Fresh and high yield plateable Hu-Liver cells can be used routinely in various *in vitro* preclinical studies, including P450 induction-mediated drug interactions, hepatic metabolism, and drug-induced hepatotoxicity. In this review, we present the P450 mRNA expression level, drug-metabolizing activity, and P450 induction following hepatocyte exposure to typical P450 inducers as assessed by P450 enzyme mRNA expression/activity in Hu-Liver cells. Hu-Liver cells and hepatocytes from other type of human liver chimeric mice generated using urokinase-type plasminogen activator/severe combined immunodeficiency and Fah −/−/Rag2 −/−/Il2rg −/− mice have been recently used as models in drug metabolism and pharmacokinetics and HBV infection studies (Azuma et al., 2007; Uehara, Higuchi, et al., 2022; Uehara et al., 2019; Yamasaki et al., 2010).

2. Preparation of hepatocytes (from chimeric mice)

TK-NOG or NOG-TKm30 mice (6- to 8-week-old) were given 0.2 mg/mL Val-ganciclovir in drinking water for 2 days to ablate hepatocytes expressing the HSVtk/tk mutant30 transgene. Ten days after the administration of Val-ganciclovir, liver-injured mice with high aminotransferase levels (exceeding 600 U/L) in plasma received human hepatocyte transplantation. Humanized liver mice were generated by transplantation of cryopreserved primary human hepatocytes (1.0×10^6 cells/mouse) into the spleen of TK-NOG or NOG-TKm30 mice (Fig. 1) (Hasegawa et al., 2011; Uehara, Higuchi, et al., 2022). We found that the ratio of the area occupied by human CK8/18-positive liver cells relative to the total area in a stained liver section (replacement index) was highly correlated with the plasma albumin concentration (Hasegawa et al., 2011). The degree of chimerism by human hepatocytes in the humanized liver was estimated by measuring plasma human albumin levels. Hu-Liver cells were isolated from 16- to 20-week-old humanized liver mice with high plasma human albumin levels (estimated replacement indexes >80%) using collagen perfusion method (Uehara et al., 2019). For hepatocytes preparations in our recent experiments ($n = 16$), fresh Hu-Liver cells exhibited a high ratio of HLA-positive cells (92% on average), with a mean viability exceeding 73%. Monolayer-cultured Hu-Liver cells had a cobblestone morphology

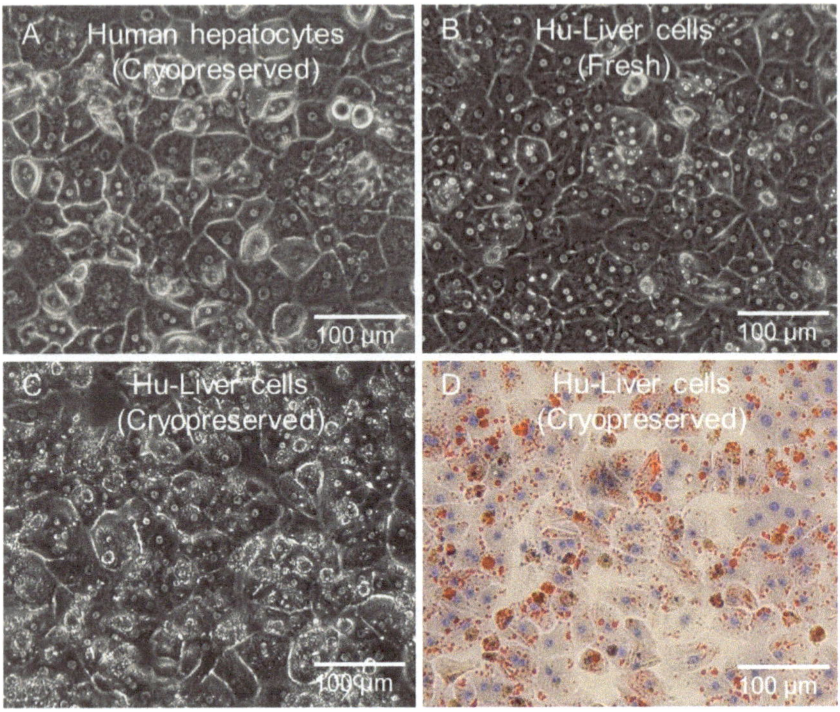

Fig. 2 Morphology of Hu-Liver cells. Phase contrast images show cryopreserved primary human hepatocytes (A), fresh Hu-Liver cells (donor A) (B), and cryopreserved Hu-Liver cells (donor D) (C) 24 h after plating. Intracytoplasmic lipid droplets in Hu-Liver cells (donor D) were stained with oil red O (D).

and showed many bi-nucleated cells, similar to primary human hepatocytes (Fig. 2A–C). Human hepatocytes from humanized TK-NOG mice have shown accumulation of lipid droplets (Fig. 2D) similarly to those observed in liver chimeric mice models (Tateno et al., 2015; Uehara, Higuchi, et al., 2022). Cryopreserved Hu-Liver cells exhibited a high ratio of HLA-positive cells (97% on average), with mean viability exceeding 86% (Table 1). Thus, residual mouse cells (including parenchymal and non-parenchymal cells) in Hu-Liver cells decreased by the freezing and thawing cycle. Notably, all fresh Hu-Liver cells were highly plateable, even those originating from poorly plateable human hepatocytes (donor C). This is in agreement with a previous study showing an improved plating efficiency of hepatocytes from humanized liver (Michailidis et al., 2020). This suggests that the passage culture *via* cell expansion in humanized liver normalizes the subsequent plateability.

Table 1 Preparation of Hu-Liver cells.

Human hepatocytes (as transplantation donor cells)						Hu-Liver mice (as liver cell donors)			Fresh Hu-Liver cells				Cryopreserved Hu-Liver cells		
									Ratio of cells (%)				Ratio of cells (%)		
ID	Race	Age	Gender	Patient information	CYP3A5 genotype	ID	BW (g)	Strain	Mouse[a]	Human[b]	Viability (%)	Cell yield ($\times 10^7$)	Mouse[a]	Human[b]	Viability (%)
A	Asian	35 years	Male	Death from fall Tobacco Use: 1 ppd.; Alcohol Use: 2 beers/day	*1/*3	A	NA	TK-NOG	4.97	92.3	96.0	4.90	NA	NA	NA
B	African	31 years	Male	Smoking; Alcohol Use: None	Unknown	B1	NA	TK-NOG	5.61	88.9	62.2	7.40	3.87	95.5	79.6
						B2	18.3	TK-NOG	4.84	91.4	47.4	10.2	2.39	97.2	74.1
						B3	17.7	TK-NOG	6.64	89.1	73.3	13.2	2.34	97.1	87.4
C	Hispanic	11 months	Male	Cytomegalovirus: positive	Unknown	C1	17.9	TK-NOG	4.53	91.6	62.3	14.4	1.13	98.0	90.4
						C2	20.8	TK-NOG	7.17	86.7	64.0	6.40	2.23	95.2	93.7
						C3	19.2	TK-NOG	7.15	88.5	75.2	9.70	1.91	97.2	92.3
						C4	21.1	TK-NOG	8.09	85.9	82.0	10.0	4.23	93.7	94.2
						C5	16.4	TK-NOG	3.42	93.9	78.0	4.60	0.65	98.0	84.3
						C6	17.3	TK-NOG	4.73	93.1	72.0	10.8	0.67	98.3	91.6
D	Caucasian	12 years	Female	Tobacco Use: None; Alcohol Use: None	*3/*3	D1	18.5	TK-NOG	4.66	94.5	77.8	7.00	1.90	97.5	83.3
						D2	13.7	TK-NOG	4.44	94.3	71.8	9.40	2.26	96.9	84.3
						D3	17.5	TK-NOG	3.78	94.8	90.5	7.60	1.72	96.9	84.6
						D4	18.0	NOG-TKm30	1.09	97.2	85.5	10.6	0.18	99.1	82.6
						D5	21.4	NOG-TKm30	4.74	92.5	84.3	19.3	1.44	97.8	91.9
E	Caucasian	2 years	Male	Death from drowning	*3/*3	E	NA	TK-NOG	6.50	93.5	78.4	8.00	NA	NA	NA

[a]The ratio of mouse liver cells stained with monoclonal mouse anti-mouse H-2kd antibody.
[b]The ratio of human liver cells stained with monoclonal mouse anti-HLA antibody.
Cryopreserved human hepatocytes (35-year-old Asian male [donor A], 11-months-old Hispanic male [donor C], 12-year-old Caucasian female [donor D], 2-year-old Caucasian male [donor E]) were provided by Lonza Walkersville, Inc. (Walkersville, MD, USA). Cryopreserved human hepatocytes (31-year-old African male [donor B]) were provided by Biopredic International (Rennes, France). NA, Not available.

3. Expression and activity of human P450 enzymes

Global expression patterns of 24 pharmacokinetic-related genes, including P450s, uridine 5′-diphospho-glucuronosyltransferases, and transporters were assessed in Hu-Liver cell suspensions (Fig. 3). The expression levels of 19 genes in Hu-Liver cell suspensions were comparable or greater to those of primary human hepatocyte suspensions (pool of 20). Similarly, the expression levels of the 13 CYP1–4 subfamily genes (CYP2A6, CYP2C8, CYP2C9, CYP2C19, CYP2D6, CYP2J2, CYP3A4, CYP3A5, CYP4A11, CYP4F2, CYP4F3B, CYP4F11 and CYP4F12) were similar (within 5-fold differences) between fresh Hu-Liver cells and cryopreserved donor hepatocytes after 48 h incubation with Dulbecco's modified Eagle's medium containing 10% fetal bovine serum after plating (Uehara et al., 2019). However, higher gene expression level (~40-fold) of CYP1A2 was found in Hu-Liver cells cultured for 48 h after plating. Metabolic activities of typical P450 and UGT substrates in primary human hepatocytes (pool of 20) and Hu-Liver cells were shown in Fig. 4. All metabolic activities in Hu-Liver cells were similar to or higher than those in human hepatocytes. Large inter-individual variations (>4-fold differences) for bupropion hydroxylation, omeprazole 5-hydroxylation, and T-1032 N-oxygenation activities were observed among Hu-Liver cells from different donors. In our recent study, T-1032 N-oxygenation activity in Hu-Liver cells (donor D, *CYP3A5 *3/*3* genotype) was lower than that of Hu-Liver cells harboring *CYP3A5 *1/*3* and *CYP3A5 *1/*7* genotypes (Uehara et al., 2022), potentially reflecting the function of CYP3A5 polymorphism in donor hepatocytes.

4. P450 enzyme-dependent drug metabolism

Our previous studies reported the formation of human-specific or disproportionate metabolites by Hu-Liver cells. In humans, tolbutamide is first oxidized by CYP2C9 into 4-hydroxytolbutamide and subsequently into 4-carboxytolbutamide (Lee et al., 2003). Substantial 4-hydroxytolbutamide and 4-carboxytolbutamide production was observed in cryopreserved Hu-Liver cells and cryopreserved human hepatocytes, whereas 4-carboxytolbutamide production was not detected in cryopreserved mouse hepatocytes (Fig. 5) (Uehara et al., 2021).

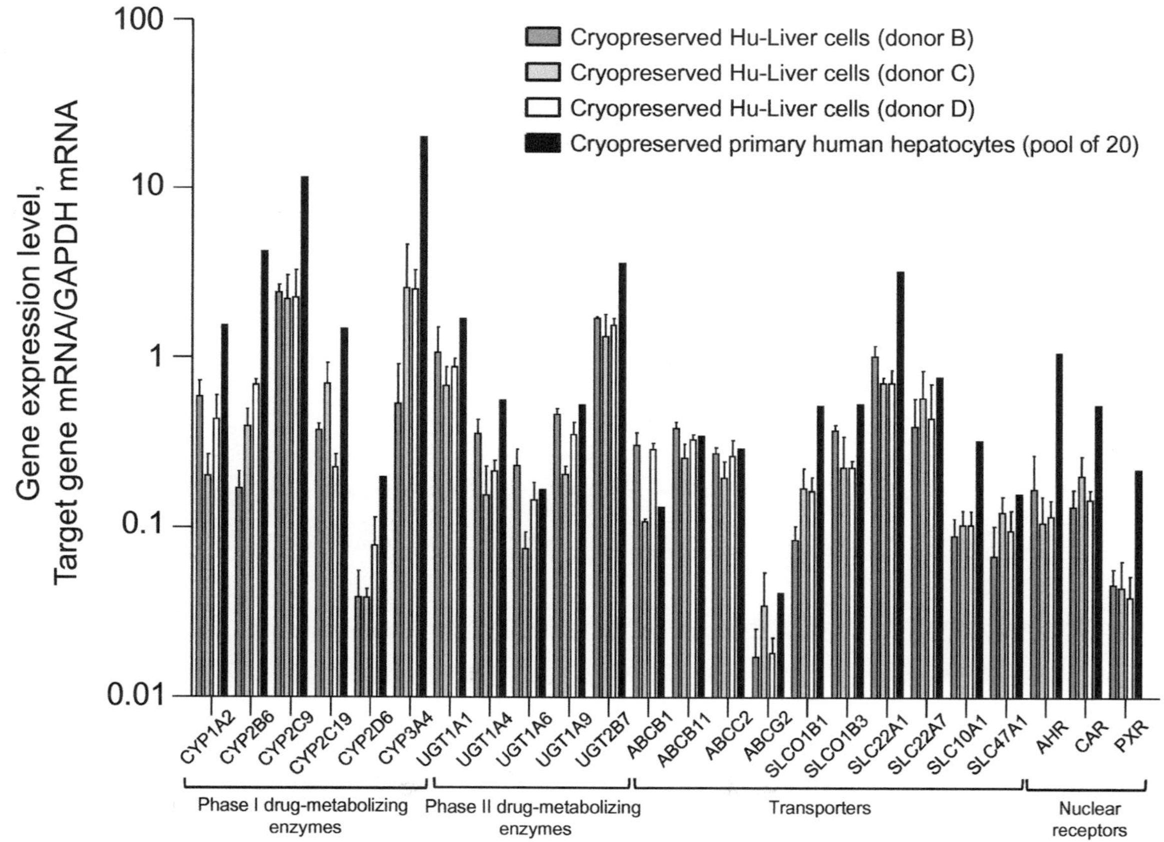

Fig. 3 Expression levels of pharmacokinetics-related genes in Hu-Liver cells. Human P450, UGT, transporter, and nuclear receptor mRNAs in cryopreserved primary human hepatocytes (pool of 20, 19003-TA05, Lonza Walkersville, Inc.) and cryopreserved Hu-Liver cells (donor B: B1–A3; donor C: C1–C3; donor D: D1–D3) were measured by quantitative reverse transcription-polymerase chain reaction using TaqMan probe and primers as previously described (Uehara, Yoneda, Higuchi, Yamazaki, & Suemizu, 2022). Each human P450 mRNA level was normalized to that of the human GAPDH.

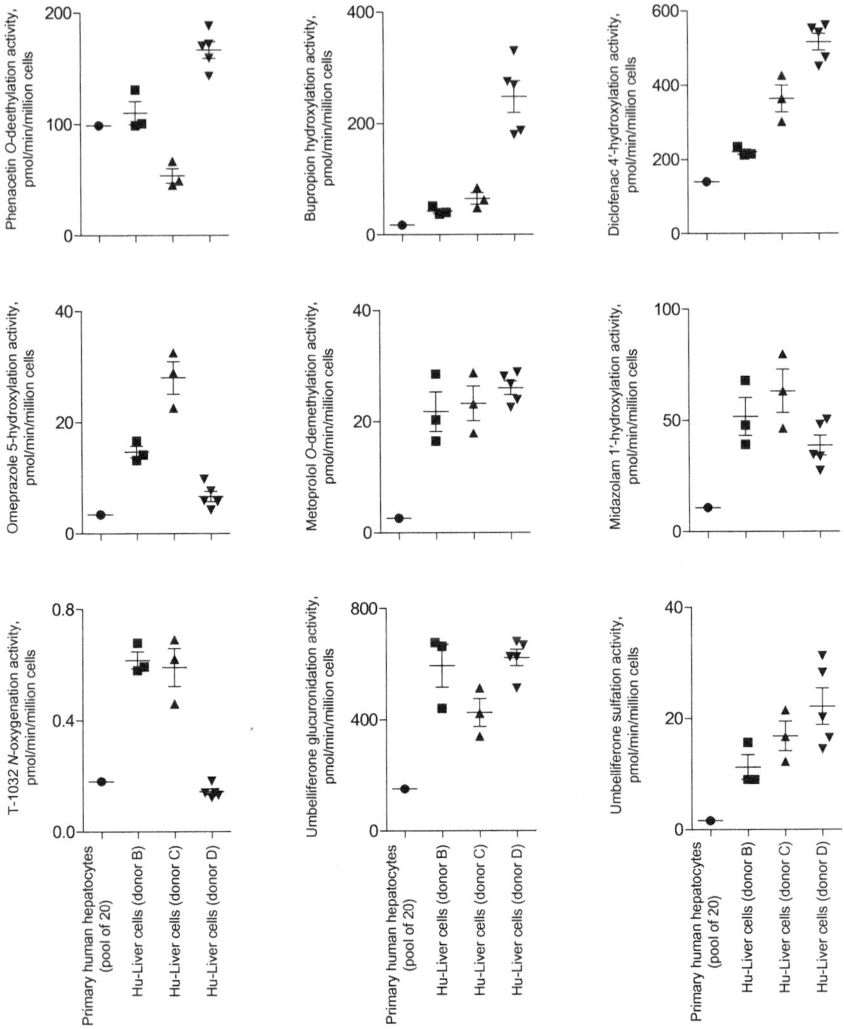

Fig. 4 Drug oxidation activities in Hu-Liver cells. Cryopreserved primary human hepatocytes (pool of 20) and cryopreserved Hu-Liver cells (donor B: B1–A3; donor C: C1–C3; donor D: D1–D3) were incubated with any of the eight typical human P450 substrates (50 μM phenacetin, 50 μM bupropion, 40 μM diclofenac, 10 μM omeprazole, 5 μM metoprolol, 5 μM midazolam, 5 μM T-1032, and 5 μM umbelliferon) at 37 °C for 30 min. Metabolites in media were measured by liquid chromatography–tandem mass spectrometry (LC-MS/MS).

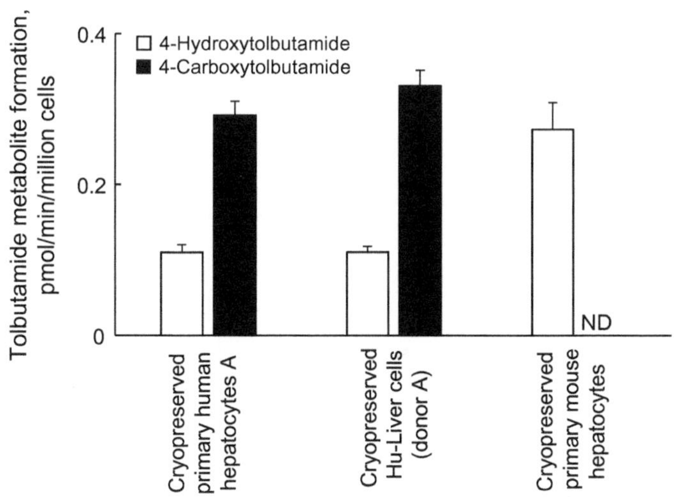

Fig. 5 Metabolic analysis of tolbutamide in primary human hepatocytes, Hu-Liver cells, and primary mouse hepatocytes. Cryopreserved primary human hepatocytes (donor A), cryopreserved Hu-Liver cells (donor A), and cryopreserved primary mouse hepatocytes were incubated with 100 μM tolbutamide at 37 °C for 60 min. Hydroxy- and carboxy-metabolites in media collected were measured by LC-MS/MS. Data show means with SD values (Uehara, Yoneda, Higuchi, Yamazaki, & Suemizu, 2021).

Diclofenac is metabolized into 4′-hydroxydiclofenac by CYP2C9. 3′-Hydroxy-4′-methoxydiclofenac was found in human plasma (Faigle et al., 1988). Interestingly, this metabolite was detected in plasma of baboons, but not mice, rats, or marmosets (Faigle et al., 1988, unpublish data). Production of 3′-hydroxy-4′-methoxydiclofenac was not detected neither in human hepatocyte suspensions (cell concentration: ~750,000 cells/mL; incubation time: 2 h), human hepatocytes cultured in three-dimensional spheroid system (2.0×10^4 cells/well on 96 format Cell-able; Incubation time, 7 days), S-9 fractions (protein concentration, 1 mg/mL; incubation time, 2 h), nor in human liver microsomes (protein concentration: 2 mg/mL; incubation time: 2 h) incubated with 10 μM diclofenac (Dalvie et al., 2009; Ohkura et al., 2014). Detection of 3′-hydroxy-4′-methoxydiclofenac in hepatocytes and S9 fractions might depend on the differences of the enzyme assay conditions, the lot-to-lot differences of enzyme sources, or the sensitivity of quantification methods. However, cryopreserved

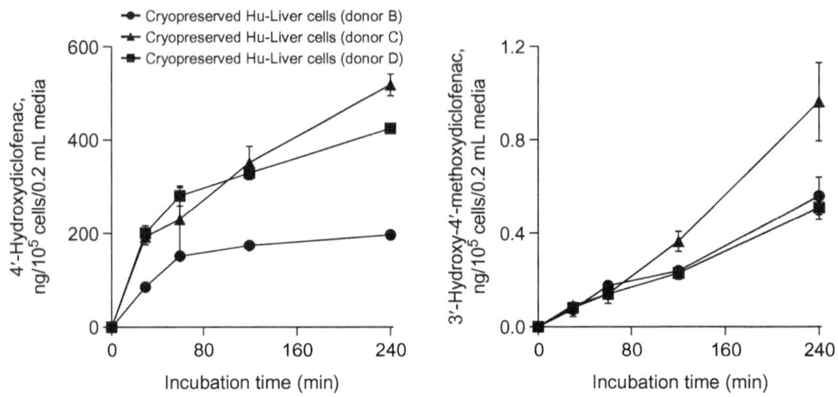

Fig. 6 Formation of diclofenac metabolites in Hu-Liver cells. Cryopreserved Hu-Liver cells (donor B, C, D) were incubated with 100 μM diclofenac at 37 °C for 240 min. 4′-Hydroxydiclofenac and human-specific 3′-hydroxy-4′-methoxydiclofenac in media collected at 0, 30, 60, 120, and 240 min were measured by LC-MS/MS.

Hu-Liver cell suspensions produced 3′-hydroxy-4′-methoxydiclofenac following the incubation with 100 μM diclofenac at 37 °C for at least 30 min (Fig. 6). The generation of human-specific diclofenac metabolite in Hu-Liver cells reflects the robust catalytic function of multiple human drug metabolizing enzymes.

5. Human hepatocytes during 1- to 4-weeks of culture

Hepatocyte morphology is a useful indicator of monolayer integrity status in *in vitro* liver models. In 4–24 h after plating, Hu-Liver cells exhibited the characteristic cobblestone morphology. As time goes by, its morphology showed confluent monolayers around day 2–14, the cells started to pile up and formed the foci of small cell aggregates by day 28 (Fig. 7). Human albumin secretion levels in Hu-Liver cells were maintained (220–360 ng/10^5 cells/24 h) for at least 28 days (Fig. 8A). Similar to primary human hepatocytes, midazolam 1′-hydroxylation activity in Hu-Liver cells was maintained (within approximately threefold differences) for 4–28 days after plating, in agreement with the stable expression of CYP3A4 mRNA (within approximately sevenfold differences) (Fig. 8A and B). We found a lack of correlation between mRNA expression and

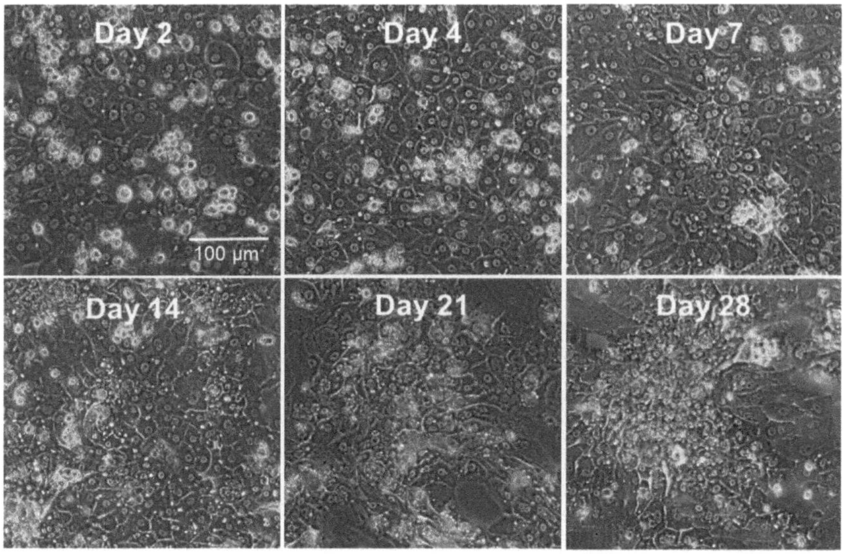

Fig. 7 Phase images of Hu-Liver cell morphology during 4weeks. Fresh Hu-Liver cells collected from humanized liver of chimeric mice transplanted with cells of donor A were plated at 5.0×10^5 cells/well in 24-well plate and cultured for up to 28days using Cellartis Power Primary HEP Medium (Takara Bio, Shiga, Japan) at 37 °C under a gas mixture of 5% CO_2 and 95% O_2. Culture medium was changed every 2–3 day.

functional parameters in Hu-Liver cells during day 2–7: the increase in midazolam 1′-hydroxylation activity (CYP3A4/5 activity) is <10-fold whereas the change in CYP3A4 mRNA expression is approximately 10- to 100-fold. Further studies investigating CYP3A4/5 mRNA and protein levels are needed to further support the findings from enzyme activity assessments. The increase in midazolam during day 2–4 in Hu-Liver cells human hepatocytes cultured in commercially available Cellartis Power Primary HEP Medium (Takara Bio, Shiga, Japan) contrasts with the usual decline in CYP3A4 activity seen in primary human hepatocytes over the first days in culture. It was reported the differences of P450 activity of human hepatocytes cultured in different medium with various composition (Toba et al., 2020). Therefore, it is important to select the optimal medium for specific application when carrying out *in vitro* pharmaceutical experiments using human hepatocytes. CYP1A2, CYP2B6, and CYP3A4 mRNAs in monolayer-cultured Hu-Liver cells were induced (~12-, ~1.8-, and ~10-fold, respectively) by 48h-exposure to typical human

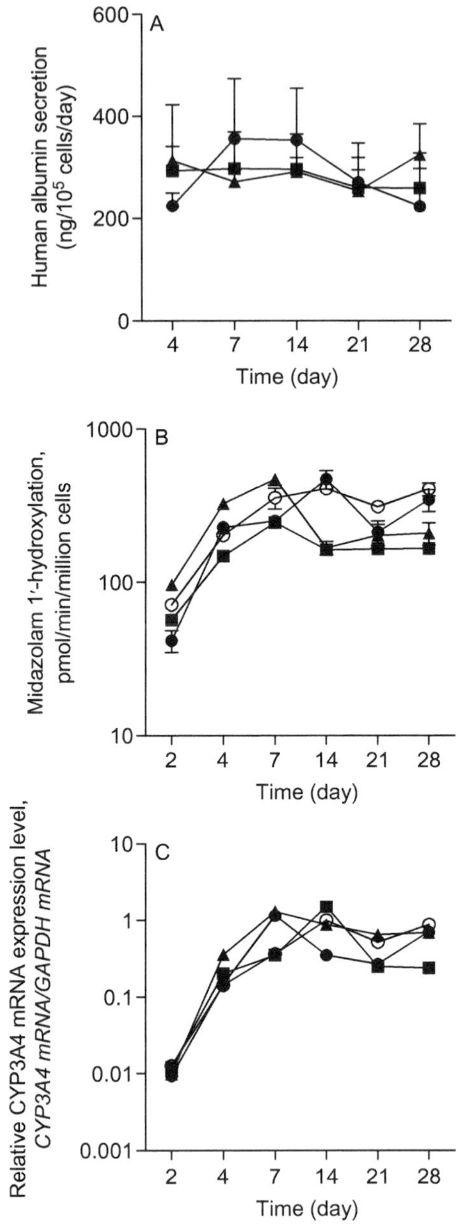

Fig. 8 See figure legend on opposite page.

P450 inducers omeprazole (50 μM), phenobarbital (1 mM), and rifampicin (10 μM), respectively, as reported previously (Uehara et al., 2019). Rifampicin-mediated CYP3A4 mRNA induction response was reproducible in three lots of Hu-Liver cells, with EC_{50} values of 2.3 μM and E_{max} values of 8.8-fold, roughly comparable to those in human hepatocytes (EC_{50}, 1.1 μM; E_{max}, 6.0-fold) as reported previously (Uehara et al., 2019). Drug-oxidation activities in Hu-Liver cells were also increased by typical P450 inducers (Table 2). Midazolam 1′-/4-hydroxylation activity (CYP3A4/5 activity) was induced by phenobarbital (2 mM) and rifampicin. Bupropion hydroxylation activity (CYP2B6 activity) was induced by omeprazole (100 μM), phenobarbital (2 mM), and rifampicin (20 μM). Ethoxyresorufin *O*-deethylation activity (CYP1A1/2 activity) was induced by omeprazole (100 μM). Omeprazole 5-hydroxylation activity (CYP2C19 activity) was induced by phenobarbital (2 mM) and rifampicin (20 μM). In addition, inducibility of P450 in Hu-Liver cells was maintained for 4–28 days after plating (Fig. 9). These results suggest that hepatocyte functions of Hu-Liver cells were stable for a long period of time allowing the use of these cells for long-term cultures and chronic and repetitive exposures.

Fig. 8 Change in human albumin secretion, midazolam 1′-hydroxylation activities and CYP3A4 mRNA levels during 4 weeks-long culture of Hu-liver cells and human hepatocytes. (A) Human albumin concentrations in the cultured medium of fresh Hu-Liver cells (donor A) collected from different three humanized liver mice were measured with a human albumin ELISA quantitation kit (Bethyl Laboratories, Montgomery, TX, USA). Data represent the mean ± SD of three independent experiments. (B) Midazolam 1′-hydroxylation activities in cultured fresh Hu-Liver cells (donor A) collected from three different humanized liver mice during 4-weeks. Monolayer-cultured primary human hepatocytes (open circles) and Hu-Liver cells (closed circles, triangles, and squares) were incubated with midazolam (5 μM) for 60 min. The 1′-hydroxymidazolam in culture media was quantified by LC/MS/MS system. (C) CYP3A4 mRNA levels in cultured primary human hepatocytes and Hu-Liver cells (donor A) during 4-weeks. CYP3A4 mRNA level was measured by qPCR using TaqMan probe and primers. Data are expressed as the ratio of the CYP3A4 mRNA to GAPDH mRNA. Data represent the mean of duplicate determinations.

Table 2 P450 induction assay using Hu-Liver cells.

Condition	Drug oxidation activities, pmol products/h/1.0×10^5 cells: Midazolam 1′-hydroxylation	Midazolam 4-hydroxylation	Omeprazole 5-hydroxylation	Diclofenac 4′-hydroxylation	Bupropion hydroxylation	Ethoxyresorufin O-deethylation
Control	850 ± 120	8.1 ± 1.7	2.8 ± 1.0	0.02 ± 0.01	7.0 ± 0.6	0.014 ± 0.005
Omeprazole	720 (630, 800)	18 (15, 21)	5.3 (4.9, 5.7)	0.03 (0.01, 0.05)	46 (42, 49)	2.4 (2.1, 2.6)
Phenobarbital	4100 (3600, 4500)	75 (56, 94)	14 (14, 13)	0.02 (0.02, 0.02)	61 (62, 60)	0.011 (0.012, 0.009)
Rifampicin	3600 (3900, 3300)	60 (57, 63)	9.7 (9.4,10)	0.02 (0.02, 0.02)	27 (25, 28)	0.011 (0.010, 0.011)

Monolayer-cultured Hu-Liver cells were then incubated separately with one of the following P450 inducers: omeprazole (100 μM), phenobarbital (2 mM), and rifampicin (20 μM) for 72 h. The medium was replaced every 24 h. P450-dependent drug oxidation activities of the hepatocytes were determined using 2.0 μM ethoxyresorufin, 50 μM bupropion, 50 μM diclofenac, 20 μM omeprazole, and 5.0 μM midazolam. After a 1 h incubation at 37 °C (5% CO_2, *v*/v), the media were collected. The rates of metabolite formation were determined. Results are expressed as mean values (± SD) obtained from three wells of cultured cells, except for the induction study with parentheses (two individual values).

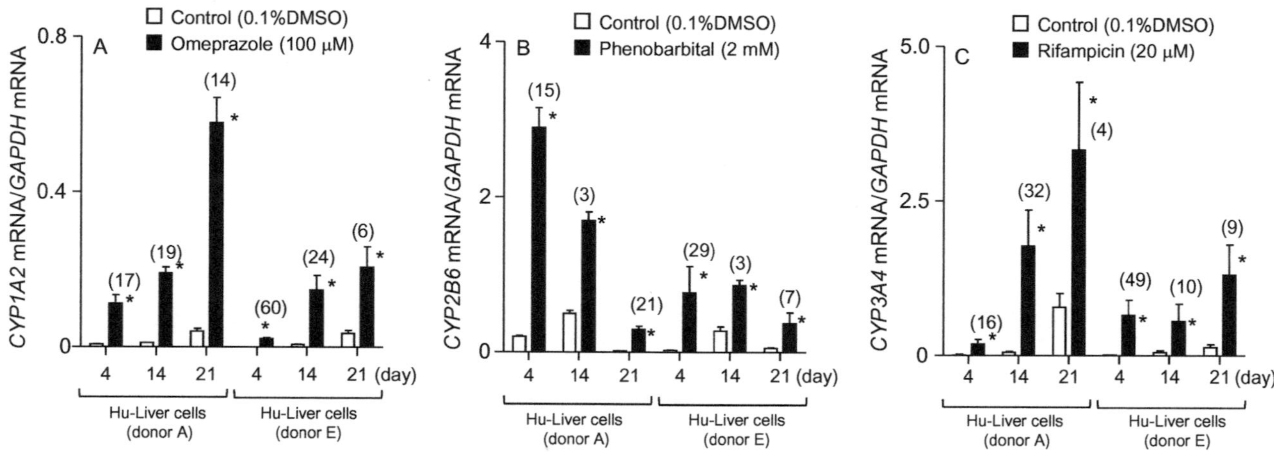

Fig. 9 Induction of CYP1A2, CYP2B6, and CYP3A4 by typical inducers in Hu-liver cells during 4 weeks-long culture. Monolayer-cultured Hu-Liver cells (donor A, E) were incubated with 0.1% DMSO (open bars) and typical human P450 inducers, 100 μM omeprazole (A), 2 mM phenobarbital, and 20 μM rifampicin for 48 h. CYP1A2 (A), CYP2B6 (B), and CYP3A4 (C) mRNA levels in Hu-Liver cells were measured by qPCR and normalized to GAPDH mRNA level. Data represent the mean ± SD of three independent experiments. Fold induction was shown in parentheses. *, $P < 0.05$.

6. Conclusion

Considering the main drawbacks of the primary human hepatocyte model, particularly those related to their restricted availability and rapid functionality decline either in suspension or in monolayer, an adequate *in vitro* model for hepatotoxicity and metabolism studies has been long awaited. So far, the HepaRG cell line is considered the best surrogate of the primary human hepatocytes but since they originate from one donor, similar systems that could be derived from multiple donors would be of great value. Recently, *in vivo* cell expansion technology using humanized mouse liver has enabled the obtention of hepatocytes from multiple donors and an abundant supply of hepatocytes from a same donor. This review provides evidence demonstrating the functionality of Hu-Liver cells, including human gene expression levels, catalytic activity, and inducibility of P450. Hu-Liver cells include a slight proportion of residual mouse cells (hepatocytes and non-parenchymal liver cells). Impact of those residual mouse cells in Hu-Liver cells on assessments of the metabolism and toxicity of drugs needs to be elucidated. Considering their sustainability and robustness as an *in vitro* liver cell model from the same hepatocyte donor, Hu-Liver cells would be a valuable tool for the characterization of metabolic pathways and cytochrome P450 induction potential of drug candidates. It would be interesting to extensively validate the previous results using hepatocytes originating from more donors, in suspension and plateable grades, in fresh cultures and in cryopreserved hepatocytes. Moreover, proving that a same lot of hepatocytes can be amplified using different mice to produce large batches of sustainable hepatocytes would be of great value.

Acknowledgments

This work was supported by the Platform Project for Supporting Drug Discovery and Life Science Research (Basis for Supporting Innovative Drug Discovery and Life Science Research [BINDS]) from the Japanese Agency for Medical Research and Development (AMED) under grant number 21am0101121j0005, The authors acknowledge the technical expertise of Dr. Yuichiro Higuchi, and Ms. Nao Yoneda and the helpful advice of Drs. Hiroshi Yamazaki, Norie Murayama, Mamoru Ito, Hiroshi Suemizu, and Yasuyuki Ohnishi.

Conflict of interest

The authors declare no conflict of interest.

Author contributions

(1) Study conception and design: CC, SU.
(2) Acquisition, analysis, and/or interpretation of data: CC, SU.
(3) Drafting/revision of the work for intellectual content and context: CC, SU, PBE.
(4) Final approval and overall responsibility for the published work: CC, SU, PBE.

References

Alexandre, E., Baze, A., Parmentier, C., Desbans, C., Pekthong, D., Gerin, B., et al. (2012). Plateable cryopreserved human hepatocytes for the assessment of cytochrome P450 inducibility: Experimental condition-related variables affecting their response to inducers. *Xenobiotica*, *42*(10), 968–979. https://doi.org/10.3109/00498254.2012.676693.

Aninat, C., Piton, A., Glaise, D., Le Charpentier, T., Langouet, S., Morel, F., et al. (2006). Expression of cytochromes P450, conjugating enzymes and nuclear receptors in human hepatoma HepaRG cells. *Drug Metabolism and Disposition*, *34*(1), 75–83. https://doi.org/10.1124/dmd.105.006759.

Antherieu, S., Chesne, C., Li, R., Camus, S., Lahoz, A., Picazo, L., et al. (2010). Stable expression, activity, and inducibility of cytochromes P450 in differentiated HepaRG cells. *Drug Metabolism and Disposition*, *38*(3), 516–525. https://doi.org/10.1124/dmd.109.030197.

Azuma, H., Paulk, N., Ranade, A., Dorrell, C., Al-Dhalimy, M., Ellis, E., et al. (2007). Robust expansion of human hepatocytes in fah−/−/Rag2−/−/Il2rg−/− mice. *Nature Biotechnology*, *25*(8), 903–910. https://doi.org/10.1038/nbt1326.

Bouma, M. E., Rogier, E., Verthier, N., Labarre, C., & Feldmann, G. (1989). Further cellular investigation of the human hepatoblastoma-derived cell line HepG2: Morphology and immunocytochemical studies of hepatic-secreted proteins. *In Vitro Cellular & Developmental Biology*, *25*(3 Pt 1), 267–275. https://doi.org/10.1007/BF02628465.

Dalvie, D., Obach, R. S., Kang, P., Prakash, C., Loi, C. M., Hurst, S., et al. (2009). Assessment of three human in vitro systems in the generation of major human excretory and circulating metabolites. *Chemical Research in Toxicology*, *22*(2), 357–368. https://doi.org/10.1021/tx8004357.

Faigle, J. W., Bottcher, I., Godbillon, J., Kriemler, H. P., Schlumpf, E., Schneider, W., et al. (1988). A new metabolite of diclofenac sodium in human plasma. *Xenobiotica*, *18*(10), 1191–1197. https://doi.org/10.3109/00498258809042242.

Gao, X., & Liu, Y. (2017). A transcriptomic study suggesting human iPSC-derived hepatocytes potentially offer a better in vitro model of hepatotoxicity than most hepatoma cell lines. *Cell Biology and Toxicology*, *33*(4), 407–421. https://doi.org/10.1007/s10565-017-9383-z.

Gerets, H. H., Tilmant, K., Gerin, B., Chanteux, H., Depelchin, B. O., Dhalluin, S., et al. (2012). Characterization of primary human hepatocytes, HepG2 cells, and HepaRG cells at the mRNA level and CYP activity in response to inducers and their predictivity for the detection of human hepatotoxins. *Cell Biology and Toxicology*, *28*(2), 69–87. https://doi.org/10.1007/s10565-011-9208-4.

Godoy, P., Hewitt, N. J., Albrecht, U., Andersen, M. E., Ansari, N., Bhattacharya, S., et al. (2013). Recent advances in 2D and 3D in vitro systems using primary hepatocytes, alternative hepatocyte sources and non-parenchymal liver cells and their use in investigating mechanisms of hepatotoxicity, cell signaling and ADME. *Archives of Toxicology*, *87*(8), 1315–1530. https://doi.org/10.1007/s00204-013-1078-5.

Hariparsad, N., Carr, B. A., Evers, R., & Chu, X. (2008). Comparison of immortalized Fa2N-4 cells and human hepatocytes as in vitro models for cytochrome P450 induction. *Drug Metabolism and Disposition*, *36*(6), 1046–1055. https://doi.org/10.1124/dmd.108.020677.

Hasegawa, M., Kawai, K., Mitsui, T., Taniguchi, K., Monnai, M., Wakui, M., et al. (2011). The reconstituted 'humanized liver' in TK-NOG mice is mature and functional. *Biochemical and Biophysical Research Communications*, *405*(3), 405–410. https://doi.org/10.1016/j.bbrc.2011.01.042.

Josse, R., Aninat, C., Glaise, D., Dumont, J., Fessard, V., Morel, F., et al. (2008). Long-term functional stability of human HepaRG hepatocytes and use for chronic toxicity and genotoxicity studies. *Drug Metabolism and Disposition*, *36*(6), 1111–1118. https://doi.org/10.1124/dmd.107.019901.

Lee, C. R., Pieper, J. A., Frye, R. F., Hinderliter, A. L., Blaisdell, J. A., & Goldstein, J. A. (2003). Tolbutamide, flurbiprofen, and losartan as probes of CYP2C9 activity in humans. *Journal of Clinical Pharmacology*, *43*(1), 84–91. https://doi.org/10.1177/0091270002239710.

Li, A. P. (2007). Human hepatocytes: Isolation, cryopreservation and applications in drug development. *Chemico-Biological Interactions*, *168*(1), 16–29. https://doi.org/10.1016/j.cbi.2007.01.001.

Luce, E., Messina, A., Duclos-Vallée, J. C., & Dubart-Kupperschmitt, A. (2021). Advanced techniques and awaited clinical applications for human pluripotent stem cell differentiation into hepatocytes. *Hepatology*, *74(2)*, 1101–1116. https://doi.org/10.1002/hep.31705.

Michailidis, E., Vercauteren, K., Mancio-Silva, L., Andrus, L., Jahan, C., Ricardo-Lax, I., et al. (2020). Expansion, in vivo-ex vivo cycling, and genetic manipulation of primary human hepatocytes. *Proceedings of the National Academy of Sciences of the United States of America*, *117*(3), 1678–1688. https://doi.org/10.1073/pnas.1919035117.

Mills, J. B., Rose, K. A., Sadagopan, N., Sahi, J., & de Morais, S. M. (2004). Induction of drug metabolism enzymes and MDR1 using a novel human hepatocyte cell line. *The Journal of Pharmacology and Experimental Therapeutics*, *309*(1), 303–309. https://doi.org/10.1124/jpet.103.061713.

Ohkura, T., Ohta, K., Nagao, T., Kusumoto, K., Koeda, A., Ueda, T., et al. (2014). Evaluation of human hepatocytes cultured by three-dimensional spheroid systems for drug metabolism. *Drug Metabolism and Pharmacokinetics*, *29*(5), 373–378. https://doi.org/10.2133/dmpk.dmpk-13-rg-105.

Raab, S., Klingenstein, M., Liebau, S., & Linta, L. (2014). A comparative view on human somatic cell sources for iPSC generation. *Stem Cells International*, *2014*, 768391. https://doi.org/10.1155/2014/768391.

Suter-Dick, L., Alves, P. M., Blaauboer, B. J., Bremm, K. D., Brito, C., Coecke, S., et al. (2015). Stem cell-derived systems in toxicology assessment. *Stem Cells and Development*, *24*(11), 1284–1296. https://doi.org/10.1089/scd.2014.0540.

Tateno, C., Kawase, Y., Tobita, Y., Hamamura, S., Ohshita, H., Yokomichi, H., et al. (2015). Generation of novel chimeric mice with humanized livers by using hemizygous cDNA-uPA/SCID mice. *PLoS One*, *10*(11), e0142145. https://doi.org/10.1371/journal.pone.0142145.

Toba, Y., Deguchi, S., Mimura, N., Sakamoto, A., Harada, K., Hirata, K., et al. (2020). Comparison of commercially available media for hepatic differentiation and hepatocyte maintenance. *PLoS One*, *15*(2), e0229654. https://doi.org/10.1371/journal.pone.0229654.

Turpeinen, M., Tolonen, A., Chesne, C., Guillouzo, A., Uusitalo, J., & Pelkonen, O. (2009). Functional expression, inhibition and induction of CYP enzymes in HepaRG cells. *Toxicology In Vitro*, *23*(4), 748–753. https://doi.org/10.1016/j.tiv.2009.03.008.

Uehara, S., Higuchi, Y., Yoneda, N., Kawai, K., Yamamoto, M., Kamimura, H., et al. (2022). An improved TK-NOG mouse as a novel platform for humanized liver that overcomes limitations in both male and female animals. *Drug Metabolism and Pharmacokinetics*, *42*, 100410. https://doi.org/10.1016/j.dmpk.2021.100410.

Uehara, S., Higuchi, Y., Yoneda, N., Yamazaki, H., & Suemizu, H. (2019). Expression and inducibility of cytochrome P450s in human hepatocytes isolated from chimeric mice with humanised livers. *Xenobiotica*, *49*(6), 678–687. https://doi.org/10.1080/00498254.2018.1495346.

Uehara, S., Shimizu, M., Plé, K., Routier, S., Yoneda, N., Higuchi, Y., et al. (2022). Probe drug T-1032 N-oxygenation mediated by cytochrome P450 3A5 in human hepatocytes in vitro and in humanized-liver mice in vivo. *Drug Metabolism and Pharmacokinetics*, (in press).

Uehara, S., Yoneda, N., Higuchi, Y., Yamazaki, H., & Suemizu, H. (2021). Methyl-hydroxylation and subsequent oxidation to produce carboxylic acid is the major metabolic pathway of tolbutamide in chimeric TK-NOG mice transplanted with human hepatocytes. *Xenobiotica*, *51*(5), 582–589. https://doi.org/10.1080/00498254.2021.1875515.

Uehara, S., Yoneda, N., Higuchi, Y., Yamazaki, H., & Suemizu, H. (2022). Cytochrome P450-dependent drug oxidation activities and their expression levels in liver microsomes of chimeric TK-NOG mice with humanized livers. *Drug Metabolism and Pharmacokinetics*, (in press).

Wilkening, S., Stahl, F., & Bader, A. (2003). Comparison of primary human hepatocytes and hepatoma cell line Hepg2 with regard to their biotransformation properties. *Drug Metabolism and Disposition*, *31*(8), 1035–1042. https://doi.org/10.1124/dmd.31.8.1035.

Yamasaki, C., Kataoka, M., Kato, Y., Kakuni, M., Usuda, S., Ohzone, Y., et al. (2010). In vitro evaluation of cytochrome P450 and glucuronidation activities in hepatocytes isolated from liver-humanized mice. *Drug Metabolism and Pharmacokinetics*, *25*(6), 539–550. https://doi.org/10.2133/dmpk.dmpk-10-rg-047.

CHAPTER TEN

Cytochrome P450s in chimeric mice with humanized liver

Shotaro Uehara[a,*], Hiroshi Suemizu[a], and Hiroshi Yamazaki[b]
[a]Central Institute for Experimental Animals, Kawasaki, Kanagawa, Japan
[b]Showa Pharmaceutical University, Machida, Tokyo, Japan
*Corresponding author: e-mail address: s-uehara@ciea.or.jp

Contents

Abstract

Chimeric mice with humanized livers (humanized liver mice) are attractive experimental animal models for drug metabolism and pharmacokinetic studies. The "humanized liver" is a mature and functional liver with zonal position-specific expressions of human cytochrome P450 (P450) enzymes and a global gene expression pattern consistent with that of the mature human liver. Most P450-dependent drug oxidation activities were comparable between microsomes from livers of human and humanized liver mice based on similar expression levels of human P450 enzymes; however, some differences were observed between the two species, including considerable variations in activities of bufuralol 1′-hydroxylation and propafenone 4′-hydroxylation. Human

Advances in Pharmacology, Volume 95
ISSN 1054-3589
https://doi.org/10.1016/bs.apha.2022.05.004

disproportionate and/or unique metabolites of P450 substrate drugs were produced in humanized liver mice. Plasma concentration profiles of typical P450 substrate drugs in humans could be extrapolated from the corresponding data in humanized liver mice using simplified physiologically based pharmacokinetic modeling. Drug-drug interaction-mediated hepatic human CYP3A/2C induction by rifampicin (a human pregnane X receptor agonist) was observed in humanized liver mice. The major role of human CYP2C9 in *in vivo* diclofenac 4′-hydroxylation were determined using human CYP2C9-inactivated chimeric mice using a mechanism-based inhibitor, tienilic acid. Overall, based on the functional characteristics of hepatic human P450 enzymes, humanized liver mice are valuable experimental animals for studying metabolite profiling, pharmacokinetics, and drug interactions.

Abbreviations

ADH	alcohol dehydrogenase
ALDH	aldehyde dehydrogenase
AOX	aldehyde oxidase
AUC	area under curve
C_{max}	minimum plasma concentration
GAPDH	glyceraldehyde-3-phosphate dehydrogenase
HSVtk	herpes simplex virus type 1 thymidine kinase
LC-MS/MS	liquid chromatography–tandem mass spectrometry
NADPH	nicotinamide adenine dinucleotide phosphate reduced form
NOG	NOD/Shi-scid IL2 receptor gamma-null mice
P450	general term for cytochrome P450 (EC 1.14.14.1)
SD	standard deviation
TK	HSVtk
TKm30	HSVtk mutant 30 clone
UGT	uridine 5′-diphospho-glucuronosyltransferases
XO	xanthine oxidase

1. Introduction

Preclinical animal models are widely used to evaluate metabolism and disposition of drug candidates. However, interspecies differences in drug metabolism have been reported because humans differ from animals in terms of isoform composition and expression, regulation, and catalytic activities of drug-metabolizing enzymes, including cytochrome P450s (P450s) and uridine 5′-diphospho-glucuronosyltransferases (UGTs). Therefore, species selection for preclinical studies should consider the similarity in the properties of drug metabolism between humans and animals. Chimeric mice with humanized livers (humanized liver mice) are an attractive experimental model for predicting human drug metabolism and pharmacokinetics because more than 70% of the liver is repopulated by human hepatocytes. This chimeric mouse was established by transplanting human hepatocytes into NOG mice expressing the herpes simplex virus type 1 thymidine kinase (HSVtk) transgene (TK-NOG) or HSVtk mutant30 transgenic NOG mice (NOG-TKm30) at the Central Institute for Experimental Animals (Hasegawa et al., 2011; Uehara et al., 2022). Briefly, exposure of these mice to a nontoxic dose of ganciclovir causes gradual ablation of mouse liver cells expressing the transgene and creates space for engraftment and maintenance of human hepatocytes. Human hepatocytes that are transplanted into ganciclovir-treated mice develop into mature and functional liver tissues. The serum concentration of human albumin has been used as a marker to estimate the replacement index. Transplanted human liver cells can stably maintain hepatic biosynthetic function for a prolonged period (8 months) (Hasegawa et al., 2011). Over the past few years, in several studies using humanized liver TK-NOG mice, we have accumulated data on P450-dependent drug oxidation activities and their protein expression in liver microsomes and *in vivo* drug metabolism/pharmacokinetics and drug interaction studies. Here, we summarized important information supporting the effective use of humanized liver TK-NOG mice.

2. Characterization of humanized liver from chimeric mice

2.1 Zonal expression of human P450 in the repopulated humanized liver

In a highly repopulated humanized liver, human leukocyte antigen-positive liver cells (brown-colored area) occupied most areas of the liver sections (Fig. 1, left). A typical lobular structure, which is a portal triad comprising the portal vein, bile duct, and hepatic artery, was conserved within humanized livers of chimeric mice (Fig. 1, right). Immunohistochemical staining using human P450 specific antibodies indicated that CYP3A4 (Fig. 1, right) and CYP1A2 were localized in the perivenous regions (Uehara, Higuchi, et al., 2022), whereas CYP2C9/CYP2D6 and CYP2E1 were distributed homogeneously across hepatic lobules and weakly around the perivenous region (Uehara, Higuchi, et al., 2022). These results indicated that the distribution pattern of major human P450 proteins in humanized livers of chimeric mice was similar to that of the mature human liver.

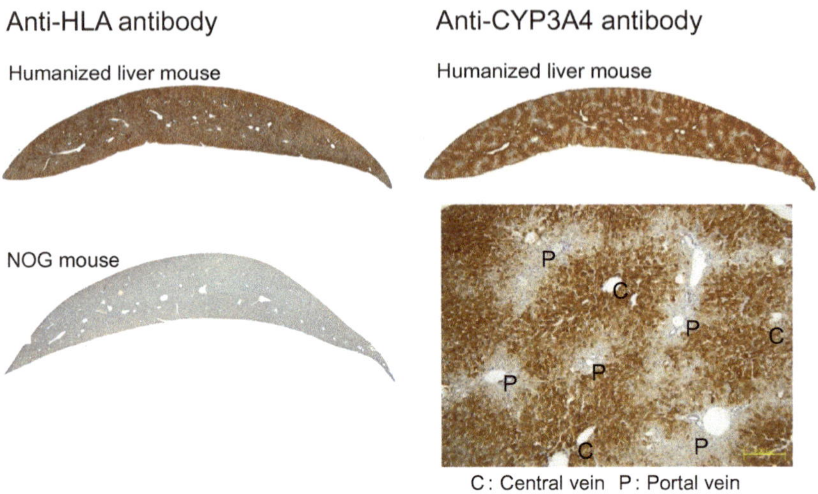

Fig. 1 Characterization of liver tissues in humanized liver mouse. Liver tissues of humanized liver from mice aged 16 weeks were stained with antibodies—antihuman leukocyte antigen and antihuman CYP3A4. C, central vein; P, portal tract.

2.2 Levels of gene expression of drug metabolizing enzymes and transporters

Gene expression levels of human phase I and phase II drug-metabolizing enzymes and transporters in humanized liver were comparable (within 2.3-fold) to those in the livers of humans (Fig. 2) (Uehara, Yoneda, et al., 2022). Large individual differences were observed in gene expression levels of *CYP2B6* and *CYP3A5* (more than 10-fold difference) among livers of humanized mice with different donor hepatocytes (Fig. 2). Low *CYP3A5* expression levels due to a single nucleotide polymorphism were observed in homozygous *CYP3A5*3/*3* individuals (donors D and E) compared with those in *CYP3A5*1* allele carriers (donors B and C) (Fig. 2). These findings suggested that the overall pattern of pharmacokinetics-related gene expression in the liver was similar between humans and humanized liver mice, and that the expression levels of *P450* genes in humanized liver substantially reflected the inter-individual variability of gene expression levels in donor human hepatocytes.

2.3 Content of human P450 protein in liver microsomes

Liquid chromatograph-tandem mass spectrometry (LC-MS/MS)-quantified human CYP1–3 family proteins in liver microsomes were compared between human and humanized liver mice. The content of each P450

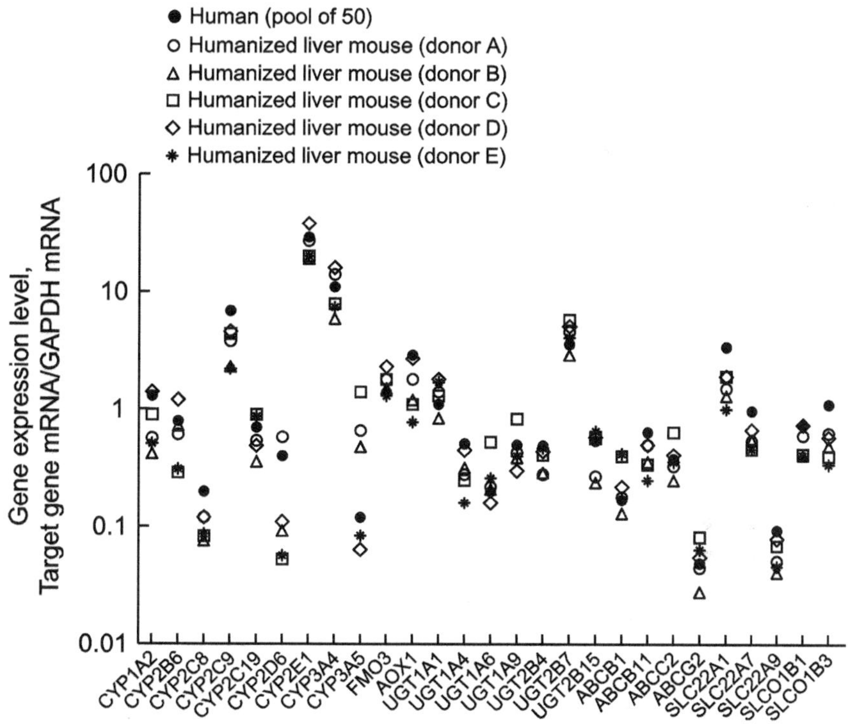

Fig. 2 Expression levels of pharmacokinetics-related genes in the liver of humanized liver mice. Expression levels of mRNA of target genes in livers of humanized liver mice and humans were measured using real-time reverse transcription-polymerase chain reaction. Raw data were normalized to expression level of glyceraldehyde-3-phosphate dehydrogenase (GAPDH) mRNA. Data are reported means for three humanized mice (Uehara, Yoneda, Higuchi, Yamazaki, & Suemizu, 2022).

was expressed as a percentage of the total quantified CYP1–3 proteins; 26% (CYP3A4), 23% (CYP2C9), 15% (CYP2E1), 12% (CYP1A2), 10% (CYP2C8), 7.3% (CYP2A6), 2.9% (CYP2C19), 2.4% (CYP2D6), 1.3% (CYP3A5), and 0.4% (CYP2B6) (Fig. 3) (Uehara, Yoneda, et al., 2022). The content of most P450 proteins showed a 3-fold difference between liver microsomes from humans and those from humanized liver mice; however, only CYP2B6 revealed an approximately 6-fold difference. Abundant expression of CYP3A4 and CYP2C9 proteins corresponding to the hepatic P450 expression profile in humanized liver mice has been reported in the human liver (Achour, Barber, & Rostami-Hodjegan, 2014; Shimada, Yamazaki, Mimura, Inui, & Guengerich, 1994). Overall, the individual P450 abundances in the liver were similar between humans and humanized liver mice.

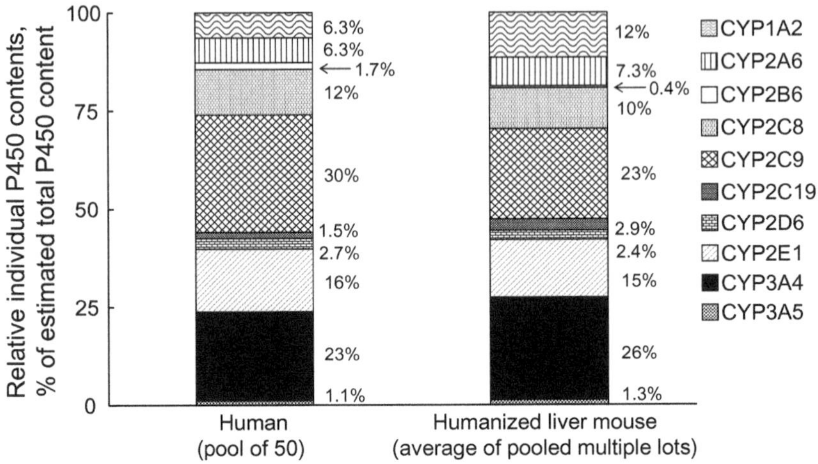

Fig. 3 Human P450 contents in liver microsomes from humanized liver mice. Estimated total P450 contents were 299 and 191 pmol/mg protein, respectively. Data are reported means for pooled liver microsomes from humanized liver mice (donor A, B, and C: pool of 16, 9, and 10, respectively) (Uehara, Yoneda, et al., 2022).

2.4 Drug oxidation activity in liver microsomes

The drug oxidation activities in pooled liver microsomes from humans, humanized liver mice, and mice on the nine P450 substrates are shown in Fig. 4. Activities of ethoxyresorufin *O*-deethylation, coumarin 7-hydroxylation, pentoxyresorufin *O*-depentylation, flurbiprofen 4′-hydroxylation, *S*-mephenytoin 4′-hydroxylation, propafenone 5-hydroxylation, chlorzoxazone 6-hydroxylation, and midazolam 1′-/4-hydroxylation in liver microsomes from humanized liver mice were comparable (approximately 3-fold difference) to those of liver microsomes from humans (Fig. 4). In contrast, liver microsomes from mouse showed low catalytic activities for coumarin 7-hydroxylation with low capacity and flurbiprofen 4′-hydroxylation/*S*-mephenytoin 4′-hydroxylation with low substrate affinity (Fig. 4, Table 1). These results indicate that activities of coumarin, flurbiprofen, and *S*-mephenytoin oxidation in liver microsomes from humanized liver mice substantially reflect the catalytic function of human CYP2A6, CYP2C9, and CYP2C19 expressed in humanized livers. In contrast, bufuralol 1′-hydroxylation and propafenone 4′-hydroxylation activities in liver microsomes from humanized liver mice were higher (approximately 9- and 50-fold differences, respectively) than in those in liver microsome

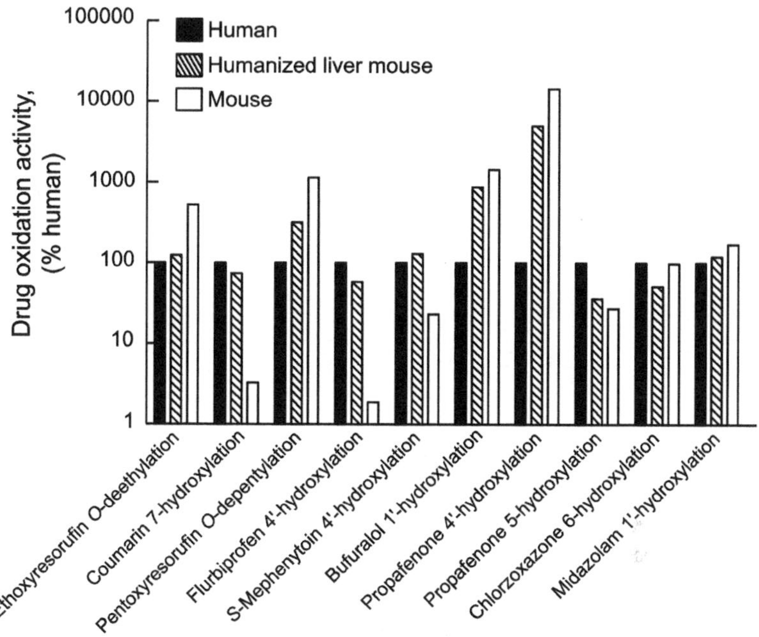

Fig. 4 Drug oxidation activities in liver microsomes from humanized liver mice. Pooled liver microsomes from human, humanized liver mice (donor A, B, and C: pool of 16, 9, and 10, respectively), and TK-NOG mice (pool of 4) were incubated with any one of nine typical human P450 substrates (0.2 μM ethoxyresorufin, 1.2 μM coumarin, 10 μM pentoxyresorufin, 20 μM flurbiprofen, 20 μM *S*-mephenytoin, 1.5 μM bufuralol, 5 μM propafenone, 100 μM chlorzoxazone, and 5 μM midazolam) at 37 °C for 10–20 min. The percentage of drug oxidation activities in humanized liver mice and normal mice when compared with that in humans (Uehara, Yoneda, et al., 2022).

from humans (Fig. 4), which was due to a higher capacity for these reactions in liver microsomes from humanized liver mice (Table 1). These findings suggest that mouse P450 enzymes expressed in a few residual mouse liver cells in humanized livers might contribute to drug oxidation. Overall, the typical human CYP1A/2B/2A/2C/3A enzyme-catalyzed drug oxidation activities were similar between liver microsomes from humans and humanized liver mice, but the typical human CYP2D enzyme-catalyzed drug oxidation activities (bufuralol 1′-hydroxylation and propafenone 4′-hydroxylation) were different between the two, probably because of the high rodent CYP2C/2D enzyme activities (Mimura et al., 1994; Uehara, Murayama, Yamazaki, & Suemizu, 2019).

Table 1 Kinetic parameters for P450-dependent drug oxidation in microsomes from livers of humans, humanized liver mice, and mice.

		K_m	V_{max}	V_{max}/K_m	K_s
Drug oxidation	**Liver microsomes**	**μM**	**nmol·min^{-1}·mg^{-1} protein**	**mL·min^{-1}·mg^{-1} protein**	**μM**
7-Ethoxyresorufin	Human	0.77	0.19	0.25	–
O-deethylation	Humanized liver mouse	0.28–1.0	0.078–0.24	0.24–0.60	–
	Mouse	0.22	0.44	2.0	–
Coumarin	Human	1.3	0.38	0.29	–
7-Hydroxylation	Humanized liver mouse	1.1–1.3	0.14–0.32	0.12–0.29	–
	Mouse	2.5	0.0093	0.0037	–
7-Pentoxyresorufin	Human	36	0.015	0.00042	–
O-depentylation	Humanized liver mouse	4.1–4.9	0.014–0.025	0.0029–0.0061	–
	Mouse	0.87	0.043	0.049	–
Flurbiprofen	Human	14	0.34	0.024	–
4′-Hydroxylation	Humanized liver mouse	10–17	0.11–0.24	0.011–0.015	–
	Mouse	>250	0.019[a]	NA	–
S-mephenytoin	Human	64	0.026	0.00041	–
4′-Hydroxylation	Humanized liver mouse	52–120	0.018–0.035	0.00023–0.00054	–
	Mouse	>200	0.0066[b]	NA	–
Bufuralol	Human	0.42	0.29	0.69	–
1′-Hydroxylation	Humanized liver mouse	0.50–1.1	2.0–2.2	1.8–4.0	–
	Mouse	0.80	5.2	6.5	–

Propafenone	Human	0.73	0.0027	0.0037	–
4′-Hydroxylation	Humanized liver mouse	0.32–0.51	0.080–0.17	0.16–0.33	–
	Mouse	0.67	0.37	0.55	–
Propafenone	Human	0.040	0.034	0.85	–
5-Hydroxylation	Humanized liver mouse	0.21–0.58	0.019–0.0079	0.014–0.053	–
	Mouse	1.4	0.017	0.012	–
Chlorzoxazone	Human	130	1.7	0.013	–
6-Hydroxylation	Humanized liver mouse	100–160	0.77–1.3	0.013–0.0064	–
	Mouse	140	2.0	0.014	–
Midazolam	Human	6.2	2.1	0.34	1.3
1′-Hydroxylation	Humanized liver mouse	2.6–2.8	1.0–2.1	0.38–0.75	0.46–2.1
	TK-NOG mouse	4.2	2.7	0.64	0.13
Midazolam	Human	67	0.98	0.015	–
4-Hydroxylation	Humanized liver mouse	25–34	0.31–0.70	0.012–0.021	–
	TK-NOG mouse	26	0.64	0.025	–

[a]Activities at 250 μM.
[b]Activities at 200 μM.
NA, Not available. Each value represents data obtained with pooled liver microsomes from humans (pool of 50), humanized liver mice (donor A, B, and C: pool of 16, 9, and 10, respectively), TK-NOG mice (pool of 4) (Uehara, Yoneda, et al., 2022).

3. *In vivo* drug metabolism by humanized liver mouse

Drug metabolism studies can provide a wealth of information on the metabolic routes of the drug, the enzymes involved in the metabolism, and the drug metabolites generated. Identification and characterization of metabolites of drug candidates provides an opportunity to assess the contribution of metabolites to the efficacy, toxicity, or drug–drug interactions. Humanized liver mice have been validated for their drug-metabolizing properties for a wide range of drugs and chemicals. They have been shown to be clearly differentiated metabolically from the recipient mouse. Furthermore, P450-mediated metabolic pathways in humanized liver mice have been demonstrated to be similar to those in humans. Extensive phase I and II human drug-metabolizing enzymes are expressed in humanized livers from chimeric mice. Therefore, humanized liver mice are a valuable animal model for predicting human drug metabolism mediated by multiple enzymes with relatively small amounts of test substances.

3.1 Tolbutamide

Tolbutamide is an oral sulfonylurea hypoglycemic agent widely used to treat non-insulin-dependent diabetes mellitus. In humans, tolbutamide is first oxidized by CYP2C9 to 4-hydroxytolbutamide (Knodell, Hall, Wilkinson, & Guengerich, 1987; Miners & Birkett, 1996) and then, 4-hydroxytolbutamide is oxidized to 4-carboxytolbutamide by several enzymes, including alcohol dehydrogenase, aldehyde dehydrogenase, aldehyde oxidase, and xanthine oxidase (Kitamura, Sugihara, & Ohta, 2006; McDaniel, Podgainy, & Bressler, 1969). The major metabolites produced in humans, rats, and dogs are 4-hydroxytolbutamide, 4-carboxytolbutamide, and *p*-tolylsulfonylurea/*p*-tolylsulfonamide, respectively (Mohnike, Wittenhagen, & Langenbeck, 1958; Thomas & Ikeda, 1966). After a single oral dose of tolbutamide (10 mg/kg), the mean values of the area under the curve (AUC) for plasma concentrations of 4-hydroxytolbutamide and 4-carboxytolbutamide were 1.3- and 48-fold higher in humanized liver mice than in control mice, respectively (Uehara, Yoneda, Higuchi, Yamazaki, & Suemizu, 2021). The 4-carboxytolbutamide was the most abundant metabolite in humanized liver mouse urine (Fig. 5) (Uehara et al., 2021), similar to that reported in humans, whereas 4-hydroxytolbutamide was predominantly excreted in the urine of the control mice.

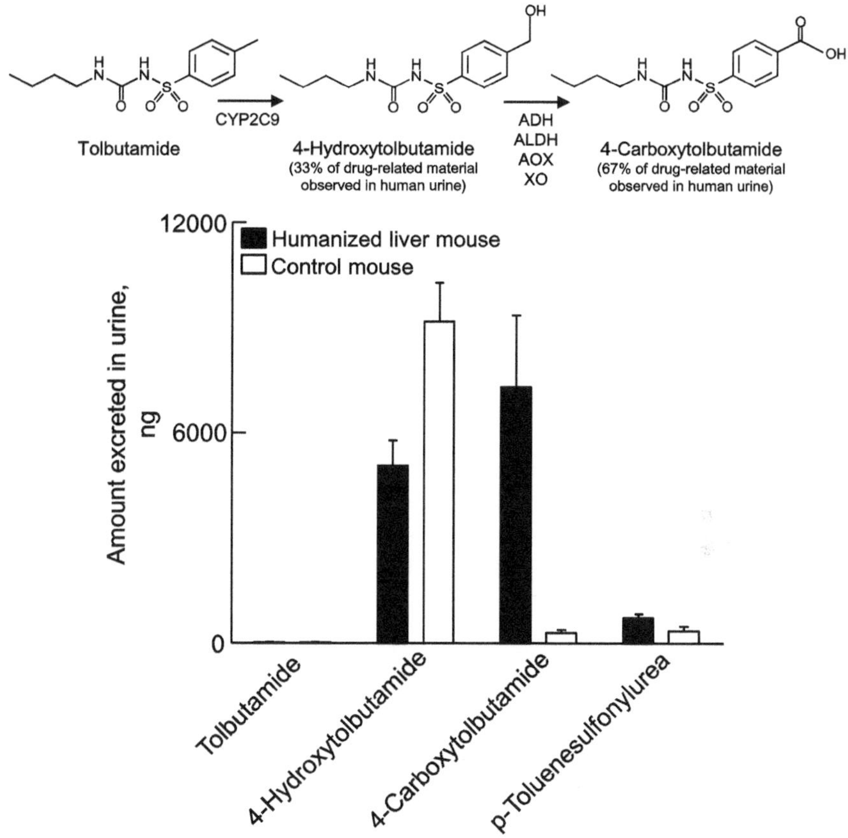

Fig. 5 Cumulative urinary excretions of tolbutamide and its metabolites for 72 h after oral administration in humanized liver mice and control mice. Tolbutamide and its metabolites were observed in urine of humanized liver mice and control mice after oral administrations of tolbutamide 10 mg/kg body weight. Data are reported means with SD values for four humanized liver mice and four control mice (Uehara et al., 2021). ADH, alcohol dehydrogenase; ALDH, aldehyde dehydrogenase; AOX, aldehyde oxidase; XO, xanthine oxidase.

3.2 Desloratadine

Desloratadine is a long-acting tricyclic antihistamine with selective peripheral histamine H1-receptor antagonistic activity. In humans, the major *in vivo* metabolic pathway for desloratadine is 3-hydroxydesloratadine, which is subsequently converted to 3-hydroxydesloratadine *O*-glucuronide. Both metabolites are excreted in roughly equal amounts in the urine and feces of humans (Ramanathan et al., 2007). The conversion of desloratadine to 3-hydroxydesloratadine is mediated by CYP2C8, with

N-glucuronidation catalyzed by UGT2B10 (Kazmi, Barbara, Yerino, & Parkinson, 2015). In contrast, these metabolites are detectable only at trace levels in non-clinical species such as mice, rats, and monkeys (Kazmi et al., 2015; Ramanathan et al., 2005). After a single oral administration of desloratadine (10 mg/kg), the mean AUC values for plasma concentrations of 3-hydroxydesloratadine and its *O*-glucuronide in humanized-liver mice were higher (>6-fold) than those in control mice (Fig. 6), whereas

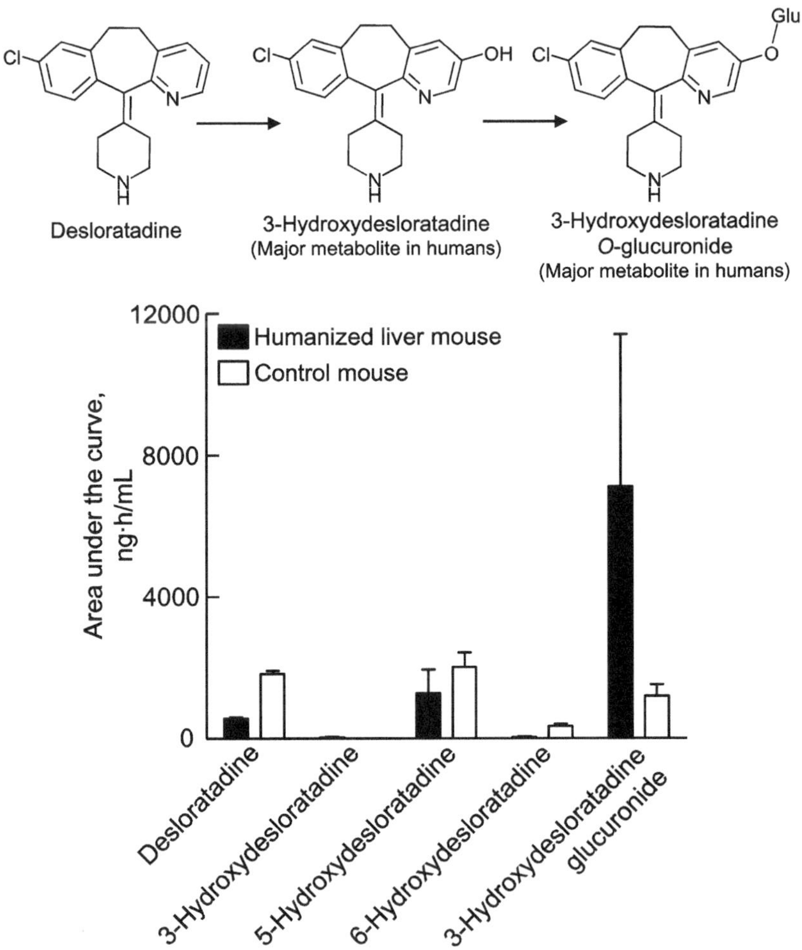

Fig. 6 Areas under the curve for plasma concentrations of desloratadine and its metabolites observed in humanized liver mice and control mice after oral administrations of desloratadine 10 mg/kg body weight. Data are reported means with SD values for four animals (Uehara, Yoneda, Higuchi, Yamazaki, & Suemizu, 2020).

the AUC values of 5- and 6-hydroxydesloratadine in humanized-liver mice were lower than those in control mice (Fig. 6) (Uehara et al., 2020). Overall, desloratadine metabolism mediated by P450 and UGT enzymes in humanized-liver mice was similar to that reported in humans.

3.3 Thalidomide

Thalidomide was previously withdrawn due to its teratogenic effects in humans but has been used for the treatment of leprosy, multiple myeloma, and cancers (Vargesson, 2015). Thalidomide causes limb defects in humans, monkeys, and rabbits, but not in rodents. Thalidomide is metabolized *via* two major pathways: 5′-hydroxythalidomide (a major product in rodents) and 5-hydroxythalidomide (human disproportionate phenyl ring-based metabolites). CYP3A4 and CYP3A5 catalyze thalidomide 5-hydroxylation that undergoes further oxidation, resulting in the formation of a glutathione conjugate (Chowdhury et al., 2010), which may be related to pharmacological and toxicological actions. In 2 h after oral administration of thalidomide (100 mg/kg), the plasma concentration ratios of 5-hydroxythalidomide to 5′-hydroxythalidomide were correlated with the ratio of human hepatocytes replaced in humanized liver mice (Miura, Uehara, Shimizu, Suemizu, & Yamazaki, 2021), suggesting the generation of 5-hydroxythalidomide by the transplanted human hepatocytes. After oral administration of thalidomide (100 mg/kg), plasma concentrations of 5-hydroxythalidomide, dihydroxythalidomide, and 5-hydroxythalidomide glutathione conjugate were higher in humanized liver mice than in control mice (Yamazaki et al., 2011), suggesting that humanized liver models are useful for studying thalidomide activation by CYP3A enzymes in humans.

3.4 Diclofenac

Diclofenac is a non-steroidal anti-inflammatory drug that exerts its effects by inhibition of prostaglandin synthesis (Gan, 2010). Diclofenac is metabolized to 4′-hydroxydiclofenac (the major pathway of diclofenac), 3′-hydroxydiclofenac, and 3′-hydroxy-4′-methoxydiclofenac by CYP2C9. Hydroxylation of diclofenac at the 3-position has only been reported in nonhuman primates and humans. 3′-Hydroxy-4′-methoxydiclofenac has not been found in mouse, rat, or marmoset plasma, but in human and baboon plasma only (unpublished data) (Faigle et al., 1988). After oral administration of diclofenac (10 mg/kg) to humanized chimeric mice, levels of 4′-hydroxydiclofenac were 3–4-fold significantly higher than those in the control mice, whereas 3-hydroxydiclofenac and 3′-hydroxy-4-methoxydiclofenac were completely absent or were found in only in trace amount in the plasma of control mice (Kamimura et al., 2015). Moreover, a single monochlorinated conjugate [M4 (2-hydroxy-3-(glutathion-S-yl) monoclofenac)], a human-specific metabolite formed by CYP2C9 (Yan et al., 2005), was detected in the bile of humanized liver mice after dosing with diclofenac. Overall, humanized mice produced human-specific metabolites of diclofenac, suggesting a functional animal model for studying diclofenac metabolism in humans.

4. Pharmacokinetic study using humanized liver mouse

The main role of preclinical pharmacokinetic studies is to characterize drug candidates to predict exposures and determine the dose and dosing regimen for initial clinical trials. The utility of humanized liver mice for predicting human pharmacokinetics has been validated. The pharmacokinetic data for cytochrome P450 substrates (caffeine, warfarin, omeprazole, metoprolol, and midazolam) in humans can be extrapolated from the corresponding data in humanized liver mice using simplified physiologically based pharmacokinetic modeling (Utoh et al., 2016). In contrast, a large fold error in clearance predicted by diazepam and quinidine calculated using physiological and empirical methods, including single-species allometry, was observed (Nakayama et al., 2020), probably resulting in P450-dependent diazepam oxidation activity in residual mouse hepatocytes. Marked differences in the *in vitro* intrinsic clearance of diazepam and quinidine by liver microsomes from other humanized liver mice due to differences in replacement indices were observed in the presence of β-NADPH (Sanoh et al., 2015). Overall, humanized liver mice may be useful pharmacokinetic models for drug development.

5. Drug interaction study using humanized liver mouse

Drug-drug interactions can either markedly reduce or enhance therapeutic or adverse effects of drugs by altering their pharmacokinetics or pharmacodynamics. The pharmacokinetics of five P450 substrates (caffeine, warfarin, omeprazole, metoprolol, and midazolam) were investigated in humanized liver mice following repeated oral administration of rifampicin, a typical human pregnane X receptor ligand. The mean AUC values for plasma concentrations of omeprazole and midazolam (unlike caffeine,

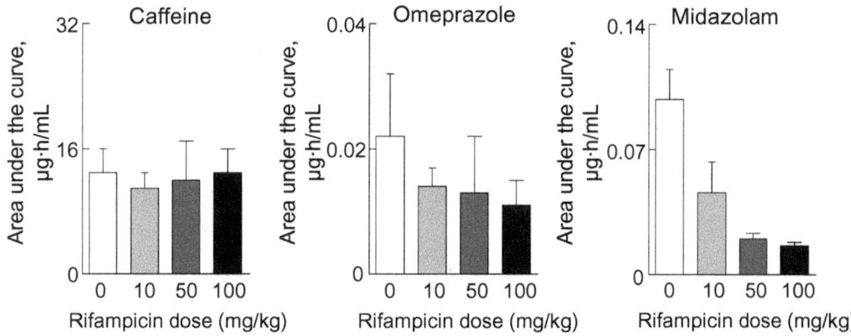

Fig. 7 Effects of rifampicin on areas under the curve for plasma concentrations of caffeine, omeprazole, and midazolam observed in humanized liver mice after oral administrations. Areas under the curve for plasma concentrations of caffeine, omeprazole, and midazolam observed in humanized liver mice and control mice after oral administrations (5.0mg/kg body weight) in untreated humanized liver mice and in those pretreated for 3 days with rifampicin (10, 50, and 100mg/kg). Bars are reported means with SD values for three animals (Uehara, Higuchi, et al., 2022).

warfarin, and metoprolol) decreased in a dose-dependent manner with respect to rifampicin, based on the induction of hepatic CYP2C19 and CYP3A4 in humanized liver mice (Fig. 7) (Uehara, Higuchi, et al., 2022). Therefore, humanized liver mice are a useful animal model for evaluating *in vivo* drug-drug interactions mediated by CYP3A/2C induction. In addition, a drug-gene interaction is an association between a drug and a genetic variant that may affect a patient's response to drug treatment. The pharmacokinetic profiles of T-1032, an *in vitro* CYP3A5 probe substrate, were investigated in humanized liver mice with hepatocytes of different *CYP3A5* genotypes, *CYP3A5** *1*/* 7, and *CYP3A5** *3*/* *3* (poor expressers). After a single oral dose of T-1032 (10mg/kg) in humanized liver mice, the mean maximum concentration (C_{max}) of T-1032 *N*-oxide in plasma was approximately 2-fold higher in humanized liver mice with *CYP3A5** *1*/* 7 hepatocytes than in those with *CYP3A5** *3*/* *3* hepatocytes (Uehara et al., 2022). These results suggested that polymorphic CYP3A5-dependent T-1032 *N*-oxidation was observed in humanized liver mice *in vivo*. Moreover, *in vivo* drug interactions between the teratogen thalidomide and midazolam (a CYP3A substrate) were observed in humanized liver mice (Yamazaki et al., 2013). The mean clearance of midazolam (administered intravenously, 10mg/kg) for plasma concentrations of thalidomide was increased by oral co-administration of thalidomide (100mg/kg). A larger AUC of the major metabolite 1′-hydroxymidazolam

(1.7-fold) was observed after daily pretreatment with thalidomide for 3 days, presumably because of the heterotropic cooperativity of human CYP3A enzymes (Okada et al., 2009). The occurrence of drug-drug interactions between clemizole and ritonavir (a CYP3A4 inhibitor) in humans was predicted in a study using humanized liver mice (Nishimura et al., 2013). The human CYP2C19 or CYP2C9 genotype of the transplanted human hepatocytes affects the rate of production of human-predominant drug metabolites for *S*-mephenytoin and diclofenac in humanized liver mice (Hu, Wu, Nishimura, Zheng, & Peltz, 2013).

6. Human P450-inactivated chimeric mouse model using mechanism-based inhibitor

Determination of the P450 enzymes involved in drug metabolism helps predict potential drug interactions *in vivo* during drug disposal. Diclofenac is a nonsteroidal anti-inflammatory drug that is metabolized by liver cytochrome P450 enzymes. CYP2C9 is responsible for 4′-hydroxylation, whereas CYP2C and CYP3A4 mediate 5′-hydroxylation (Bort et al., 1999; Leemann, Transon, & Dayer, 1993). After diclofenac administration to humanized liver mice, plasma levels of diclofenac and the mean values of C_{max} and AUC for plasma concentrations of 4′-hydroxydiclofenac were significantly lower (38% and 53% of the untreated group, respectively) in the tienilic acid (a mechanism-based inhibitor of CYP2C9)-treated group (Fig. 8) (Miura et al., 2020). In contrast, 5-hydroxydiclofenac and diclofenac acyl glucuronide levels were similar in pretreated and untreated mice. Humanized liver mice orally pretreated with tienilic acid could be a possible model for metabolically inactivated CYP2C9 in human hepatocytes. In addition, coumarin is a natural product with aromatic and fragrant characteristics from various plants, and exhibits marked species differences in metabolism and toxicity (Fentem & Fry, 1993). The major metabolic pathway for coumarin metabolism in humans is 7-hydroxylation (Moran, O'Kennedy, & Thornes, 1987; Shilling, Crampton, & Longland, 1969), whereas coumarin causes hepatotoxicity in rats *via* the reactive metabolite coumarin 3,4-epoxide (Lake et al., 1989). Coumarin metabolism in rat liver microsomes occurs mainly *via* 3,4-epoxidation, predominantly mediated by CYP1A and CYP2E1 (Born, Caudill, Fliter, & Purdon, 2002), which ultimately leads to the formation of *o*-hydroxyphenylacetic acid (Born, Hu, & Lehman-McKeeman, 2000). The *in vivo* biotransformation of coumarin to conjugated and unconjugated 7-hydroxycoumarin after oral administration of coumarin

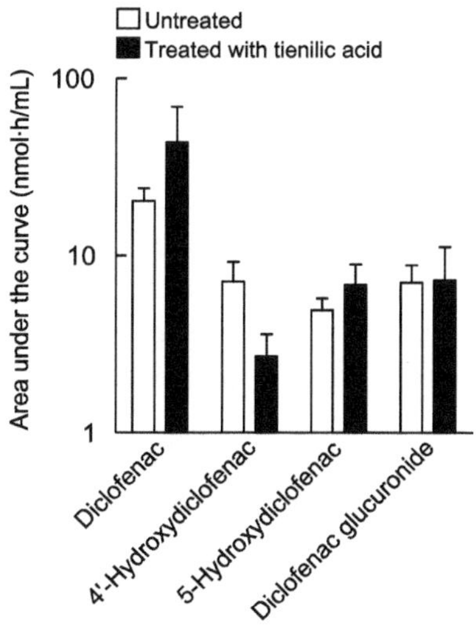

Fig. 8 Areas under the curve for plasma concentrations of diclofenac and its metabolites observed in humanized liver mice after oral administrations in untreated humanized-liver mice and in those pretreated for 3 days with tienilic acid (15 mg/kg). Areas under the curve for plasma concentrations of diclofenac and its metabolites observed in humanized liver mice and control mice after intravenous administrations (10 mg/kg body weight) in untreated humanized-liver mice and in those pretreated for 3 days with tienilic acid (15 mg/kg). Data are reported means with SD values for three (untreated) or four (pretreated with tienilic acid) animals (Miura et al., 2020).

was higher in humanized liver mice than in control mice (Miura et al., 2021), reflecting the rapid 7-hydroxylation of coumarin by liver microsomes from humanized liver mice (Uehara, Yoneda, et al., 2022). After intravenous administration of coumarin to humanized liver mice, the mean C_{max} and AUC for plasma concentrations of *o*-hydroxyphenylacetic acid were significantly lower in the group orally pretreated with furafylline (57% and 45% of the untreated values, respectively) (Miura, Uehara, Shimizu, Murayama, et al., 2021). These results suggested that the metabolic activation of coumarin in humans was mainly mediated by CYP1A2. Thus, *in vivo* P450 identification strategies for drug metabolism using humanized liver mice with selectively inactivated liver CYP2C9, CYP1A2, and other P450 enzymes may provide important information for drug interaction studies.

7. Conclusion

This review presents a comprehensive overview of cytochrome P450 enzymes in humanized liver mice. The expression levels of hepatic human P450 genes/proteins and liver microsomal drug oxidation activities were similar in humans and humanized liver mice. *In vivo* drug metabolism and drug interactions mediated by multiple human drug-metabolizing enzymes, including P450 and UGT, have been observed in humanized liver mice. The human P450-inactivated chimeric mouse model using a mechanism-based inhibitor is a novel tool for understanding important information regarding *in vivo* drug interactions in humans. However, the utility of humanized liver mice as experimental models depends on the degree of humanization of chimeric mouse liver with transplanted human hepatocytes, because residual mouse hepatocytes hinder determination of the phenotypes and functions of human hepatocytes. Indeed, a few kinds of drug oxidation activities in liver microsomes (bufuralol 1′-hydroxylation and propafenone 4′-hydroxylation) were much higher in humanized liver mice than humans. An ideal solution to this problem is to functionally inactivate mouse drug-metabolizing enzymes. The humanized liver mice lacking murine P450 oxidoreductase would be advanced preclinical models for studying human drug metabolism (Barzi et al., 2017). This information on the fundamental characteristics of P450 in humanized livers from chimeric mice should be useful in the application of humanized liver mice for *in vivo* studies on drug metabolism/pharmacokinetics and drug interactions.

Conflict of interest

The authors declare no conflict of interest.

Acknowledgments

This work was supported by the Platform Project for Supporting Drug Discovery and Life Science Research (Basis for Supporting Innovative Drug Discovery and Life Science Research [BINDS]) from the Japanese Agency for Medical Research and Development (AMED) under grant number 21am0101121j0005, the METI Artificial Intelligence-based Substance Hazard Integrated Prediction System project, Japan, and the Japan Society for the Promotion of Science Grant-in-Aid for Scientific Research 20K06463 and 20K07164. We thank the helpful advice of Drs. Mamoru Ito, Yasuyuki Ohnishi, Hidetaka Kamimura and the technical expertise of Drs. Yuichiro Higuchi and Nao Yoneda for their assistance.

Author contributions

(1) Study conception and design: SU, HS, and HY.

(2) Acquisition, analysis, and/or interpretation of data: SU and HS.

(3) Drafting/revision of the work for intellectual content and context: SU, HS, and HY.

(4) Final approval and overall responsibility for the published work: HY.

References

Achour, B., Barber, J., & Rostami-Hodjegan, A. (2014). Expression of hepatic drug-metabolizing cytochrome p450 enzymes and their intercorrelations: A meta-analysis. *Drug Metabolism and Disposition*, *42*(8), 1349–1356. https://doi.org/10.1124/dmd.114.058834.

Barzi, M., Pankowicz, F. P., Zorman, B., Liu, X., Legras, X., Yang, D., et al. (2017). A novel humanized mouse lacking murine P450 oxidoreductase for studying human drug metabolism. *Nature Communications*, *8*(1), 39. https://doi.org/10.1038/s41467-017-00049-x.

Born, S. L., Caudill, D., Fliter, K. L., & Purdon, M. P. (2002). Identification of the cytochromes P450 that catalyze coumarin 3,4-epoxidation and 3-hydroxylation. *Drug Metabolism and Disposition*, *30*(5), 483–487. https://doi.org/10.1124/dmd.30.5.483.

Born, S. L., Hu, J. K., & Lehman-McKeeman, L. D. (2000). o-Hydroxyphenylacetaldehyde is a hepatotoxic metabolite of coumarin. *Drug Metabolism and Disposition*, *28*(2), 218–223. Retrieved from https://www.ncbi.nlm.nih.gov/pubmed/10640521.

Bort, R., Mace, K., Boobis, A., Gomez-Lechon, M. J., Pfeifer, A., & Castell, J. (1999). Hepatic metabolism of diclofenac: Role of human CYP in the minor oxidative pathways. *Biochemical Pharmacology*, *58*(5), 787–796. https://doi.org/10.1016/s0006-2952(99)00167-7.

Chowdhury, G., Murayama, N., Okada, Y., Uno, Y., Shimizu, M., Shibata, N., et al. (2010). Human liver microsomal cytochrome P450 3A enzymes involved in thalidomide 5-hydroxylation and formation of a glutathione conjugate. *Chemical Research in Toxicology*, *23*(6), 1018–1024. https://doi.org/10.1021/tx900367p.

Faigle, J. W., Bottcher, I., Godbillon, J., Kriemler, H. P., Schlumpf, E., Schneider, W., et al. (1988). A new metabolite of diclofenac sodium in human plasma. *Xenobiotica*, *18*(10), 1191–1197. https://doi.org/10.3109/00498258809042242.

Fentem, J. H., & Fry, J. R. (1993). Species differences in the metabolism and hepatotoxicity of coumarin. *Comparative Biochemistry and Physiology Part C Comparative Pharmacology and Toxicology*, *104*(1), 1–8. https://doi.org/10.1016/0742-8413(93)90102-q.

Gan, T. J. (2010). Diclofenac: An update on its mechanism of action and safety profile. *Current Medical Research and Opinion*, *26*(7), 1715–1731. https://doi.org/10.1185/03007995.2010.486301.

Hasegawa, M., Kawai, K., Mitsui, T., Taniguchi, K., Monnai, M., Wakui, M., et al. (2011). The reconstituted 'humanized liver' in TK-NOG mice is mature and functional. *Biochemical and Biophysical Research Communications*, *405*(3), 405–410. https://doi.org/10.1016/j.bbrc.2011.01.042.

Hu, Y., Wu, M., Nishimura, T., Zheng, M., & Peltz, G. (2013). Human pharmacogenetic analysis in chimeric mice with 'humanized livers'. *Pharmacogenetics and Genomics*, *23*(2), 78–83. https://doi.org/10.1097/FPC.0b013e32835cb2c7.

Kamimura, H., Ito, S., Nozawa, K., Nakamura, S., Chijiwa, H., Nagatsuka, S., et al. (2015). Formation of the accumulative human metabolite and human-specific glutathione conjugate of diclofenac in TK-NOG chimeric mice with humanized livers. *Drug Metabolism and Disposition*, *43*(3), 309–316. https://doi.org/10.1124/dmd.114.061689.

Kazmi, F., Barbara, J. E., Yerino, P., & Parkinson, A. (2015). A long-standing mystery solved: The formation of 3-hydroxydesloratadine is catalyzed by CYP2C8 but prior glucuronidation of desloratadine by UDP-glucuronosyltransferase 2B10 is an obligatory requirement. *Drug Metabolism and Disposition: The Biological Fate of Chemicals*, *43*(4), 523–533. https://doi.org/10.1124/dmd.114.062620.

Kitamura, S., Sugihara, K., & Ohta, S. (2006). Drug-metabolizing ability of molybdenum hydroxylases. *Drug Metabolism and Pharmacokinetics*, *21*(2), 83–98. https://doi.org/10.2133/dmpk.21.83.

Knodell, R. G., Hall, S. D., Wilkinson, G. R., & Guengerich, F. P. (1987). Hepatic metabolism of tolbutamide: Characterization of the form of cytochrome P-450 involved in methyl hydroxylation and relationship to in vivo disposition. *Journal of Pharmacology And Experimental Therapeutics*, *241*(3), 1112–1119. Retrieved from https://www.ncbi.nlm.nih.gov/pubmed/3598900.

Lake, B. G., Gray, T. J., Evans, J. G., Lewis, D. F., Beamand, J. A., & Hue, K. L. (1989). Studies on the mechanism of coumarin-induced toxicity in rat hepatocytes: Comparison with dihydrocoumarin and other coumarin metabolites. *Toxicology and Applied Pharmacology*, *97*(2), 311–323. https://doi.org/10.1016/0041-008x(89)90336-0.

Leemann, T., Transon, C., & Dayer, P. (1993). Cytochrome P450TB (CYP2C): A major monooxygenase catalyzing diclofenac 4′-hydroxylation in human liver. *Life Sciences*, *52*(1), 29–34. https://doi.org/10.1016/0024-3205(93)90285-b.

McDaniel, H. G., Podgainy, H., & Bressler, R. (1969). The metabolism of tolbutamide in rat liver. *Journal of Pharmacology and Experimental Therapeutics*, *167*(1), 91–97. Retrieved from https://www.ncbi.nlm.nih.gov/pubmed/5772753. https://jpet.aspetjournals.org/content/167/1/91.long.

Mimura, M., Yamazaki, H., Sugahara, C., Hiroi, T., Funae, Y., & Shimada, T. (1994). Differential roles of cytochromes P450 2D1, 2C11, and 1A1/2 in the hydroxylation of bufuralol by rat liver microsomes. *Biochemical Pharmacology*, *47*(11), 1957–1963. https://doi.org/10.1016/0006-2952(94)90069-8.

Miners, J. O., & Birkett, D. J. (1996). Use of tolbutamide as a substrate probe for human hepatic cytochrome P450 2C9. *Methods in Enzymology*, *272*, 139–145. https://doi.org/10.1016/s0076-6879(96)72017-7.

Miura, T., Uehara, S., Shimizu, M., Murayama, N., Suemizu, H., & Yamazaki, H. (2021). Roles of human cytochrome P450 1A2 in coumarin 3,4-epoxidation mediated by untreated hepatocytes and by those metabolically inactivated with furafylline in previously transplanted chimeric mice. *The Journal of Toxicological Sciences*, *46*(11), 525–530. https://doi.org/10.2131/jts.46.525.

Miura, T., Uehara, S., Shimizu, M., Murayama, N., Utoh, M., Suemizu, H., et al. (2020). Different roles of human cytochrome P450 2C9 and 3A enzymes in diclofenac 4′- and 5-hydroxylations mediated by metabolically inactivated human hepatocytes in previously transplanted chimeric mice. *Chemical Research in Toxicology*, *33*(2), 634–639. https://doi.org/10.1021/acs.chemrestox.9b00446.

Miura, T., Uehara, S., Shimizu, M., Suemizu, H., & Yamazaki, H. (2021). Pharmacokinetics of primary oxidative metabolites of thalidomide in rats and in chimeric mice humanized with different human hepatocytes. *The Journal of Toxicological Sciences*, *46*(7), 311–317. https://doi.org/10.2131/jts.46.311.

Mohnike, G., Wittenhagen, G., & Langenbeck, W. (1958). Uber des Ausscheidengsprodukt von N-(4-Mathyl-benzolsulfonyl)- Nt-butyl harnstoff beim Hunt. *Naturwissenschaften*, *45*, 13.

Moran, E., O'Kennedy, R., & Thornes, R. D. (1987). Analysis of coumarin and its urinary metabolites by high-performance liquid chromatography. *Journal of Chromatography*, *416*(1), 165–169. https://doi.org/10.1016/0378-4347(87)80499-1.

Nakayama, K., Kamimura, H., Suemizu, H., Yoneda, N., Nishiwaki, M., Iwamoto, K., et al. (2020). Predicted values for human total clearance of a variety of typical compounds with differently humanized-liver mouse plasma data. *Drug Metabolism and Pharmacokinetics*, *35*(4), 389–396. https://doi.org/10.1016/j.dmpk.2020.05.004.

Nishimura, T., Hu, Y., Wu, M., Pham, E., Suemizu, H., Elazar, M., et al. (2013). Using chimeric mice with humanized livers to predict human drug metabolism and a drug-drug interaction. *The Journal of Pharmacology and Experimental Therapeutics*, *344*(2), 388–396. https://doi.org/10.1124/jpet.112.198697.

Okada, Y., Murayama, N., Yanagida, C., Shimizu, M., Guengerich, F. P., & Yamazaki, H. (2009). Drug interactions of thalidomide with midazolam and cyclosporine A: Heterotropic cooperativity of human cytochrome P450 3A5. *Drug Metabolism and Disposition*, *37*(1), 18–23. https://doi.org/10.1124/dmd.108.024679.

Ramanathan, R., Alvarez, N., Su, A. D., Chowdhury, S., Alton, K., Stauber, K., et al. (2005). Metabolism and excretion of loratadine in male and female mice, rats and monkeys. *Xenobiotica, 35*(2), 155–189. https://doi.org/10.1080/00498250500038906.
Ramanathan, R., Reyderman, L., Su, A. D., Alvarez, N., Chowdhury, S. K., Alton, K. B., et al. (2007). Disposition of desloratadine in healthy volunteers. *Xenobiotica, 37*(7), 770–787. https://doi.org/10.1080/00498250701463325.
Sanoh, S., Naritomi, Y., Fujimoto, M., Sato, K., Kawamura, A., Horiguchi, A., et al. (2015). Predictability of plasma concentration-time curves in humans using single-species allometric scaling of chimeric mice with humanized liver. *Xenobiotica, 45*(7), 605–614. https://doi.org/10.3109/00498254.2015.1007112.
Shilling, W. H., Crampton, R. F., & Longland, R. C. (1969). Metabolism of coumarin in man. *Nature, 221*(5181), 664–665. https://doi.org/10.1038/221664b0.
Shimada, T., Yamazaki, H., Mimura, M., Inui, Y., & Guengerich, F. P. (1994). Interindividual variations in human liver cytochrome P-450 enzymes involved in the oxidation of drugs, carcinogens and toxic chemicals: Studies with liver microsomes of 30 Japanese and 30 Caucasians. *The Journal of Pharmacology and Experimental Therapeutics, 270*(1), 414–423. Retrieved from https://www.ncbi.nlm.nih.gov/pubmed/8035341.
Thomas, R. C., & Ikeda, G. J. (1966). The metabolic fate of tolbutamide in man and in the rat. *Journal of Medicinal Chemistry, 9*(4), 507–510. https://doi.org/10.1021/jm00322a014.
Uehara, S., Higuchi, Y., Yoneda, N., Kawai, K., Yamamoto, M., Kamimura, H., et al. (2022). An improved TK-NOG mouse as a novel platform for humanized liver that overcomes limitations in both male and female animals. *Drug Metabolism and Pharmacokinetics, 42*, 100410. https://doi.org/10.1016/j.dmpk.2021.100410.
Uehara, S., Murayama, N., Yamazaki, H., & Suemizu, H. (2019). Regioselective hydroxylation of an antiarrhythmic drug, propafenone, mediated by rat liver cytochrome P450 2D2 differs from that catalyzed by human P450 2D6. *Xenobiotica, 49*(11), 1323–1331. https://doi.org/10.1080/00498254.2018.1564401.
Uehara, S., Shimizu, M., Plé, K., Routier, S., Yoneda, N., Higuchi, Y., et al. (2022). Probe drug T-1032 N-oxygenation mediated by cytochrome P450 3A5 in human hepatocytes in vitro and in humanized-liver mice in vivo. *Drug Metabolism and Pharmacokinetics, 44*, 100453. https://doi.org/10.1016/j.dmpk.2022.100453.
Uehara, S., Yoneda, N., Higuchi, Y., Yamazaki, H., & Suemizu, H. (2020). Metabolism of desloratadine by chimeric TK-NOG mice transplanted with human hepatocytes. *Xenobiotica, 50*(6), 733–740. https://doi.org/10.1080/00498254.2019.1688892.
Uehara, S., Yoneda, N., Higuchi, Y., Yamazaki, H., & Suemizu, H. (2021). Methyl-hydroxylation and subsequent oxidation to produce carboxylic acid is the major metabolic pathway of tolbutamide in chimeric TK-NOG mice transplanted with human hepatocytes. *Xenobiotica, 51*(5), 582–589. https://doi.org/10.1080/00498254.2021.1875515.
Uehara, S., Yoneda, N., Higuchi, Y., Yamazaki, H., & Suemizu, H. (2022). Cytochrome P450-dependent drug oxidation activities and their expression levels in liver microsomes of chimeric TK-NOG mice with humanized livers. *Drug Metabolism and Pharmacokinetics, 44*, 100454. https://doi.org/10.1016/j.dmpk.2022.100454.
Utoh, M., Suemizu, H., Mitsui, M., Kawano, M., Toda, A., Uehara, S., et al. (2016). Human plasma concentrations of cytochrome P450 probe cocktails extrapolated from pharmacokinetics in mice transplanted with human hepatocytes and from pharmacokinetics in common marmosets using physiologically based pharmacokinetic modeling. *Xenobiotica, 46*(12), 1049–1055. https://doi.org/10.3109/00498254.2016.1147102.
Vargesson, N. (2015). Thalidomide-induced teratogenesis: History and mechanisms. *Birth Defects Research. Part C, Embryo Today, 105*(2), 140–156. https://doi.org/10.1002/bdrc.21096.

Yamazaki, H., Suemizu, H., Igaya, S., Shimizu, M., Shibata, N., Nakamura, M., et al. (2011). In vivo formation of a glutathione conjugate derived from thalidomide in humanized uPA-NOG mice. *Chemical Research in Toxicology*, *24*(3), 287–289. https://doi.org/10.1021/tx200005g.

Yamazaki, H., Suemizu, H., Murayama, N., Utoh, M., Shibata, N., Nakamura, M., et al. (2013). In vivo drug interactions of the teratogen thalidomide with midazolam: Heterotropic cooperativity of human cytochrome P450 in humanized TK-NOG mice. *Chemical Research in Toxicology*, *26*(3), 486–489. https://doi.org/10.1021/tx400008g.

Yan, Z., Li, J., Huebert, N., Caldwell, G. W., Du, Y., & Zhong, H. (2005). Detection of a novel reactive metabolite of diclofenac: Evidence for CYP2C9-mediated bioactivation via arene oxides. *Drug Metabolism and Disposition*, *33*(6), 706–713. https://doi.org/10.1124/dmd.104.003095.

CHAPTER ELEVEN

Polymorphic cytochromes P450 in non-human primates

Yasuhiro Uno[a,*], Shotaro Uehara[b], and Hiroshi Yamazaki[b]
[a]Joint Faculty of Veterinary Medicine, Kagoshima University, Kagoshima, Japan
[b]Showa Pharmaceutical University, Machida, Tokyo, Japan
*Corresponding author: e-mail address: unoxx001@vet.kagoshima-u.ac.jp

Contents

Abstract

Cynomolgus macaques (*Macaca fascicularis*, an Old World monkey) are widely used in drug development because of their genetic and physiological similarities to humans, and this trend has continued with the use of common marmosets (*Callithrix jacchus*, a New World monkey). Information on the major drug-metabolizing cytochrome P450 (CYP, P450) enzymes of these primate species indicates that multiple forms of their

Advances in Pharmacology, Volume 95
ISSN 1054-3589
https://doi.org/10.1016/bs.apha.2022.05.005

P450 enzymes have generally similar substrate selectivities to those of human P450 enzymes; however, some differences in isoform, activity, and substrate specificity account for limited species differences in drug oxidative metabolism. This review provides information on the P450 enzymes of cynomolgus macaques and marmosets, including cDNA, tissue expression, substrate specificity, and genetic variants, along with age differences and induction. Typical examples of important P450s to be considered in drug metabolism studies include cynomolgus CYP2C19, which is expressed abundantly in liver and metabolizes numerous drugs. Moreover, genetic variants of cynomolgus CYP2C19 affect the individual pharmacokinetic data of drugs such as *R*-warfarin. These findings provide a foundation for understanding each P450 enzyme and the individual pharmacokinetic and toxicological results in cynomolgus macaques and marmosets as preclinical models. In addition, the effects of induction on some drug clearances mediated by P450 enzymes are also described. In summary, this review describes genetic and acquired individual differences in cynomolgus and marmoset P450 enzymes involved in drug oxidation that may be associated with pharmacological and/or toxicological effects.

Abbreviations

AUC	areas under the plasma concentration curve
CYP or P450	cytochrome P450
EROD	7-ethoxyresorufin *O*-deethylation
Glu-P-1	2-amino-6-methyldipyrido[1,2-*a*:3′,2′-*d*]imidazole
IQ	2-amino-3-methylimidazo[4,5-*f*]quinoline
MeIQx	2-amino-3,8-dimethylimidazo[4,5-*f*]quinoxaline
PhIP	2-amino-1-methyl-6-phenylimidazo[4,5-*b*]pyridine
SRS	substrate recognition site
TCDD	2,3,7,8-tetrachlorodibenzo-*p*-dioxin
Trp-P-2	3-amino-l-methyl-5*H*-pyrido[4,3-*b*]-indole

1. Introduction

The cytochromes P450 (CYP or P450) form a superfamily of heme-thiolate enzymes that mediate the biotransformation and metabolism of endogenous steroid hormones, xenobiotics, and drugs. In humans, 57 functional genes and 58 pseudogenes are known (Nelson et al., 2004), and the CYP1A, CYP2B, CYP2C, CYP2D, CYP2E, and CYP3A isoforms are major drug-metabolizing enzymes, whereas CYP4 isoforms metabolize endogenous and exogenous compounds. Various enzymatic reactions are catalyzed by P450 enzymes, including hydroxylation, dealkylation, sulfoxidation, epoxidation, and *N*-oxidation (Danielson, 2002). Species differences of P450-mediated drug metabolism have been noted in mice, rats, dogs, pigs, and cynomolgus macaques (Martignoni, Groothuis, & de Kanter, 2006). Consequently, to select appropriate animal species for drug metabolism and pharmacokinetic studies, it is of great importance to understand the orthologous relationships and functional characteristics of their P450 isoforms.

The cynomolgus macaque (*Macaca fascicularis*) is an Old World primate species widely used in preclinical studies, including drug metabolism studies, due to their close genetic and physiological similarities to humans (Bogaards et al., 2000). Common marmosets (*Callithrix jacchus*), a New World primate species, recently has received attention as an animal model in various biomedical investigations, including those on drug metabolism (Uno, Uehara, & Yamazaki, 2016). These two non-human primate species might help to minimize the problems of species differences, which constitute an important issue during drug development. For cynomolgus macaques and marmosets, a number of P450s that are major xenobiotic-metabolizing enzymes have been identified and characterized (Table 1). These P450s generally have high sequence identities to their human counterparts (Table 1). A majority of these P450s have similar enzyme characteristics to those of human P450s (Table 2); however, some differences have been noted.

For example, cynomolgus CYP2C76, which is not orthologous to any human P450, is abundantly expressed in liver, metabolizes numerous P450 substrates, and accounts for species differences in the metabolism of drugs such as pitavastatin (Uno et al., 2016). Similarly, cynomolgus CYP2C8, CYP2C9, and CYP2C19 metabolize substrates of human CYP2Cs, but also those of human CYP2B6 and CYP3A4 (Hosaka et al., 2015). Cynomolgus CYP3A enzymes show similar substrate selectivities to human CYP3A enzymes, but also exhibit wider substrate selectivity toward human CYP2D substrates (Iwasaki, Murayama, Koizumi, Uno, & Yamazaki, 2010), resulting in higher CYP2D-related drug clearance in cynomolgus macaques than in humans. In marmosets, CYP2C58 and CYP2C8 are highly homologous to human CYP2C8; however, marmoset CYP2C58, unlike human and marmoset CYP2C8, does not catalyze paclitaxel 6α-hydroxylation, but has the highest metabolic activities among the five marmoset CYP2Cs for oxidations of 7-ethoxycoumarin and chlorzoxazone, which are not human CYP2C substrates (Uehara, Uno, Inoue, Kawano, et al., 2015). These findings collectively suggest that cynomolgus and marmoset CYP2Cs have similar substrate recognition and functionality as human CYP2Cs, but there are also a few specific differences in drug oxidative metabolism among the three species.

Table 1 Homologous P450 cDNAs in humans, cynomolgus macaques, and marmosets with the amino acid sequence identities of cynomolgus and marmoset P450s to human P450s.

Marmoset			Cynomolgus			Human	
P450	GenBank accession no.	Sequence identity (%)	P450	GenBank accession no.	Sequence identity (%)	P450	GenBank accession no.
1A1	KJ922553	90	1A1	D17575	94	1A1	NM_000499
1A2	NM_001204434	88	1A2	D86474	93	1A2	NM_000761
1B1	KX231947	92	1B1	KX231946	94	1B1	NM_000104
–		–	1D1	GU289741	91[a]	1D1P	N/A
2A6	KJ922555	89	2A23	DQ074790	92	2A6	NM_000762
		86			89	2A7	NM_000764
		93			94	2A13	NM_000766
–		–	2A24	DQ074792	95	2A6	
–		–			93	2A7	
–		–			94	2A13	
–		–	2A26	GU289744	93	2A6	
–		–			91	2A7	
–		–			93	2A13	
2B6	KJ922556	86	2B6	DQ074793	91	2B6	NM_000767
2C8	NM_001204437	88	2C8(20)	S53046	92	2C8	NM_000770
2C18	KJ922558	93	2C18	DQ297685	96	2C18	NM_000772
2C19	KJ922561	86	2C9(43)	DQ074806	93	2C9	NM_000771

		86			91	2C19	NM_000769
–		–	2C19(75)	DQ074805	93	2C9	
–		–			92	2C19	
2C58	KJ922559	87	–		–	2C8	
		79	–		–	2C9	
		78	–		–	2C18	
		78	–		–	2C19	
2C76	KJ922560	68	2C76	DQ074807	70	2C8	
		68			71	2C9	
		79			72	2C18	
		69			72	2C19	
2D6 (19)	NM_001204438	91	2D6(17)	GU981762	93	2D6	NM_000106
2D8	KJ922562	85	2D8(44)	DQ297684	91	2D6	
2E1	NM_001267751	89	2E1	HQ162318	94	2E1	NM_000773
2F1	MF457786	93	2F1	MF457780	95	2F1	NP_000765
			2G2	GU289743	93[a]	2G2P	N/A
2J2	KX231948	91	2J2	DQ074794	95	2J2	NM_000775
3A4 (21)	NM_001204440	90	3A4(8)	S53047	94	3A4	NM_017460
3A5	NM_001204442	89	3A5	DQ074795	91	3A5	NM_000777

Continued

Table 1 Homologous P450 cDNAs in humans, cynomolgus macaques, and marmosets with the amino acid sequence identities of cynomolgus and marmoset P450s to human P450s.—cont'd

Marmoset			**Cynomolgus**			**Human**	
P450	**GenBank accession no.**	**Sequence identity (%)**	**P450**	**GenBank accession no.**	**Sequence identity (%)**	**P450**	**GenBank accession no.**
–		–	3A43	DQ074796	97	3A43	NM_022820
3A90	NM_001204443	82	–		–	3A4	
		88	–		–	3A5	
		78	–		–	3A7	NM_000765
		74	–		–	3A43	
4A11	KX231949	88	4A11	DQ074797	95	4A11	NM_000778
4F2	KX231950	93	4F2(45)	DQ074798	94	4F2	NM_001082
4F3 (3B)	KX231951	93	4F3v2	DQ074799	95	4F3B	
	NM_001199208	4F71(11)		KX231952	89	4F11	DQ074800
91	4F11						NM_021187
4F12	KX231953	87	4F12	DQ074801	92	4F12	NM_023944

For P450 enzymes that have been renamed, the original names are indicated in parentheses. N/A, not available.

Table 2 Representative substrates for marmoset, cynomolgus, and human P450 enzymes.

Species	P450	Substrate
Marmoset	1A2	Caffeine, phenacetin
	2C19	*S*-Warfarin, omeprazole
	2D6(19), 2D8	Metoprolol
	3A4(21), 3A5, 3A90	Midazolam, caffeine
Cynomolgus	1A2	Phenacetin
	2C9(43)	Caffeine
	2C19(75)	*R,S*-Warfarin, omeprazole
	2D6(17), 2D8(44)	Metoprolol
	3A4(8), 3A5	Midazolam
Human	1A2	Caffeine, phenacetin, *R*-warfarin
	2C9	*S*-Warfarin
	2C19	Omeprazole
	2D6	Metoprolol
	3A4, 3A5	Midazolam

2. Molecular characteristics of P450s

Among humans, cynomolgus macaques, and marmosets, the locations and directions of *CYP1–CYP4* genes in gene clusters are well conserved; however, the gene arrangements of the *CYP2ABFGST*, *CYP2C*, *CYP2D*, *CYP3A*, *CYP4ABXZ*, and *CYP4F* clusters are slightly different (Uehara, Uno, & Yamazaki, 2020; Uno, Iwasaki, Yamazaki, & Nelson, 2011). *CYP1D1* is pseudogenized in humans and marmosets but is expressed in cynomolgus liver and kidney and encodes a functional enzyme (Uno, Uehara, Murayama, & Yamazaki, 2011a). Human *CYP2G2* is a pseudogene, whereas cynomolgus *CYP2G2* contains a complete open reading frame, is expressed in the nasal mucosa, and encodes a functional drug-metabolizing enzyme (Uno, Uehara, Murayama, & Yamazaki, 2011b). In contrast, no *CYP2G2* has been found in the marmoset genome

(Uehara, Uno, & Yamazaki, 2020). Interestingly, unlike the human and macaque genomes, the marmoset genome contains the additional human *CYP2C8*-like gene *CYP2C58* (which has a complete open reading frame) but no human *CYP2C9* ortholog (Uehara, Uno, & Yamazaki, 2020). *CYP2C76* is present in the macaque and marmoset genomes, but not in the human genome (Uehara, Uno, & Yamazaki, 2020; Uno, Iwasaki, et al., 2011). *CYP2D* genes are arranged in the human genome differently than in the macaque and marmoset genomes, and *CYP2D8*, a pseudogene in humans, encodes a functional enzyme in macaques and marmosets (Uehara, Uno, & Yamazaki, 2020; Uno, Iwasaki, et al., 2011). For *CYP3A* genes, the number and arrangements of genes in the genome are well-conserved between humans and macaques, but not between humans and marmosets (Uehara, Uno, & Yamazaki, 2020; Uno, Iwasaki, et al., 2011). Marmoset CYP3A5 and CYP3A90, which are highly homologous to human CYP3A5, are functional enzymes, whereas the marmoset genome does not contain a *CYP3A43* ortholog. The gene arrangements in the marmoset *CYP4ABXZ* and *CYP4F* clusters are slightly different to those in the human and/or macaque clusters (Uehara, Uno, & Yamazaki, 2020). A total of 36 marmoset and 27 cynomolgus P450s in the CYP1–CYP4 families have been identified to date and generally have high sequence identities to human P450s (Table 1).

The relative levels of hepatic P450 expressions show similarities in humans, cynomolgus macaques, and marmosets (Fig. 1). Except for CYP2E1, which is abundant at mRNA level, CYP3A expression is most abundant and CYP2C is moderately abundant in human and cynomolgus macaque liver in terms of protein levels; in marmosets in terms of mRNA levels, CYP3A expression is dominant and CYP2C is expressed to a lesser extent. In contrast, cynomolgus CYP2As and marmoset CYP2Ds are more abundant, and cynomolgus and marmoset CYP1As are less abundant compared with their human counterparts. It should be noted that expression levels are not always comparable between mRNA and protein levels.

2.1 CYP1A subfamily

Cynomolgus CYP1A1 and CYP1A2 are highly identical to human CYP1A1 and CYP1A2 (Table 1). Cynomolgus CYP1A1 and CYP1A2 mRNAs are expressed in liver, and the former is much more abundant than the latter (Sakuma et al., 1998; Uno, Uehara, et al., 2011a). Cynomolgus

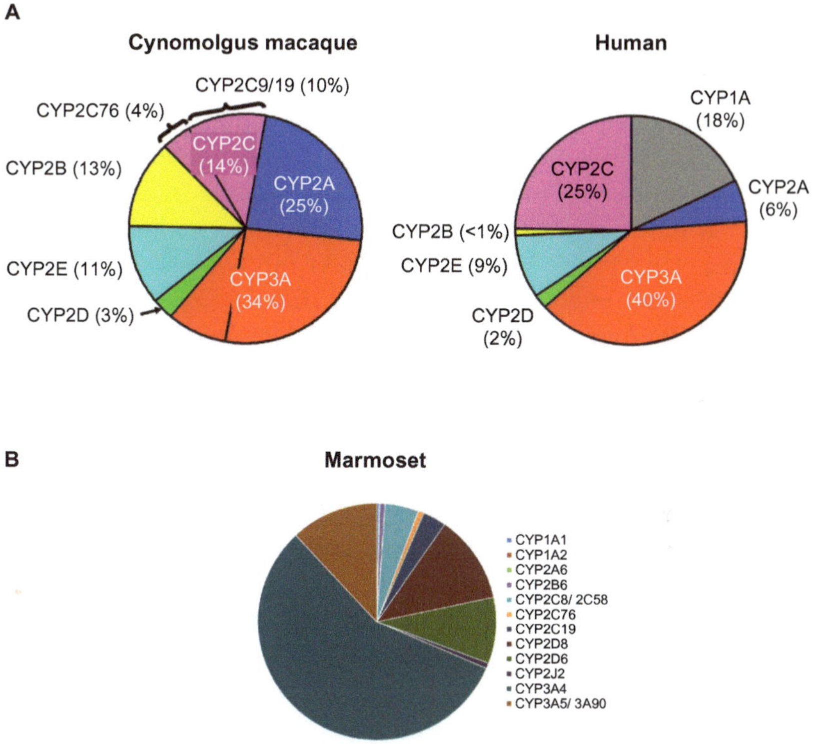

Fig. 1 Hepatic expression levels of human and cynomolgus P450 proteins (A) and of marmoset P450 mRNAs (B) in the CYP1–CYP3 family. To allow better comparison of the other P450s, marmoset CYP2E1 is not shown; its mRNA expression level is approximately 4.1 times that of CYP3A4.

CYP1A1 catalyzes benzo(*a*)pyrene hydroxylation; 7-ethoxycoumarin *O*-deethylation; and the activation of heterocyclic amines, including 2-amino-6-methyldipyrido[1,2-*a*:3′,2′-*d*]imidazole (Glu-P-1), 2-amino-3-methylimidazo[4,5-*f*]quinoline (IQ), and 3-amino-l-methyl-5*H*-pyrido [4,3-*b*]-indole (Trp-P-2) (Komori, Kikuchi, Kitada, & Kamataki, 1992). Cynomolgus CYP1A2 also catalyzes 7-ethoxycoumarin *O*-deethylation and metabolizes the heterocyclic amines, IQ, 2-amino-3,8-dimethylimidazo [4,5-*f*]quinoxaline (MeIQx), and less efficiently 2-amino-1-methyl-6-phenylimidazo[4,5-*b*]pyridine (PhIP) (Sakuma et al., 1998). Similarly, human CYP1As are involved in 7-ethoxycoumarin *O*-deethylation and activation of the heterocyclic amines IQ, Trp-P-2, Glu-P-1, MeIQx, and PhIP (Kim & Guengerich, 2005). These results suggest functional similarities of cynomolgus macaque and human CYP1As.

Marmoset CYP1A1 and CYP1A2, which are highly identical to human CYP1A1 and CYP1A2 (Table 1), catalyze 7-ethoxycoumarin *O*-deethylation, 7-ethoxyresorufin *O*-deethylation (EROD), and phenacetin *O*-deethylation, in a similar way to their human and cynomolgus CYP1A orthologs (Uno et al., 2016) (Table 2). Marmoset CYP1A2 efficiently activates heterocyclic amines IQ and MeIQx and also activates PhIP, but at relatively lower rates than human and cynomolgus CYP1A2 do (Sakuma et al., 1997). Marmoset CYP1A1 mRNA is mainly expressed in lung and small intestine (Uehara, Uno, Inoue, Sasaki, & Yamazaki, 2016), similar to human CYP1A1 mRNA, which is mainly expressed in extrahepatic tissues such as lung, trachea, and small intestine (Bieche et al., 2007). Marmoset CYP1A2 mRNA is predominantly expressed in liver (Sakuma et al., 1997; Uehara, Uno, Inoue, Sasaki, & Yamazaki, 2016), similar to human CYP1A2 mRNA (Bieche et al., 2007). Tissue expression patterns of marmoset CYP1A1 and CYP1A2 proteins are largely similar to those of CYP1A1 and CYP1A2 mRNAs (Uehara, Uno, Inoue, Sasaki, & Yamazaki, 2016). In marmoset liver, CYP1A1 protein expression is greatly increased by treatment with 2,3,7,8-tetrachlorodibenzo-*p*-dioxin (TCDD), which is associated with EROD and methoxyresorufin *O*-demethylation, whereas CYP1A2 shows only slight induction by TCDD (Schulz, Neubert, Davies, & Edwards, 1996). A similar slight induction has been noted for cynomolgus CYP1A2 (Edwards et al., 1994). Similarly, CYP1A1 mRNA and protein levels increased in human liver slices treated with TCDD, resulting in increased enzyme activity; in contrast, the induction of CYP1A2 mRNA was modest (Drahushuk et al., 1996). In marmosets and cynomolgus macaques, CYP1A2 mRNA is induced by 3-methylcholanthrene (Sakuma et al., 1997, 1998), similar to human CYP1A2 in primary hepatocytes (Rhodes, Otten, Hingorani, Hartley, & Franklin, 2011). In hepatocytes, marmoset CYP1A1 and CYP1A2 mRNAs are induced strongly by β-naphthoflavone and omeprazole (Uehara, Uno, Suzuki, et al., 2017), similar to their human orthologs (Daujat et al., 1992; Lnenickova, Skalova, Stuchlikova, Szotakova, & Matouskova, 2018). These results suggest similarities of the catalytic properties, tissue expression patterns, and inducibility levels of human, cynomolgus, and marmoset CYP1As.

2.2 CYP1B subfamily

Cynomolgus and marmoset CYP1B1 are highly identical with human CYP1B1 (Table 1). Cynomolgus and marmoset CYP1B1 catalyze EROD and 7-ethoxycoumarin *O*-deethylation, similar to human CYP1B1

(Uehara, Uno, Inoue, Sasaki, & Yamazaki, 2016). Human, cynomolgus, and marmoset CYP1B1 preferentially catalyze estradiol 4-hydroxylation (Uehara, Uno, Inoue, Sasaki, & Yamazaki, 2016), and share V395, a key residue for regioselective estradiol hydroxylation (Nishida, Everett, & Ortiz de Montellano, 2013). Marmoset CYP1B1 mRNA and protein are expressed more abundantly in kidney and lung, and less abundantly in liver, small intestine, and brain (Uehara, Uno, Inoue, Sasaki, & Yamazaki, 2016). Similarly, human CYP1B1 mRNA is expressed in extrahepatic tissues, particularly in the prostate, uterus, trachea, lung, and kidney (Bieche et al., 2007). These findings suggest enzymatic similarities of CYP1B1 in humans, cynomolgus macaques, and marmosets.

2.3 CYP1D subfamily

Cynomolgus CYP1D1 amino acid sequences are highly identical to the inferred sequences of human CYP1D1P (Table 1). Cynomolgus CYP1D1 mRNA is expressed most abundantly in liver, followed by kidney and jejunum (Uno, Uehara, et al., 2011a). Cynomolgus CYP1D1 is a functional enzyme, catalyzing EROD, similar to human and cynomolgus CYP1A1 and CYP1A2. Therefore, cynomolgus CYP1D1, orthologous to human *CYP1D1P*, a pseudogene, could potentially account for species differences in the metabolism of selective substrates.

2.4 CYP2A subfamily

Cynomolgus CYP2A23, CYP2A24, and CYP2A26 are highly identical to human CYP2A6, CYP2A7, and CYP2A13 (Table 1). Similar to human CYP2A6, cynomolgus CYP2A23, CYP2A24, and CYP2A26 substantially catalyze coumarin 7-hydroxylation, and their mRNAs are predominantly expressed in liver (Uehara, Murayama, Yamazaki, & Uno, 2010; Uno et al., 2007). In contrast, marmoset CYP2A6 catalyzes coumarin 7-hydroxylation much less efficiently than human CYP2A6 does (Pelkonen, Rautio, Raunio, & Pasanen, 2000; Uehara, Uno, Inoue, Sasaki, & Yamazaki, 2015), although marmoset CYP2A6 is highly identical to human CYP2A6 (Table 1). This finding explains why marmosets excrete less than 5% of the administered doses of coumarin as urinary 7-hydroxycoumarin (Lake, Walters, & Gangolli, 1989), whereas in humans, the figure is approximately 79% (Shilling, Crampton, & Longland, 1969). In contrast, marmoset CYP2A6 efficiently catalyzes phenacetin *O*-deethylation (Uehara, Uno, Inoue, Sasaki, & Yamazaki, 2015), which is catalyzed by human CYP1A2 and CYP2A13 (Fukami, Nakajima, Sakai, Katoh, & Yokoi, 2007), but not by human CYP2A6 (Fukami et al., 2007; Uehara, Uno, Inoue, Sasaki, & Yamazaki, 2015). This discrepancy is possibly accounted for by the amino acid substitution Val117Ala in marmoset CYP2A6, because this substitution (mutation) reduces the catalytic activity of human CYP2A6 (He et al., 2004).

Marmoset CYP2A6 mRNA and protein are mainly expressed in liver (Uehara, Uno, Inoue, Sasaki, & Yamazaki, 2015), similar to human CYP2A6 (Koskela et al., 1999). Phenobarbital and rifampicin increased coumarin 7-hydroxylation activities in marmoset liver (Schulz et al., 2001), but CYP2A protein levels did not change, indicating a possible contribution of other P450 enzymes to this reaction, similar to rats (Raunio et al., 1988). Therefore, the substrate selectivity of CYP2A6 is different between marmosets and humans, suggesting that marmosets might not be a suitable animal model for CYP2A-dependent drug metabolism studies.

2.5 CYP2B subfamily

Cynomolgus CYP2B6 is highly identical to human CYP2B6 (Table 1). Cynomolgus CYP2B6, predominantly expressed in liver at the mRNA level, catalyzes testosterone 16β-hydroxylation and bupropion hydroxylation (Uno, Matsuno, Nakamura, Utoh, & Yamazaki, 2009b), similar to human CYP2B6. Cynomolgus CYP2B protein is undetectable in liver, but becomes detectable when the animal is treated with phenobarbital (Bullock et al., 1995), indicating the induction of CYP2B by phenobarbital in cynomolgus macaques, similar to humans. Cynomolgus CYP2B6, therefore, has similarities in tissue expression pattern and enzymatic properties to human CYP2B6.

Marmoset CYP2B6 is highly similar to human CYP2B6 (Table 1) and catalyzes 7-ethoxycoumarin *O*-deethylation, pentoxyresorufin *O*-depentylation, propofol 4-hydroxylation, and testosterone 16β-hydroxylation, similar to human and cynomolgus CYP2B6 (Mayumi et al., 2013; Oshio et al., 2019). Unlike human and cynomolgus CYP2B6, however, marmoset CYP2B6 does not exhibit detectable activity for bupropion hydroxylation or efavirenz 8-hydroxylation (Mayumi et al., 2013). Marmoset CYP2B6 mRNA is predominantly expressed in liver (Oshio et al., 2019), similar to human CYP2B6 (Nishimura, Yaguti, Yoshitsugu, Naito, & Satoh, 2003). Hepatic CYP2B6 levels increase in marmosets and cynomolgus macaques treated with phenobarbital (Bullock et al., 1995; Oshio et al., 2019), but phenobarbital does not induce

CYP2B6 mRNA in marmoset and cynomolgus hepatocytes (Uehara, Uno, Suzuki, et al., 2017). This discrepancy might be caused by individual variabilities and/or the *in vitro* experimental conditions. These results suggest that the substrate selectivity of CYP2B6 might be different in humans and marmosets.

2.6 CYP2C subfamily

In cynomolgus macaques, CYP2C8, CYP2C9, CYP2C18, and CYP2C19 are highly identical to human CYP2Cs, but cynomolgus CYP2C76 is not orthologous to any human CYP2C (Table 1). Cynomolgus CYP2C8, predominantly expressed in liver at the mRNA level, substantially catalyzes paclitaxel 6α-hydroxylation, a human CYP2C8 marker reaction (Uno et al., 2007; Uno, Fujino, Kito, Kamataki, & Nagata, 2006). Expression of cynomolgus CYP2C18 mRNA in liver is much lower than for other CYP2C mRNAs (Uno, Matsuno, Nakamura, Utoh, & Yamazaki, 2010). Moreover, cynomolgus CYP2C18 does not metabolize human CYP2C substrates such as paclitaxel and diclofenac, and it only slightly catalyzes *S*-mephenytoin 4′-hydroxylation (Uno, Matsuno, et al., 2010). Although human CYP2C18 protein metabolizes human CYP2C substrates, the expression of human CYP2C18 in liver is undetectable (Gerbal-Chaloin et al., 2001). Therefore, neither cynomolgus nor human CYP2C18 contributes to overall drug metabolism in liver.

Cynomolgus CYP2C9 and CYP2C19 are highly identical to both human CYP2C9 and CYP2C19 (Table 1), and their mRNAs are highly expressed in liver (Uno et al., 2006). Cynomolgus CYP2C9 catalyzes *S*-mephenytoin 4′-hydroxylation, progesterone 21-hydroxylation, and testosterone 17-hydroxylation, similar to human CYP2C19 (Mitsuda, Iwasaki, & Asahi, 2006; Uno et al., 2006; Uno, Kumano, et al., 2007). Cynomolgus CYP2C19 catalyzes *S*-mephenytoin 4′-hydroxylation and tolbutamide methyl-hydroxylation, which are catalyzed by human CYP2C9 and CYP2C19, respectively (Uno et al., 2006; Uno, Kumano, et al., 2007). Therefore, cynomolgus CYP2C9 and CYP2C19 share similar metabolic properties with human CYP2C9 and CYP2C19 (Matsunaga et al., 2002; Mitsuda et al., 2006), although their substrate specificities do not correspond perfectly to human CYP2Cs.

Among cynomolgus CYP2Cs, CYP2C76 has the lowest amino acid sequence identity (70–72%) to human CYP2Cs (Table 1). CYP2C76 mRNA is predominantly expressed in liver, and its expression in liver is the most abundant among cynomolgus CYP2C mRNAs (Uno et al., 2006). Cynomolgus CYP2C76 protein, expressed in liver, substantially catalyzes testosterone 2α- and 16α-hydroxylation and tolbutamide methyl hydroxylation, but not *S*-mephenytoin 4′-hydroxylation or paclitaxel 6α-hydroxylation, indicating substrate specificity different from other cynomolgus and human CYP2Cs (Uno et al., 2006). The *CYP2C76* gene is located at a genomic region corresponding to an intergenic region in the human genome, and expression of CYP2C76 protein is not detected by immunoblotting in human liver, indicating that no CYP2C76 ortholog is present in humans (Uno et al., 2006). In pitavastatin metabolism, cynomolgus CYP2C76 catalyzes the reaction catalyzed by human CYP3A and is involved in the formation of a metabolite that is not found in humans (Uno, Kumano, et al., 2007). Screening with 89 compounds found that various human P450 substrates are metabolized by cynomolgus CYP2C76, including bupropion and nifedipine, which are probe drugs of human CYP2B6 and CYP3A4, respectively (Hosaka, Murayama, Satsukawa, Shimizu, et al., 2015). Therefore, CYP2C76 accounts for the differences in drug metabolism between cynomolgus macaques and humans.

In marmosets, CYP2C8, CYP2C18, CYP2C19, and CYP2C58 are highly similar to human CYP2Cs, but CYP2C76 is not orthologous to any human CYP2C (Table 1). All marmoset CYP2C mRNAs are predominantly expressed in liver, just as human CYP2C mRNAs are (Bieche et al., 2007). Marmoset CYP2C8 and CYP2C58 are highly similar to human CYP2C8 (Table 1). Marmoset CYP2C8 modestly catalyzes paclitaxel 6α-hydroxylation (a human CYP2C8 probe reaction) and effectively catalyzes tolbutamide methyl hydroxylation (with a similar activity level to that of human CYP2C) (Narimatsu et al., 2006; Uehara, Uno, Inoue, Kawano, et al., 2015). Marmoset CYP2C58 has 86% amino acid sequence identity with marmoset CYP2C8, but its enzyme activities are negligible or undetectable for paclitaxel 6α-hydroxylation and tolbutamide methyl hydroxylation (Uehara, Uno, Inoue, Kawano, et al., 2015). Although marmoset CYP2C58 has no or negligible enzyme activities for paclitaxel 6α-hydroxylation and tolbutamide methyl hydroxylation, it does exhibit high metabolic activities for 7-ethoxycoumarin and chlorzoxazone, which human CYP2Cs do not metabolize (Uehara, Uno, Inoue, Kawano, et al., 2015).

Among marmoset CYP2Cs, CYP2C19 effectively catalyzes human CYP 2C9 and CYP2C19 probe reactions, including diclofenac 4′-hydroxylation, flurbiprofen 4′-hydroxylation, omeprazole 5-hydroxylation, tolbutamide methyl hydroxylation, and *S*-warfarin 7-hydroxylation (Table 2) (Nakanishi et al., 2018; Uehara, Uno, Inoue, Kawano, et al., 2015). In warfarin metabolism, marmoset CYP2C19 and human CYP2C9 preferentially catalyze *S*-warfarin 7-hydroxylation, whereas cynomolgus macaque CYP2C19 preferentially catalyzes *R*-warfarin hydroxylation (Uehara, Uno, Inoue, Kawano, et al., 2015). This result suggests a similar stereoselectivity in warfarin metabolism in humans and marmosets. In marmosets, slow *S*-warfarin and *R*-omeprazole clearances are observed in animals with the CYP2C19 p.[(F7L; S254L; T469I)] variant compared with wild-type animals, which can be partly accounted for by the low metabolic activities of the variant CYP2C19 enzyme (Uehara et al., 2016, 2020).

Marmoset CYP2C18 and CYP2C76 mRNAs are expressed in liver, but at much lower levels than other marmoset CYP2C mRNAs (Uehara, Uno, Inoue, Kawano, et al., 2015). Marmoset CYP2C18 catalyzes *S*-warfarin 7-hydroxylation and tolbutamide methyl hydroxylation, but the catalytic activity is much lower than that for human CYP2C9 (Uehara, Uno, Inoue, Kawano, et al., 2015). Similarly, human CYP2C18, a functional enzyme, is not detected in human hepatocytes (Gerbal-Chaloin et al., 2001). Marmoset CYP2C76 catalyzes tolbutamide methyl hydroxylation, just as cynomolgus CYP2C76 does (Uno et al., 2006), but the catalytic activity is much lower than that of human CYP2C9 (Uehara, Uno, Inoue, Kawano, et al., 2015). Consequently, the contribution of marmoset CYP2C18 and CYP2C76 to hepatic drug metabolism is extremely limited.

Both the rate of tolbutamide methyl hydroxylation and the levels of CYP2C in marmoset liver increase after treatment with rifampicin and phenobarbital (Schulz et al., 2001). Rifampicin induces CYP2C8 and CYP2C19 in marmoset hepatocytes (Uehara, Uno, Suzuki, et al., 2017). Therefore, marmoset CYP2C19 is functionally similar to human CYP2C9, and CYP2C19 and plays important roles in inter-individual differences of CYP2C-dependent drug metabolism in marmosets.

2.7 CYP2D subfamily

Cynomolgus CYP2D6 and CYP2D8 are highly homologous to human CYP2D6 (Table 1). Cynomolgus CYP2D6 and CYP2D8 are expressed predominantly in liver at the mRNA level and catalyze dextromethorphan *O*-deethylation and bufuralol 1′-hydroxylation, similar to human CYP2D6

(Mankowski et al., 1999; Uno, Uehara, Kohara, Murayama, & Yamazaki, 2010). Both cynomolgus CYP2D enzymes catalyze dextromethorphan *N*-demethylation more efficiently than human CYP2D6 does (Uno et al., 2010). These results suggest that cynomolgus macaques are similar to humans in terms of the metabolic properties of their CYP2Ds, with some differences, *e.g.*, dextromethorphan *N*-demethylation. The protein levels of cynomolgus CYP2Ds in liver are much greater than in humans (Weaver, Dickins, & Burke, 1999). Moreover, cynomolgus CYP2D6 and CYP2D8 show higher intrinsic clearances of bufuralol and dextromethorphan than human CYP2D6 (Mankowski et al., 1999; Uno, Matsushita, et al., 2010). Therefore, cynomolgus macaques generally have higher metabolic activities of CYP2D proteins in liver than humans do.

Marmoset CYP2D6 and CYP2D8 are highly similar to human CYP2D6 (Table 1) and efficiently catalyze typical human CYP2D6 probe reactions such as bufuralol 1′-hydroxylation, dextromethorphan *O*-demethylation, and metoprolol *O*-demethylation; however, marmoset CYP2D8 exhibits lower catalytic activities than those seen in human and marmoset CYP2D6 (Uehara, Uno, Inoue, Sasaki, & Yamazaki, 2015). Similarly, cynomolgus CYP2D6 and CYP2D8 catalyze dextromethorphan *O*-demethylation and bufuralol 1′-hydroxylation (Uno, Matsushita, et al., 2010). The enantioselectivity of propranolol oxidation by CYP2D6 enzymes is similar in humans, cynomolgus macaques, and marmosets (Narimatsu et al., 2011). *R*-metoprolol *O*-demethylation is catalyzed in human and marmoset liver microsomes, whereas *S*-metoprolol *O*-demethylation and *R*-metoprolol α-hydroxylation are effectively catalyzed in cynomolgus liver microsomes (Table 2). These findings indicate that regio- and stereo-selectivity of metoprolol oxidation is similar in human and marmoset CYP2D6 (Uehara, Ishii, Uno, et al., 2017). Furthermore, human and marmoset CYP2D6 play similar roles in deactivating and activating the potential proneurotoxin 1-methyl-4-phenyl-1,2,3,6-tetrahydropyridine in liver (Uehara et al., 2015). Marmoset CYP2D6 and CYP2D8 mRNAs are expressed in liver, although the level of the latter is much lower than the former (Uehara et al., 2015). Human CYP2D6 mRNA is also predominantly expressed in liver (Bieche et al., 2007; Uno, Matsushita, et al., 2010). Marmoset CYP2D mRNA is also expressed in various brain regions, including the cerebral cortex, hippocampus, substantia nigra, and cerebellum, similar to the observations in human brain (Shimamoto, Niimi, Kitamura, Tsubakishita, & Takahashi, 2016). Taken together, these results suggest the functional similarity of human and marmoset CYP2D6.

2.8 CYP2E subfamily

Cynomolgus and marmoset CYP2E1 are highly identical to human CYP2E1 (Table 1). Cynomolgus and marmoset CYP2E1 substantially catalyze chlorzoxazone 6-hydroxylation, *p*-nitrophenol 2-hydroxylation, and theophylline 8-hydroxylation, just as human CYP2E1 does (Hanioka et al., 2007; Uehara, Uno, Tomioka, et al., 2017; Uno, Hosaka, et al., 2007). Isoniazid, a known inducer of human CYP2E1, also increases CYP2E1 activity for chlorzoxazone 6-hydroxylation in marmoset liver microsomes (Schulz, Thiel, Davies, & Edwards, 1998). Marmoset CYP2E1 mRNA and protein are predominantly expressed in liver (Uehara, Uno, Tomioka, et al., 2017). Furthermore, human and cynomolgus CYP2E1 mRNA are also abundantly expressed in liver (Nishimura et al., 2003; Uno, Hosaka, et al., 2007). These results suggest that the substrate specificities and catalytic activities of CYP2E1 are similar in humans, cynomolgus macaques, and marmosets.

2.9 CYP2F subfamily

Cynomolgus and marmoset CYP2F1 are highly identical to human CYP2F1 (Table 1). Cynomolgus and marmoset CYP2F1 mRNAs are predominantly expressed in lung where marmoset CYP2F1 protein is also expressed (Uehara et al., 2018). Cynomolgus and marmoset CYP2F1 catalyze biphenyl hydroxylation, chlorzoxazone 6-hydroxylation, coumarin 7-hydroxylation, and 7-ethoxycoumarin *O*-deethylation (Uehara, Uno, et al., 2018). Human CYP2F1, which is mainly expressed in lung and trachea at the mRNA level, metabolizes classic P450 substrates and environmental toxicants, including biphenyl, 7-ethoxycoumarin, propoxycoumarin, and pentoxyresorufin (Nhamburo et al., 1990; Uehara, Uno, et al., 2018). These results suggest similar tissue expression patterns and catalytic functions of CYP2F1 in humans, cynomolgus macaques, and marmosets.

2.10 CYP2G subfamily

Cynomolgus CYP2G2 is highly identical to the sequence inferred from human CYP2G2P (Table 1). Cynomolgus CYP2G2 mRNA is predominantly expressed in nasal mucosa (Uno, Uehara, et al., 2011b). Cynomolgus CYP2G2 metabolizes coumarin in a similar manner to that of cynomolgus CYP2A23, CYP2A24, and CYP2A26 (Uno, Uehara, et al., 2011b) and is, therefore, a functional enzyme. Human CYP2A13 is also expressed in nasal mucosa (Su et al., 2000). Therefore, cynomolgus CYP2G2 may play a role similar to that of human CYP2A13 in nasal mucosa.

2.11 CYP2J subfamily

Cynomolgus and marmoset CYP2J2 are highly identical to human CYP2J2 (Table 1). Cynomolgus and marmoset CYP2J2 mRNAs are preferentially expressed in jejunum and liver (Uno, Hosaka, et al., 2007) where their proteins are also expressed (Uehara et al., 2015, 2016). Human CYP2J2 mRNA is mainly expressed in small intestine, liver, and heart, where the human protein is also expressed (Wu, Moomaw, Tomer, Falck, & Zeldin, 1996). Cynomolgus and marmoset CYP2J2 efficiently catalyze astemizole *O*-demethylation and terfenadine *t*-butyl hydroxylation, similar to human CYP2J2 (Uehara, Uno, Inoue, Okamoto, et al., 2016). Therefore, human, cynomolgus, and marmoset CYP2J2 are similar in terms of tissue expression patterns and enzymatic properties.

2.12 CYP3A subfamily

Cynomolgus CYP3A4 and CYP3A5 are highly homologous to human CYP3A4 and CYP3A5 (Table 1). Cynomolgus CYP3A4 mRNA is expressed abundantly in liver and to a lesser extent in jejunum, whereas cynomolgus CYP3A5 mRNA shows abundant expression in both liver and jejunum (Uno, Hosaka, et al., 2007). Alprazolam 4-hydroxylation, midazolam 1′-hydroxylation, nifedipine oxidation, and testosterone 6β-hydroxylation are all substantially catalyzed by cynomolgus CYP3A4 and CYP3A5 (Ohtsuka et al., 2010; Uno, Hosaka, et al., 2007; Uno, Matsushita, et al., 2010), just as they are by human CYP3A4 and CYP3A5 (Table 2). Rifampicin induces cynomolgus CYP3A4 mRNA in hepatocytes (Nishimura et al., 2007) and also *in vivo via* a pregnane X receptor-mediated mechanism in a similar manner to that in humans (Kim et al., 2010). These results suggest functional similarities of CYP3A4 and CYP3A5 in cynomolgus macaques and humans. Cynomolgus CYP3A43 is highly identical to human CYP3A43 (Table 1). Cynomolgus CYP3A43 shows low mRNA expression in liver and minimal catalytic activity for midazolam 1′-hydroxylation (Uno, Matsuno, Nakamura, Utoh, & Yamazaki, 2009a). Therefore, the contribution of cynomolgus CYP3A43 to hepatic drug metabolism is extremely limited, which is also true for human CYP3A43.

Marmoset CYP3A4 and CYP3A5/3A90 are highly identical to human CYP3A4 and CYP3A5, respectively (Table 1). Marmoset CYP3A4 mRNA is more abundant in liver and small intestine than marmoset CYP3A5 and CYP3A90 mRNAs are (Uehara, Uno, Nakanishi, et al., 2017), and both marmoset CYP3A4 and CYP3A5/CYP3A90 proteins are expressed in liver (Uehara, Uno, Nakanishi, et al., 2017), similar to human and cynomolgus CYP3A4 and CYP3A5 mRNAs (Bieche et al., 2007; Uno, Hosaka, et al., 2007). These three marmoset CYP3A enzymes catalyze typical human CYP3A probe reactions, *e.g.*, alprazolam 4-hydroxylation, midazolam 1′- and 4-hydroxylations, nifedipine oxidation, and testosterone 6β-hydroxylation (Table 2) (Uehara, Uno, Nakanishi, et al., 2017). Marmoset CYP3A4 catalyzes midazolam 1′-hydroxylation more efficiently than marmoset CYP3A5 and CYP3A90 do (Uehara, Uno, Nakanishi, et al., 2017), and the substrate inhibition kinetics are similar in human, cynomolgus, and marmoset CYP3A4 (Uehara, Uno, Nakanishi, et al., 2017).

In liver microsomes from 23 individual marmosets, the mean CYP3A4 content was 150 pmol/mg protein (64% of total CYP3A proteins) and was correlated with midazolam 1′-hydroxylation and bufuralol 1′-hydroxylation activities (Uehara, Uno, Nakanishi, et al., 2017). Moreover, in liver microsomes from different individuals, midazolam 1′-hydroxylation activities were correlated with the CYP3A-dependent reactions bufuralol 1′-hydroxylation and *R*-metoprolol *O*-demethylation (Uehara et al., 2019). Therefore, marmoset CYP3A enzymes contribute to typical human CYP2D/CYP3A probe reactions. The bioavailability of midazolam based on single-dose pharmacokinetic analysis is lower in marmosets (4%) (Uehara, Uno, Inoue, Sasaki, & Yamazaki, 2016) than in humans (23%) (Lappin et al., 2006), suggesting some first-pass metabolism of hepatic and intestinal CYP3A4 (Uehara et al., 2016). The roles of CYP3A4 in progesterone 6β-hydroxylation, omeprazole sulfoxidation, and diclofenac 5-hydroxylation in liver are generally similar in humans and marmosets (Nakanishi et al., 2018; Nakanishi, Uehara, Kusama, et al., 2018; Uehara et al., 2016).

In hepatocyte cultures, marmoset CYP3A4 mRNA is induced by rifampicin, phenobarbital, and omeprazole (Uehara, Uno, Suzuki, et al., 2017), and the protein is also induced by phenobarbital in liver (Schulz et al., 2001). Promoter assays indicated pronounced and moderate responses of marmoset CYP3A4 to rifampicin and dexamethasone, respectively, similar to human CYP3A4 (Koehler et al., 2006). These results indicate that there are similarities in expression and gene regulation of marmoset and human CYP3A4, and these are likely accounted for by the presence of similar gene regulatory modules in promoter regions (Koehler et al., 2006). There are, therefore, similarities in expression and gene regulation between marmoset and human CYP3A4. In summary, CYP3A4, CYP3A5, and CYP3A90 are functional enzymes in marmosets, and the tissue expression patterns, enzymatic properties, and the contributions of marmoset CYP3A4 to drug metabolism in liver and small intestine are similar to those of human CYP3A4.

2.13 CYP4A subfamily

Cynomolgus and marmoset CYP4A11 are highly identical to human CYP4A11 and CYP4A22 (Table 1), and, as in humans, cynomolgus and marmoset CYP4A11 mRNAs are preferentially expressed in liver and kidney (Uehara, Uno, Ishii, et al., 2017; Uno, Hosaka, et al., 2007). Cynomolgus and marmoset CYP4A11 catalyze the ω-hydroxylation of lauric acid and arachidonic acid, similar to human CYP4A11 (Powell, Wolf, Jin, & Lasker, 1998; Powell, Wolf, & Lasker, 1996; Uehara, Uno, Ishii, et al., 2017). Marmoset CYP4A11 shares with human CYP4A11 the glutamic acid residues EGHDTT321–326 in the heme-binding region (Hoch & Ortiz De Montellano, 2001) and also shares the key residues important for fatty acid ω-hydroxylation with human CYP4A11 (Chang & Loew, 1999). These results indicate that marmoset CYP4A11 might have heme binding and catalytic properties similar to human CYP4A11.

2.14 CYP4F subfamily

Cynomolgus CYP4F2, CYP4F3v2, CYP4F11, and CYP4F12 and marmoset CYP4F2, CYP4F3, CYP4F71, and CYP4F12 are highly similar to human CYP4F2, CYP4F3v2, CYP4F11, and CYP4F12, respectively (Table 1). Cynomolgus CYP4F2 mRNA is preferentially expressed in liver, kidney, and jejunum, and cynomolgus CYP4F3v2 mRNA is preferentially expressed in liver and kidney (Uno, Hosaka, et al., 2007).

Marmoset CYP4F3 and CYP4F71 mRNAs are predominantly expressed in liver, whereas marmoset CYP4F2 and CYP4F12 mRNAs are mainly expressed in small intestine and liver (Uehara et al., 2016). Similarly, human CYP4F2 and CYP4F12 mRNAs are expressed in liver and liver/small intestine, respectively (Christmas et al., 2001; Hashizume et al., 2001), and human CYP4F11 mRNA is mainly expressed in liver

(Cui, Nelson, & Strobel, 2000). All cynomolgus CYP4F enzymes are functional and metabolize arachidonic acid, carebastine, and/or ebastine (Uehara, Uno, Yuki, Inoue, et al., 2016; Uno, Matsuno, Nakamura, Utoh, & Yamazaki, 2011), whereas all marmoset CYP4Fs catalyze leukotriene B_4 20-hydroxylation (Uehara, Uno, Yuki, Inoue, et al., 2016). Ebastine hydroxylation and terfenadine *t*-butyl hydroxylation are efficiently catalyzed by marmoset and human CYP4F12 (Uehara et al., 2018; Uehara, Uno, Yuki, Inoue, et al., 2016), suggesting that the contribution of CYP4Fs to the metabolism of endogenous and exogenous compounds in marmosets are similar to those in humans.

3. Genetic polymorphisms

3.1 Genetic variants identified

Numerous genetic variants have been identified in cynomolgus macaques (Ferguson et al., 2007; Hernandez et al., 2007; Street, Kyes, Grant, & Ferguson, 2007), which, like humans, have a diverse genetic background. Various variants have been found in CYP1A1, CYP1A2, CYP1B1, CYP1D1, CYP2B6, CYP2C9, CYP2C19, CYP2C76, CYP2D6, CYP2D8, CYP2G2, CYP3A4, and CYP3A5, including the functionally relevant variants such as seven nonsense mutations (in CYP1A2, CYP2D8, CYP2G2, and CYP3A5) and five frameshift mutations (in CYP1A2, CYP2C76, CYP2D8, and CYP3A4) (Uno et al., 2016) (Table 3). The frequencies of some P450 genetic variants are different depending on the location of origin of the cynomolgus macaques, indicating that the source of the animals could be an important factor in successful drug metabolism studies using cynomolgus macaques. The *in vitro* and/or *in vivo* function of these cynomolgus P450 variants have been investigated.

Cynomolgus CYP2C9 I112L and CYP2C19 compound variant [F100N; A103V; I112L] result in significant functional changes both *in vitro* and *in vivo* (Table 3) (Uno, Uehara, & Yamazaki, 2018). Cynomolgus CYP2D6 compound variant [I297M; N337D] is responsible for significant catalytic changes in bufuralol 1′-hydroxylation and dextromethorphan *O*-demethylation (Uno, Uehara, & Yamazaki, 2018). Notably, null mutations of cynomolgus CYP2C76 (L150fs156X), CYP3A4 (G73fs89X), and CYP3A5 (K209X) (Table 3) do not exhibit peaks at 450 nm on carbon monoxide difference spectra and their recombinant proteins show no drug-metabolizing catalytic activities (Uno, Uehara, & Yamazaki, 2018). A high prevalence of null variants has been found in cynomolgus *CYP1A2* and *CYP2D8*, suggesting

Table 3 Cynomolgus P450 genetic variants relevant to enzyme function.

P450	Variant	Amino acid change	Allele frequency							Site	Function	
			Indochina	Indonesia	Cambodia	Philippines	Vietnam	Malaysia	Mauritius		*In vitro*	*In vivo*
2C9(43)	c.334A>C	I112L	1/76	0/20; 0/78	1/20	0/20	2/20	0/14	0/42	SRS1	↓ (1,2) R	↓ (8*)
2C19(75)	c.298TT>AA (c.308C>T; c.334ATC>CTT)	F100N (A103V; I112L)	20/76	0/20; 3/78	6/20	0/20	4/20	0/14	16/42	SRS1	↓ (1,3,4,5) L,R	↓ (5**)
2C76	c.449TG>A	L150fs156X	0/78	0/20; 8/204	0/20	4/20	0/20	N/A	N/A		Null	
2D6(17)	c.891A>G	I297M (; N337D)	0/78	2/20; 25/96	0/20	20/20	0/20	14/14	1/42	SRS4		
3A4(8)	IVS3 + 1G>del	G73fs89X	0/76	0/20; 2/478	0/20	0/20	0/20	0/14	0/42		BDL (6, 7)	
3A5	c.625A>T	K209X	0/76	0/20; 3/516	0/20	0/20	0/20	0/14	0/42	SRS2	BDL (6, 7)	

For P450 enzymes that have been renamed, the original names are indicated in parentheses. ↓, activity reduced; and BDL, below detection limit. SRS, substrate recognition site; L, liver microsomes; R, recombinant protein; N/A, not available. Reactions used to determine function were: (1) flurbiprofen 4′-hydroxylation, (2) caffeine 7-*N*-demethylation, (3) omeprazole 5-hydroxylation, (4) *S*-warfarin 7-hydroxylation, (5) *R*-warfarin 7-hydroxylation, (6) midazolam 1′-/4-hydroxylation, (7) nifedipine oxidation, and (8) efavirenz 8-hydroxylation. Statistically significant $^{**}P<0.01$, $^{*}P<0.05$.

that these genes might be in the process of pseudogenization (Uno, Uehara, & Yamazaki, 2018). In contrast, *CYP1D1* and *CYP2G2* are pseudogenized in humans due to several nonsense mutations that are not found at all or are found only at very low frequencies in cynomolgus macaques; therefore, cynomolgus *CYP1D1* and *CYP2G2* are functional (Uno, Uehara, & Yamazaki, 2018).

3.2 Characterization of polymorphic P450s *in vitro*

Some non-synonymous variants are located in the regions important for enzyme function [*e.g.*, the substrate recognition site (SRS) and heme-binding region] and have been analyzed *in vitro* using liver microsomes and/or recombinant proteins. CYP2C76 variants L65F, M310L, and N364S result in lower rates of progesterone 16α-hydroxylation than the wild-type protein (Uehara, Murayama, Yamazaki, & Uno, 2012) and, in addition to the null mutation L150fs156X, influence the catalytic activity of CYP2C76 (Uno et al., 2009). CYP2C76 variants L65F, Y236F, M310L, and N364S have been found in Indochinese and Indonesian cynomolgus macaques (Uehara et al., 2012; Uno, Sakuraba, et al., 2009). CYP2C9 I112L substantially decreases the rates of flurbiprofen 4′-hydroxylation and caffeine 7-*N*-demethylation, which are mainly catalyzed by CYP2C9 (Iwasaki et al., 2016). This variant has been found in Indochinese cynomolgus macaques, but not in Indonesian cynomolgus macaques (Uno, Matsushita, Murayama, & Yamazaki, 2015, 2017); it was also found in cynomolgus macaques bred in Cambodia and Vietnam of the Indochinese linage (Uno et al., 2018).

For cynomolgus CYP2C19, the rates of flurbiprofen 4′-hydroxylation and omeprazole 5-hydroxylation are significantly lower in liver microsomes from homozygotes and heterozygotes of the compound variant [F100N; A103V; I112L] than in those from wild-type animals (Table 3) (Uno et al., 2014). Similarly, the rates of *R*- and *S*-warfarin 7-hydroxylation and diclofenac 4-hydroxylation are lower for the homozygotes and heterozygotes, but not significantly so (Uno, Matsushita, et al., 2014; Utoh et al., 2015). Moreover, the rates of flurbiprofen 4′-hydroxylation, omeprazole 5-hydroxylation, and *S*/*R*- warfarin 7-hydroxylation are substantially lower for the recombinant protein of CYP2C19 variants F100N, A103V, and I112L, and activity for these reactions is absent in the compound variant [F100N; A103V; I112L] (Uno, Matsushita, et al., 2014). These low catalytic activities might be at least partly accounted for by A103V, which has been shown by structural analysis to diminish homotropic cooperativity of the enzyme with *R*-warfarin (Uno, Matsushita, et al., 2014). This compound variant has been found at relatively high frequency in Indochinese, Cambodian, Mauritian, and Vietnamese cynomolgus macaques (Uno, Osada, et al., 2018; Uno & Yamazaki, 2016).

For liver microsomes from cynomolgus macaques homozygous or heterozygous for the CYP2D6 compound variant [I297M; N337D], bufuralol 1′-hydroxylation and dextromethorphan *O*-demethylation rates were significantly higher than for the wild-type (Uno, Uehara, Kohara, Murayama, & Yamazaki, 2014), indicating that the compound variant [I297M; N337D] influences the catalytic activity of CYP2D6 (Table 3). This variant has been found in Indonesian cynomolgus macaques at a high frequency and also in Mauritian, Philippine, and Malaysian cynomolgus macaques, but not in Indochinese cynomolgus macaques; all 10 Philippine and all seven Malaysian cynomolgus macaques analyzed were homozygous for CYP2D6 [I297M; N337D] (Table 3) (Uno, Osada, et al., 2018).

For recombinant CYP3A4 V296M protein, nifedipine oxidation activity is higher than for the wild-type protein, but for midazolam 1′-/4-hydroxylation, the variant protein activity is comparable to the wild type (Uno, Matsushita, et al., 2010). Therefore, in addition to the null variants of CYP3A4 and CYP3A5, the CYP3A4 V296M variant might also influence the catalytic activity of the enzyme.

3.3 Drug elimination mediated by polymorphic P450s *in vivo*

The *in vivo* metabolic clearances of typical human P450 cocktail probes, namely caffeine, warfarin, omeprazole, metoprolol, and midazolam (Turpault et al., 2009), administered individually or in combination, were investigated in cynomolgus macaques (Koyanagi et al., 2015; Utoh et al., 2015, 2018) and marmosets (Kusama et al., 2018; Toda et al., 2018; Uehara, Uno, Inoue, Kawano, et al., 2015; Utoh et al., 2016). Reported areas under the plasma concentration curve (AUCs) after oral administrations of the five probes normalized by mg doses per kg body weights in humans, cynomolgus macaques, and marmosets are indicated in Fig. 2. Although cynomolgus macaques and marmosets are generally expected to show similar drug-metabolizing properties to humans, some attention should be paid to the slight differences in levels of unmetabolized probe substrates in plasma shown in Fig. 2. The dose-normalized AUCs after oral

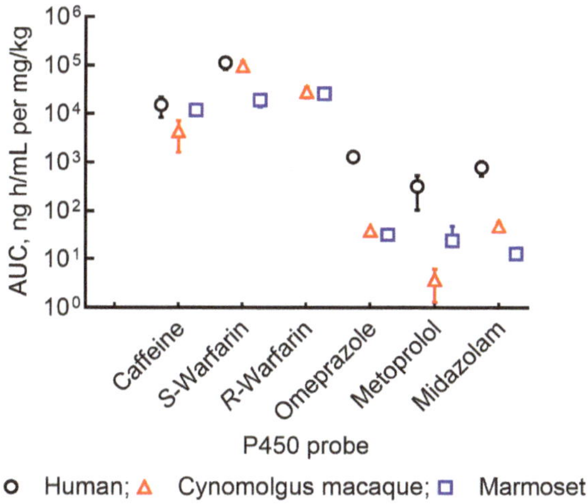

Fig. 2 Reported areas under the plasma concentration curve (AUC) with standard deviations after oral administrations of five probe substances normalized by mg dose per kg body weight. Plasma concentrations of caffeine, chirally separated *R/S*-warfarin, omeprazole, metoprolol, and midazolam in humans, cynomolgus macaques, and marmosets were taken from previous reports (Koyanagi et al., 2015; Toda et al., 2018; Turpault et al., 2009; Uehara, Inoue, Utoh, Toda, et al., 2016; Utoh et al., 2016).

administrations of caffeine were generally similar among humans, cynomolgus macaques, and marmosets (Fig. 2). However, caffeine (Table 2) is metabolized differently in the three species, *i.e.*, by human CYP1A2 to the N_3-demethylated metabolite paraxanthine (Turpault et al., 2009), by cynomolgus CYP2C9 to the N_7-demethylated metabolite theophylline (Utoh et al., 2016), and by marmoset CYP1A2 and CYP3A4 to N_3-demethylated and 8-hydroxylated metabolites, respectively (Uehara et al., 2016).

Faster *in vivo* *S*-warfarin clearance than *R*-warfarin clearance (resulting in low AUC values for *S*-warfarin) was observed after oral administration of racemic warfarin in marmosets (Uehara, Uno, Inoue, Kawano, et al., 2015), which finding is consistent with the stereoselectivity of warfarin in humans (Turpault et al., 2009). In contrast, in cynomolgus macaques, faster *in vivo* clearance of *R*-warfarin than *S*-warfarin was seen (Utoh et al., 2015, 2018). Faster clearances of omeprazole were observed in cynomolgus macaques and marmosets than in humans (Fig. 2). *S*-Omeprazole has been developed as a single enantiomer medicine, which is reportedly not associated with polymorphic human CYP2C19 phenotypes. Liver microsomes from humans and cynomolgus macaques preferentially mediated

R-omeprazole 5-hydroxylations; however, those from marmosets preferentially mediated *S*-omeprazole 5-hydroxylations *in vitro* (Uehara, Kawano, Murayama, Uno, et al., 2016). Moreover, *S*-omeprazole depletion was faster than that of *R*-omeprazole in marmosets *in vivo* (Kusama et al., 2018).

Faster clearance of metoprolol was observed in cynomolgus macaques than in humans or marmosets. This faster clearance in cynomolgus macaques may be related to our findings that cynomolgus CYP2D and CYP3A enzymes metabolize nearly all the human CYP2D and 3A substrates known to date (Emoto et al., 2011, 2013; Iwasaki & Uno, 2009; Uno, Matsushita, et al., 2010). Faster clearances of midazolam, a common CYP3A substrate (Table 2), were observed in cynomolgus macaques and marmosets than in humans (Fig. 2).

Cynomolgus CYP2C enzymes metabolize most human CYP2C substrates and also some non-CYP2C substrates, such as efavirenz and nifedipine, which, respectively, are metabolized by cynomolgus CYP2C9 and CYP2C76 and by human CYP2B6 and CYP3A4 (Hosaka et al., 2015; Hosaka, Murayama, Satsukawa, Shimizu, et al., 2015; Iwasaki et al., 2016; Uno et al., 2016). The effects on *in vivo* pharmacokinetics of genetic polymorphisms in some CYP2C enzymes in cynomolgus macaques and marmosets have been noted. For example, slow efavirenz and *R*-warfarin clearances from plasma were evident in cynomolgus macaques genotyped for CYP2C9 I112L (Iwasaki et al., 2016) and for the compound variant CYP2C19 [F100N; A103V; I112L], respectively (Uno & Yamazaki, 2016). Furthermore, slow *S*-warfarin, *R*-omeprazole, cilomilast, phenytoin, repaglinide, and tolbutamide clearances were observed in marmosets genotyped for the compound variant CYP2C19 [F7L; S254L; T469I] (Kusama et al., 2018; Matsumoto et al., 2021; Uehara, Uno, Inoue, et al., 2020; Uehara, Uno, Inoue, Kawano, et al., 2016).

To predict the human age-related changes of pharmacokinetics and physiological parameters, the use of cynomolgus macaques aged 16 years or marmosets aged 10–14 years may be suitable because of their similarities to humans in terms of their age-dependent physiological parameter changes and/or reduced hepatic clearances of some human P450 substrates (Koyanagi et al., 2015; Koyanagi, Yamaura, Yano, Kim, & Yamazaki, 2014; Toda et al., 2018). Animal models that reflect the age-related pharmacokinetic changes in humans would highlight important aspects of the development of drugs suitable for elderly patients.

4. Conclusion

Polymorphic P450 variants, aging, and induction by xenobiotics partly account for the inter-individual variability of P450-dependent drug clearances in cynomolgus macaques, marmosets, and humans. Information on the inter-individual variability in cynomolgus macaque or marmoset P450 enzymes should help to clarify apparent species differences in drug metabolism and disposition and thereby improve extrapolations to humans of the preclinical data obtained in cynomolgus macaques or marmosets. Polymorphic CYP2C19 variants are responsible for much of the inter-individual variability of CYP2C-dependent drug clearances in cynomolgus macaques and marmosets, just as they are in humans. The number, expression, and metabolic property of CYP2C and other P450 enzymes greatly differ between humans and non-primate species such as rats. Thus, cynomolgus macaques and marmosets would be useful animal models in drug metabolism studies, for which ethical issues need to be considered as done for other animal species. It would likely be beneficial to genotype the drug-metabolizing enzyme genes in cynomolgus macaques and marmosets before and after drug metabolism studies.

Acknowledgments

We thank Drs. Masahiro Utoh, Makiko Shimizu, Norie Murayama, Takashi Inoue, and Erika Sasaki for their support in experiments and David Smallbones for copyediting a draft of this chapter. This work was supported partly by the Japan Society for the Promotion of Science Grant-in-Aid for Scientific Research 20K06434.

Conflicts of interest

The authors declare that there are no conflicts of interest.

References

Bieche, I., Narjoz, C., Asselah, T., Vacher, S., Marcellin, P., Lidereau, R., et al. (2007). Reverse transcriptase-PCR quantification of mRNA levels from cytochrome (CYP) 1, CYP2 and CYP3 families in 22 different human tissues. *Pharmacogenetics and Genomics*, *17*(9), 731–742. https://doi.org/10.1097/FPC.0b013e32810f2e58.

Bogaards, J. J., Bertrand, M., Jackson, P., Oudshoorn, M. J., Weaver, R. J., van Bladeren, P. J., et al. (2000). Determining the best animal model for human cytochrome P450 activities: A comparison of mouse, rat, rabbit, dog, micropig, monkey and man. *Xenobiotica*, *30*(12), 1131–1152. https://doi.org/10.1080/00498250010021684.

Bullock, P., Pearce, R., Draper, A., Podval, J., Bracken, W., Veltman, J., et al. (1995). Induction of liver microsomal cytochrome P450 in cynomolgus monkeys. *Drug Metabolism and Disposition*, *23*(7), 736–748. Retrieved from https://www.ncbi.nlm.nih.gov/pubmed/7587963.

Chang, Y. T., & Loew, G. H. (1999). Homology modeling and substrate binding study of human CYP4A11 enzyme. *Proteins*, *34*(3), 403–415. Retrieved from https://www.ncbi.nlm.nih.gov/pubmed/10024026.

Christmas, P., Jones, J. P., Patten, C. J., Rock, D. A., Zheng, Y., Cheng, S. M., et al. (2001). Alternative splicing determines the function of CYP4F3 by switching substrate specificity. *The Journal of Biological Chemistry*, *276*(41), 38166–38172. https://doi.org/10.1074/jbc.M104818200.

Cui, X., Nelson, D. R., & Strobel, H. W. (2000). A novel human cytochrome P450 4F isoform (CYP4F11): cDNA cloning, expression, and genomic structural characterization. *Genomics*, *68*(2), 161–166. https://doi.org/10.1006/geno.2000.6276.

Danielson, P. B. (2002). The cytochrome P450 superfamily: Biochemistry, evolution and drug metabolism in humans. *Current Drug Metabolism*, *3*(6), 561–597. https://doi.org/10.2174/1389200023337054.

Daujat, M., Peryt, B., Lesca, P., Fourtanier, G., Domergue, J., & Maurel, P. (1992). Omeprazole, an inducer of human CYP1A1 and 1A2, is not a ligand for the Ah receptor. *Biochemical and Biophysical Research Communications*, *188*(2), 820–825. https://doi.org/10.1016/0006-291x(92)91130-i.

Drahushuk, A. T., McGarrigle, B. P., Tai, H. L., Kitareewan, S., Goldstein, J. A., & Olson, J. R. (1996). Validation of precision-cut liver slices in dynamic organ culture as an in vitro model for studying CYP1A1 and CYP1A2 induction. *Toxicology and Applied Pharmacology*, *140*(2), 393–403. https://doi.org/10.1006/taap.1996.0236.

Edwards, R. J., Murray, B. P., Murray, S., Schulz, T., Neubert, D., Gant, T. W., et al. (1994). Contribution of CYP1A1 and CYP1A2 to the activation of heterocyclic amines in monkeys and human. *Carcinogenesis*, *15*(5), 829–836. https://doi.org/10.1093/carcin/15.5.829.

Emoto, C., Iwasaki, K., Koizumi, R., Utoh, M., Murayama, N., Uno, Y., et al. (2011). Species difference between cynomolgus monkeys and humans on cytochromes P450 2D and 3A-dependent drug oxidation activities in liver microsomes. *Journal of Health Science*, *57*, 164–170.

Emoto, C., Yoda, N., Uno, Y., Iwasaki, K., Umehara, K., Kashiyama, E., et al. (2013). Comparison of P450 enzymes between cynomolgus monkeys and humans: P450 identities, protein contents, kinetic parameters, and potential for inhibitory profiles. *Current Drug Metabolism*, *14*, 239–252. https://doi.org/10.2174/138920013804870664.

Ferguson, B., Street, S. L., Wright, H., Pearson, C., Jia, Y., Thompson, S. L., et al. (2007). Single nucleotide polymorphisms (SNPs) distinguish Indian-origin and Chinese-origin rhesus macaques (Macaca mulatta). *BMC Genomics*, *8*, 43. https://doi.org/10.1186/1471-2164-8-43.

Fukami, T., Nakajima, M., Sakai, H., Katoh, M., & Yokoi, T. (2007). CYP2A13 metabolizes the substrates of human CYP1A2, phenacetin, and theophylline. *Drug Metabolism and Disposition*, *35*(3), 335–339. https://doi.org/10.1124/dmd.106.011064.

Gerbal-Chaloin, S., Pascussi, J. M., Pichard-Garcia, L., Daujat, M., Waechter, F., Fabre, J. M., et al. (2001). Induction of CYP2C genes in human hepatocytes in primary culture. *Drug Metabolism and Disposition*, *29*(3), 242–251. Retrieved from https://www.ncbi.nlm.nih.gov/pubmed/11181490.

Hanioka, N., Yamamoto, M., Iwabu, H., Jinno, H., Tanaka-Kagawa, T., Naito, S., et al. (2007). Functional characterization of human and cynomolgus monkey cytochrome P450 2E1 enzymes. *Life Sciences*, *81*(19–20), 1436–1445. https://doi.org/10.1016/j.lfs.2007.09.002.

Hashizume, T., Imaoka, S., Hiroi, T., Terauchi, Y., Fujii, T., Miyazaki, H., et al. (2001). cDNA cloning and expression of a novel cytochrome p450 (cyp4f12) from human small intestine. *Biochemical and Biophysical Research Communications*, *280*(4), 1135–1141. https://doi.org/10.1006/bbrc.2000.4238.

He, X. Y., Shen, J., Hu, W. Y., Ding, X., Lu, A. Y., & Hong, J. Y. (2004). Identification of Val117 and Arg372 as critical amino acid residues for the activity difference between human CYP2A6 and CYP2A13 in coumarin 7-hydroxylation. *Archives of Biochemistry and Biophysics*, *427*(2), 143–153. https://doi.org/10.1016/j.abb.2004.03.016.

Hernandez, R. D., Hubisz, M. J., Wheeler, D. A., Smith, D. G., Ferguson, B., Rogers, J., et al. (2007). Demographic histories and patterns of linkage disequilibrium in Chinese and Indian rhesus macaques. *Science*, *316*(5822), 240–243. https://doi.org/10.1126/science.1140462.

Hoch, U., & Ortiz De Montellano, P. R. (2001). Covalently linked heme in cytochrome p4504a fatty acid hydroxylases. *The Journal of Biological Chemistry*, *276*(14), 11339–11346. https://doi.org/10.1074/jbc.M009969200.

Hosaka, S., Murayama, N., Satsukawa, M., Shimizu, M., Uehara, S., Fujino, H., et al. (2015). Evaluation of 89 compounds for identification of substrates for cynomolgus monkey CYP2C76, a new bupropion/nifedipine oxidase. *Drug Metabolism and Disposition*, *43*(1), 27–33. https://doi.org/10.1124/dmd.114.061275.

Hosaka, S., Murayama, N., Satsukawa, M., Uehara, S., Shimizu, M., Iwasaki, K., et al. (2015). Comprehensive evaluation for substrate selectivity of cynomolgus monkey cytochrome P450 2C9, a new efavirenz oxidase. *Drug Metabolism and Disposition*, *43*(7), 1119–1122. https://doi.org/10.1124/dmd.115.063925.

Iwasaki, K., Kitsugi, Y., Ikeda, K., Yoshikawa, T., Hosaka, S., Uehara, S., et al. (2016). In vivo individual variations in pharmacokinetics of efavirenz in cynomolgus monkeys genotyped for cytochrome P450 2C9. *Biopharmaceutics & Drug Disposition*, *37*(6), 379–383. https://doi.org/10.1002/bdd.2021.

Iwasaki, K., Murayama, N., Koizumi, R., Uno, Y., & Yamazaki, H. (2010). Comparison of cytochrome P450 3A enzymes in cynomolgus monkeys and humans. *Drug Metabolism and Pharmacokinetics*, *25*(4), 388–391. https://doi.org/10.2133/dmpk.dmpk-10-nt-022.

Iwasaki, K., & Uno, Y. (2009). Cynomolgus monkey CYPs: A comparison with human CYPs. *Xenobiotica*, *39*(8), 578–581. https://doi.org/10.1080/00498250903003135.

Kim, S., Dinchuk, J. E., Anthony, M. N., Orcutt, T., Zoeckler, M. E., Sauer, M. B., et al. (2010). Evaluation of cynomolgus monkey pregnane X receptor, primary hepatocyte, and in vivo pharmacokinetic changes in predicting human CYP3A4 induction. *Drug Metabolism and Disposition*, *38*(1), 16–24. https://doi.org/10.1124/dmd.109.029637.

Kim, D., & Guengerich, F. P. (2005). Cytochrome P450 activation of arylamines and heterocyclic amines. *Annual Review of Pharmacology and Toxicology*, *45*, 27–49. https://doi.org/10.1146/annurev.pharmtox.45.120403.100010.

Koehler, S. C., Von Ahsen, N., Schlumbohm, C., Asif, A. R., Goedtel-Armbrust, U., Oellerich, M., et al. (2006). Marmoset CYP3A21, a model for human CYP3A4: Protein expression and functional characterization of the promoter. *Xenobiotica*, *36*(12), 1210–1226. https://doi.org/10.1080/00498250600962831.

Komori, M., Kikuchi, O., Kitada, M., & Kamataki, T. (1992). Molecular cloning of monkey P450 1A1 cDNA and expression in yeast. *Biochimica et Biophysica Acta*, *1131*(1), 23–29. https://doi.org/10.1016/0167-4781(92)90093-f.

Koskela, S., Hakkola, J., Hukkanen, J., Pelkonen, O., Sorri, M., Saranen, A., et al. (1999). Expression of CYP2A genes in human liver and extrahepatic tissues. *Biochemical Pharmacology*, *57*(12), 1407–1413. https://doi.org/10.1016/s0006-2952(99)00015-5.

Koyanagi, T., Nakanishi, Y., Murayama, N., Yamaura, Y., Ikeda, K., Yano, K., et al. (2015). Age-related changes of hepatic clearances of cytochrome P450 probes, midazolam and R-/S-warfarin in combination with caffeine, omeprazole and metoprolol in cynomolgus monkeys using in vitro-in vivo correlation. *Xenobiotica*, *45*(4), 312–321. https://doi.org/10.3109/00498254.2014.979271.

Koyanagi, T., Yamaura, Y., Yano, K., Kim, S., & Yamazaki, H. (2014). Age-related pharmacokinetic changes of acetaminophen, antipyrine, diazepam, diphenhydramine, and ofloxacin in male cynomolgus monkeys and beagle dogs. *Xenobiotica*, *44*(10), 893–901. https://doi.org/10.3109/00498254.2014.903532.

Kusama, T., Toda, A., Shimizu, M., Uehara, S., Inoue, T., Uno, Y., et al. (2018). Association with polymorphic marmoset cytochrome P450 2C19 of in vivo hepatic clearances of chirally separated R-omeprazole and S-warfarin using individual marmoset physiologically based pharmacokinetic models. *Xenobiotica*, *48*(10), 1072–1077. https://doi.org/10.1080/00498254.2017.1393121.

Lake, B. G., Walters, D. G., & Gangolli, S. D. (1989). Comparison of the metabolism and disposition of [3-14C]coumarin in the rat and marmoset (Callithrix jacchus). *Toxicology Letters*, *45*(2–3), 299–306. https://doi.org/10.1016/0378-4274(89)90021-0.

Lappin, G., Kuhnz, W., Jochemsen, R., Kneer, J., Chaudhary, A., Oosterhuis, B., et al. (2006). Use of microdosing to predict pharmacokinetics at the therapeutic dose: Experience with 5 drugs. *Clinical Pharmacology and Therapeutics*, *80*(3), 203–215. https://doi.org/10.1016/j.clpt.2006.05.008.

Lnenickova, K., Skalova, L., Stuchlikova, L., Szotakova, B., & Matouskova, P. (2018). Induction of xenobiotic-metabolizing enzymes in hepatocytes by beta-naphthoflavone: Time-dependent changes in activities, protein and mRNA levels. *Acta Pharmaceutica*, *68*(1), 75–85. https://doi.org/10.2478/acph-2018-0005.

Mankowski, D. C., Laddison, K. J., Christopherson, P. A., Ekins, S., Tweedie, D. J., & Lawton, M. P. (1999). Molecular cloning, expression, and characterization of CYP2D17 from cynomolgus monkey liver. *Archives of Biochemistry and Biophysics*, *372*(1), 189–196. https://doi.org/10.1006/abbi.1999.1506.

Martignoni, M., Groothuis, G. M., & de Kanter, R. (2006). Species differences between mouse, rat, dog, monkey and human CYP-mediated drug metabolism, inhibition and induction. *Expert Opinion on Drug Metabolism & Toxicology*, *2*(6), 875–894. https://doi.org/10.1517/17425255.2.6.875.

Matsumoto, S., Uehara, S., Kamimura, H., Ikeda, H., Maeda, S., Hattori, M., et al. (2021). Human total clearance values and volumes of distribution of typical human cytochrome P450 2C9/19 substrates predicted by single-species allometric scaling using pharmacokinetic data sets from common marmosets genotyped for P450 2C19. *Xenobiotica*, *51*(4), 479–493. https://doi.org/10.1080/00498254.2020.1871113.

Matsunaga, T., Ohmori, S., Ishida, M., Sakamoto, Y., Nakasa, H., & Kitada, M. (2002). Molecular cloning of monkey CYP2C43 cDNA and expression in yeast. *Drug Metabolism and Pharmacokinetics*, *17*(2), 117–124. https://doi.org/10.2133/dmpk.17.117.

Mayumi, K., Hanioka, N., Masuda, K., Koeda, A., Naito, S., Miyata, A., et al. (2013). Characterization of marmoset CYP2B6: cDNA cloning, protein expression and enzymatic functions. *Biochemical Pharmacology*, *85*(8), 1182–1194. https://doi.org/10.1016/j.bcp.2013.01.024.

Mitsuda, M., Iwasaki, M., & Asahi, S. (2006). Cynomolgus monkey cytochrome P450 2C43: cDNA cloning, heterologous expression, purification and characterization. *Journal of Biochemistry*, *139*(5), 865–872. https://doi.org/10.1093/jb/mvj093.

Nakanishi, K., Uehara, S., Kusama, T., Inoue, T., Shimura, K., Kamiya, Y., et al. (2018). In vivo and in vitro diclofenac 5-hydroxylation mediated primarily by cytochrome P450 3A enzymes in common marmoset livers genotyped for P450 2C19 variants. *Biochemical Pharmacology*, *152*, 272–278. https://doi.org/10.1016/j.bcp.2018.04.002.

Nakanishi, K., Uehara, S., Uno, Y., Inoue, T., Sasaki, E., & Yamazaki, H. (2018). Progesterone hydroxylation by cytochromes P450 2C and 3A enzymes in marmoset liver microsomes. *Xenobiotica*, *48*(8), 757–763. https://doi.org/10.1080/00498254.2017.1363444.

Narimatsu, S., Nakata, T., Shimizudani, T., Nagaoka, K., Nakura, H., Masuda, K., et al. (2011). Regio- and stereoselective oxidation of propranolol enantiomers by human CYP2D6, cynomolgus monkey CYP2D17 and marmoset CYP2D19. *Chemico-Biological Interactions*, *189*(3), 146–152. https://doi.org/10.1016/j.cbi.2010.12.014.

Narimatsu, S., Torigoe, F., Tsuneto, Y., Saito, K., Hanioka, N., Masuda, K., et al. (2006). Cloning of a cDNA encoding a novel marmoset CYP2C enzyme, expression in yeast cells and characterization of its enzymatic functions. *Biochemical Pharmacology*, *72*(12), 1738–1748. https://doi.org/10.1016/j.bcp.2006.08.025.

Nelson, D. R., Zeldin, D. C., Hoffman, S. M., Maltais, L. J., Wain, H. M., & Nebert, D. W. (2004). Comparison of cytochrome P450 (CYP) genes from the mouse and human genomes, including nomenclature recommendations for genes, pseudogenes and alternative-splice variants. *Pharmacogenetics*, *14*(1), 1–18. https://doi.org/10.1097/00008571-200401000-00001.

Nhamburo, P. T., Kimura, S., McBride, O. W., Kozak, C. A., Gelboin, H. V., & Gonzalez, F. J. (1990). The human CYP2F gene subfamily: Identification of a cDNA encoding a new cytochrome P450, cDNA-directed expression, and chromosome mapping. *Biochemistry*, *29*(23), 5491–5499. https://doi.org/10.1021/bi00475a012.

Nishida, C. R., Everett, S., & Ortiz de Montellano, P. R. (2013). Specificity determinants of CYP1B1 estradiol hydroxylation. *Molecular Pharmacology*, *84*(3), 451–458. https://doi.org/10.1124/mol.113.087700.

Nishimura, M., Koeda, A., Suganuma, Y., Suzuki, E., Shimizu, T., Nakayama, M., et al. (2007). Comparison of inducibility of CYP1A and CYP3A mRNAs by prototypical inducers in primary cultures of human, cynomolgus monkey, and rat hepatocytes. *Drug Metabolism and Pharmacokinetics*, *22*(3), 178–186. https://doi.org/10.2133/dmpk.22.178.

Nishimura, M., Yaguti, H., Yoshitsugu, H., Naito, S., & Satoh, T. (2003). Tissue distribution of mRNA expression of human cytochrome P450 isoforms assessed by high-sensitivity real-time reverse transcription PCR. *Yakugaku Zasshi*, *123*(5), 369–375. https://doi.org/10.1248/yakushi.123.369.

Ohtsuka, T., Yoshikawa, T., Kozakai, K., Tsuneto, Y., Uno, Y., Utoh, M., et al. (2010). Alprazolam as an in vivo probe for studying induction of CYP3A in cynomolgus monkeys. *Drug Metabolism and Disposition*, *38*(10), 1806–1813. https://doi.org/10.1124/dmd.110.032656.

Oshio, T., Uehara, S., Uno, Y., Inoue, T., Sasaki, E., & Yamazaki, H. (2019). Marmoset cytochrome P450 2B6, a propofol hydroxylase expressed in liver. *Xenobiotica*, *49*(3), 265–269. https://doi.org/10.1080/00498254.2018.1439204.

Pelkonen, O., Rautio, A., Raunio, H., & Pasanen, M. (2000). CYP2A6: A human coumarin 7-hydroxylase. *Toxicology*, *144*(1–3), 139–147. https://doi.org/10.1016/s0300-483x(99)00200-0.

Powell, P. K., Wolf, I., Jin, R., & Lasker, J. M. (1998). Metabolism of arachidonic acid to 20-hydroxy-5,8,11, 14-eicosatetraenoic acid by P450 enzymes in human liver: Involvement of CYP4F2 and CYP4A11. *The Journal of Pharmacology and Experimental Therapeutics*, *285*(3), 1327–1336. Retrieved from https://www.ncbi.nlm.nih.gov/pubmed/9618440.

Powell, P. K., Wolf, I., & Lasker, J. M. (1996). Identification of CYP4A11 as the major lauric acid omega-hydroxylase in human liver microsomes. *Archives of Biochemistry and Biophysics*, *335*(1), 219–226. https://doi.org/10.1006/abbi.1996.0501.

Raunio, H., Syngelma, T., Pasanen, M., Juvonen, R., Honkakoski, P., Kairaluoma, M. A., et al. (1988). Immunochemical and catalytical studies on hepatic coumarin 7-hydroxylase in man, rat, and mouse. *Biochemical Pharmacology*, *37*(20), 3889–3895. https://doi.org/10.1016/0006-2952(88)90070-6.

Rhodes, S. P., Otten, J. N., Hingorani, G. P., Hartley, D. P., & Franklin, R. B. (2011). Simultaneous assessment of cytochrome P450 activity in cultured human hepatocytes for compound-mediated induction of CYP3A4, CYP2B6, and CYP1A2. *Journal of Pharmacological and Toxicological Methods*, *63*(3), 223–226. https://doi.org/10.1016/j.vascn.2010.11.002.

Sakuma, T., Hieda, M., Igarashi, T., Ohgiya, S., Nagata, R., Nemoto, N., et al. (1998). Molecular cloning and functional analysis of cynomolgus monkey CYP1A2. *Biochemical Pharmacology*, *56*, 131–139. https://doi.org/10.1016/S0006-2952(98)00100-2.

Sakuma, T., Igarashi, T., Hieda, M., Ohgiya, S., Isogai, M., Ninomiya, S., et al. (1997). Marmoset CYP1A2: Primary structure and constitutive expression in livers. *Carcinogenesis*, *18*(10), 1985–1991. https://doi.org/10.1093/carcin/18.10.1985.

Schulz, T. G., Neubert, D., Davies, D. S., & Edwards, R. J. (1996). Induction of cytochromes P450 by dioxins in liver and lung of marmoset monkeys (Callithrix jacchus). *Advances in Experimental Medicine and Biology*, *387*, 443–446. https://doi.org/10.1007/978-1-4757-9480-9_53.

Schulz, T. G., Thiel, R., Davies, D. S., & Edwards, R. J. (1998). Identification of CYP2E1 in marmoset monkey. *Biochimica et Biophysica Acta*, *1382*(2), 287–294. https://doi.org/10.1016/s0167-4838(97)00170-2.

Schulz, T. G., Thiel, R., Neubert, D., Brassil, P. J., Schulz-Utermoehl, T., Boobis, A. R., et al. (2001). Assessment of P450 induction in the marmoset monkey using targeted anti-peptide antibodies. *Biochimica et Biophysica Acta*, *1546*(1), 143–155. https://doi.org/10.1016/s0167-4838(01)00134-0.

Shilling, W. H., Crampton, R. F., & Longland, R. C. (1969). Metabolism of coumarin in man. *Nature*, *221*(5181), 664–665. https://doi.org/10.1038/221664b0.

Shimamoto, Y., Niimi, K., Kitamura, H., Tsubakishita, S., & Takahashi, E. (2016). In situ hybridization study of CYP2D mRNA in the common marmoset brain. *Experimental Animals*, *65*(4), 465–471. https://doi.org/10.1538/expanim.16-0045.

Street, S. L., Kyes, R. C., Grant, R., & Ferguson, B. (2007). Single nucleotide polymorphisms (SNPs) are highly conserved in rhesus (Macaca mulatta) and cynomolgus (Macaca fascicularis) macaques. *BMC Genomics*, *8*, 480. https://doi.org/10.1186/1471-2164-8-480.

Su, T., Bao, Z., Zhang, Q. Y., Smith, T. J., Hong, J. Y., & Ding, X. (2000). Human cytochrome P450 CYP2A13: Predominant expression in the respiratory tract and its high efficiency metabolic activation of a tobacco-specific carcinogen, 4-(methylnitrosamino)-1-(3-pyridyl)-1-butanone. *Cancer Research*, *60*(18), 5074–5079. Retrieved from https://www.ncbi.nlm.nih.gov/pubmed/11016631.

Toda, A., Uehara, S., Inoue, T., Utoh, M., Kusama, T., Shimizu, M., et al. (2018). Effects of aging and rifampicin pretreatment on the pharmacokinetics of human cytochrome P450 probes caffeine, warfarin, omeprazole, metoprolol and midazolam in common marmosets genotyped for cytochrome P450 2C19. *Xenobiotica*, *48*(7), 720–726. https://doi.org/10.1080/00498254.2017.1353716.

Turpault, S., Brian, W., Van Horn, R., Santoni, A., Poitiers, F., Donazzolo, Y., et al. (2009). Pharmacokinetic assessment of a five-probe cocktail for CYPs 1A2, 2C9, 2C19, 2D6 and 3A. *British Journal of Clinical Pharmacology*, *68*(6), 928–935. https://doi.org/10.1111/j.1365-2125.2009.03548.x.

Uehara, S., Inoue, T., Utoh, M., Toda, A., Shimizu, M., Uno, Y., et al. (2016). Simultaneous pharmacokinetics evaluation of human cytochrome P450 probes, caffeine, warfarin, omeprazole, metoprolol and midazolam, in common marmosets (Callithrix jacchus). *Xenobiotica*, *46*(2), 163–168. https://doi.org/10.3109/00498254.2015.1057270.

Uehara, S., Ishii, S., Uno, Y., Inoue, T., Sasaki, E., & Yamazaki, H. (2017). Regio- and stereo-selective oxidation of a cardiovascular drug, metoprolol, mediated by cytochrome P450 2D and 3A enzymes in marmoset livers. *Drug Metabolism and Disposition, 45*(8), 896–899. https://doi.org/10.1124/dmd.117.075630.

Uehara, S., Kawano, M., Murayama, N., Uno, Y., Utoh, M., Inoue, T., et al. (2016). Oxidation of R- and S-omeprazole stereoselectively mediated by liver microsomal cytochrome P450 2C19 enzymes from cynomolgus monkeys and common marmosets. *Biochemical Pharmacology, 120*, 56–62. https://doi.org/10.1016/j.bcp.2016.09.010.

Uehara, S., Murayama, N., Nakanishi, Y., Nakamura, C., Hashizume, T., Zeldin, D. C., et al. (2015). Immunochemical quantification of cynomolgus CYP2J2, CYP4A and CYP4F enzymes in liver and small intestine. *Xenobiotica, 45*(2), 124–130. https://doi.org/10.3109/00498254.2014.952800.

Uehara, S., Murayama, N., Yamazaki, H., & Uno, Y. (2010). A novel CYP2A26 identified in cynomolgus monkey liver metabolizes coumarin. *Xenobiotica, 40*(9), 621–629. https://doi.org/10.3109/00498254.2010.501118.

Uehara, S., Murayama, N., Yamazaki, H., & Uno, Y. (2012). CYP2C76 non-synonymous variants in cynomolgus and rhesus macaques. *Drug Metabolism and Pharmacokinetics, 27*(3), 344–348. https://doi.org/10.2133/dmpk.dmpk-11-nt-118.

Uehara, S., Oshio, T., Nakanishi, K., Tomioka, E., Suzuki, M., Inoue, T., et al. (2019). Survey of drug oxidation activities in hepatic and intestinal microsomes of individual common marmosets, a new nonhuman primate animal model. *Current Drug Metabolism, 20*(2), 103–113. https://doi.org/10.2174/1389200219666181003143312.

Uehara, S., Uno, Y., Hagihira, Y., Murayama, N., Shimizu, M., Inoue, T., et al. (2015). Marmoset cytochrome P450 2D8 in livers and small intestines metabolizes typical human P450 2D6 substrates, metoprolol, bufuralol and dextromethorphan. *Xenobiotica, 45*(9), 766–772. https://doi.org/10.3109/00498254.2015.1019595.

Uehara, S., Uno, Y., Inoue, T., Kawano, M., Shimizu, M., Toda, A., et al. (2015). Novel marmoset cytochrome P450 2C19 in livers efficiently metabolizes human P450 2C9 and 2C19 substrates, S-warfarin, tolbutamide, flurbiprofen, and omeprazole. *Drug Metabolism and Disposition, 43*(10), 1408–1416. https://doi.org/10.1124/dmd.115.066100.

Uehara, S., Uno, Y., Inoue, T., Kawano, M., Shimizu, M., Toda, A., et al. (2016). Individual differences in metabolic clearance of S-warfarin efficiently mediated by polymorphic marmoset cytochrome P450 2C19 in livers. *Drug Metabolism and Disposition, 44*(7), 911–915. https://doi.org/10.1124/dmd.116.070383.

Uehara, S., Uno, Y., Inoue, T., Kawano, M., Shimizu, M., Toda, A., et al. (2020). Correction to "individual differences in metabolic clearance of S-warfarin efficiently mediated by polymorphic marmoset cytochrome P450 2C19 in livers". *Drug Metabolism and Disposition, 48*(8), 723. https://doi.org/10.1124/dmd.120.000141.

Uehara, S., Uno, Y., Inoue, T., Murayama, N., Shimizu, M., Sasaki, E., et al. (2015). Activation and deactivation of 1-methyl-4-phenyl-1,2,3,6-tetrahydropyridine by cytochrome P450 enzymes and flavin-containing monooxygenases in common marmosets (Callithrix jacchus). *Drug Metabolism and Disposition, 43*(5), 735–742. https://doi.org/10.1124/dmd.115.063594.

Uehara, S., Uno, Y., Inoue, T., Okamoto, E., Sasaki, E., & Yamazaki, H. (2016). Marmoset cytochrome P450 2J2 mainly expressed in small intestines and livers effectively metabolizes human P450 2J2 probe substrates, astemizole and terfenadine. *Xenobiotica, 46*(11), 977–985. https://doi.org/10.3109/00498254.2016.1146366.

Uehara, S., Uno, Y., Inoue, T., Sasaki, E., & Yamazaki, H. (2015). Substrate selectivities and catalytic activities of marmoset liver cytochrome P450 2A6 differed from those of human P450 2A6. *Drug Metabolism and Disposition, 43*(7), 969–976. https://doi.org/10.1124/dmd.115.063909.

Uehara, S., Uno, Y., Inoue, T., Sasaki, E., & Yamazaki, H. (2016). Molecular cloning, tissue distribution, and functional characterization of marmoset cytochrome P450 1A1, 1A2, and 1B1. *Drug Metabolism and Disposition, 44*(1), 8–15. https://doi.org/10.1124/dmd.115.067561.

Uehara, S., Uno, Y., Inoue, T., Suzuki, T., Utoh, M., Sasaki, E., et al. (2016). Caffeine 7-N-demethylation and C-8-oxidation mediated by liver microsomal cytochrome P450 enzymes in common marmosets. *Xenobiotica, 46*(7), 573–578. https://doi.org/10.3109/00498254.2015.1096980.

Uehara, S., Uno, Y., Ishii, S., Inoue, T., Sasaki, E., & Yamazaki, H. (2017). Marmoset cytochrome P450 4A11, a novel arachidonic acid and lauric acid omega-hydroxylase expressed in liver and kidney tissues. *Xenobiotica, 47*(7), 553–561. https://doi.org/10.1080/00498254.2016.1206673.

Uehara, S., Uno, Y., Nakanishi, K., Ishii, S., Inoue, T., Sasaki, E., et al. (2017). Marmoset cytochrome P450 3A4 ortholog expressed in liver and small-intestine tissues efficiently metabolizes midazolam, alprazolam, nifedipine, and testosterone. *Drug Metabolism and Disposition, 45*(5), 457–467. https://doi.org/10.1124/dmd.116.074898.

Uehara, S., Uno, Y., Oshio, T., Inoue, T., Sasaki, E., & Yamazaki, H. (2018). Marmoset pulmonary cytochrome P450 2F1 oxidizes biphenyl and 7-ethoxycoumarin and hepatic human P450 substrates. *Xenobiotica, 48*(7), 656–662. https://doi.org/10.1080/00498254.2017.1354138.

Uehara, S., Uno, Y., Suzuki, T., Inoue, T., Utoh, M., Sasaki, E., et al. (2017). Strong induction of cytochrome P450 1A/3A, but not P450 2B, in cultured hepatocytes from common marmosets and cynomolgus monkeys by typical human P450 inducing agents. *Drug Metabolism Letters, 10*(4), 244–253. https://doi.org/10.2174/1872312810666161114144412.

Uehara, S., Uno, Y., Tomioka, E., Inoue, T., Sasaki, E., & Yamazaki, H. (2017). Functional characterization and tissue expression of marmoset cytochrome P450 2E1. *Biopharmaceutics & Drug Disposition, 38*(6), 394–397. https://doi.org/10.1002/bdd.2080.

Uehara, S., Uno, Y., & Yamazaki, H. (2020). The marmoset cytochrome P450 superfamily: Sequence/phylogenetic analyses, genomic structure, and catalytic function. *Biochemical Pharmacology, 171*, 113721. https://doi.org/10.1016/j.bcp.2019.113721.

Uehara, S., Uno, Y., Yuki, Y., Inoue, T., Sasaki, E., & Yamazaki, H. (2016). A new marmoset P450 4F12 enzyme expressed in small intestines and livers efficiently metabolizes antihistaminic drug ebastine. *Drug Metabolism and Disposition, 44*(6), 833–841. https://doi.org/10.1124/dmd.116.070367.

Uehara, S., Yuki, Y., Uno, Y., Inoue, T., Sasaki, E., & Yamazaki, H. (2018). Terfenadine t-butyl hydroxylation catalyzed by human and marmoset cytochrome P450 3A and 4F enzymes in livers and small intestines. *Xenobiotica, 48*(4), 342–347. https://doi.org/10.1080/00498254.2017.1321811.

Uno, Y., Fujino, H., Kito, G., Kamataki, T., & Nagata, R. (2006). CYP2C76, a novel cytochrome P450 in cynomolgus monkey, is a major CYP2C in liver, metabolizing tolbutamide and testosterone. *Molecular Pharmacology, 70*(2), 477–486. https://doi.org/10.1124/mol.106.022673.

Uno, Y., Hosaka, S., Matsuno, K., Nakamura, C., Kito, G., Kamataki, T., et al. (2007). Characterization of cynomolgus monkey cytochrome P450 (CYP) cDNAs: Is CYP2C76 the only monkey-specific CYP gene responsible for species differences in drug metabolism? *Archives of Biochemistry and Biophysics, 466*(1), 98–105. https://doi.org/10.1016/j.abb.2007.07.003.

Uno, Y., Iwasaki, K., Yamazaki, H., & Nelson, D. R. (2011). Macaque cytochromes P450: Nomenclature, transcript, gene, genomic structure, and function. *Drug Metabolism Reviews, 43*(3), 346–361. https://doi.org/10.3109/03602532.2010.549492.

Uno, Y., Kumano, T., Kito, G., Nagata, R., Kamataki, T., & Fujino, H. (2007). CYP2C76-mediated species difference in drug metabolism: A comparison of pitavastatin metabolism between monkeys and humans. *Xenobiotica*, *37*(1), 30–43. Retrieved from PM:17178632.

Uno, Y., Matsuno, K., Nakamura, C., Utoh, M., & Yamazaki, H. (2009a). Cloning, expression, and characterization of CYP3A43 cDNA in cynomolgus macaque (Macaca fascicularis). *Drug Metabolism Letters*, *3*(4), 228–233. https://doi.org/10.2174/187231209790218127.

Uno, Y., Matsuno, K., Nakamura, C., Utoh, M., & Yamazaki, H. (2009b). Identification and characterization of CYP2B6 cDNA in cynomolgus macaques (Macaca fascicularis). *The Journal of Veterinary Medical Science*, *71*(12), 1653–1656. https://doi.org/10.1292/jvms.001653.

Uno, Y., Matsuno, K., Nakamura, C., Utoh, M., & Yamazaki, H. (2010). Identification and characterization of CYP2C18 in the cynomolgus macaque (Macaca fascicularis). *The Journal of Veterinary Medical Science*, *72*(2), 225–228. https://doi.org/10.1292/jvms.09-0341.

Uno, Y., Matsuno, K., Nakamura, C., Utoh, M., & Yamazaki, H. (2011). Cynomolgus macaque CYP4 isoforms are functional, metabolizing arachidonic acid. *The Journal of Veterinary Medical Science*, *73*(4), 487–490. https://doi.org/10.1292/jvms.10-0333.

Uno, Y., Matsushita, A., Murayama, N., & Yamazaki, H. (2015). Genetic polymorphism of cynomolgus and rhesus macaque CYP2C9. *Drug Metabolism and Pharmacokinetics*, *30*(1), 130–132. https://doi.org/10.1016/j.dmpk.2014.10.002.

Uno, Y., Matsushita, A., Murayama, N., & Yamazaki, H. (2017). Corrigendum to "genetic polymorphism of cynomolgus and rhesus macaque CYP2C9" [Drug Metab Pharmacokinet 30 (2015) 130-132]. *Drug Metabolism and Pharmacokinetics*, *32*(3), 192. https://doi.org/10.1016/j.dmpk.2017.04.001.

Uno, Y., Matsushita, A., Osada, N., Uehara, S., Kohara, S., Nagata, R., et al. (2010). Genetic variants of CYP3A4 and CYP3A5 in cynomolgus and rhesus macaques. *Drug Metabolism and Disposition*, *38*(2), 209–214. https://doi.org/10.1124/dmd.109.029710.

Uno, Y., Matsushita, A., Shukuya, M., Matsumoto, Y., Murayama, N., & Yamazaki, H. (2014). CYP2C19 polymorphisms account for inter-individual variability of drug metabolism in cynomolgus macaques. *Biochemical Pharmacology*, *91*(2), 242–248. https://doi.org/10.1016/j.bcp.2014.07.004.

Uno, Y., Osada, N., Sakurai, S., Shimozawa, N., Iwata, T., Ikeo, K., et al. (2018). Development of genotyping method for functionally relevant variants of cytochromes P450 in cynomolgus macaques. *Journal of Veterinary Pharmacology and Therapeutics*, *41*(1), e30–e34. https://doi.org/10.1111/jvp.12443.

Uno, Y., Sakuraba, H., Uehara, S., Kumano, T., Matsuno, K., Nakamura, C., et al. (2009). A null allele impairs function of CYP2C76 gene in cynomolgus monkeys: A possible genetic tool for generation of a better animal model in drug metabolism. *Drug Metabolism and Disposition*, *37*(1), 14–17. https://doi.org/10.1124/dmd.108.023622.

Uno, Y., Uehara, S., Kohara, S., Murayama, N., & Yamazaki, H. (2010). Cynomolgus monkey CYP2D44 newly identified in liver, metabolizes bufuralol, and dextromethorphan. *Drug Metabolism and Disposition*, *38*(9), 1486–1492. https://doi.org/10.1124/dmd.110.033274.

Uno, Y., Uehara, S., Kohara, S., Murayama, N., & Yamazaki, H. (2014). Polymorphisms of CYP2D17 in cynomolgus and rhesus macaques: An evidence of the genetic basis for the variability of CYP2D-dependent drug metabolism. *Drug Metabolism and Disposition*, *42*(9), 1407–1410. https://doi.org/10.1124/dmd.114.059220.

Uno, Y., Uehara, S., Murayama, N., & Yamazaki, H. (2011a). CYP1D1, pseudogenized in human, is expressed and encodes a functional drug-metabolizing enzyme in cynomolgus monkey. *Biochemical Pharmacology*, *81*(3), 442–450. https://doi.org/10.1016/j.bcp.2010.11.003.

Uno, Y., Uehara, S., Murayama, N., & Yamazaki, H. (2011b). CYP2G2, pseudogenized in human, is expressed in nasal mucosa of cynomolgus monkey and encodes a functional drug-metabolizing enzyme. *Drug Metabolism and Disposition*, *39*(4), 717–723. https://doi.org/10.1124/dmd.110.036574.

Uno, Y., Uehara, S., & Yamazaki, H. (2016). Utility of non-human primates in drug development: Comparison of non-human primate and human drug-metabolizing cytochrome P450 enzymes. *Biochemical Pharmacology*, *121*, 1–7. https://doi.org/10.1016/j.bcp.2016.06.008.

Uno, Y., Uehara, S., & Yamazaki, H. (2018). Genetic polymorphisms of drug-metabolizing cytochrome P450 enzymes in cynomolgus and rhesus monkeys and common marmosets in preclinical studies for humans. *Biochemical Pharmacology*, *153*, 184–195. https://doi.org/10.1016/j.bcp.2017.12.015.

Uno, Y., & Yamazaki, H. (2016). Development of a genotyping tool for a functionally relevant CYP2C19 allele (Phe100Asn, Ala103Val and Ile112Leu) in cynomolgus macaques. *The Journal of Veterinary Medical Science*, *78*(1), 147–148. https://doi.org/10.1292/jvms.15-0416.

Utoh, M., Kusama, T., Miura, T., Mitsui, M., Kawano, M., Hirano, T., et al. (2018). R-warfarin clearances from plasma associated with polymorphic cytochrome P450 2C19 and simulated by individual physiologically based pharmacokinetic models for 11 cynomolgus monkeys. *Xenobiotica*, *48*(2), 206–210. https://doi.org/10.1080/00498254.2017.1288945.

Utoh, M., Suemizu, H., Mitsui, M., Kawano, M., Toda, A., Uehara, S., et al. (2016). Human plasma concentrations of cytochrome P450 probe cocktails extrapolated from pharmacokinetics in mice transplanted with human hepatocytes and from pharmacokinetics in common marmosets using physiologically based pharmacokinetic modeling. *Xenobiotica*, *46*(12), 1049–1055. https://doi.org/10.3109/00498254.2016.1147102.

Utoh, M., Yoshikawa, T., Hayashi, Y., Shimizu, M., Iwasaki, K., Uno, Y., et al. (2015). Slow R-warfarin 7-hydroxylation mediated by P450 2C19 genetic variants in cynomolgus monkeys in vivo. *Biochemical Pharmacology*, *95*(2), 110–114. https://doi.org/10.1016/j.bcp.2015.03.008.

Weaver, R. J., Dickins, M., & Burke, M. D. (1999). A comparison of basal and induced hepatic microsomal cytochrome P450 monooxygenase activities in the cynomolgus monkey (Macaca fascicularis) and man. *Xenobiotica*, *29*(5), 467–482. https://doi.org/10.1080/004982599238489.

Wu, S., Moomaw, C. R., Tomer, K. B., Falck, J. R., & Zeldin, D. C. (1996). Molecular cloning and expression of CYP2J2, a human cytochrome P450 arachidonic acid epoxygenase highly expressed in heart. *The Journal of Biological Chemistry*, *271*(7), 3460–3468. https://doi.org/10.1074/jbc.271.7.3460.

CHAPTER TWELVE

Cytochrome P450 enzymes in the pediatric population: Connecting knowledge on P450 expression with pediatric pharmacokinetics

Chie Emoto[a,b,*] and Trevor N. Johnson[c]
[a]Laboratory of Drug Metabolism and Pharmacokinetics, Showa Pharmaceutical University, Tokyo, Japan
[b]Translational Research Division, Chugai Pharmaceutical Co., Ltd., Tokyo, Japan
[c]Certara UK Limited, Sheffield, United Kingdom
*Corresponding author: e-mail address: c-emoto@umin.ac.jp

Contents

Advances in Pharmacology, Volume 95
ISSN 1054-3589
https://doi.org/10.1016/bs.apha.2022.05.006

Abstract

Cytochrome P450 enzymes play an important role in the pharmacokinetics, efficacy, and toxicity of drugs. Age-dependent changes in P450 enzyme expression have been studied based on several detection systems, as well as by deconvolution of *in vivo* pharmacokinetic data observed in pediatric populations. The age-dependent changes in P450 enzyme expression can be important determinants of drug disposition in childhood, in addition to the changes in body size and the other physiological parameters, and effects of pharmacogenetics and disease on organ functions. As a tool incorporating drug-specific and body-specific factors, physiologically-based pharmacokinetic (PBPK) models have become increasingly used to characterize and explore mechanistic insights into drug disposition. Thus, PBPK models can be a bridge between findings from basic science and utilization in predictive science. Pediatric PBPK models incorporate additional system specific information on developmental physiology and ontogeny and have been used to predict pharmacokinetic parameters from preterm neonates onwards. These models have been advocated by regulatory authorities in order to support pediatric clinical trials.

The purpose of this chapter is to highlight accumulated knowledge and findings from basic research focusing on P450 enzymes, as well as the current status and future challenges of expanding the utilization of pediatric PBPK modeling.

1. Introduction

Metabolism is the main elimination pathway for the majority of drugs (Wienkers & Heath, 2005). Approximately 75% of the top 200 drugs prescribed in the United States (U.S.) in 2002 were eliminated by metabolism (Williams et al., 2004). Cytochrome P450s (P450s, CYPs) are the enzymes most responsible for the oxidation of many drugs and endogenous substrates. P450 enzymes contribute to drug metabolism, mainly as detoxifying agents. They are also known to work on activation and detoxification in the case of organophosphorus pesticides such as chlorpyrifos (Timchalk, Kousba, & Poet, 2007). P450s exist mainly in the liver, and expression is also observed in extrahepatic tissues such as the intestine, lungs, and kidneys (Krishna & Klotz, 1994; Paine et al., 2006). Of FDA-approved drugs between 2005 and 2016, 54% were metabolized by P450 enzymes, while 28% were metabolized by non-P450 enzymes (Saravanakumar, Sadighi, Ryu, & Akhlaghi, 2019). Three CYP families, namely CYP1, CYP2, and CYP3, primarily participate in drug metabolism in humans (Zanger et al., 2014).

The ontogeny of these P450 enzymes has been studied over the years and classified based on the developmental patterns of the expression (Hines, 2013). These data have been an integral part in the understanding of drug metabolism in the pediatric population.

The general understanding is that determination of sensitivity to drug effects, including adverse drug reactions, for any age group or population is dependent on multiple factors, such as genetic influences, pharmacokinetics and pharmacodynamics, and exposure (Hines et al., 2010). Age-dependent changes in the pharmacokinetics of drugs during childhood are attributable to two aspects: one is growth in body size as well as anatomical organ size; and the other is the developmental changes in organ functions (Anderson & Holford, 2008; Vinks, Emoto, & Fukuda, 2015). An age-dependent change in clearance of drugs metabolized by P450 enzymes has been observed in pediatric populations, including neonates and infants. Overall changes in the liver elimination function in the pediatric population are reflected by the developmental changes in expression and activity of drug-metabolizing enzymes, as well as transporters. Age-dependent changes were also observed in the other determinants of hepatic clearance, such as liver size, hepatic blood flow, microsomal concentrations, serum protein concentrations, and hematocrit (Salem, Abduljalil, Kamiyama, & Rostami-Hodjegan, 2016). In order to quantitatively address the age-dependent effects of multiple factors, a physiologically-based pharmacokinetic (PBPK) model has been used to predict the pharmacokinetics of drugs in pediatric populations (Johnson & Rostami-Hodjegan, 2011).

PBPK models are not only used in evaluating pharmaceuticals for regulatory purposes but are also supporting tools for chemical safety assessment. A study by Bagley et al. highlighted the use of PBPK modeling in the assessment of bisphenol A exposure in children and adults following treatment with dental composite restoratives (Bagley, Smith, & Teeguarden, 2021). As with pharmaceuticals, the contribution of each P450 isoform to metabolic elimination pathways of new and existing chemicals needs to be determined in order to apply PBPK modeling to predict pharmacokinetics and/or toxicokinetics. The use of PBPK modeling has been accelerated by availability of parameters incorporated in the model, as well as an increase in user-friendly PBPK modeling software. General standards for publishing PBPK models will further enhance model reproducibility.

The current chapter intends to provide an overview of the developmental change of P450 enzyme expression as a key factor to predict PK in the pediatric population. Subsequently, applications of PBPK modeling and simulation using developmental changes in P450 enzyme expression are introduced through several case studies.

2. Developmental changes in cytochrome P450 enzyme expression

Changes in the pharmacokinetics (PK) of drugs in pediatric are not monotonic in nature but generated by a range of age-related factors, such as changes in body size and composition, and the development of drug elimination pathways. For children, drug doses, estimated using a simplistic allometric scaling with body size, resulted in over-prediction, particularly in neonates and infants (Johnson, 2008; Johnson & Ke, 2021). This may be due to age-dependent changes in the expression of drug-metabolizing enzymes and transporters, which play a key role in the drug elimination pathways. Age-dependent quantitative changes in P450 expression, as well as transporters, are involved in the accuracy of predicted clearance in children.

P450 expression for each isoform in children has been studied using mRNA and/or protein and activity levels (van Groen et al., 2021). The same paper also provides age-dependent changes in P450 expression in animals, which could support understanding of species differences in P450 ontogeny. The *in vitro* findings classified each P450 isoform into three classes, according to their developmental trajectory (Table 1). Class 1 enzymes were expressed at their highest levels in the fetus during the first trimester and low or absent after birth. Class 2 enzymes were expressed at relatively constant levels throughout gestation and into adulthood. Class 3 enzymes were expressed at negligible or low levels in the fetus. The onset of expression can be

Table 1 Classification of developmental changes in hepatic P450 enzymes.

Class 1	**Class 2**	**Class 3**
CYP3A7	CYP2B6	CYP1A2
	CYP2C19	CYP2C9
	CYP3A5	CYP2D6
		CYP2E1
		CYP3A4

The P450 data were extracted from the previous report (Hines, 2013).

observed in either the second or third trimester, in which the expression level is less than the fully-matured level. The period of reaching fully-matured expression varies depending on the P450 isoforms.

In addition to *in vitro* studies, age-dependent changes in size-normalized clearance have been studied as a reflection of P450 expression development. To describe the *in vivo* developmental changes in clearance, Salem et al. demonstrated a novel approach involving the creation of enzyme ontogeny models by deconvolution of *in vivo* drug clearance values across the pediatric age range. Particularly in younger pediatric populations, the relationship between age and size-normalized clearance was originally described by a Hill model as follows (Tod, Jullien, & Pons, 2008):

$$Factor\ of\ adult\ (maturation\ level) = \frac{Age^s}{Age_{50}{}^s + Age^s}$$

where Age_{50}, the age to reach 50% of mature function; s, a sigmoidicity coefficient.

In order to consider a baseline of the expression, the equation was further modified as follows (Johnson, Rostami-Hodjegan, & Tucker, 2006; Upreti & Wahlstrom, 2016):

$$Factor\ of\ adult = \frac{Age^s}{Age_{50}{}^s + Age^s} \times (Adult_{Max} - F_{birth}) + F_{birth}$$

where $Adult_{Max}$ is the maximal response from adult samples and F_{birth} is the fraction of adult response at birth. For some P450 substrates, pediatric clearances at a certain age range may exceed adult values. To describe these observations, a linear or exponential function was used with the above formula depending on the age range. These equations are implemented in the pediatric PBPK model to take into account the maturation of P450 enzymes (please see the third paragraph). Details on age-dependent changes in P450 expression, as well as clearance observed in pediatric patients, are described below for each P450 isoform contributing drug metabolism.

2.1 CYP1A1

In adults, CYP1A1 exists largely extrahepatically, such as in the lung and placenta, and is known to be induced by cigarette smoking and/or other inducers mediated through an aryl hydrocarbon receptor (Zevin & Benowitz, 1999). However, the mRNA of CYP1A1 has been identified in fetal livers aged as early as 45 days of gestation and its expression was higher in older gestational ages (Omiecinski, Redlich, & Costa, 1990;

Yang, Namkung, & Juchau, 1995). Interestingly, its immunoreactive expression in fetal livers showed no apparent zonal distribution (Murray et al., 1992). Another paper reported there was no mRNA expression of CYP1A1 in fetal livers at 11–24 weeks of gestation (Hakkola et al., 1994). The reason for the gap among *in vitro* observations remains to be addressed.

2.2 CYP1A2

The expression was absent in microsomes prepared from fetal and neonatal livers and the levels increased in infants aged 1–3 months to reach 50% of the adult value at 1 year (Sonnier & Cresteil, 1998). CYP1A2 protein expression in the perinatal to the infant group (gestational 37 weeks to postnatal 10 months) was much lower compared to the older age groups (2–72 years) (Tateishi et al., 1997). Using an *in vivo* approach where data on the total clearance of CYP1A2 substrates such as caffeine and theophylline, collected across the pediatric age range, is deconvoluted back to intrinsic metabolic clearance relative to adults. The relative activity of CYP1A2 reached adult levels at 63 weeks post menstrual age (PMA), then rose above adult values up to 196 weeks PMA (i.e., 3 years) followed by a decline to adult levels by 25 years (Salem, Johnson, Abduljalil, Tucker, & Rostami-Hodjegan, 2014, 2015). This *in vivo* CYP1A2 ontogeny was conformed in a later study (Upreti & Wahlstrom, 2016) and shown to perform better than the *in vitro* derived ontogeny patterns.

2.3 CYP2A6

Many alleles of CYP2A6 have been identified to show a wide interethnic variability of the allele-carrying individuals (Lopez-Flores, Perez-Rubio, & Falfan-Valencia, 2017). There was no correlation between age (2–64 years) and CYP2A6 protein in wild-type livers, which were chosen to minimize any potential genetic bias (Al Koudsi, Hoffmann, Assadzadeh, & Tyndale, 2010). Considering ages less than 2 years, the CYP2A6 protein expression in the perinatal to the infant group was slightly lower compared to the older age group, although there was no consideration of genetic alleles (Tateishi et al., 1997). Regarding the fetal expression, the findings were not consistent, CYP2A6 mRNA levels were detected in 17- to 37-week fetal liver samples and were elevated eightfold in postnatal samples (5–65 years) (Nagata et al., 2003). However, another study reported that none of the

CYP2A enzymes appeared to be expressed in fetal livers (Maenpaa, Rane, Raunio, Honkakoski, & Pelkonen, 1993).

2.4 CYP2B6

Detectable CYP2B6 protein was observed in most liver microsomes from pediatric donors ($n=217$) with the age range from 10 weeks gestation to 17 years (Croom, Stevens, Hines, Wallace, & Hodgson, 2009). This paper demonstrated a twofold, increase in the median of CYP2B6 protein expression after the neonatal period (10 weeks gestation to 30 postnatal days, compared to >30 days to 17 years). Another study also reported that the CYP2B6 expression in the perinatal-infant age group (>37 weeks gestation but <10 months of age) was approximately 10-fold lower compared to the older age group (Tateishi et al., 1997). After infancy, there was no obvious dependency of the CYP2B6 expression on ages between 5 and 85 years; however, considerable interindividual variation was observed, partly due to its polymorphisms (Lang et al., 2001). A further study has verified this finding and concluded that CYP2B6 increases through infancy and by 1 year of age reaches adult expression and activity (Pearce et al., 2016).

Developmental changes in the oral clearance of efavirenz, which was a substrate of CYP2B6 (Ward et al., 2003), were observed in HIV-infected pediatric patients from 2 to 202 months old ($n=96$) (Salem, Fletcher, & Brundage, 2014). The oral clearance of efavirenz after size normalization with allometric scaling reached 90% of its maturity level by the age of 9 months. Regarding the pharmacogenetic effect of CYP2B6, it was reported that the median oral clearance was significantly lower in children with the CYP2B6-516-T/T genotype ($3.0\,L/h/m^2$, $n=13$) than in children with the G/T genotype ($5.7\,L/h/m^2$, $n=30$; $P=0.02$) or the G/G genotype ($7.0\,L/h/m^2$, $n=31$; $P=0.003$) (Saitoh et al., 2007). This indicated the contribution of metabolic activity driven by the CYP2B6 genotype to oral clearance. In contrast to this finding *in vivo*, the *in vitro* study by Pearce et al. (2016) found CYP2B6 inter-individual variability was not associated with genetic variation. This illustrates the importance of studying ontogeny in relation to genotype/phenotype in the pediatric population (Leeder, Kearns, Spielberg, & van den Anker, 2010).

2.5 CYP2C8

CYP2C8 expression in livers from fetuses and individuals less than 35 days old post age were significantly lower compared to postnatal individuals aged between 35 days and 11 years (Song et al., 2017). The CYP2C8 expression among individuals in the latter age group was not statistically different from that in the group greater than 11 years, although the overall distribution of CYP2C8 content for the entire sample varied approximately 80-fold. The authors mentioned that the age differential appeared to be driven by the onset of CYP2C8 expression after birth, and progressive increase at 35 days of age. Another report also demonstrated that CYP2C8 expression in the perinatal to the infant group (gestational 37 weeks to postnatal 10 months) was 3.6-fold lower compared to the older age group (2–72 years) (Tateishi et al., 1997). CYP2C8 expression did not change in donors aged 7–70 years (Naraharisetti et al., 2010), which was also found in another study (Rodriguez-Antona et al., 2008).

2.6 CYP2C9

CYP2C9 mRNA levels were detected in 17- to 37-week fetal liver samples and were elevated 13-fold in postnatal samples (ages 5–65 years) (Nagata et al., 2003). CYP2C9 expression was shown to be, at 1–2% of mature values during the first trimester, with progressive increases during the second and third trimesters to approximately 30% of mature values (Koukouritaki et al., 2004). From birth to 5 months, CYP2C9 protein values varied 35-fold and were significantly higher than those observed during the late fetal period, with 51% of samples exhibiting values commensurate with mature levels. From 5 months to 18 years, expression levels were greater than other age groups and approached adult values, but interestingly exhibited less variability.

CYP2C9 has at least 71 variant alleles which have been defined by the human CYP Allele Nomenclature Committee (https://www.pharmvar.org/gene/CYP2C9). It was reported that carriers of the *CYP2C9 *1/*2*, **1/*3*, **2/*2*, **2/*3*, and **3/*3* genotypes required warfarin doses that are 19.6%, 33.7%, 36.0%, 56.7%, and 78.1% lower than in carriers of the wild-type *CYP2C9 *1/*1* genotype, respectively (Lindh, Holm, Andersson, & Rane, 2009). In Japanese pediatric and adult patients (prepubertal group, 1–11 years; pubertal, 12–18 years; and adult, 37–76 years), no differences were observed in the liver weight–normalized unbound oral clearance of (*S*)-warfarin, which has 3–5 times more potent anticoagulation effect than its (*R*)-congener (Takahashi et al., 2000). That means that liver weight may be a better parameter than body weight in order to estimate warfarin doses for prepubertal patients on the basis of the corresponding adult values. This study also reported that the liver weight–normalized unbound oral clearance of (*S*)-warfarin in adult patients with heterozygous *CYP2C9*3* appeared approximately 50% less than that in prepubertal patients with the corresponding genotype (158 ± 52 vs 302 ± 137 mL/min, respectively), although the difference between the groups was not significant (Takahashi et al., 2000). Again, understanding the genotype-dependent developmental changes are important for this enzyme.

2.7 CYP2C19

CYP2C19 protein expression was detectable as early as 8 weeks of gestation, and it was similar among all gestational ages (Koukouritaki et al., 2004). In contrast to CYP2C9 expression, CYP2C19 expression did not change at birth but increased linearly over the first 5 postnatal months, and varied greatly, i.e., a 21-fold difference from 5 months to 10 years. During infancy—which was defined as being greater than 30 days, but less than 1 year of age—there was an approximately twofold increase in mean CYP2C19 expression to levels that were nearly 50% of those observed in adults (Hines, 2007). From 10 years through 18 years postnatal age, a significant but modest increase in CYP2C19-specific content was observed (Koukouritaki et al., 2004). Comparing CYP2C9 and CYP2C19, there was no relationship in the expression during either the fetal or early infancy period (postnatal 0–5 months) (Koukouritaki et al., 2004). The comparison between these two isoforms also demonstrated that CYP2C19 is the dominant enzyme in most individuals during fetal development, and it is only after birth that CYP2C9 expression becomes the dominant CYP2C enzyme (Hines, 2007).

CYP2C19 is the major CYP isoforms involved in drug metabolism of proton pump inhibitors (PPIs), such as lansoprazole, omeprazole, and pantoprazole, along with CYP3A4 (Ishizaki & Horai, 1999). In pediatric patients from 0.375 to 2.25 years, allometrically-scaled omeprazole clearance after intravenous administration seemed to increase with age (Faure et al., 2001; Ward & Kearns, 2013). However, there is no age-dependent change in the apparent terminal elimination rate constant of omeprazole from 2 to 16 years old (Kearns et al., 2003). The clearance of pantoprazole after size normalization with allometric scaling was best described by a sigmoid Emax model in pediatric patients aged 0.025–16 years old (Knebel et al., 2011). The clearance reached 50% of adult level at 0.153 years old in full-term infants, then rapidly approached adult level by the age of 1 year.

In addition to the effects of age and body weight, variability in pantoprazole clearance was explained by CYP2C19 metabolizer status. The Clinical Pharmacogenetics Implementation Consortium (CPIC) provides therapeutic recommendations for PPIs' prescriptions, based on the CYP2C19 genotype (Lima et al., 2021). The most common loss-of-function alleles, *CYP2C19*2* and *CYP2C19*3*, were more frequent in Chinese, compared to African-Americans and Caucasians (Desta, Zhao, Shin, & Flockhart, 2002).

2.8 CYP2D6

The CYP2D6 mRNA was detectable in at least some of the fetal livers at 11 weeks of gestation (Hakkola et al., 1994). A clear increase in the CYP2D6 protein expression was found during the first postnatal week (Treluyer, Jacqz-Aigrain, Alvarez, & Cresteil, 1991). Similarly, the CYP2D6 protein expression in liver samples from neonates less than 7 days of age was higher than that observed in the first and second-trimester samples, but not significantly higher than the third-trimester fetal samples (Stevens et al., 2008). Expression in postnatal samples greater than 7 days of age was substantially higher than that for an earlier age category. Like CYP2C9, the CYP2D6 protein expression increased significantly after birth, independent of gestational age, and continued upward to levels about 50–75% of adult values during the neonatal period (Hines & McCarver, 2002). The protein level increased steadily in neonates of 7–28 days and infants over 28 days of age (Treluyer et al., 1991). There is no significant difference in CYP2D6 protein expression between perinatal to the infant group (gestational 37 weeks to postnatal 10 months) and older age group (2–72 years old) (Tateishi et al., 1997). CYP2D6 is known as a polymorphism isoform and more than 80 alleles have been defined by the Cytochrome P450 Nomenclature Committee (https://www.pharmvar.org/gene/CYP2D6). Stevens and colleagues suggested that CYP2D6 variability in individuals older than 1–2 weeks of age is largely due to genetic variability (Stevens et al., 2008).

As a clinical observation, clearance for the formation of *O*-desmethyltramadol (CYP2D6 metabolite of tramadol, M1) in extreme and preterm neonates was very low, independent of the CYP2D6 genotype, while from term age onwards CYP2D6 polymorphisms became a relevant covariate of *O*-demethylation activity (Allegaert et al., 2008). Subsequently, the complex interplay between ontogeny, CYP2D6 polymorphisms and renal elimination clearance was illustrated as relevant covariates of the phenotypical variability in time–concentration profiles of tramadol and its pharmacodynamic relevant metabolite M1 (Allegaert, Rochette, & Veyckemans, 2011). For the youngest populations, it should be noted that the urinary drug/metabolite ratio may be relatively constant, since the development of renal function from birth is parallel to the development of the enzyme (Johnson, Tucker, & Rostami-Hodjegan, 2008).

2.9 CYP2E1

The CYP2E1 protein was detected in fetuses in the second and third-trimester (Oesterheld, 1998), although some scientific groups reported that they were unable to detect the expression (Hakkola et al., 1994; Vieira, Sonnier, & Cresteil, 1996). The variability among *in vitro* observations was considered to be involved in prenatal alcohol metabolism (Oesterheld, 1998). At birth and during the neonatal period (the first 30 days after birth), there was a two- to threefold increase in CYP2E1 expression relative to the third trimester (Hines, 2007). CYP2E1 in neonatal samples was low and less than that of infants 31–90 days of age, which was less than that of older infants, children, and young adults (Johnsrud et al., 2003). That study suggested that an increase in CYP2E1 protein expression was associated with increasing postnatal age, but it is less clear with increasing gestational age.

2.10 CYP3A7, CYP3A5, and CYP3A4

CYP3A4 and CYP3A5 are mainly expressed in the adult liver and intestine (Paine et al., 2006; Zanger et al., 2014). Among CYP3A enzymes, CYP3A7 is known as a fetal isoform (Komori et al., 1990; Nelson et al., 1996) and its expression was found to exist from the first trimester and remained at relatively high expression throughout gestation (Hines, 2007). On the other hand, CYP3A4 was not expressed or is expressed at low levels in the fetus, with the onset of expression generally in either the second or third trimester. The expression of CYP3A7 declines after the first postnatal week and falls to very low levels or disappears by 1 year of age, whereas CYP3A4 expression begins to increase dramatically at about 1 week of age (Lacroix, Sonnier, Moncion, Cheron, & Cresteil, 1997). This suggests that CYP3A7 expression is replaced by CYP3A4 shortly after birth, with a possible reason being that CYP3A7 appears to have a role in protecting the fetus against endogenous substrates such as dehydroepiandrosterone and retinoic acid. CYP3A7 appears to have a low capacity for eliminating exogenous drugs (Williams et al., 2002). The CYP3A4 expression was reported to reach 30% of the adult level by 1 month after birth, but it was highly variable (Stevens et al., 2003). Unlike CYP3A4, CYP3A5 expression remains at relatively constant levels throughout gestation (Hines, 2007). After birth, the CYP3A5 level showed no apparent increase as a function of age, only a very high degree of inter-individual variability (Blake, Castro, Leeder, & Kearns, 2005; Stevens et al., 2003).

Regarding the intestinal CYP3A expression, the information is more limited. CYP3A4 was almost absent in fetal duodenum and was expressed at relatively low levels in neonates (Johnson, Tanner, Taylor, & Tucker, 2001). The CYP3A4 expression in neonates was lower compared to that in children over 5 years. A recent study has confirmed these observations with lower expression found in the 0–2 year age group compared to older groups (Kiss et al., 2021).

As a clinical observation, relative intrinsic metabolic clearance, as a function of hepatic CYP3A, reached half of adult levels at 71 weeks post-menstrual age, based on the deconvolution of *in vivo* pharmacokinetic data of midazolam (a CYP3A substrate) after intravenous administration (Salem, Johnson, et al., 2014, 2015). This finding was supported by another report based on clearance of intravenous-administered clindamycin, which is primarily metabolized by CYP3A enzymes (Wynalda, Hutzler, Koets, Podoll, & Wienkers, 2003). Allometrically size-normalized clearance with body weight demonstrated that half of adult value was reached at a post-menstrual age of 43.6 weeks (Gonzalez et al., 2014). In contrast, another *in vivo* derived ontogeny function for hepatic CYP3A4 based on sufentanil clearance changes with age, showed an increase in activity going above adult values during childhood (Upreti & Wahlstrom, 2016).

3. Utilization of P450 ontogeny for predicting pharmacokinetics of drugs in the pediatric population: Physiologically-based pharmacokinetic (PBPK) modeling and simulations

The long-standing achievements regarding developmental changes in P450 enzyme expression have been leveraged to predict drug pharmacokinetics in a pediatric population through PBPK modeling and simulations.

Compared to traditional clinical trials in adults, pediatric studies are more challenging due to logistical and ethical reasons, such as low study consent rates from parents of subject children, limited blood volume available to conduct pharmacokinetic studies, and difficulties associated with blood sample timing, etc. (Laughon et al., 2011). In addition, pediatric clinical trials with a limited age group are difficult to evaluate, so when feasible, the trials should have a wide range of age groups. In reality, there are often age gaps in pediatric clinical data and this is an area where predictive science is needed to both help in optimal pediatric trial design (Dumont et al., 2013) as well as support the conclusions made from the trials.

PBPK models are one of the tools that can quantitatively take into account the effects of the contribution of multiple physiological factors on drug pharmacokinetics (Fig. 1). PBPK models can also potentially address the individual differences in drug disposition by including realistic physiological variability based on a correlated Monte Carlo approach. To predict the drug pharmacokinetic profile in the pediatric population, information on developmental changes in physiology (e.g., liver size and glomerular filtration rate, GFR), as well as ontogeny profiles of P450 enzymes and transporters, are included in the PBPK model. In this approach, predictive science is supported by basic science such as studies investigating the ontogeny of P450 enzymes.

Regulations aimed at promoting pediatric drug development in the U.S. and Europe are also associated with the increasing use of the pediatric PBPK models. A pharmacometrics approach, including PBPK modeling and

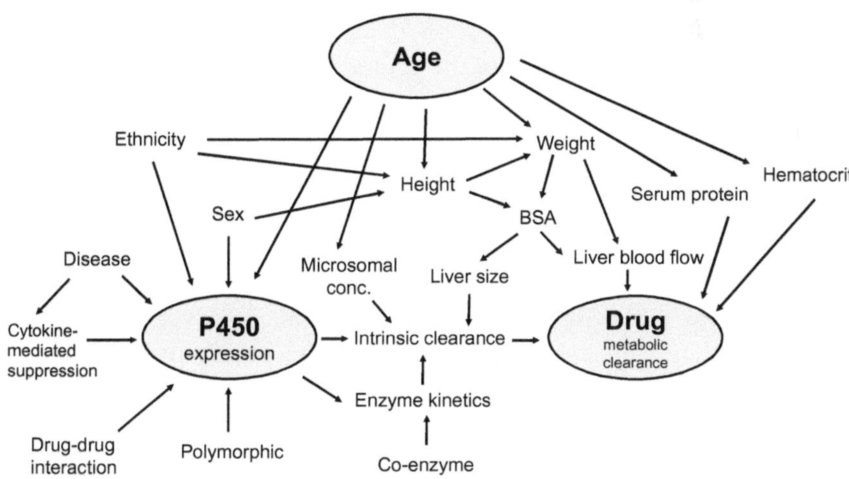

Fig. 1 Relationship between covariates specific to age, P450 expression, and metabolic clearance. BSA, body surface area.

simulation, is proposed in order to support global regulatory strategies for pediatric drug development programs. Among the applications in which the PBPK model was used in the Investigational New Drug (IND)/New Drug Application (NDA) submitted from 2008 to 2012, pediatric submissions were 18%, the second-highest percentage after use for the evaluation of drug interactions (Huang, Abernethy, Wang, Zhao, & Zineh, 2013). A similar trend in utility was maintained in subsequent survey reports from 2008 to 2017 (Grimstein et al., 2019) and from 2018 to 2019 (Zhang et al., 2020).

Leong and the FDA colleagues advocated the workflow for pediatric PBPK model development and verification (Leong et al., 2012). The PBPK model for adults should first be developed using drug-specific parameters (e.g., physicochemical properties; kinetic characteristics of P450 and/or transporter-mediated reactions; protein binding; membrane permeability, etc.) and system-dependent parameters in adults (e.g., abundance of P450 and/or transporter in each tissue; cardiac output; tissue composition; and organ and body sizes, etc.). After verification and refinement of the developed model using available clinical PK data, the adult model should be adapted to a pediatric model by replacing adult physiological parameters with pediatric ones. The predictive performance of the pediatric model should be assessed through a stepwise approach from older to younger pediatric age groups. First it is desirable to evaluate the effect of body size on PK using older children, and then evaluate the effect of developmental changes using younger children separately. Although having a 2-year age cut-off for pediatric age groups is generalized, for certain dosing scenarios, this age cut off for the use of PBPK does not necessarily apply in all cases (Johnson & Ke, 2021).

The predictive performance of the pediatric PBPK model implementing ontogeny profiles of P450 enzymes has been evaluated using clinical PK data. The use of *in vitro* derived ontogeny profiles for some P450 enzymes in a pediatric PBPK model have given acceptable performance with valuable scientific insights (Johnson et al., 2006). On the other hand, some cases did not capture the developmental changes in clearance observed clinically (Leong et al., 2012). Further investigational activities are needed to bridge the gap between *in vitro* and *in vivo* ontogeny profiles of P450 enzymes. However, in many cases the implementation of *in vivo* data derived ontogeny profiles in PBPK models has demonstrated improved predictive performance as a practical alternative to *in vitro* derived profiles (Salem, Johnson, et al., 2014, 2015).

An advantage of a pediatric PBPK model is the ability to demonstrate possible changes in contributing elimination pathways. For example, acetaminophen is known to be metabolized by multiple enzymes such as P450s,

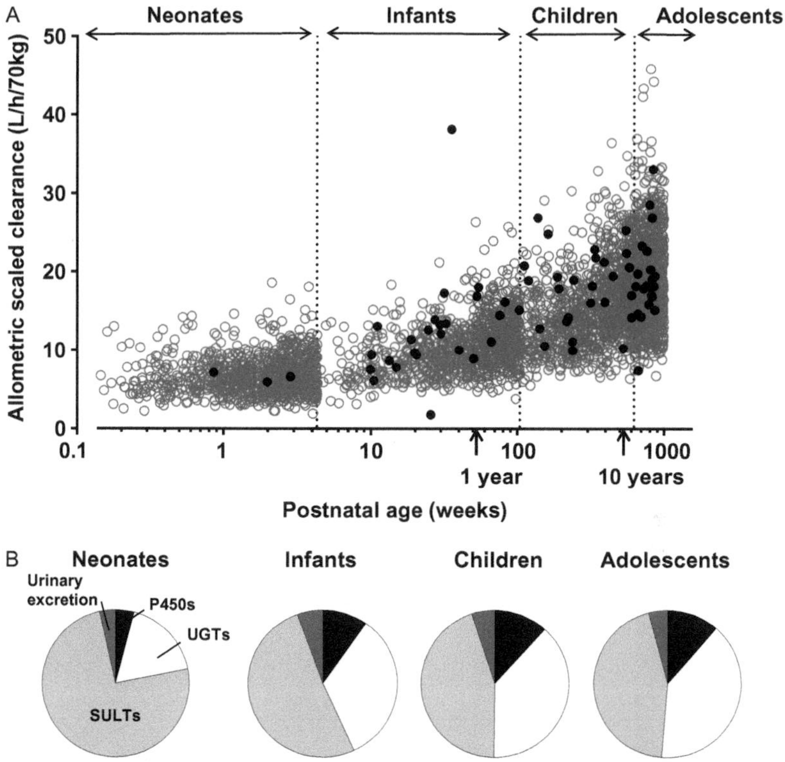

Fig. 2 Age-dependent changes in acetaminophen clearance (A) and elimination pathways (B). The PBPK model was used to simulate concentration-time profiles for 8 h after a 15-min infusion of 12.5 mg/kg acetaminophen ($N = 1000$ virtual subjects with a same ratio for male and female). The clearances were allometrically scaled to a standard adult weight of 70 kg. PBPK model-predicted allometric scaled clearances (open circles) were overlaid with the observed data (closed circles) (Zuppa et al., 2011). The age groups were defined as follows: newborns, birth to <1 month old; infants, 1 month to <2 years old; school children, 2–12 years old; and adolescents, 12–20 years old. SULT, sulfotransferase; UGT, Uridine 5′-diphospho-glucuronosyltransferase. *Adapted from Emoto, C., & Fukuda, T. (2018). Physiologically-based pharmacokinetic (PBPK)-pharmacodynamic (PD) model of acetaminophen: Development and its potential clinical applications.* The Japanese Journal of Developmental Pharmacology and Therapeutics, 31*(1), 14–21.*

Uridine 5′-diphospho-glucuronosyltransferases, and sulfotransferases, in addition to renal elimination (Fig. 2) (Emoto & Fukuda, 2018). The pediatric PBPK model, implementing multiple elimination pathways with their ontogeny profiles, was able to demonstrate not only age-dependent changes in clearances but also changes in contributing elimination pathways during growth. This can be important is predicting drug-drug interactions in pediatrics as discussed below.

It is generally difficult to conduct clinical trials with a sufficient sample size for neonates and early infants. Lessons learned, from available PK data across several probe drugs having similar ADME characteristics and/or elimination pathways with the investigational drug, can be valuable to reduce the uncertainty and complexity. The acceptability of simulation results is usually assessed by the predicted to observed ratio, traditionally within twofold was considered acceptable based on *in vitro* to *in vivo* extrapolation. However, with the refinement of models and based on input data and application 1.5-fold or even 0.8 to 1.25-fold may be a more acceptable target. For simulations where results show poor prediction it is worth considering the best- and worst-case scenarios through sensitivity analyses, focusing on parameters of interest. Continuous accumulation of experiences and knowledge from various sources is necessary to support the rationale of assumptions built into the pediatric PBPK models. Building model confidence from extensive verification and qualification is important moving forward so that, both from a regulatory and clinical prospective, they can be used to their full potential. This may include, negating the need to perform some pediatric studies and their application to predicting drug behavior in individuals.

4. Future challenges

Research on P450 ontogeny has been applied into PBPK models to predict PK in pediatric populations in the drug development process. The characteristics of a typical pediatric population may differ from those in a patient population of interest, as well as an individual patient. In this section, we would like to raise several suggestions and future challenges in order to make further progress in this field.

4.1 Performing more comprehensive basic science and clinical studies in children

An ongoing challenge, mainly due to ethical and logistical reasons, is obtaining tissue samples and comprehensive PK data from across the age range in both healthy children and those with disease. Obtaining intestinal, liver and kidney biopsies from pediatric subjects is very difficult as well as invasive; however, new less invasive methodology is constantly evolving. For example, in terms of quantification of the abundance and inter-individual variability of hepatic enzymes and transporters, a "liquid biopsy" test has been developed based on analysis in plasma exosomes isolated from blood samples (Achour et al., 2021). This is relatively non-invasive and could be developed further for use in pediatrics. The "liquid biopsy" approach has some challenges which remain to be addressed, most importantly the need for verification of the quantitative link between liquid biopsy and tissue biopsy in wider patient groups and repeated samples from the same individuals.

More comprehensive PK studies in pediatric populations are needed for better understanding of drug behavior and for supporting model validation; however, it is unrealistic especially in neonate and small infants to conduct an intensive PK study. In order to solve the difficulty in obtaining PK data from the youngest pediatric populations, a pediatric opportunistic pharmacokinetics study (POPS) was proposed to utilize scavenged blood samples which are collected from children already receiving drugs as a part of their standard of care (Laughon et al., 2011). With this approach, the risk for pediatric patients could be minimalized. Furthermore, the dried blood spot (DBS) method has also received a lot of attention in recent years (Edelbroek, van der Heijden, & Stolk, 2009), since relatively non-invasive blood sampling with small volumes is the most suitable method for pediatric patients. The POPS with DBS can help enrich the limited blood concentration data from pediatric populations. This will lead to accelerating the evaluation of the PBPK models.

4.2 Disease effects on pediatric P450 expression

In adults, the effects of disease on P450-mediated PKs and/or their expression have been studied. It was reported that interleukin-6 (IL-6), induced during inflammation, suppresses the expression of P450 enzymes (Morgan, 2009). A decrease in P450 expression has been observed in adult patients with liver cirrhosis (George, Liddle, Murray, Byth, & Farrell, 1995) and in renal impairment (Deri et al., 2020). Regarding the liver cirrhosis, the decreased CYP3A expression level was considered to correspond with disease severity, based on the Child-Pugh score (Johnson, Boussery, Rowland-Yeo, Tucker, & Rostami-Hodjegan, 2010). To utilize these findings in adults into the pediatric PBPK model, it is assumed that the disease effects are the same in adults and children but this may not always the case.

Theophylline toxicity due to a decrease in its clearance was observed in pediatric patients with serologic evidence of influenza B, which is a very common childhood disease (Kraemer et al., 1982). This could be associated with reduced CYP1A2 expression and/or activity due to inflammation (de Jong, Jiskoot, Swen, & Manson, 2020). Recently, it was reported that active regional inflammation in Crohn's disease was associated with both villous lengths blunting and decreased mRNA/protein expression of CYP3A4 in the small intestine from pediatric patients aged 1–19 years (Vyhlidal et al., 2021). There are few examples of the use of specific PBPK models in pediatrics where disease is considered, one study reported on a cystic fibrosis (Cicali, Long, Kim, & Cristofoletti, 2020) and another on a pediatric renal impairment in Asian children (Yoon et al., 2019).

Simultaneous characterization of age-related and disease-related changes in physiological parameters will directly enhance the development of a virtual target pediatric patient population used in PBPK modeling.

4.3 Effects of pharmacogenetics and drug-drug interactions on pediatric P450 enzymes

In the sections above (i.e., Section 2) on the individual enzymes the importance of considering the genotype/phenotype when studying ontogeny has been emphasized. The ontogeny should ideally be on the wild type or extensive metabolizer (EM) phenotype with other genotypes/phenotypes generated based on population frequency within the mechanistic PBPK model. As more research is done in this area and simpler more routine tests become available for genotyping this will allow more comprehensive ontogeny studies in pediatrics that fully account for genotype/phenotype effects. Even within the same genotype, individual difference in the expression level of a target protein unexplained by genotype are observed, more research is needed in this area, the liquid biopsy approach, highlighted above, will help improve the characterization of a target population.

In addition to genotype, it is important to consider the effects of co-administered drugs, foods, and herbs on drug metabolizing enzymes. In pediatric dentistry, Goho mentioned excessive sedation could be due to increased exposure after administration of midazolam with grapefruit juice (Goho, 2001). Regarding co-administered drugs, certain drugs are mechanism-based inhibitors of CYP enzymes and will lower expression (e.g., erythromycin), while other such as rifampicin may increase expression due to induction. As well as drug-drug interactions (DDI), influencing ontogeny studies the converse of this is also true in that the pattern of ontogeny is crucial in the accurate prediction of pediatric DDI (Lang, Vincent, Chenel, Ogungbenro, & Galetin, 2021). In the case of neonates and infants, the differential ontogeny may change the contribution of P450 enzymes compared to that in adults (Salem, Johnson, Barter,

Leeder, & Rostami-Hodjegan, 2013), consequently a significant DDI in adults may not be significant in neonates and *vice-versa*. The use of pediatric PBPK models to predict DDIs in children is an emerging area of research (Gonzalez & Sinha, 2021) and has been used as part of regulatory submission (Cleary et al., 2021). Pediatric PBPK model-based simulations can facilitate the discussion on the potential effect of polymorphism or DDI risk in each age group of pediatric populations.

4.4 Pediatric PK prediction in an individual

In order to apply PBPK simulations to individuals, some of the representative anatomical and physiological data of a population—including demographics, co-medications, the genotype and the expression level of P450 enzymes, and level of organ function—need to be adapted with individual values for a target patient. Matching virtual patients to the characteristics of those that are being simulated is a field of study is currently attracting attention and is often referred to a virtual twin approach (Polasek & Rostami-Hodjegan, 2020). A study reported that the PBPK model of olanzapine successfully predicted the systemic exposure in individual patients with reasonable accuracy (Polasek et al., 2018). In this study, a "virtual twin" profile for each study subject was constructed by individualizing a healthy volunteer population for ethnicity, gender, age, height, weight, CYP2C8 genotype and CYP1A2 phenotype. Proof-of-concept for model-informed precision dosing was demonstrated by adapting individual parameters to an available PBPK platform, although further study is required to examine clinical potential. This approach relies on additional data becoming available, not routinely found in most electronic medical records, such as genetic polymorphisms. An interdisciplinary approach is required to move forward in this area, which has the potential to improve therapeutic use of drugs and allow more cost-effective prescribing.

5. Conclusion

This chapter has summarized the age-dependent changes in the expression of P450 enzymes that are utilized as part of the pediatric PBPK model, in order to predict drug disposition in these populations. The feasibility of the pediatric PBPK model has been demonstrated for many drugs and drug development candidates, where there are several uncertainties and assumptions in some physiological parameters. PBPK modeling providers and users should acknowledge the uncertainties behind the model, and then discuss with basic researchers how to fill in the research gaps as needed. Collaborations between basic and clinical scientists will make the models more robust and improve our confidence in their predictability.

Finally, as with the P450s highlighted in this chapter, age-related changes in expression of drug transporters and receptors are also essential to better understand differences in drug disposition, efficacy, and toxicity between pediatric and adult populations. This is because sensitivity of effect or risk is assessed by combined effects of susceptibility (i.e., biological factors for pharmacology and toxicity) and exposure levels of target drugs and chemicals. In addition, developing more specific PBPK models, such as mechanistic kidney or brain for predicting concentrations in different areas of these organs, respectively, would enhance understanding of the behavior of drugs and chemicals in terms of their efficacy and safety. Further scientific advances in these fields will promote the accurate use of pediatric drugs.

Acknowledgments

Chie Emoto thanks Dr. Tsuyoshi Fukuda for providing scientific discussion on pediatric clinical pharmacology.

Conflict of interest

Chie Emoto is an employee of Chugai Pharmaceutical Co. Ltd., but is working outside the subject area of the submitted work. Trevor N. Johnson is an employee of Certara UK Limited (Simcyp Division), a company that develops and supplies modeling and simulation software and services to the pharmaceutical industry.

References

Achour, B., Al-Majdoub, Z. M., Grybos-Gajniak, A., Lea, K., Kilford, P., Zhang, M., et al. (2021). Liquid biopsy enables quantification of the abundance and interindividual variability of hepatic enzymes and transporters. *Clinical Pharmacology and Therapeutics, 109*(1), 222–232. https://doi.org/10.1002/cpt.2102.

Al Koudsi, N., Hoffmann, E. B., Assadzadeh, A., & Tyndale, R. F. (2010). Hepatic CYP2A6 levels and nicotine metabolism: Impact of genetic, physiological, environmental, and epigenetic factors. *European Journal of Clinical Pharmacology, 66*(3), 239–251. https://doi.org/10.1007/s00228-009-0762-0.

Allegaert, K., Rochette, A., & Veyckemans, F. (2011). Developmental pharmacology of tramadol during infancy: Ontogeny, pharmacogenetics and elimination clearance. *Paediatric Anaesthesia, 21*(3), 266–273. https://doi.org/10.1111/j.1460-9592.2010.03389.x.

Allegaert, K., van den Anker, J. N., de Hoon, J. N., van Schaik, R. H., Debeer, A., Tibboel, D., et al. (2008). Covariates of tramadol disposition in the first months of life. *British Journal of Anaesthesia, 100*(4), 525–532. https://doi.org/10.1093/bja/aen019.

Anderson, B. J., & Holford, N. H. (2008). Mechanism-based concepts of size and maturity in pharmacokinetics. *Annual Review of Pharmacology and Toxicology, 48*, 303–332. https://doi.org/10.1146/annurev.pharmtox.48.113006.094708.

Bagley, B. D., Smith, J. N., & Teeguarden, J. G. (2021). Risk assessment of predicted serum concentrations of bisphenol A in children and adults following treatment with dental composite restoratives, dental sealants, or orthodontic adhesives using physiologically based pharmacokinetic modeling. *Regulatory Toxicology and Pharmacology, 120*, 104839. https://doi.org/10.1016/j.yrtph.2020.104839.

Blake, M. J., Castro, L., Leeder, J. S., & Kearns, G. L. (2005). Ontogeny of drug metabolizing enzymes in the neonate. *Seminars in Fetal & Neonatal Medicine, 10*(2), 123–138. https://doi.org/10.1016/j.siny.2004.11.001.

Cicali, B., Long, T., Kim, S., & Cristofoletti, R. (2020). Assessing the impact of cystic fibrosis on the antipyretic response of ibuprofen in children: Physiologically-based modeling as a candle in the dark. *British Journal of Clinical Pharmacology, 86*(11), 2247–2255. https://doi.org/10.1111/bcp.14326.

Cleary, Y., Gertz, M., Grimsey, P., Gunther, A., Heinig, K., Ogungbenro, K., et al. (2021). Model-based drug-drug interaction extrapolation strategy from adults to children: Risdiplam in pediatric patients with spinal muscular atrophy. *Clinical Pharmacology and Therapeutics, 110*(6), 1547–1557. https://doi.org/10.1002/cpt.2384.

Croom, E. L., Stevens, J. C., Hines, R. N., Wallace, A. D., & Hodgson, E. (2009). Human hepatic CYP2B6 developmental expression: The impact of age and genotype. *Biochemical Pharmacology, 78*(2), 184–190. https://doi.org/10.1016/j.bcp.2009.03.029.

de Jong, L. M., Jiskoot, W., Swen, J. J., & Manson, M. L. (2020). Distinct effects of inflammation on cytochrome P450 regulation and drug metabolism: Lessons from experimental models and a potential role for pharmacogenetics. *Genes (Basel), 11*(12), 1509. https://doi.org/10.3390/genes11121509.

Deri, M. T., Kiss, A. F., Toth, K., Paulik, J., Sarvary, E., Kobori, L., et al. (2020). End-stage renal disease reduces the expression of drug-metabolizing cytochrome P450s. *Pharmacological Reports, 72*(6), 1695–1705. https://doi.org/10.1007/s43440-020-00127-w.

Desta, Z., Zhao, X., Shin, J. G., & Flockhart, D. A. (2002). Clinical significance of the cytochrome P450 2C19 genetic polymorphism. *Clinical Pharmacokinetics, 41*(12), 913–958. https://doi.org/10.2165/00003088-200241120-00002.

Dumont, C., Mentre, F., Gaynor, C., Brendel, K., Gesson, C., & Chenel, M. (2013). Optimal sampling times for a drug and its metabolite using SIMCYP((R)) simulations as prior information. *Clinical Pharmacokinetics, 52*(1), 43–57. https://doi.org/10.1007/s40262-012-0022-9.

Edelbroek, P. M., van der Heijden, J., & Stolk, L. M. (2009). Dried blood spot methods in therapeutic drug monitoring: Methods, assays, and pitfalls. *Therapeutic Drug Monitoring, 31*(3), 327–336. https://doi.org/10.1097/FTD.0b013e31819e91ce.

Emoto, C., & Fukuda, T. (2018). Physiologically-based pharmacokinetic (PBPK)-pharmacodynamic (PD) model of acetaminophen: Development and its potential clinical applications. *The Japanese Journal of Developmental Pharmacology and Therapeutics, 31*(1), 14–21.

Faure, C., Michaud, L., Shaghaghi, E. K., Popon, M., Turck, D., Navarro, J., et al. (2001). Intravenous omeprazole in children: Pharmacokinetics and effect on 24-hour intragastric pH. *Journal of Pediatric Gastroenterology and Nutrition, 33*(2), 144–148. https://doi.org/10.1097/00005176-200108000-00009.

George, J., Liddle, C., Murray, M., Byth, K., & Farrell, G. C. (1995). Pre-translational regulation of cytochrome P450 genes is responsible for disease-specific changes of individual P450 enzymes among patients with cirrhosis. *Biochemical Pharmacology, 49*(7), 873–881. https://doi.org/10.1016/0006-2952(94)00515-n.

Goho, C. (2001). Oral midazolam-grapefruit juice drug interaction. *Pediatric Dentistry, 23*(4), 365–366. Retrieved from https://www.ncbi.nlm.nih.gov/pubmed/11572503.

Gonzalez, D., Melloni, C., Yogev, R., Poindexter, B. B., Mendley, S. R., Delmore, P., et al. (2014). Use of opportunistic clinical data and a population pharmacokinetic model to support dosing of clindamycin for premature infants to adolescents. *Clinical Pharmacology and Therapeutics*, *96*(4), 429–437. https://doi.org/10.1038/clpt.2014.134.

Gonzalez, D., & Sinha, J. (2021). Pediatric drug-drug interaction evaluation: Drug, patient population, and methodological considerations. *Journal of Clinical Pharmacology*, *61*(Suppl. 1), S175–S187. https://doi.org/10.1002/jcph.1881.

Grimstein, M., Yang, Y., Zhang, X., Grillo, J., Huang, S. M., Zineh, I., et al. (2019). Physiologically based pharmacokinetic modeling in regulatory science: An update from the U.S. Food and Drug Administration's Office of Clinical Pharmacology. *Journal of Pharmaceutical Sciences*, *108*(1), 21–25. https://doi.org/10.1016/j.xphs.2018.10.033.

Hakkola, J., Pasanen, M., Purkunen, R., Saarikoski, S., Pelkonen, O., Maenpaa, J., et al. (1994). Expression of xenobiotic-metabolizing cytochrome P450 forms in human adult and fetal liver. *Biochemical Pharmacology*, *48*(1), 59–64. https://doi.org/10.1016/0006-2952(94)90223-2.

Hines, R. N. (2007). Ontogeny of human hepatic cytochromes P450. *Journal of Biochemical and Molecular Toxicology*, *21*(4), 169–175. https://doi.org/10.1002/jbt.20179.

Hines, R. N. (2013). Developmental expression of drug metabolizing enzymes: Impact on disposition in neonates and young children. *International Journal of Pharmaceutics*, *452*(1–2), 3–7. https://doi.org/10.1016/j.ijpharm.2012.05.079.

Hines, R. N., & McCarver, D. G. (2002). The ontogeny of human drug-metabolizing enzymes: Phase I oxidative enzymes. *The Journal of Pharmacology and Experimental Therapeutics*, *300*(2), 355–360. https://doi.org/10.1124/jpet.300.2.355.

Hines, R. N., Sargent, D., Autrup, H., Birnbaum, L. S., Brent, R. L., Doerrer, N. G., et al. (2010). Approaches for assessing risks to sensitive populations: Lessons learned from evaluating risks in the pediatric population. *Toxicological Sciences*, *113*(1), 4–26. https://doi.org/10.1093/toxsci/kfp217.

Huang, S. M., Abernethy, D. R., Wang, Y., Zhao, P., & Zineh, I. (2013). The utility of modeling and simulation in drug development and regulatory review. *Journal of Pharmaceutical Sciences*, *102*(9), 2912–2923. https://doi.org/10.1002/jps.23570.

Ishizaki, T., & Horai, Y. (1999). Review article: Cytochrome P450 and the metabolism of proton pump inhibitors—Emphasis on rabeprazole. *Alimentary Pharmacology & Therapeutics*, *13*(Suppl. 3), 27–36. https://doi.org/10.1046/j.1365-2036.1999.00022.x.

Johnson, T. N. (2008). The problems in scaling adult drug doses to children. *Archives of Disease in Childhood*, *93*(3), 207–211. https://doi.org/10.1136/adc.2006.114835.

Johnson, T. N., Boussery, K., Rowland-Yeo, K., Tucker, G. T., & Rostami-Hodjegan, A. (2010). A semi-mechanistic model to predict the effects of liver cirrhosis on drug clearance. *Clinical Pharmacokinetics*, *49*(3), 189–206. https://doi.org/10.2165/11318160-000000000-00000.

Johnson, T. N., & Ke, A. B. (2021). Physiologically based pharmacokinetic modeling and allometric scaling in pediatric drug development: Where do we draw the line? *Journal of Clinical Pharmacology*, *61*(Suppl. 1), S83–S93. https://doi.org/10.1002/jcph.1834.

Johnson, T. N., & Rostami-Hodjegan, A. (2011). Resurgence in the use of physiologically based pharmacokinetic models in pediatric clinical pharmacology: Parallel shift in incorporating the knowledge of biological elements and increased applicability to drug development and clinical practice. *Paediatric Anaesthesia*, *21*(3), 291–301. https://doi.org/10.1111/j.1460-9592.2010.03323.x.

Johnson, T. N., Rostami-Hodjegan, A., & Tucker, G. T. (2006). Prediction of the clearance of eleven drugs and associated variability in neonates, infants and children. *Clinical Pharmacokinetics*, *45*(9), 931–956. https://doi.org/10.2165/00003088-200645090-00005.

Johnson, T. N., Tanner, M. S., Taylor, C. J., & Tucker, G. T. (2001). Enterocytic CYP3A4 in a paediatric population: Developmental changes and the effect of coeliac disease and cystic fibrosis. *British Journal of Clinical Pharmacology*, *51*(5), 451–460. https://doi.org/10.1046/j.1365-2125.2001.01370.x.

Johnson, T. N., Tucker, G. T., & Rostami-Hodjegan, A. (2008). Development of CYP2D6 and CYP3A4 in the first year of life. *Clinical Pharmacology and Therapeutics*, *83*(5), 670–671. https://doi.org/10.1038/sj.clpt.6100327.

Johnsrud, E. K., Koukouritaki, S. B., Divakaran, K., Brunengraber, L. L., Hines, R. N., & McCarver, D. G. (2003). Human hepatic CYP2E1 expression during development. *The Journal of Pharmacology and Experimental Therapeutics*, *307*(1), 402–407. https://doi.org/10.1124/jpet.102.053124.

Kearns, G. L., Andersson, T., James, L. P., Gaedigk, A., Kraynak, R. A., Abdel-Rahman, S. M., et al. (2003). Omeprazole disposition in children following single-dose administration. *Journal of Clinical Pharmacology*, *43*(8), 840–848. https://doi.org/10.1177/0091270003256122.

Kiss, M., Mbasu, R., Nicolai, J., Barnouin, K., Kotian, A., Mooij, M. G., et al. (2021). Ontogeny of small intestinal drug transporters and metabolizing enzymes based on targeted quantitative proteomics. *Drug Metabolism and Disposition*, *49*(12), 1038–1046. https://doi.org/10.1124/dmd.121.000559.

Knebel, W., Tammara, B., Udata, C., Comer, G., Gastonguay, M. R., & Meng, X. (2011). Population pharmacokinetic modeling of pantoprazole in pediatric patients from birth to 16 years. *Journal of Clinical Pharmacology*, *51*(3), 333–345. https://doi.org/10.1177/0091270010366146.

Komori, M., Nishio, K., Kitada, M., Shiramatsu, K., Muroya, K., Soma, M., et al. (1990). Fetus-specific expression of a form of cytochrome P-450 in human livers. *Biochemistry*, *29*(18), 4430–4433. https://doi.org/10.1021/bi00470a024.

Koukouritaki, S. B., Manro, J. R., Marsh, S. A., Stevens, J. C., Rettie, A. E., McCarver, D. G., et al. (2004). Developmental expression of human hepatic CYP2C9 and CYP2C19. *The Journal of Pharmacology and Experimental Therapeutics*, *308*(3), 965–974. https://doi.org/10.1124/jpet.103.060137.

Kraemer, M. J., Furukawa, C. T., Koup, J. R., Shapiro, G. G., Pierson, W. E., & Bierman, C. W. (1982). Altered theophylline clearance during an influenza B outbreak. *Pediatrics*, *69*(4), 476–480. Retrieved from https://www.ncbi.nlm.nih.gov/pubmed/7070895.

Krishna, D. R., & Klotz, U. (1994). Extrahepatic metabolism of drugs in humans. *Clinical Pharmacokinetics*, *26*(2), 144–160. https://doi.org/10.2165/00003088-199426020-00007.

Lacroix, D., Sonnier, M., Moncion, A., Cheron, G., & Cresteil, T. (1997). Expression of CYP3A in the human liver—Evidence that the shift between CYP3A7 and CYP3A4 occurs immediately after birth. *European Journal of Biochemistry*, *247*(2), 625–634. https://doi.org/10.1111/j.1432-1033.1997.00625.x.

Lang, T., Klein, K., Fischer, J., Nussler, A. K., Neuhaus, P., Hofmann, U., et al. (2001). Extensive genetic polymorphism in the human CYP2B6 gene with impact on expression and function in human liver. *Pharmacogenetics*, *11*(5), 399–415. https://doi.org/10.1097/00008571-200107000-00004.

Lang, J., Vincent, L., Chenel, M., Ogungbenro, K., & Galetin, A. (2021). Impact of hepatic CYP3A4 ontogeny functions on drug-drug interaction risk in pediatric physiologically-based pharmacokinetic/pharmacodynamic modeling: Critical literature review and ivabradine case study. *Clinical Pharmacology and Therapeutics*, *109*(6), 1618–1630. https://doi.org/10.1002/cpt.2134.

Laughon, M. M., Benjamin, D. K., Jr., Capparelli, E. V., Kearns, G. L., Berezny, K., Paul, I. M., et al. (2011). Innovative clinical trial design for pediatric therapeutics. *Expert Review of Clinical Pharmacology*, *4*(5), 643–652. https://doi.org/10.1586/ecp.11.43.

Leeder, J. S., Kearns, G. L., Spielberg, S. P., & van den Anker, J. (2010). Understanding the relative roles of pharmacogenetics and ontogeny in pediatric drug development and regulatory science. *Journal of Clinical Pharmacology*, *50*(12), 1377–1387. https://doi.org/10.1177/0091270009360533.

Leong, R., Vieira, M. L., Zhao, P., Mulugeta, Y., Lee, C. S., Huang, S. M., et al. (2012). Regulatory experience with physiologically based pharmacokinetic modeling for pediatric drug trials. *Clinical Pharmacology and Therapeutics*, *91*(5), 926–931. https://doi.org/10.1038/clpt.2012.19.

Lima, J. J., Thomas, C. D., Barbarino, J., Desta, Z., Van Driest, S. L., El Rouby, N., et al. (2021). Clinical pharmacogenetics implementation consortium (CPIC) guideline for CYP2C19 and proton pump inhibitor dosing. *Clinical Pharmacology and Therapeutics*, *109*(6), 1417–1423. https://doi.org/10.1002/cpt.2015.

Lindh, J. D., Holm, L., Andersson, M. L., & Rane, A. (2009). Influence of CYP2C9 genotype on warfarin dose requirements—A systematic review and meta-analysis. *European Journal of Clinical Pharmacology*, *65*(4), 365–375. https://doi.org/10.1007/s00228-008-0584-5.

Lopez-Flores, L. A., Perez-Rubio, G., & Falfan-Valencia, R. (2017). Distribution of polymorphic variants of CYP2A6 and their involvement in nicotine addiction. *EXCLI Journal*, *16*, 174–196. https://doi.org/10.17179/excli2016-847.

Maenpaa, J., Rane, A., Raunio, H., Honkakoski, P., & Pelkonen, O. (1993). Cytochrome P450 isoforms in human fetal tissues related to phenobarbital-inducible forms in the mouse. *Biochemical Pharmacology*, *45*(4), 899–907. https://doi.org/10.1016/0006-2952(93)90175-v.

Morgan, E. T. (2009). Impact of infectious and inflammatory disease on cytochrome P450-mediated drug metabolism and pharmacokinetics. *Clinical Pharmacology and Therapeutics*, *85*(4), 434–438. https://doi.org/10.1038/clpt.2008.302.

Murray, G. I., Foster, C. O., Barnes, T. S., Weaver, R. J., Snyder, C. P., Ewen, S. W., et al. (1992). Cytochrome P450IA expression in adult and fetal human liver. *Carcinogenesis*, *13*(2), 165–169. https://doi.org/10.1093/carcin/13.2.165.

Nagata, T., Takahashi, Y., Ishii, Y., Asai, S., Sugahara, M., Nishida, Y., et al. (2003). Profiling of genes differentially expressed between fetal liver and postnatal liver using high-density oligonucleotide DNA array. *International Journal of Molecular Medicine*, *11*(6), 713–721. Retrieved from https://www.ncbi.nlm.nih.gov/pubmed/12736711.

Naraharisetti, S. B., Lin, Y. S., Rieder, M. J., Marciante, K. D., Psaty, B. M., Thummel, K. E., et al. (2010). Human liver expression of CYP2C8: Gender, age, and genotype effects. *Drug Metabolism and Disposition*, *38*(6), 889–893. https://doi.org/10.1124/dmd.109.031542.

Nelson, D. R., Koymans, L., Kamataki, T., Stegeman, J. J., Feyereisen, R., Waxman, D. J., et al. (1996). P450 superfamily: Update on new sequences, gene mapping, accession numbers and nomenclature. *Pharmacogenetics*, *6*(1), 1–42. https://doi.org/10.1097/00008571-199602000-00002.

Oesterheld, J. R. (1998). A review of developmental aspects of cytochrome P450. *Journal of Child and Adolescent Psychopharmacology*, *8*(3), 161–174. https://doi.org/10.1089/cap.1998.8.161.

Omiecinski, C. J., Redlich, C. A., & Costa, P. (1990). Induction and developmental expression of cytochrome P450IA1 messenger RNA in rat and human tissues: Detection by the polymerase chain reaction. *Cancer Research*, *50*(14), 4315–4321. Retrieved from https://www.ncbi.nlm.nih.gov/pubmed/1694720.

Paine, M. F., Hart, H. L., Ludington, S. S., Haining, R. L., Rettie, A. E., & Zeldin, D. C. (2006). The human intestinal cytochrome P450 "pie". *Drug Metabolism and Disposition*, *34*(5), 880–886. https://doi.org/10.1124/dmd.105.008672.

Pearce, R. E., Gaedigk, R., Twist, G. P., Dai, H., Riffel, A. K., Leeder, J. S., et al. (2016). Developmental expression of CYP2B6: A comprehensive analysis of mRNA expression, protein content and bupropion hydroxylase activity and the impact of genetic variation. *Drug Metabolism and Disposition*, *44*(7), 948–958. https://doi.org/10.1124/dmd.115.067546.

Polasek, T. M., & Rostami-Hodjegan, A. (2020). Virtual twins: Understanding the data required for model-informed precision dosing. *Clinical Pharmacology and Therapeutics*, *107*(4), 742–745. https://doi.org/10.1002/cpt.1778.

Polasek, T. M., Tucker, G. T., Sorich, M. J., Wiese, M. D., Mohan, T., Rostami-Hodjegan, A., et al. (2018). Prediction of olanzapine exposure in individual patients using physiologically based pharmacokinetic modelling and simulation. *British Journal of Clinical Pharmacology*, *84*(3), 462–476. https://doi.org/10.1111/bcp.13480.

Rodriguez-Antona, C., Niemi, M., Backman, J. T., Kajosaari, L. I., Neuvonen, P. J., Robledo, M., et al. (2008). Characterization of novel CYP2C8 haplotypes and their contribution to paclitaxel and repaglinide metabolism. *The Pharmacogenomics Journal*, *8*(4), 268–277. https://doi.org/10.1038/sj.tpj.6500482.

Saitoh, A., Fletcher, C. V., Brundage, R., Alvero, C., Fenton, T., Hsia, K., et al. (2007). Efavirenz pharmacokinetics in HIV-1-infected children are associated with CYP2B6-G516T polymorphism. *Journal of Acquired Immune Deficiency Syndromes*, *45*(3), 280–285. https://doi.org/10.1097/QAI.0b013e318040b29e.

Salem, F., Abduljalil, K., Kamiyama, Y., & Rostami-Hodjegan, A. (2016). Considering age variation when coining drugs as high versus low hepatic extraction ratio. *Drug Metabolism and Disposition*, *44*(7), 1099–1102. https://doi.org/10.1124/dmd.115.067595.

Salem, A. H., Fletcher, C. V., & Brundage, R. C. (2014). Pharmacometric characterization of efavirenz developmental pharmacokinetics and pharmacogenetics in HIV-infected children. *Antimicrobial Agents and Chemotherapy*, *58*(1), 136–143. https://doi.org/10.1128/AAC.01738-13.

Salem, F., Johnson, T. N., Abduljalil, K., Tucker, G. T., & Rostami-Hodjegan, A. (2014). A re-evaluation and validation of ontogeny functions for cytochrome P450 1A2 and 3A4 based on in vivo data. *Clinical Pharmacokinetics*, *53*(7), 625–636. https://doi.org/10.1007/s40262-014-0140-7.

Salem, F., Johnson, T. N., Abduljalil, K., Tucker, G. T., & Rostami-Hodjegan, A. (2015). Erratum to: A re-evaluation and validation of ontogeny functions for cytochrome P450 1A2 and 3A4 based on in vivo data. *Clinical Pharmacokinetics*, *54*(6), 671. https://doi.org/10.1007/s40262-015-0284-0.

Salem, F., Johnson, T. N., Barter, Z. E., Leeder, J. S., & Rostami-Hodjegan, A. (2013). Age related changes in fractional elimination pathways for drugs: Assessing the impact of variable ontogeny on metabolic drug-drug interactions. *Journal of Clinical Pharmacology*, *53*(8), 857–865. https://doi.org/10.1002/jcph.100.

Saravanakumar, A., Sadighi, A., Ryu, R., & Akhlaghi, F. (2019). Physicochemical properties, biotransformation, and transport pathways of established and newly approved medications: A systematic review of the top 200 most prescribed drugs vs. the FDA-approved drugs between 2005 and 2016. *Clinical Pharmacokinetics*, *58*(10), 1281–1294. https://doi.org/10.1007/s40262-019-00750-8.

Song, G., Sun, X., Hines, R. N., McCarver, D. G., Lake, B. G., Osimitz, T. G., et al. (2017). Determination of human hepatic CYP2C8 and CYP1A2 age-dependent expression to support human health risk assessment for early ages. *Drug Metabolism and Disposition*, *45*(5), 468–475. https://doi.org/10.1124/dmd.116.074583.

Sonnier, M., & Cresteil, T. (1998). Delayed ontogenesis of CYP1A2 in the human liver. *European Journal of Biochemistry*, *251*(3), 893–898. https://doi.org/10.1046/j.1432-1327.1998.2510893.x.

Stevens, J. C., Hines, R. N., Gu, C., Koukouritaki, S. B., Manro, J. R., Tandler, P. J., et al. (2003). Developmental expression of the major human hepatic CYP3A enzymes. *The Journal of Pharmacology and Experimental Therapeutics*, *307*(2), 573–582. https://doi.org/10.1124/jpet.103.054841.

Stevens, J. C., Marsh, S. A., Zaya, M. J., Regina, K. J., Divakaran, K., Le, M., et al. (2008). Developmental changes in human liver CYP2D6 expression. *Drug Metabolism and Disposition*, *36*(8), 1587–1593. https://doi.org/10.1124/dmd.108.021873.

Takahashi, H., Ishikawa, S., Nomoto, S., Nishigaki, Y., Ando, F., Kashima, T., et al. (2000). Developmental changes in pharmacokinetics and pharmacodynamics of warfarin enantiomers in Japanese children. *Clinical Pharmacology and Therapeutics*, *68*(5), 541–555. https://doi.org/10.1067/mcp.2000.110977.

Tateishi, T., Nakura, H., Asoh, M., Watanabe, M., Tanaka, M., Kumai, T., et al. (1997). A comparison of hepatic cytochrome P450 protein expression between infancy and postinfancy. *Life Sciences*, *61*(26), 2567–2574. https://doi.org/10.1016/s0024-3205(97)01011-4.

Timchalk, C., Kousba, A. A., & Poet, T. S. (2007). An age-dependent physiologically based pharmacokinetic/pharmacodynamic model for the organophosphorus insecticide chlorpyrifos in the preweanling rat. *Toxicological Sciences*, *98*(2), 348–365. https://doi.org/10.1093/toxsci/kfm119.

Tod, M., Jullien, V., & Pons, G. (2008). Facilitation of drug evaluation in children by population methods and modelling. *Clinical Pharmacokinetics*, *47*(4), 231–243. https://doi.org/10.2165/00003088-200847040-00002.

Treluyer, J. M., Jacqz-Aigrain, E., Alvarez, F., & Cresteil, T. (1991). Expression of CYP2D6 in developing human liver. *European Journal of Biochemistry*, *202*(2), 583–588. https://doi.org/10.1111/j.1432-1033.1991.tb16411.x.

Upreti, V. V., & Wahlstrom, J. L. (2016). Meta-analysis of hepatic cytochrome P450 ontogeny to underwrite the prediction of pediatric pharmacokinetics using physiologically based pharmacokinetic modeling. *Journal of Clinical Pharmacology*, *56*(3), 266–283. https://doi.org/10.1002/jcph.585.

van Groen, B. D., Nicolai, J., Kuik, A. C., Van Cruchten, S., van Peer, E., Smits, A., et al. (2021). Ontogeny of hepatic transporters and drug-metabolizing enzymes in humans and in nonclinical species. *Pharmacological Reviews*, *73*(2), 597–678. https://doi.org/10.1124/pharmrev.120.000071.

Vieira, I., Sonnier, M., & Cresteil, T. (1996). Developmental expression of CYP2E1 in the human liver. Hypermethylation control of gene expression during the neonatal period. *European Journal of Biochemistry*, *238*(2), 476–483. https://doi.org/10.1111/j.1432-1033.1996.0476z.x.

Vinks, A. A., Emoto, C., & Fukuda, T. (2015). Modeling and simulation in pediatric drug therapy: Application of pharmacometrics to define the right dose for children. *Clinical Pharmacology and Therapeutics*, *98*(3), 298–308. https://doi.org/10.1002/cpt.169.

Vyhlidal, C. A., Chapron, B. D., Ahmed, A., Singh, V., Casini, R., & Shakhnovich, V. (2021). Effect of Crohn's disease on villous length and CYP3A4 expression in the pediatric small intestine. *Clinical and Translational Science*, *14*(2), 729–736. https://doi.org/10.1111/cts.12938.

Ward, B. A., Gorski, J. C., Jones, D. R., Hall, S. D., Flockhart, D. A., & Desta, Z. (2003). The cytochrome P450 2B6 (CYP2B6) is the main catalyst of efavirenz primary and secondary metabolism: Implication for HIV/AIDS therapy and utility of efavirenz as a substrate marker of CYP2B6 catalytic activity. *The Journal of Pharmacology and Experimental Therapeutics*, *306*(1), 287–300. https://doi.org/10.1124/jpet.103.049601.

Ward, R. M., & Kearns, G. L. (2013). Proton pump inhibitors in pediatrics: Mechanism of action, pharmacokinetics, pharmacogenetics, and pharmacodynamics. *Paediatric Drugs*, *15*(2), 119–131. https://doi.org/10.1007/s40272-013-0012-x.

Wienkers, L. C., & Heath, T. G. (2005). Predicting in vivo drug interactions from in vitro drug discovery data. *Nature Reviews. Drug Discovery*, *4*(10), 825–833. https://doi.org/10.1038/nrd1851.

Williams, J. A., Hyland, R., Jones, B. C., Smith, D. A., Hurst, S., Goosen, T. C., et al. (2004). Drug-drug interactions for UDP-glucuronosyltransferase substrates: A pharmacokinetic explanation for typically observed low exposure (AUCi/AUC) ratios. *Drug Metabolism and Disposition*, *32*(11), 1201–1208. https://doi.org/10.1124/dmd.104.000794.

Williams, J. A., Ring, B. J., Cantrell, V. E., Jones, D. R., Eckstein, J., Ruterbories, K., et al. (2002). Comparative metabolic capabilities of CYP3A4, CYP3A5, and CYP3A7. *Drug Metabolism and Disposition, 30*(8), 883–891. https://doi.org/10.1124/dmd.30.8.883.

Wynalda, M. A., Hutzler, J. M., Koets, M. D., Podoll, T., & Wienkers, L. C. (2003). In vitro metabolism of clindamycin in human liver and intestinal microsomes. *Drug Metabolism and Disposition, 31*(7), 878–887. https://doi.org/10.1124/dmd.31.7.878.

Yang, H. Y., Namkung, M. J., & Juchau, M. R. (1995). Expression of functional cytochrome P4501A1 in human embryonic hepatic tissues during organogenesis. *Biochemical Pharmacology, 49*(5), 717–726. https://doi.org/10.1016/0006-2952(94)00493-6.

Yoon, S., Yi, S., Rhee, S. J., Lee, H. A., Kim, Y., Yu, K. S., et al. (2019). Development of a physiologically-based pharmacokinetic model for cyclosporine in Asian children with renal impairment. *Translational and Clinical Pharmacology, 27*(3), 107–114. https://doi.org/10.12793/tcp.2019.27.3.107.

Zanger, U. M., Klein, K., Thomas, M., Rieger, J. K., Tremmel, R., Kandel, B. A., et al. (2014). Genetics, epigenetics, and regulation of drug-metabolizing cytochrome p450 enzymes. *Clinical Pharmacology and Therapeutics, 95*(3), 258–261. https://doi.org/10.1038/clpt.2013.220.

Zevin, S., & Benowitz, N. L. (1999). Drug interactions with tobacco smoking. An update. *Clinical Pharmacokinetics, 36*(6), 425–438. https://doi.org/10.2165/00003088-199936060-00004.

Zhang, X., Yang, Y., Grimstein, M., Fan, J., Grillo, J. A., Huang, S. M., et al. (2020). Application of PBPK modeling and simulation for regulatory decision making and its impact on US prescribing information: An update on the 2018-2019 submissions to the US FDA's Office of Clinical Pharmacology. *Journal of Clinical Pharmacology, 60*(Suppl. 1), S160–S178. https://doi.org/10.1002/jcph.1767.

Zuppa, A. F., Hammer, G. B., Barrett, J. S., Kenney, B. F., Kassir, N., Mouksassi, S., et al. (2011). Safety and population pharmacokinetic analysis of intravenous acetaminophen in neonates, infants, children, and adolescents with pain or fever. *Journal of Pediatric Pharmacology and Therapeutics, 16*(4), 246–261. https://doi.org/10.5863/1551-6776-16.4.246.

CHAPTER THIRTEEN

Cytochrome P450 polymorphism: From evolution to clinical use

Magnus Ingelman-Sundberg*
Department of Physiology and Pharmacology, Section of Pharmacogenetics, Karolinska Institute, Stockholm, Sweden
*Corresponding author: e-mail address: magnus.ingelman-sundberg@ki.se

Contents

Abstract

The cytochromes P450s can be divided in two groups, those of high importance for endogenous functions being evolutionary quite stable and those participating in detoxification of drugs and other xenobiotics having less important endogenous functions. In the latter group extensive genetic diversity has been allowed and in addition this is of high importance for survival in different environments. The genetic polymorphisms in these genes have evolved to some extent based on dietary restrictions and environmental factors and have not been subject of conservation due to less importance for survival. In cases of high dietary selection events, gene multiplication and

Advances in Pharmacology, Volume 95
ISSN 1054-3589
https://doi.org/10.1016/bs.apha.2022.04.004

amplification events have been seen. The different variants in genes encoding drug metabolizing enzymes can be used as genetic biomarkers (pharmacogenomic labels) for adjustment of drug treatment leading to less adverse drug reactions and better response. Indeed, this has improved the use of personalized medicine, although the missing heredity seen based on twin studies indicates that there are indeed many more genetic variants to be discovered before one can achieve a satisfactory relationship between genotype and phenotype with respect to drug metabolism and toxicity.

Abbreviations

ADME absorption distribution metabolism excretion
CNV copy number variation
CPIC Clinical Pharmacogenetics Implementation Consortium
CYP cytochrome P450
DPWG Dutch Pharmacogenetics Working Group
EMA European Medicines Agency
ExAC Exome Aggregation Consortium
FDA U.S. Food and Drug Administration
GWAS genome-wide association study
NFIB Nuclear Factor 1B
NGS next generation sequencing
P450 cytochrome P450
SNP single nucleotide polymorphism
WES whole exon sequencing

1. Introduction

The origin of the P450 superfamily lies in prokaryotes about 3 billion years ago, before the advent of eukaryotes and before molecular oxygen in the atmosphere (Werck-Reichhart & Feyereisen, 2000). Thus cytochrome P450s (P450s) were early present in bacteria and probably also in algae, the oldest green seaweed on record, the ancestor of all land plants, lived about 1 billion years ago, https://www.livescience.com/oldest-green-algae-discovered.html

Life on Earth is dependent on photosynthesizing plants and algae for food, yet land plants did not evolve until about 450 million years ago, whereas the oldest algae developed about 1 billion years ago. The first cytochrome P450 gene might have arisen as much as three and a half billion years ago (Loomis, 1988). It has been suggested that one and a half billion years ago, the first families of cytochrome P450s were formed, mainly involved in the metabolism of fatty acids, cholesterol and their derivatives (e.g., CYP11 and CYP4 families). Animals living in the sea became terrestrial about 450 million years ago. The earliest known terrestrial animals were arthropods (Little, 1983) members of the Myriapoda (millipedes, centipedes), Arachnida (spiders, scorpions, and relatives), and Hexapoda (insects and three smaller, primitively wingless groups). https://evolution-outreach.biomedcentral.com/articles/10.1007/s12052-011-0357-y. During this period the P450 genes were subject to repeated rounds of expansion by gene and genome duplication and conversions well as sequence alterations. The *CYP1A2* gene may arise via duplication of CYP1A1 about 350 million years ago during the evolution of mammals and birds, based on the phylogenetic analysis of CYP1A genes (Morrison, Oleksiak, Cornell, Sogin, & Stegeman, 1995) It is also likely that there was a high selection pressure for this of dietary origin, with plant toxins probably playing a major role (Ingelman-Sundberg, Oscarson, & McLellan, 1999). As of 2018, more than 300,000 distinct CYP proteins are known Nelson (2018) found in all kingdoms of life: animals, plants, fungi, protists, bacteria, and archaea (Danielson (2002).

In this chapter it is described how different P450 genes have been changed during evolution and how selection of some of the of P450 gene variants have been attributed to environmental and dietary factors. The polymorphic nature of the P450 genes has been a great advantage in the adaptation of different animals and humans to various diets and environments. However, the polymorphism of certain important genes encoding drug metabolizing P450 enzymes now constitutes a problem for efficient drug treatment of human populations due to the altered pharmacokinetics between different individuals based on the accommodation of specific gene variants.

2. Selection of CYP gene variants in relation to environmental and dietary factors

Adoption of the CYP-genes to diet and environment has involved modifications in the regulatory region, selection of variants carrying specific amino acid substitutions and gene duplication. A similar situation has occurred in insects where dietary adaptation of *Drosophila mettleri* to the isoquinoline alkaloids secreted by the *Senita cactus* is caused by extensive induction of CYP28 and CYP6 as a response to these compounds (Danielson, MacIntyre, & Fogleman, 1997). By contrast, *Drosophila melanogaster* does not survive in this environment because of the lack of CYP-mediated dietary adaptation (Frank & Fogleman, 1992). Furthermore, CYP6G1 is linked to insecticide resistance in DDT-resistant *Drosophila melanogaster* (McCart &

Ffrench-Constant, 2008) and CYP6M2 in the mosquito malaria vector *Anopheles gambiae* is capable of directly metabolizing pyrethroids (Ismail et al., 2013). In insecticide resistant Drosophila strains a transposome (Accord) is inserted, which most probably causes up to 100-fold higher gene expression of Cyp6g1, (Daborn et al., 2002). Also, selection for specific mutations in *Cyp6a2* has caused resistance to DDT since the R335S, L336V and V476L mutations cause changes the CYP6A2 enzyme from being inactive to active in the metabolism of DDT (Amichot et al., 2004).

An interesting selection has been seen in *Myzus persicae*. This insect originally living on potato plants have during evolution shifted host to be harboring on the tobacco plant thus exposed to toxic nicotine. As a response of this host shift the insect has genetically adapted by overexpression of the nicotine metabolizing CYP6CY3 by expansion of a dinucleotide microsatellite in the promoter region and a recent up to 100-fold gene amplification (Fig. 1). This indicates that gene amplification and microsatellite polymorphism are evolutionary drivers in insect host adaptation. From (Bass et al., 2013).

The information given then accentuate the relationship between active CYP genes and the environment. If one compares the evolution of *CYP2D* genes between mice and humans (Fig. 2) where 75 million years ago both species carried 4 active genes in this locus, but when during evolution 2 genes in the human *CYP2D* locus were inactivated and one became polymorphic (*CYP2D6*), whereas in mice 9 genes developed, all active. Since the CYP2D enzymes are very active in the metabolism of plant toxins like different alkaloids, one could interpret this as a need for the mice for a high detoxification potential for survival, whereas dietary regimens among humans have been transferred intellectually between generations making this aspect of less importance.

3. Genetic selection in humans

Alleles containing multiple CYP gene copies have been formed, indicating that the population recently has been exposed to a selection pressure, probably of dietary origin. According to Clark (1994), gene duplication can invade only if it provides a direct advantage to the organism. One example of CYP gene duplication is in Ethiopia, where alleles carrying 1, 2, 3, 4 and 5 active *CYP2D6* genes have been identified (Aklillu et al., 1996). There is evidence for a dietary selection here and dietary adaptation by means of induction has not been possible because CYP2D6 is a non-inducible enzyme. It is likely

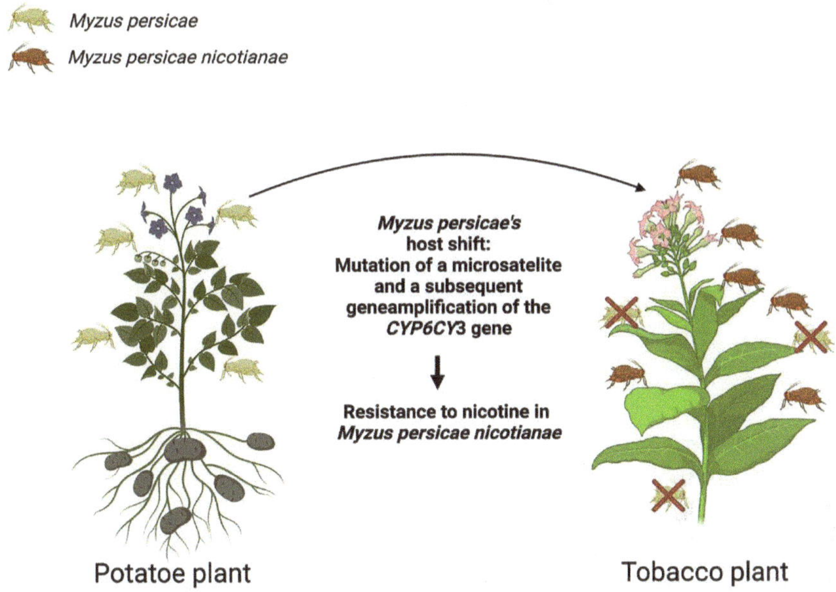

Fig. 1 Dietary stress induced *CYP6CY3* gene amplification in *Myzus persicae's* following shift in host from the potato plant to the tobacco plant. The host shift of *Myzus persicae* to the tobacco plant harboring the toxic nicotine causes an adaptation of the insect which results in overexpression of the nicotine metabolizing CYP6CY3 results from the expansion of a dinucleotide microsatellite in the promoter region and a recent gene amplification, with some aphid clones carrying up to 100 copies. The data indicate that gene amplification and microsatellite polymorphism are evolutionary drivers in insect host adaptation. *From Bass, C., Zimmer, C.T., Riveron, J.M., Wilding, C.S., Wondji, C.S., Kaussmann, M., et al., (2013) Gene amplification and microsatellite polymorphism underlie a recent insect host shift.* Proceedings of the National Academy of Sciences of the United States of America 110, *19460–5. Figure created with BioRender.com.*

that alkaloids, which display a nanomolar affinity for CYP2D6 (Fonne-Pfister and Meyer (1988), have exerted this pressure and that survival has, in part, been based on adaptation to dietary compounds. Thus, this adaptation has instead occurred through recombination events creating alleles with multiple gene copies and selection of individuals carrying duplicated or multiduplicated *CYP2D6* genes over those carrying alleles with deleted or inactive genes. This *CYP2D6* gene duplication has after this selection about 10,000–5000 years ago migrated to other parts of the globe as illustrated in Fig. 3. The *CYP2D6* gene duplications worldwide are then mostly originated from duplication of *CYP2D6*2B*, whereas some contributions have been found from Micronesia where a similar duplication event occurred, but then encompassing the *CYP2D6*1* allele (Ingelman-Sundberg, 2005).

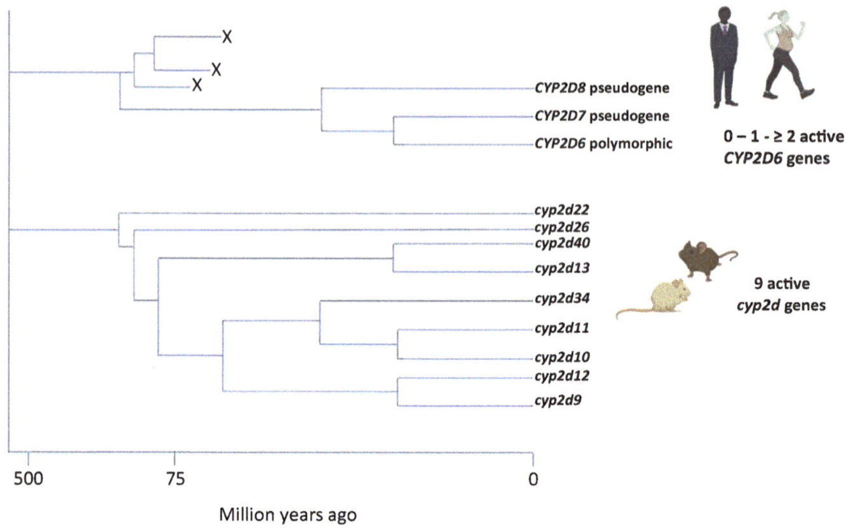

Fig. 2 Parallel evolution in the *CYP2D* locus in humans (top) and mice. Four active *CYP2D* genes were present about 75 million years ago but subsequent evolution included full inactivation of two genes and partial inactivation in one gene in humans, whereas in mice the evolution resulted in 9 active *Cyp2d* genes, forming a much higher protections of toxic alkaloids in plants in mice than in humans. *From Nelson, D.R., Zeldin, D.C., Hoffman, S.M.G., Maltais, L.J., Wain, H.M., Nebert, DW. (2004) Comparison of cytochrome P450 (CYP) genes from the mouse and human genomes, including nomenclature recommendations for genes, pseudogenes, and alternative-splice variants.* Pharmacogenetics, 14, *1–18. and Ingelman-Sundberg, M. (2005) Genetic polymorphisms of cytochrome P450 2D6 (CYP2D6): Clinical consequences, evolutionary aspects and functional diversity.* The Pharmacogenomics Journal, 5, *6–13. Figure partly created with BioRender.com*

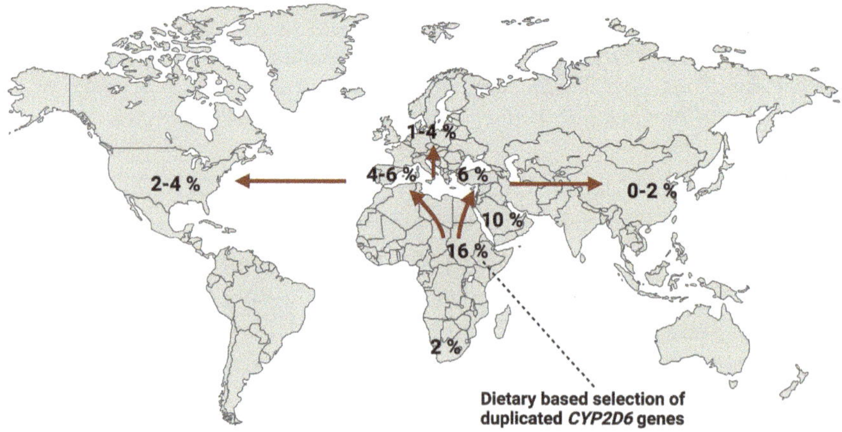

Fig. 3 Global distribution of duplicated *CYP2D6* alleles. Duplicated active *CYP2D6**2* alleles have been found at a high frequency in North East Africa. In Ethiopia alleles carrying 1, 2, 3, 4 and 5 active *CYP2D6* genes have been identified (Aklillu et al., 2002). These have been proposed to have been formed caused by dietary selection because of severe starvation periods in Ethiopia causing extensive death in the population would favor subjects carrying a higher number of active *CYP2D6* allele being able to detoxify alkaloids in plants at a higher extent thereby extending the number of plants useful as diet. *Figure created with BioRender.com.*

Mechanistically it appears that alleles with duplicated or multi-duplicated *CYP2D6* genes have occurred through unequal crossover at a specific breakpoint in the 3′-flanking region of the *CYP2D6*2B* allele with a specific repetitive sequence (Lundqvist, Johansson, & Ingelman-Sundberg, 1999). By contrast, alleles with 13 copies of the *CYP2D6* gene have been formed by unequal segregation and extrachromosomal replication of the acentric DNA (Lundqvist et al., 1999).

In order to validate the possibility that this selection of duplicated *CYP2D6* genes in North East Africa might have occurred due to dietary selection we hypothesized that the plant-based diet in Ethiopia would contain substances inhibiting the CYP2D6 enzyme contributing to this dietary stress. Accordingly, we carried out a study where we compared the debrisoquine MR (indicative for CYP2D6 activity) among Ethiopian individuals of the same *CYP2D6* genotype but living in Sweden or in Ethiopia compared with Swedes living in Sweden (Aklillu, Herrlin, Gustafsson, Bertilsson, & Ingelman-Sundberg, 2002). We found that Swedes exhibited the highest rate of debrisoquine metabolism, followed by Ethiopians in Sweden and Ethiopians in Ethiopia. The difference between the Ethiopian groups was significantly 50% of the magnitude of the MR difference between Swedes and last Ethiopians in Ethiopia. It is thus tempting to speculate that inhibitory dietary factors contribute to the differences seen between the two Ethiopian groups and we suggest that these components in the past might have contributed to dietary stress-mediated selection of duplicated and multi-duplicated active *CYP2D6* genes, as frequently seen in Ethiopians.

There are in Africa also another variant of CYP2D6, CYP2D6.17 harboring amino acid substitutions and exhibiting another substrate specificity as compared to CYP2D6.1. Thus, debrisoquine and dextromethorphan metabolism are decreased, and codeine or metoprolol increased in carriers of the *CYP2D6*17* variant (Wennerholm et al., 2002). It might be possible that this enrichment of *CYP2D6*17* in, e.g., Zimbabwe and Tanzania, has been based on dietary factors, although at present the components exerting such a stress are not known.

4. Genetic variants of CYP genes

The CYP genes encoding drug metabolizing P450s are to the main part very polymorphic and several hundreds of variant alleles have been identified in humans (https://www.pharmvar.org/). Principally different polymorphisms can affect the expression and functionality of CYP-genes. Those are SNPs (single nucleotide polymorphisms) causing stop codons and no expression of functional enzyme, SNPs resulting in amino acid substitutions which can be functional or silent on the enzyme level. The functional genetic variation can cause inactive enzyme or an enzyme with an altered substrates specificity (*CYP2D6*17* as an example). A third category is CNVs (copy number variations) where gene duplications or deletions can cause enhanced or abolishment of enzyme expression. Among the drug metabolizing enzymes, such CNV variability is seen mainly in the *CYP2A6* and *CYP2D6* genes. There are also partial deletions and duplications in the CYP genes seen in different populations (Santos et al., 2018). Their frequency is between 0,1 and 1% and a spectrum of different exons are subject for such partial deletions and duplication, the duplications causing non-functional enzymes because this type of duplication does not encompass the full gene. In total over 5500 such CNVs have been identified among different ADME genes (Santos et al., 2018). These deletions are subject to high interethnic differences in frequency and, e.g., in Finns almost 1% of all *CYP2C19* genes have partial deletions. In addition, functionally important SNPs can also be found in 5′-upstream regulatory region (e.g., *CYP2C19*17*) and in introns causing aberrant splicing and decreased gene expression (e.g., *CYP3A5*3* and *CYP3A4*22*). Polymorphic CYP gene expression can also be achieved due to the polymorphism of genes encoding regulatory proteins for CYPs as seen in the control of NFIB of the CYP2D6 expression, causing ultrarapid metabolisers of patients being, e.g., homozygous for *CYP2D6*1/2*) (Lenk et al., 2022).

For NGS (next generation sequencing) and GWAS (genome wide association study) based CYP genotyping these CNVs cause problems. Since the duplicated genes often are in loci very complex having pseudogenes adjacent, these CNVs are in many cases impossible to identify without selective long read PCR amplification followed by CNV determination. As an alternative for genotyping of clinical applications, recent data indicate the presence of novel endogenous biomarkers derived from solanidine as quite accurate predictors for different CYP2D6 phenotypes (Magliocco et al., 2021).

5. Examples of Functionality of CYP polymorphism

The polymorphism of P450s does indeed influence the effect of many drugs and toxic substances. This field is of substantial importance and search in PubMed for "cytochrome P450 AND pharmacogenomics OR

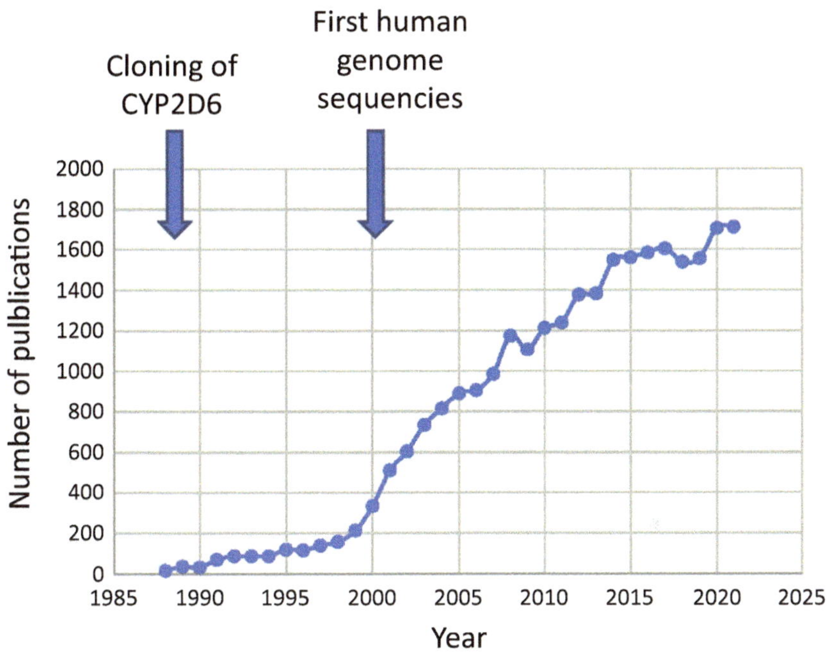

Fig. 4 Development of the area of pharmacogenomics since 1988 based on the number of publications per year.

pharmacogenetics" provides >25,000 papers as illustrated in Fig. 4. More than 7500 reviews have been written in this topic (also see Daly, 2015) where apparently the largest one specific for the CYP genes is written by Zhou, Liu, and Chowbay (2009) having >200 pages. This large field is beyond the possibility to be summarized here, rather some interesting aspects are provided below.

5.1 CYP2A6 and smoking

CYP2A6 is the main enzyme involved in the metabolism of nicotine, and the influence of CYP2A6 polymorphism on smoking behavior has been extensively studied (see (Gold & Lerman, 2012)). A GWAS study by Thorgeirsson et al. (2010) found that SNP variation in both CYP2A6 (19q3) and nicotinic acetylcholine receptors (nAchR, 15q25) containing loci significantly affected cigarette consumption. Furthermore, the highly frequent *CYP2A6*2* allele (up to 10%) causing an abolished CYP2A6 enzyme activity was found associated with a significantly lower number of cigarettes smoked per day (reduction of 0.68 cigarettes per day and

*CYP2A6*2* allele). These findings have been replicated several times, see a review by Tanner and Tyndale (2017) and the *CYP2A6* genotype modulates lung cancer risk. The absence of CYP2A6 enzyme activity could reduce the risk of lung cancer because the activation of procarcinogens found in tobacco smoke, such as NNK and NNN, would be decreased. Indeed, a recent meta-analysis has been published (Johani, Majid, Azme, & Nawi, 2020) where it is evident that among 4385 lung cancer cases and 4142 controls there is an almost 3-fold higher risk of lung cancer for carriers of functional *CYP2A6* alleles. In addition, those with CYP2A6 reduced metabolism are more likely to quit smoking than those with normal metabolism (Jones et al., 2021). See also a review in Daly (2015).

5.2 CYP2A6 and caffeine

Caffeine has long been known as one of the substrates and inducers of CYP1A2. In 2011, three independent GWA (genome wide association) studies amounting to 472,000 subjects in total, found an association between CYP1A2 variation and the habitual consumption of coffee. In a genome-wide meta-analysis of 47,341 subjects, Cornelis et al. (2016) first presented an association between the behavioral caffeine intake trait and variations in both the CYP1A1-1A2 bidirectional 5′-flanking region as well as a locus upstream the AhR gene that regulates the expression of CYP1A genes. The effect of each individual CYP1A2 and AHR allele has been estimated to about 0.2 coffee cups per day (Sulem et al., 2011). However, the identified polymorphisms at the two loci were together found to explain only a small part of the caffeine intake variation, see further Tanner and Tyndale (2017) and chapter "Cytochrome P450 enzymes and metabolism of drugs and neurotoxins within the mammalian brain" by Rachel Tyndale in this volume).

6. Missing heritability

Early analyses of twins indeed were instrumental to identify the interindividual variability as to a large extent being heritable (Lauschke & Ingelman-Sundberg, 2019). Early clinical trials in monozygotic and dizygotic twins using nortriptyline showed the inheritable part for the CYP2D6 poor metaboliser phenotype (Alexanderson, Evans, & Sjoqvist, 1969). After the cloning of the genes encoding the major polymorphic P450s in 1988–1992, the major genetic variants could be identified affecting the rate of drug metabolism. However, now it is clear that the genetic variants hitherto identified cannot predict the inherent drug metabolism to a satisfactory level. This was indeed pinpointed some years ago when Brockmöller and colleagues intravenously administered metoprolol and torsemide to 44 monozygotic and 14 dizygotic twin pairs (Matthaei et al., 2015). The results showed that the metoprolol AUC varied 4.7-fold and torsemide AUC 3.5-fold and indeed 91% of metoprolol and 86% of torsemide AUC variations were caused by additive genetic effects. However, known genetic variants of CYP2D6, CYP2C9, and OATP1B1 explained only 39%, 2%, and 39% of this variation, respectively.

The basis for this discrepancy, called the missing heritability, is not elucidated. One might suggest five different factor of importance in this respect as shown in Fig. 5: (i) contribution of genetic variants in other loci not analyzed for, (ii) influence on the drug metabolism of more than one polymorphic gene that has to be accounted for, (iii) importance of rare genetic variants not analyzed, (iv) hidden mutations requiring long read PCR techniques for detection and (v) variable haplotypes affecting the drug metabolism all carrying the same traditional allelic variant.

6.1 Variation in other loci

Traditionally the investigation for genetic variations of putative importance for the inter-individual differences in the metabolism of a drug are restricted to the candidate gene believed to be responsible for the synthesis of transporters and enzymes influencing the pharmacokinetics. However, the ADME gene of interest is regulated by factors that could exhibit genetic

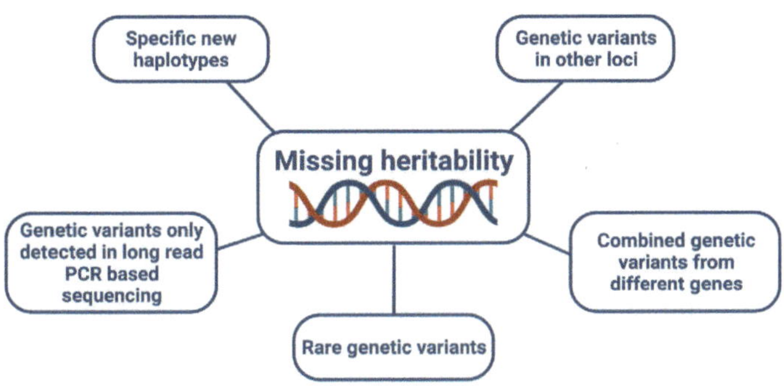

Fig. 5 Possible causes for the missing heritability in studies of phenotype- genotype correlations of drug metabolism. The figure illustrates the factors that are overseen in many clinical studies comparing the influence of different polymorphic *CYP* gene variants on drug pharmacokinetics. *Figure created with BioRender.com.*

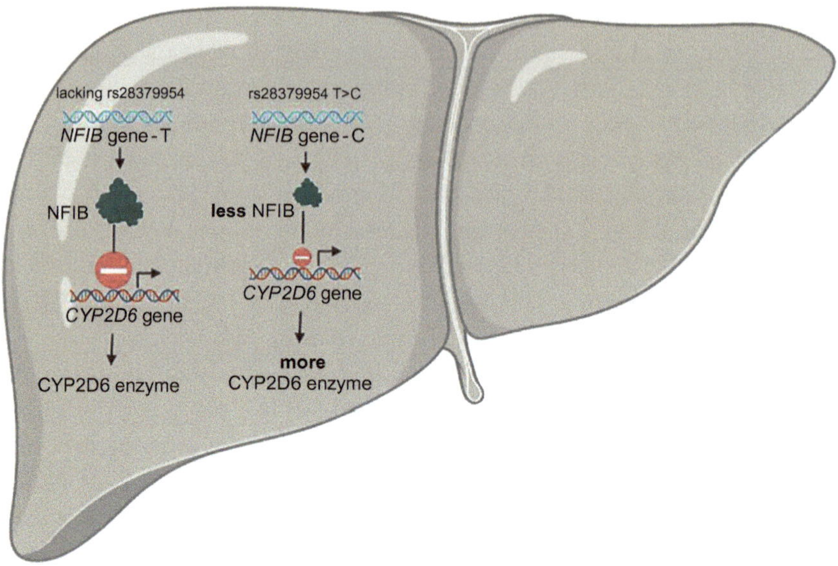

Fig. 6 Effect of NFIB polymorphism on the expression of CYP2D6 in recombinant Huh7 cells and in vivo. NFIB inhibits the expression of CYP2D6 in Huh7 cell based CYP2D6 reporter gene systems. The mutant NFIB C allele causes less expression of the protein and is then expected to have a lower capacity for repression of the *CYP2D6* gene expression in human liver. *Figure created with BioRender.com*

polymorphism and thus in a polymorphic manner influence the transport or metabolism of a certain drug. On such recent example is the role of NFIB polymorphism for expression of CYP2D6 (Fig. 6).

6.2 NFIB

Thus, polymorphisms in genes encoding nuclear regulatory proteins in control of, e.g., CYP gene expression adds to the factors of missing heritability. In this concept the Nuclear Factor 1B (NFIB) rs28379954 T > C intron polymorphism was picked up by GWAS analysis as a genetic factor associating to the serum concentrations of clozapine (Smith et al., 2020). NFIB participates in embryonic development of many organ systems and in the control of tumor cell proliferation (Becker-Santos, Lonergan, Gronostajski, & Lam, 2017). In order to elucidate any role in ADME gene expression we silenced NFIB in in vivo like human liver spheroids (Bell et al., 2016) and observed a drastic reduction of *GSTP1* expression and an important reduction of *CYP1A2, CYP2D6, CYP2C8* and *CYP2B6* gene expression (Lenk et al., 2022). NFIB overexpression in Huh7 cells caused inhibited expression of

CYP2D6 reporter constructs. Analyses of a large risperidone cohort, showed that the NFIB C variant associated strongly with increased CYP2D6 activity. The subjects homozygous for *CYP2D6*1/*2* carrying the NFIB C variant had a rate of risperidone metabolism similar as ultra-rapid metabolisers carrying duplicated active *CYP2D6* genes. In human livers we found that the NFIB C variant correlated strongly to reduced NFIB expression and if this is the case in vivo then the activatory action of NFIB C should be reduced inhibition of the CYP2D6 gene expression (Fig. 6). It remains to be elucidated to what extent other clinically important genes are affected by the NFIB polymorphism in vivo. The NFIB example indeed provides evidence that polymorphism in genes encoding regulatory nuclear proteins can contribute to the missing inheritance in pharmacogenomics.

6.3 Long read PCR for complete gene sequence

In pharmacogenomic studies mostly the most common and functionally important genetic variants are considered. Thus, within a gene many mutations might not be determined, this is in particular important for genes presence in complex loci with adjacent sequence like pseudogenes or other similar genes. In the CYP field this is most relevant for CYP2A6, CYP2B6, CYP2D6 and CYP3A4 (Lauschke, Milani, & Ingelman-Sundberg, 2017). This problem can be overcome by using long read PCR amplification where in a first step the whole gene or large part of it is amplified, followed by specific analyses for gene mutations. This technique was, e.g., applied to the *CYP2D6* gene in the Dutch CYP-TAM study. Based on 561 patients with breast cancer the method of continuous-scale (instead of categorical) assignments to predict enzyme based on long read sequencing explained 79% of interindividual variability in CYP2D6 activity compared to 54% using the conventional allele approach. For venlafaxine, which is also metabolized by CYP2C19, a lower prediction of 63% was obtained compatible with the fact that about 30% of the clearance is mediated by CYP2C19. Indeed, it can be concluded that this type of more deep sequencing combined with predictive algorithms can reduce the gap in the missing heritability to a significant extent.

6.4 Hidden haplotypes

One additional factor for the missing habitability is linked to the presence of specific haplotypes carrying specific allelic variant potentials but where these are in linkage disequilibrium to other mutations that might influence the expression of the gene in question. Such mutations might be located in elements controlling expression of regulatory proteins or regulating RNAs like lncRNAs. The interindividual differences of escitalopram metabolism and levels within a defined phenotypic group of CYP2C19 are extremely high (Jukić, Haslemo, Molden, & Ingelman-Sundberg, 2018). The subjects having a rapid metabolism of the drug have been found to carry the *CYP2C19*17* allele, but the variability within the normal metaboliser (NM) group encompass subjects exhibiting a wide range of rates for escitalopram metabolism, from UM to PM phenotype. Based on an enhanced gene sequencing effort many novel genetic variants were identified in alleles formally classified as *CYP2C19*1* carriers. From these sequence data four different haplotypes could be identified, one of them carrying rs2860840T and rs11188059G (CYP2C:TG). This variant caused ultrarapid metabolism of escitalopram somewhat higher as *CYP2C19*17* and has a similar frequency (Bråten et al., 2021). As seen from Fig. 7, the three other haplotypes carrying these mutations in other combinations caused lower activity. The data are

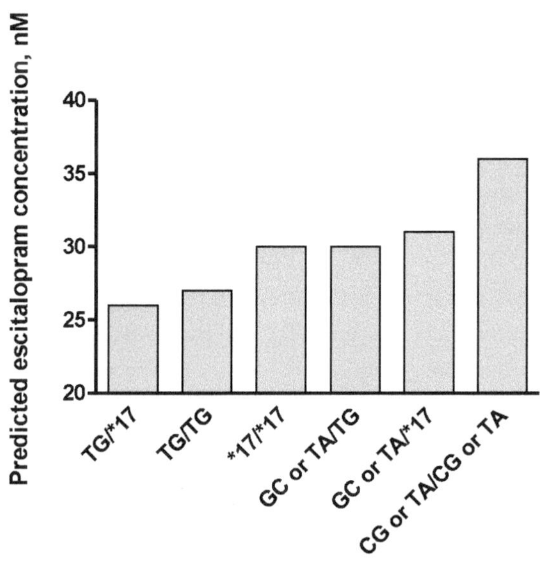

Fig. 7 Effect of the combination of different *CYP2C* haplotypes genotypes on the predicted serum concentrations of escitalopram. Three new haplotypes of the CYP2C locus (CYP2C:TG, CYP2C:TA, and CYP2C:CG) were from a cohort of 875 previously genotyped escitalopram-treated patients, carrying the *CYP2C19*1* or *CYP2C19*17* allelic variants. The mean predicted escitalopram concentrations are given in relationship to the occurrence of the specific haplotypes. *Data from Bråten, L.S., Haslemo, T., Jukic, M.M., Ivanov, M., Ingelman-Sundberg, M., Molden, E. et al., (2021) A novel CYP2C-haplotype associated with Ultrarapid metabolism of escitalopram.* Clinical Pharmacology and Therapeutics *110:786–793.*

principally important indicating that what we hitherto have defined by the current allele nomenclature is insufficient and within every allele many different haplotypes causing altered activity might be "hidden". It is anticipated that further stratification according to this line will indeed explain a lot of the hidden hereditary.

6.5 Rare variants

Another reason for the missing heritability in pharmacogenomics is due to rare genetic variants. Indeed, results presented 4–5 years ago based on the databases for sequence data like ExAC (Exome Aggregation Consortium) with WES (whole exon sequencing) sequence data from about 60,000 individuals available at that time, revealed a high number of rare variants in CYP genes (Ingelman-Sundberg, Mkrtchian, Zhou, & Lauschke, 2018; Santos et al., 2018). The stratification of rare and common genetic variants revealed that 30–40% of the ADME (absorption distribution metabolism excretion) genes carry common genetic variants, but that the genetic variability in the remaining fraction is mainly due to rare variants. Each individual carried on average a total of 40.6 putatively functional variants, where 10.8% of these were rare and the contribution of rare variants was found to be highly gene- and drug-specific. Recently, a similar analysis was done using GWAS arrays for analysis of genetic variation in 487,409 participants in the UK Biobank (McInnes et al., 2021). The investigators found that among 14 ADME genes 99.5% of individuals may have an atypical response to at least 1 drug; on average they may have an atypical response to 10.3 drugs. Nearly 24% of participants had been prescribed a drug for which they are predicted to have an atypical response (McInnes, Yee, Pershad, and Altman (2021). A recent extensive study presented the distribution of rare variants in pharmacogenes and it was shown that among the *CYP2C9, CYP2C19* and *CYP3A4* genes the contribution of rare variants to the genetic variability is as high as 19%, 18% and 27%, respectively (see Table 1) (Lauschke, Zhou, & Ingelman-Sundberg, 2019). In conclusion, the rare genetic variants have an important contribution to the missing heritability in pharmacogenomics, which however exhibit a strong gene specificity. Applied to all ADME genes the contribution of rare alleles to the variability can be estimated to 4–5%.

6.6 Polymorphic gene synergy

As a last factor of importance for the missing heritability is the fact that the metabolism of a drug might be influenced by two or more polymorphic genes. The problem is illustrated by the analyses of the influence of

Table 1 Importance of rare genetic variants for interindividual variation in CYP genes.

Enzyme	Estimated no of individuals to be screened in order to find one rare deleterious variant	Fraction of functional variability allotted to rare variants (%)
CYP1A2	49	2
CYP2C9	23	19
CYP2C19	18	12
CYP2D6	12	7
CYP3A4	44	27

Data from Lauschke V. M., Zhou Y., & Ingelman-Sundberg M. (2019) Novel genetic and epigenetic factors of importance for inter-individual differences in drug disposition, response and toxicity. *Pharmacology & Therapeutics 197*, 122–152.

CYP2C19 and CYP2D6 polymorphisms for the pharmacokinetics on venlafaxine, a substrate for both enzymes (Kringen, Bråten, Haslemo, & Molden, 2020). In many pharmacogenomic studies of genetic polymorphisms is not well taken into consideration.

7. Pharmacogenomic labels

Pharmacogenomic research for several decades has yielded an increasing amount of information about the most common and important genetic variations that can affect drug response and risk for adverse drug reactions. The field of pharmacogenomics has expanded a lot after the characterization of the human genome in 2000 (Fig. 4). In the area of P450 genes it is evident that the polymorphisms of CYP2C8, CYP2C9, CYP2C19 and CYP2D6 are the most important (see Daly, 2015 for detailed information). Much effort is placed at translating this information into a system that can be utilized in the clinics. At present direct application of genetic variability as a factor to consider in drug prescription are done by introduction of pharmacogenomic labels into the summaries of product characteristics (SmPCs). This is most common within the therapeutic area of oncology (Fig. 8). Such drug labels are provided by the EMA (European Medicines Agency), FDA (U.S. Food and Drug Administration) and other medical product agencies. In addition, two different Academic organizations, CPIC (Clinical Pharmacogenetics Implementation Consortium) and DPWG (Dutch Pharmacogenetics Working Group) do publish guidance on similar matters. A recent survey identified 55 drugs for which all these

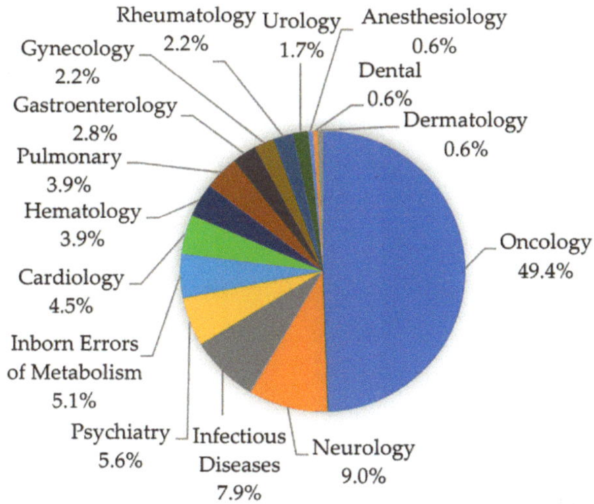

Fig. 8 Therapeutic areas of new FDA drug approvals with pharmacogenomics (PGx) labelling from 2000 to 2020. *From Kim, J.A., Ceccarelli, R., Lu, C.Y.J. (2021) Pharmacogenomic biomarkers in US FDA-approved drug labels (2000 – 2020).* Journal of Personalized Medicine, 11 *(3), 179.*

organization have provided actionable recommendations and in addition 277 drugs where FDA and or EMA had an actionable drug label (Shekhani, Steinacher, Swen, & Ingelman-Sundberg, 2020). However, the concordance between the agencies were not optimal (Fig. 9). Of 54 drugs with an actionable gene-drug interaction in the CPIC or DPGW guidelines, only 50% had actionable pharmacogenomic information in the SmPCs, and all agencies were common in their recommendation only in 18% of the cases. In Fig. 9 the 54 drugs based on CIPIC and DPGW guidelines are visualized as to which extent EMA or FDA take these information into account in the SmPCs. As seen from the Venn diagram in Fig. 9, the distribution of the actionable recommendations differs substantially between the agencies. A recent overview regarding biomarker qualification at the EMA has recently been presented. The statement that biomarkers for general use instead of drug specific biomarkers is controversial since the specificity would increase when the action of specific drugs is taken into consideration.

In the future, it is anticipated that rapid technological developments will provide us with an arsenal of novel genetic variations of importance for understanding inter-individual differences in drug metabolism and response. In order for optimal usage of this information the basis for the assignment of a specific drug label must improve and be based on solid and reproducible

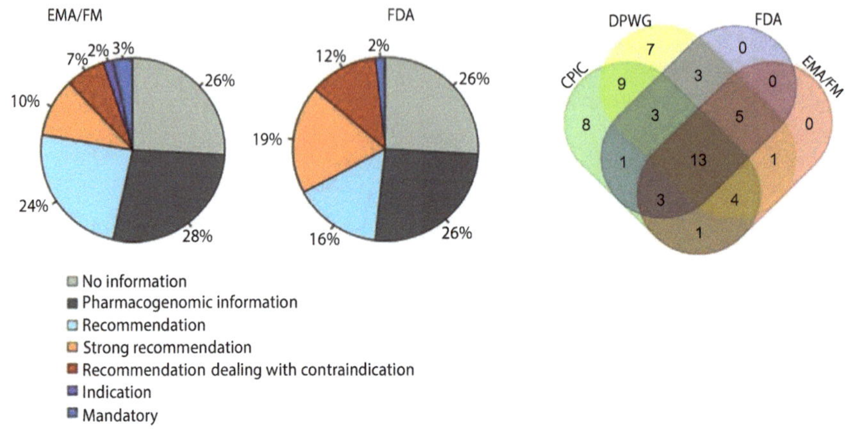

Fig. 9 Comparison of CPIC, DPWG, EMA, and FDA provided advice for pharmacogenomic drug labels among the 55 drugs approved by FDA or EMA and where such information has been provided by CPIC and DPWG guidelines. Left: Pie charts showing the distribution of different label categories between the EMA and the FDA for 55 drugs (58 gene drug interactions, GDIs) that have guidelines by the CPIC and/or DPWG. Right: Venn diagram of the same 58 GDIs that have guidelines by the CPIC and/or DPWG and are approved by both the EMA/FM and the FDA, with actionable labels (mandatory, indication, recommendation dealing with contraindication, or (strong) recommendation). *Data from Shekhani, R., Steinacher, L., Swen, J.J., & Ingelman-Sundberg, M. (2020) Evaluation of current regulation and guidelines of Pharmacogenomic drug labels: Opportunities for improvements.* Clinical Pharmacology and Therapeutics, 107, *1240–1255.*

information. As a start an initial harmonization of the drug labels between the FDA and EMA might be relevant. In addition, for the future one might consider the establishment of an International committee consisting of scientific experts, regulatory agencies, expert organizations and other stakeholders to continuously validate the appropriateness of different pharmacogenomic labels (Ingelman-Sundberg, 2020).

8. Looking into the future

There is a rapid development in equipment, methods and knowledge regarding analyses of genetic variation in large volumes of human DNA samples. In addition, specifically the bioinformatic instruments have in recent years improved tremendously. By AI based algorithms, the functionality of different types of mutations determined by whole genome sequencing or GWAS arrays can be predicted at a relatively good accuracy. Looking into the current situation and possibilities, the pharmacogenomic analyses at a broader perspective can be planned for as outlined in Fig. 10. There are

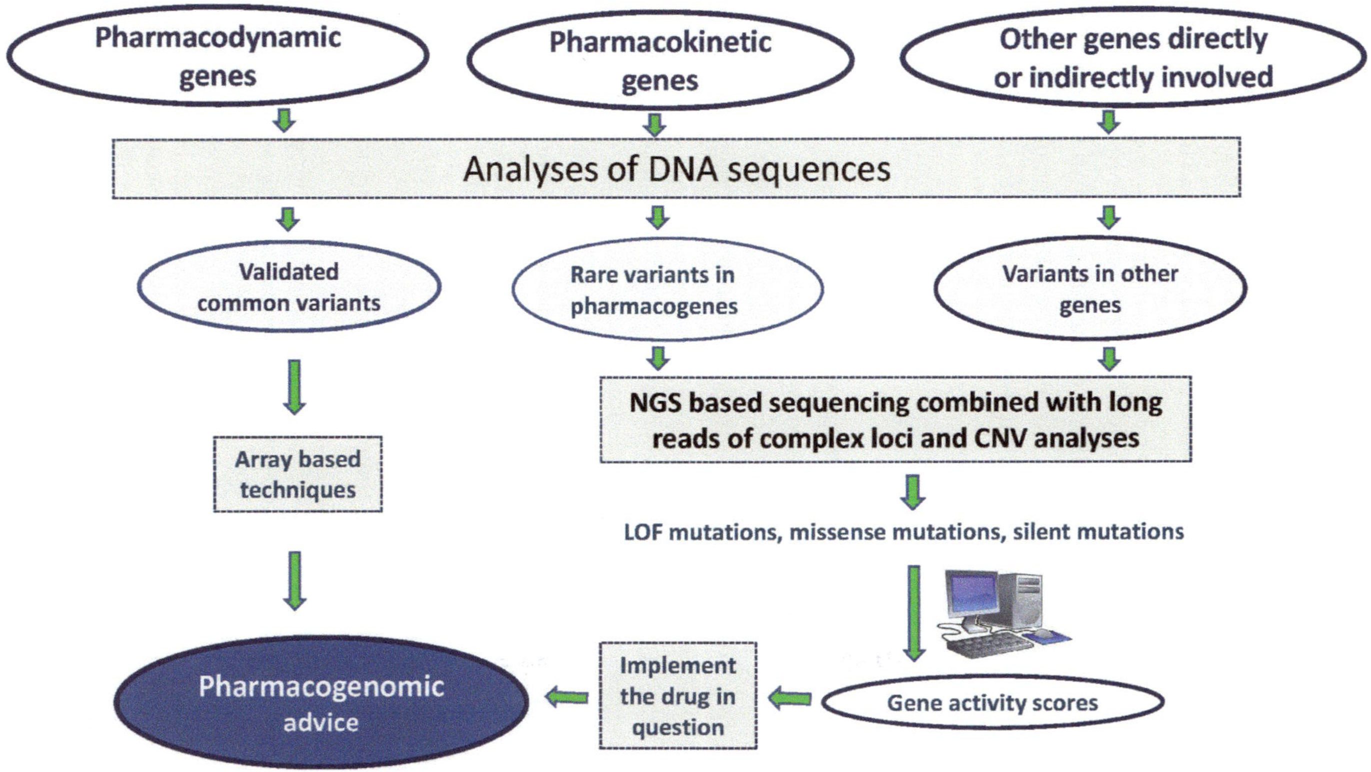

Fig. 10 See figure legend on next page.

many commercially available array platform-based methods for detection of the common and important genetic variants. These should be combined with NGS and long read PCR sequencing analyses including CNV analyses for determination of rare variants, variants in regulatory gene regions and in other genes which might influence the efficacy and metabolism of the drugs in question. The genetic data obtained can then be analyzed by AI to provide a basis for pharmacogenomic advice after including the specific drug to be analyzed. This system would be difficult to use extensively in clinical routine but can provide useful novel pharmacogenomic information during drug development and for research. The resulting data containing all critical genetic variants can be used clinically after transfer to different array-platforms.

9. Conclusion

The functionally important genetic polymorphisms of *CYP* genes have to a significant extent been evolved based on dietary restrictions and environmental factors. Such genetic variations involve CNVs, amino acid changes, stop codons, mutations causing alternate splicing and mutations leading to increased or suppressed gene expression. The current knowledge about CYP polymorphism is however not sufficient as to with high accuracy predict the consequences regarding drug pharmacokinetics, or adverse drug reactions. Much has to be considered for better predictions in the future such as taking genetic variations in other loci controlling the expression of CYPs into account, apply long read sequencing techniques to genes in complex loci, to a greater extent analyze the composition of different haplotypes, consider rare genetic variants and take synergistic action of genetic variations in different CYP genes into account when necessary. Combined with a rapid development in the content and number of genetic databases and

Fig. 10 Proposed schedule for genetic analyses of patient gDNA for genetic variants of importance for altered drug metabolism or for adverse drug reactions. Genes of importance for altered drug response are analyzed for validated common variants using array-based techniques, for rare and novel variants in pharmacogenes and variants in other genes by NGS combined with long reads of complex loci and CNV analyses. The importance of the mutations determined are functionally evaluated using relevant software's providing gene activity scores for the genes of interest. The drug of interest will then be implemented into the genetic data and the resulting genetic variants are used as a basis for pharmacogenomic advice to the patients in question. For routine clinical analyses the genetic variants generated in such systems should be transferred to different array platforms.

development of novel softwares and algorithms where AI will take a larger role, it is plausible that the true personalized drug therapy will be much improved in the decade to come.

Acknowledgments

I am indebted to Assoc Prof Inger Johansson for important input. The work in the author's lab is funded by the Swedish Cancer Society [Grant Agreement 17 0599], the European Research Council (ERC)–Advanced Grant (AdG) project HEPASPHER [Grant Agreement 742020], The Swedish Research Council (grant 2021-02732) and the European Union's Horizon 2020 research and innovation program [Grant Agreement 668353/U-PGx].

Conflict of interests

Magnus Ingelman-Sundberg is a Co-founder and Co-owner of HepaPredict AB.

References

Aklillu, E., Herrlin, K., Gustafsson, L. L., Bertilsson, L., & Ingelman-Sundberg, M. (2002). Evidence for environmental influence on CYP2D6-catalysed debrisoquine hydroxylation as demonstrated by phenotyping and genotyping of Ethiopians living in Ethiopia or in Sweden. *Pharmacogenetics*, *12*, 375–383.

Aklillu, E., Persson, I., Bertilsson, L., Johansson, I., Rodrigues, F., & Ingelman-Sundberg, M. (1996). Frequent distribution of ultrarapid metabolizers of debrisoquine in an ethiopian population carrying duplicated and multiduplicated functional CYP2D6 alleles. *The Journal of Pharmacology and Experimental Therapeutics*, *278*, 441–446.

Alexanderson, B., Evans, D. A., & Sjoqvist, F. (1969). Steady-state plasma levels of nortriptyline in twins: Influence of genetic factors and drug therapy *Br. Medizinhistorisches Journal*, *4*, 764–768.

Amichot, M., Tarès, S., Brun-Barale, A., Arthaud, L., Bride, J.-M., & Bergé, J.-P. (2004). Point mutations associated with insecticide resistance in the Drosophila cytochrome P450 Cyp6a2 enable DDT metabolism. *European Journal of Biochemistry*, *271*, 1250–1257.

Bass, C., Zimmer, C. T., Riveron, J. M., Wilding, C. S., Wondji, C. S., Kaussmann, M., et al. (2013). Gene amplification and microsatellite polymorphism underlie a recent insect host shift. *Proceedings of the National Academy of Sciences of the United States of America*, *110*, 19460–19465.

Becker-Santos, D. D., Lonergan, K. M., Gronostajski, R. M., & Lam, W. L. (2017). Nuclear factor I/B: A master regulator of cell differentiation with paradoxical roles in Cancer. *eBioMedicine*, *22*, 2–9.

Bell, C. C., Hendriks, D. F., Moro, S. M., Ellis, E., Walsh, J., Renblom, A., et al. (2016). Characterization of primary human hepatocyte spheroids as a model system for drug-induced liver injury, liver function and disease. *Scientific Reports*, *6*, 25187.

Bråten, L. S., Haslemo, T., Jukic, M. M., Ivanov, M., Ingelman-Sundberg, M., Molden, E., et al. (2021). A novel CYP2C-haplotype associated with Ultrarapid metabolism of escitalopram. *Clinical Pharmacology and Therapeutics*, *110*, 786–793.

Clark, A. G. (1994). Invasion and maintenance of a gene duplication. *Proceedings of the National Academy of Sciences of the United States of America*, *91*, 2950–2954.

Cornelis, M. C., Kacprowski, T., Menni, C., Gustafsson, S., Pivin, E., Adamski, J., et al. (2016). Genome-wide association study of caffeine metabolites provides new insights to caffeine metabolism and dietary caffeine-consumption behavior. *Human Molecular Genetics*, *25*, 5472–5482.

Daborn, P. J., Yen, J. L., Bogwitz, M. R., Le Goff, G., Feil, E., Jeffers, S., et al. (2002). A single p450 allele associated with insecticide resistance in Drosophila. *Science*, *297*, 2253–2256.

Daly, A. K. (2015). Polymorphic variants of cytochrome P450: Relevance to Cancer and other diseases. *Advances in Pharmacology*, *74*, 85–111.

Danielson, P. B. (2002). The cytochrome P450 superfamily: Biochemistry, evolution and drug metabolism in humans. *Current Drug Metabolism*, *3*, 561–597.

Danielson, P. B., MacIntyre, R. J., & Fogleman, J. C. (1997). Molecular cloning of a family of xenobiotic-inducible drosophilid cytochrome P450s: Evidence for involvement in host-plant allelochemical resistance. *Proceedings of the National Academy of Sciences of the United States of America*, *94*, 10797–10802.

Fonne-Pfister, R., & Meyer, U. A. (1988). (1988) xenobiotic and endobiotic inhibitors of cytochrome P-450dbl function, the target of the debrisoquine/sparteine type polymorphism. *Biochemical Pharmacology*, *37*, 3829–3835.

Frank, M. R., & Fogleman, J. C. (1992). Involvement of cytochrome P450 in host-plant utilization bySonoran desert Drosophila. *Proceedings of the National Academy of Sciences of the United States of America*, *89*, 11998–12002.

Gold, A. B., & Lerman, C. (2012). Pharmacogenetics of smoking cessation: Role of nicotine target and metabolism genes. *Human Genetics*, *31*. https://doi.org/10.1007/s00439-012-1143-9.

Ingelman-Sundberg, M. (2005). Genetic polymorphisms of cytochrome P450 2D6 (CYP2D6): Clinical consequences, evolutionary aspects and functional diversity. *The Pharmacogenomics Journal*, *5*, 6–13.

Ingelman-Sundberg, M. (2020). Translation of pharmacogenomic drug labels into the clinic. Current problems. *Pharmacological Research*, *153*, 104620.

Ingelman-Sundberg, M., Mkrtchian, S., Zhou, Y., & Lauschke, V. M. (2018). Integrating rare genetic variants into pharmacogenetic drug response predictions. *Human Genomics*, *12*, 26.

Ingelman-Sundberg, M., Oscarson, M., & McLellan, R. A. (1999). Polymorphic human cytochrome P450 enzymes: An opportunity for individualized drug treatment. *Trends in Pharmacological Sciences*, *20*, 342–349.

Ismail, H. M., O'Neill, P. M., Hong, D. W., Finn, R. D., Henderson, C. J., Wright, A. T., et al. (2013). Pyrethroid activity-based probes for profiling cytochrome P450 activities associated with insecticide interactions. *Proceedings of the National Academy of Sciences of the United States of America*, *110*, 19766–19771.

Johani, F. H., Majid, M. S. A., Azme, M. H., & Nawi, A. M. (2020). Cytochrome P450 2A6 whole-gene deletion (CYP2A6*4) polymorphism reduces risk of lung cancer: A meta-analysis. *Tobacco Induced Diseases*, *2020*(18), 50.

Jones, S. K., Wolf, B. J., Froeliger, B., Wallace, K., Carpenter, M. J., & Alberg, A. J. (2021). Nicotine metabolism predicted by CYP2A6 genotypes in relation to smoking cessation: A systematic review. *Nicotine & Tobacco Research*, *2021*, ntab175.

Jukić, M. M., Haslemo, T., Molden, E., & Ingelman-Sundberg, M. (2018). Impact of CYP2C19 genotype on escitalopram exposure and therapeutic failure: A retrospective study based on 2,087 patients. *The American Journal of Psychiatry*, *175*, 463–470.

Kringen, M. K., Bråten, L. S., Haslemo, T., & Molden, E. (2020). The influence of combined CYP2D6 and CYP2C19 genotypes on venlafaxine and O-Desmethylvenlafaxine concentrations in a large patient cohort. *Journal of Clinical Psychopharmacology*, *40*, 137–144.

Lauschke, V. M., & Ingelman-Sundberg, M. (2019). Prediction of drug response and adverse drug reactions: From twin studies to next generation sequencing. *European Journal of Pharmaceutical Sciences*, *130*, 65–77.

Lauschke, V. M., Milani, L., & Ingelman-Sundberg, M. (2017). Pharmacogenomic biomarkers for improved drug therapy—Recent progress and future developments. *The AAPS Journal, 20*, 4.

Lauschke, V. M., Zhou, Y., & Ingelman-Sundberg, M. (2019). Novel genetic and epigenetic factors of importance for inter-individual differences in drug disposition, response and toxicity. *Pharmacology & Therapeutics, 197*, 122–152.

Lenk, H. C., Klöditz, K., Johansson, I., Løvsletten Smith, R., Jukic, M., Molden, E., et al. (2022). The polymorphic nuclear factor NFIB regulates hepatic CYP2D6 expression and influences risperidone metabolism in psychiatric patients. *Clinical Pharmacology and Therapeutics*. https://doi.org/10.1002/cpt.2571.

Little, C. (1983). *The colonisation of land: Origins and adaptations of terrestrial animals*. Cambridge: Cambridge University Press.

Loomis, W. F. (1988). *Four billion years, an essay on the Evolution of genes and organisms* (p. 286). Sunderland, Massachusetts: Sinauer Associates, Inc.

Lundqvist, E., Johansson, I., & Ingelman-Sundberg, M. (1999). Genetic mechanisms for duplication and multiduplication of the human CYP2D6 gene and methods for detection of duplicated CYP2D6 genes. *Gene, 226*, 327–338.

Magliocco, G., Desmeules, J., Matthey, A., Quirós-Guerrero, L. M., Bararpour, N., Joye, T., et al. (2021). Metabolomics reveals biomarkers in human urine and plasma to predict cytochrome P450 2D6 (CYP2D6) activity. *British Journal of Pharmacology, 178*, 4708–4725.

Matthaei, J., Brockmöller, M. V., Tzvetkov, D., Sehrt, C., Sachse-Seeboth, J. B., et al. (2015). Heritability of metoprolol and torsemide pharmacokinetics. *Clinical Pharmacology and Therapeutics, 98*, 611–662.

McCart, C., & Ffrench-Constant, R. H. (2008). Dissecting the insecticide-resistance- associated cytochrome P450 gene Cyp6g1. *Pest Management Science, 64*, 639–645.

McInnes, G., Lavertu, A., Sangkuhl, K., Klein, T. E., Whirl-Carrillo, M., & Altman, R. B. (2021). Pharmacogenetics at scale: An analysis of the UK biobank. *Clinical Pharmacology and Therapeutics, 109*, 1528–1537.

McInnes, G., Yee, S. W., Pershad, Y., & Altman, R. B. (2021). Genome wide association studies in pharmacogenomics. *Clinical Pharmacology and Therapeutics, 110*, 637–648.

Morrison, H. G., Oleksiak, M. F., Cornell, N. W., Sogin, M. L., & Stegeman, J. J. (1995). Identification of cytochrome P-450 1A (CYP1A) genes from two teleost fish, toadfish (Opsanus tau), and scup (Stenotomus chrysops), and phylogenetic analysis of CYP1A genes. *The Biochemical Journal, 308*, 97–104.

Nelson, D. R. (2018). Cytochrome P450 diversity in the tree of life. *Biochimica et Biophysica Acta (BBA) - Proteins and Proteomics., 1866*, 141–154.

Santos, M., Niemi, M., Hiratsuka, M., Kumondai, M., Ingelman-Sundberg, M., Lauschke, V. M., et al. (2018). Novel copy-number variations in pharmacogenes contribute to interindividual differences in drug pharmacokinetics. *Genetics in Medicine, 20*, 622–629.

Shekhani, R., Steinacher, L., Swen, J. J., & Ingelman-Sundberg, M. (2020). Evaluation of current regulation and guidelines of Pharmacogenomic drug labels: Opportunities for improvements. *Clinical Pharmacology and Therapeutics, 107*, 1240–1255.

Smith, R. L., O'Connell, K., Athanasiu, L., Djurovic, S., Kringen, M. K., Andreassen, O. A., et al. (2020). Identification of a novel polymorphism associated with reduced clozapine concentration in schizophrenia patients-a genome-wide association study adjusting for smoking habits. *Translational Psychiatry, 19*(10), 198.

Sulem, P., Gudbjartsson, D. F., Geller, F., Prokopenko, I., Feenstra, B., Aben, K. K., et al. (2011). Sequence variants at CYP1A1-CYP1A2 and AHR associate with coffee consumption. *Human Molecular Genetics, 20*, 2071–2077.

Tanner, J. A., & Tyndale, R. F. (2017). Variation in CYP2A6 activity and personalized medicine. *Journal of Personalized Medicine*, *7*, 18.
Thorgeirsson, T. E., Gudbjartsson, D. F., Surakka, I., Vink, J. M., Amin, N., Geller, F., et al. (2010). Sequence variants at CHRNB3-CHRNA6 and CYP2A6 affect smoking behavior. *Nature Genetics*, *42*, 448–453.
Wennerholm, A., Dandara, C., Sayi, J., Svensson, J. O., Abdi, Y. A., Ingelman-Sundberg, M., et al. (2002). The African-specific CYP2D6*17 allele encodes an enzyme with changed substrate specificity. *Clinical Pharmacology and Therapeutics*, *71*, 77–88.
Werck-Reichhart, D., & Feyereisen. (2000). Cytochromes P450: a success story. *Genome Biology*. https://doi.org/10.1186/gb-2000-1-6-reviews3003. *PMID: 11178272.*
Zhou, S. F., Liu, J. P., & Chowbay, B. (2009). Polymorphism of human cytochrome P450 enzymes and its clinical impact. *Drug Metabolism Reviews*, *41*, 89–295.

Further reading

Crews, K. R., Gaedigk, A., Dunnenberger, H. M., Klein, T. E., Shen, D. D., Callaghan, J. T., et al. (2012). Clinical pharmacogenetics implementation consortium (CPIC) guidelines for codeine therapy in the context of cytochrome P450 2D6 (CYP2D6) genotype. *Clinical Pharmacology and Therapeutics*, *91*, 321–326.
Haeggström, S., Ingelman-Sundberg, M., Pääbo, S., & Zeberg, H. (2022). *The clinically relevant CYP2C8*3 and CYP2C9*2 alleles are inherited from Neandertals*. submitted.
Jukić, M. M., Smith, R. L., Molden, E., & Ingelman-Sundberg, M. (2021). Evaluation of the CYP2D6 haplotype activity scores based on metabolic ratios of 4,700 patients treated with three different CYP2D6 substrates. *Clinical Pharmacology and Therapeutics*, *110*, 750–758.
Loriot, M. A., Rebuissou, S., Oscarson, M., Cenee, S., Miyamoto, M., Ariyoshi, et al. (2001). Genetic polymorphisms of cytochrome P450 2A6 in a case-control study on lung cancer in a French population. *Pharmacogenetics*, *11*, 39–44.
Sim, S. C., Kacevska, M., & Ingelman-Sundberg, M. (2013). Pharmacogenomics of drug-metabolizing enzymes: A recent update on clinical implications and endogenous effects. *The Pharmacogenomics Journal*, *13*, 1–11.
Sistonen, J., Madadi, P., Ross, C. J., Yazdanpanah, M., Lee, J. W., Landsmeer, M. L., et al. (2012). Prediction of codeine toxicity in infants and their mothers using a novel combination of maternal genetic markers. *Clinical Pharmacology and Therapeutics*, *91*, 692–699.
Steele-Perkins, G., Plachez, C., Butz, K. G., Yang, G., Bachurski, C. J., Kinsman, S. L., et al. (2005). The transcription factor gene Nfib is essential for both lung maturation and brain development. *Molecular and Cellular Biology*, *25*, 685–698.
van der Lee, M., Allard, W. G., Vossen, R. H. A. M., Baak-Pablo, R. F., Menafra, R., Deiman, B. A. L. M., et al. (2021). Toward predicting CYP2D6-mediated variable drug response from CYP2D6 gene sequencing data. *Science Translational Medicine*, *13*(603), eabf3637.
Yang, H., Wu, Z., Liu, X., Chen, M., Zhang, X., & Jiang, Y. (2021). NFIB promotes the progression of gastric cancer by upregulating circMAP7D1 to stabilize HER2 mRNA. *Molecular Medicine Reports*, *23*, 269.